D0507324

BYPASS THIS BOOK

How to avoid

or survive

Cardiac Bypass Surgery

FRANK M PRICE MD

The Library of Congress has catalogued this edition as follows:

Price, Frank M, MD
Bypass This Book
How to avoid or survive Cardiac Bypass Surgery/ Frank M Price
Text and additional artwork

ISBN: 978-0-9982266-0-6

Printed in the United States of America

This Masterpiece is Dedicated to

Frank Surdakowski, M.D.

And

Maryann Stoltz, R.N.

ACKNOWLEDGEMENTS

Alan Cooper, M.D. for input and editing of cardiology topics.

Bailey Anne Cooper for illustrations.

Mike Cadogan, M.D., Chris Nickson, M.D., and Ed Burns, M.D. of Life In The Fast Lane for illustrations as noted and all EKG tracings. www.lifeinthefastlane.com

The research for many of my "You" chapters began, but never ended, with Wikipedia. Although the folks at Wikipedia prefer that they not be referenced, I feel that they do deserve a golf clap for their efforts.

My co-workers, colleagues and caregivers at John C. Lincoln North Mountain Hospital for getting me through the diagnosis, treatment and recovery from a single disease process and a slew of procedures.

The folks at Esolbiz for cleaning up my cover art.

TABLE OF CONTENTS

1. WARNING!

This book is chock full of poor taste, and many will find it extremely offensive. Here's why:

POORTASTEASE

Poortastease (poor-TASTE-ee-ace), or PT-ase, as it is known in chemistry circles, is a conceptual enzyme whose existence was first postulated in discussions with Eddie Chelist, M.D., and Ed Myers, J.D. We observed that, in certain social situations, many individuals often get the urge to say or do something which might be considered to be in poor taste. This could be something as simple as an offhand remark. Obscene gestures are a common example of poor taste, as are acts such as throwing tomatoes, honking one's horn repeatedly, or grabbing one's genitalia. Although there is a wide degree of variation, most individuals possessed of even the slightest degree of decorum can easily suppress these impulses. We attribute this ability to the presence of PT-ase, which inactivates the neural impulse to say or do something in poor taste.

After extensive research, we further observed that there are a variety of agents which appear to suppress the activity of PT-ase. This suppression becomes evident when normally well-behaved individuals do or say something in an atypically inappropriate manner. Conditions or activities which we noted to inhibit PT-ase include consumption of alcohol and other mind-altering substances, lack of sleep, physical exhaustion, and some environmental extremes including heat, but not cold. In general, PT-ase also seems to be susceptible to inhibition in certain groups of people at specific types of gatherings, including but not limited to dance parties, river trips, and the most fertile of all scenarios, hot tubs. In fact, any situation in which one encounters either full or partial nudity facilitates the rapid and complete degradation of PT-ase.

In addition, after careful consideration of available data, it became clear that there is a certain subgroup of the population who exhibit what appears to be a congenitally low level or even complete absence of the enzyme. These individuals were generally found to spend their entire lives floundering in a bottomless sea of poor taste.

-John H. Rees, M.D.

2. WHY YOU SHOULD BYPASS THIS BOOK

Bypass this book, unless you have heart disease.

And by all means, bypass this book:
Unless you know somebody with heart disease;
Unless you have a family history of heart disease;
Unless you have high blood pressure;
Unless you smoke;
Unless you are overweight;
Unless you have high cholesterol levels;
Unless you have diabetes;
Unless you do not exercise regularly.
That's a lot of unlesses. A lot of semicolons too.

I have been bumbling along with the concept of writing this book since early 2007. At the time I was on disability, mentally challenged, and still trying to recover from bypass surgery myself. I started writing to make some sense of what was happening to me, why I was feeling the way I did. I still haven't made any sense of it, but now, more than eight years later, I seem to have finished. That is to say, I've run out of things to say on the subject. Mostly I wanted to leave something behind for my daughter and her kids to look at and say, "So that's what Grandpa did for ten years of his life." Blame them.

This book has three parts to it. "They", "You", and "Me".

"They" is a collection of lamentable pieces of short fiction, most of which deal with cardiac risk factors, the medical education system or various stages in the diagnosis and treatment of coronary artery disease. I've been concocting this nonsense in my head over the course of four decades, and, until I wound up in a couple of knife fights with heart surgeons (They won. Twice.), despaired of ever finding a suitable repository for them. They come from the dark recesses of what was once a lively and inquisitive mind, clearly skewed from what passes for "normal". Don't look for peppy heartwarming stories. Kleenex will not be necessary.

"You", vaguely connected to and interspersed among the "They", is simple non-fiction written in the style of Sgt. Joe Friday: "Just the facts, Ma'am." With a dash of Bill Gannon thrown in for spice. Together they comprise a fairly accurate description of prevention and treatment of various aspects of coronary artery disease. If you can't stand the other two parts, you might at least learn some of the facts concerning heart disease. Facts are funny things though. Particularly in the field of medicine, today's indisputable time-honored truism may be relegated to the scrapheap of old wives' tales in a decade or two.

"Me" is my experience as a patient and a physician dealing with heart disease. It's not particularly fascinating, but it does shed light on how things may go when they don't go according to plan. On the upside, if I can survive, so can you.

There it is, your full-service bypass book. Just like old-timey gas stations.

"Check that oil, Ma'am?"

For the past ten years, it has been my daily challenge to differentiate reality from fantasy. First thing each morning, I reassure myself that the last dream of the night was just that, a dream. Then again, that's not so far off from baseline for most of my life. On a good day I can barely remember life before a bypass procedure changed me forever. To the best of my knowledge, the stories in this book, the "They" section, are complete fabrications, most of which came to me in the form of random observations of strangers, medical lore, or snippets of early morning dreams. If you keep your eyes, ears, and nose open and your mouth shut, you tend to absorb some pretty good stories. Should one or more of the characters in any way resemble you or someone you know, I assure you it is purely coincidental. My memory is so crappy that, even if I've known you all my life, there is a better than even chance I wouldn't recognize you if you handed me a pound of twenties. Feel free to give it a try.

Heart disease is a serious subject; from time to time I shall endeavor to treat it thusly. FDR was mostly right when he said, "the only thing we have to fear is fear itself...". It is entirely reasonable to fear the unknown, especially when it involves a masked man sticking large needles into your body or cutting open your chest. I figure if I can illuminate some of the unknown, you will have a better chance of avoiding heart surgery or, if worse comes to worse, facing it with optimism, not fear. My goal is to give you something to read as you avoid or endure the path through the land of heart disease, amuse you from time to time, provide a few travel tips, and prepare you for some of the things that may come your way. One thing for sure: you'll learn what not to do.

What took me so long?

I was born a world-class procrastinator. In addition, when you are comfortable, especially when your comfort comes courtesy of the public or private dole, you lack hunger and poverty, two of the most powerful motivators for success; there's always tomorrow. Some days I'd wait for inspiration, which is a complete waste of time. Inspiration prances in on a horse, all piss-elegant with a foppish hat and frilly cuffs. Then, like all worthless courtiers, it promptly takes a powder. After that, it is a death march through the fields of just-plain-work. Not hard work when compared to some jobs, but it sure pulls everything out of me, from my brains to my guts. Like every endeavor, the first step is the toughest. It gets easier with practice. Does it get better? In this case, I have my doubts. You be the judge.

My short term memory has been and continues to be a disaster. After a full day of writing, I'd get up the next morning, sit down at the computer, peruse my work and wonder, *Who the hell wrote this crap?* Other days I'd read something not quite finished from the day before and realize that all my momentum had disappeared during the night. I'd think, *This isn't half bad! How'd I come up with all these terrific ideas, and where did the rest of them go?*

Incidentally, I have never been very good at thinking from the female perspective. At one particularly delusional time in my life, I convinced myself that I understood women. That passed quickly. Consequently, this effort tends to be directed at males, from the perspective of a male patient and a former male health care provider who has treated far more male than female heart patients. Each decade brings new XX-specific breakthroughs in the diagnosis and treatment of diseases, including heart disease. In this, as in most areas pertaining to women, I am clueless. Undoubtedly, someone unencumbered by my limitations will come along and do justice to the subject of heart disease in women.

Especially in the "You" chapters, I have endeavored to describe how things proceed on a nice normal day. However, be advised. If you want to know how a hip replacement should normally go, ask an orthopedic surgeon. If you want to know how a cardiac bypass procedure should normally go, ask a cardiac surgeon. If you ask a hospitalist or an E.R. doc about a hip replacement or bypass surgery, you may get a different story. That's because those guys see the complications, when things don't go according to plan. They treat the one percent who don't follow the playbook.

This book will at times be repetitious. It is also full of rough edges. Repetition and rough edges. Just like me. Just like life.

Despite all the negativity that abounds in the media about American medical care, if you're going to have heart disease, this is the place to have it. While some of the most important discoveries regarding the human heart were made by many civilizations long before the United States existed, over the past century we have led the world in research, prevention and treatment of coronary artery disease. When it comes to heart disease, more money and more brains are at work here than anywhere else. While more money does not always translate to better care, it rarely hurts. More brainpower always leads to better results. No matter how superb your physical condition, you are little more than a sneeze away from a raging case of myocarditis and a subsequent lifesaving heart transplant. In most other countries, a heart transplant is not an option.

As you hike the trail of heart disease, you can forget all those phrases from the Touchy-Feely School of Medicine that are bandied about when it comes to surviving an illness:

1. "Fighting for your life". You are undergoing treatment and hopefully recovering. Your health care team is fighting for your life: you are not. Part of the time you are unconscious. Part of the time you are lying in bed. Part of the time you are walking. Most of the time you are simply hoping for the average outcome. If you walk away with the average outcome from CABG surgery in the U.S., you've done very well. The alternative is much worse. Don't bother with the "fighting" part. It takes too much energy, which you will surely need for other endeavors.

2. "Survivor". The term is trendy, truly uplifting, but what does it say about those who succumb? Are they any less noble, any weaker, any less desirous of survival, so therefore they didn't make it? Sometimes, far more often than any of us would care to admit, survival is nothing more than the good fortune that it isn't your day to die. Fate, luck, a flip of the cosmic coin. Nobody knows. You may have the simplest illness in the world, but if it's your day to go, sayonara. Likewise, a case that starts with the worst possible prognosis can go incredibly smoothly; everybody winds up with a satisfied stupid grin of surprise and a pat on the back for a job well done as you get wheeled out of the hospital in a chair, not a body bag.

3. "Hero". You are a hero when you go far beyond what is expected of you. Just doing your job, in this case recovering, is not the stuff of heroes. It is the stuff of the majority of patients. You don't have to be a hero to survive this ordeal. As a matter of fact, as soon as you are discharged, you don't want to be remembered as a "hero". You want to be erased from the collective memory of your health care team. In and out in less than a week, forgotten by all concerned as soon as your bed is empty. That is far better than having them remember you for your

incessant whining or your pushy visitors or your protracted hospital course laden with hideously disfiguring complications. So even if you're not "hero" material, don't sweat it. To recover from heart surgery, it's simply a matter of putting one foot in front of the other, both figuratively and literally, on a daily basis. That's it. If you do your best, most likely that will be enough. The vast majority of patients who don't follow even half of their physicians' recommendations recover perfectly well, another testament to the resilience of the human body.

On the other hand, to get through it all, to survive and thrive, there is one thing you will require...

3. FAITH

She sits across from me, lustrous blue eyes beaming up at the waiter. His job barely pays the bills, but that's it; with his talent, he could be making his mark in the world. Once his artwork starts to sell, he can pay off his loans and paint full-time. Some acting on the side. No more picking up egg-strewn plates and booger-laden napkins.

"The Princessa here wants the French toast. Any juice, honey?"

"Mm-hmm."

"Mm-hmm?"

"Yes, please."

"A small orange juice. I'll have the lox with chive cream cheese on a toasted poppy-seed bagel, with capers and tomatoes. No onions, please. No, no lettuce either. Just coffee, with ice on the side. Thanks."

"You don't like your coffee too hot. It burns your mouth."

She looks down at her place setting, waiting for the food to magically arrive. She is hungry. I think about the time at a Denny's near Disneyworld. While I sang the entire Anita Bryant orange juice commercial song, she downed a huge glass of fresh-squeezed Florida orange juice. Then she covered the table in the booth with fresh-puked fresh-squeezed Florida orange juice. Then we left.

"Daddy, I have to go potty."

"Excuse me, Michael. Where are the restrooms?"

"You go out that door over there, into the Drake…"

She looks up at Michael, the artist. "The Sir Francis Drake Hotel!"

The waiter notices her for the first time, looks down at her, that pair of big blues focused on him. His head recoils backward just a fraction. I can tell he's thinking what they all think, *Good God, those eyes!*

"Out the door," still staring at her eyes, mesmerized, lining up the colors he would combine on his palette, trying to focus on what he was saying, "across the lobby, up the stairs, and around the corner to the restrooms."

"Is there a potty for boys and for girls?"

"Uh, yes, one for each."

"Good. One for boys, one for girls. Boys are messy in the potty."

"So you don't have restrooms here in the restaurant?"

"No, not in the Bistro." *Bistro. We're breakfasting at a bistro.*

"OK. Let's go." Together we walk up the steps and through the door into the hotel. In the lobby, I stop.

"Honey, would you rather go up to the room to go potty? It's probably nicer than the restroom."

"No. I want to go here."

"OK, Big Girl. I'll go with you. You want me to take you to the boys' room and help?"

"No. There's a girls' room and I want to go. By. My. Self."

"Of course." We cross the lobby together. It's old but still retains a touch of old San Francisco class. "I like your outfit today. The last time you wore that much hot pink and purple, you were a little girl, maybe two. We went up to the indoor amusement park by Uncle Sam's. They had a train, a carousel, and a little pool with boats in it."

"I remember it. The train could go forward and backwards."

"Oh, yeah, that's right. I forgot about that. That's the one. I had to stop going on it with you because I got so dizzy when it went backwards.

Anyway, the first time we went to that place, you wanted to drive a boat. There was a man who worked there. He had rubber boots up to his knees."

"Yes, he had a beard like you, but he smelled like cigarettes."

"Yes, he did. He would spend all day picking up little kids and putting them in the boats and…"

"And buckling my seat belt."

"Exactly. He put you in, you had both your binks strapped to your shirt. You started toodling around in the boat. Kept both hands on the steering wheel, like a good driver. The water had a current to it, so all the boats moved around in a big circle. After going around once, you were tired of it or you got scared. You would open and close your hand to come get you and say, "Come get me."

"I wasn't scared."

"No, of course not. Every time you did that, I would say, 'I can't'. Then you would put your hand back on the steering wheel and shake your head just a little and go around again. You did that four or five times before your ride was done and the man lifted you out of the boat and put you into my arms. You didn't seem upset, had a big smile on your face."

"I was okay, Dad. I knew you'd come get me."

"That's what I figured. As soon as we started walking away, you said, 'Do again.' So we did."

We were jumping down the stairs, ending up in the basement. Here I could truly appreciate the hotel's age. Pitted concrete floors painted industrial red supporting gray concrete walls. There were shallow cavities everywhere in the walls, where old layers of paint, no doubt lead-laden, had come off unevenly. We turned to the left and walked down a narrow, dimly-lit corridor. Halfway down on the right was a doorway. As we neared, the familiar smell of drying clothes wafted around us.

"Mmmmm. Ah. That smells good. Like cotton candy at the fair."

"Yes, Honey. This is one of the places where they make cotton candy for the fair." She just looked at me, eyes wide for an instant. Then the "Hmmph" came through her nose, and I knew she was on to me.

At the end of the corridor, there was a double door with a push bar, like a school exit. I opened it into a dark damp storage room.

"This is kind of dark for a girls' room. I think we must have made a wrong turn somewhere."

"The man said to go upstairs, but we went down. Why did we go down, Dad?"

"Probably because I am not as smart as you. Okay, you show me where the girls' room is."

"Okay. I can find the boys' room for you too."

So Mr. Not-So-Smart followed the pink and purple wizard girl up one set of stairs, around a corner, and up another short flight. In the dim light of the corridor, you could vaguely see the Ladies sign on the left and the Gentlemen sign up a couple more steps to the right.

"Let's check out the girls' room."

She looked up at me. "What does that word say?"

"It says 'Ladies'."

"I'm a young lady."

"Yes you are, Honey." I pushed the door open. Brighter than the corridor, the place was empty. I held the door and my little girl walked in.

"Do you want me to come in with you?"

"I can do it."

"By yourself?"

"By. My. Self."

"Uh-huh. OK, I'll wait out here for you. Take your time."

"Dad, I can do it by myself. I'll come back down to the restaurant when I'm done. I'll be OK."

"You sure?"

"Yes."

"OK, Pea Sweet."

"Sweet Pea!"

"Oh yeah, right. Remember. Go out the door, turn left, and go down the stairs. OK?"

"OK, Dad."

"Show me your left hand."

"This one." She flipped her left hand up into the air to show me her freshly-painted fingernails, then waved at me. "Bye-BYE, D-A-D. MWUAH!" A big kiss and in she went. I held the door open.

"What's your name?"

"Pink and purple. Pink and purple Sally, Pink and purple Katie, Pink and purple Rosie, Pink and purple."

I backed out of the room, letting the door swing shut. To my left was a short hallway which ended at a set of doors. They each had a push bar and a small window at eye level. I pushed on both bars. Heavy doors. They opened out onto Sutter St. on the north side of the hotel. No way to open them from the outside. You can get out but you can't get in. Just the opposite of the Roach Motel. Good. I stepped back, let the doors shut. Then I pushed on them to see if they opened. Neither one budged.

While walking back to the staircase, I weighed the risks. Then I promptly ignored my gut.

Back inside the restaurant, I dropped a couple of ice cubes in my coffee and tried to read The Chronicle. The waiter came with her juice. I kept looking over at the door to the hotel. After a few minutes, the food arrived. *Uh-oh. Too long.*

I got up and walked as slowly as I could to the door. Then I ran across the lobby and up the stairs. Jumping up the last two steps, I nearly plowed into a short maid.

"Oh, sorry, Ma'am." I slid around her and pushed open the ladies' room door. Visions of drooling pedophiles danced in my head.

"Oh!" A woman standing at one of the sinks saw me out of the corner of her eye and backed up a couple of steps.

"Sorry, Ma'am. I'm looking for my little girl. Dressed in pink and purple. Did you see her in here?" I had shaved off my beard a few months before, so I looked a little less like a pirate, but she slowly backed away cringing. Her left hand held a mascara bottle, her right an eyelash brush.

"Uh, no. Nobody's been in here for the past five minutes."

"Shit. Sorry. Thanks." I backed out the door. To the left, the double doors were closed. I ran to the men's room. An old homeless guy shuffled out the door, looking guilty.

Oh, Christ. I rushed past him into the men's room, envisioning my little girl shoehorned into a toilet.

I checked every stall and trashcan. No kid. No dead kid.

Sweat was dripping into my eyes and down my back. I took the stairs back down, two at a time, thinking, desperately hoping that she was wandering around the lobby.

No pink, no purple.

I ran back to the restaurant. No little girl with six pigtails sitting at our table.

Idiot. About this time those two words of self-damnation from *Ninety-Two in the Shade* screamed repeatedly inside my head. I felt like such a fool.

On my way out the front door onto Powell St., I almost collided with the Beefeater on the sidewalk.

"Hi. Sorry. Did you see a little girl with pigtails in a pink and purple getup out here?"

"No, sir. I always keep an eye out for kids by themselves. Lots of kids with adults, lots of little girls with pigtails. No solo kids."

"Thanks." Great. Lots of little girls with pigtails in the company of adults.

When I was a senior in high school, I went up to take a look at NYU. It was early in the '70s, and pretty much every guy I passed in the Village looked to be either enjoying a serious buzz or sizing me up as potential sex prey. Now every guy I passed on my way south on Powell had that same creepy leer on his face. *Which one of you?*, I thought. *Which one of you just sold my little girl to a Columbian white slaver?*

Nothing doing on either side of Powell down to Post, so I turned and ran back up Powell. Now I was soaked and sucking gas, and the tourists were grumbling as I wove in and out of the crowd. I thought about how good a shower would feel, and then I had that thought that every divorced Dad has at least once: *Her mom is going to have me killed.* And I would richly deserve it.

I ran past the Beefeater, who shook his head, and turned the corner at Sutter. About twenty feet down Sutter, just past the double doors, almost but not quite in tears, stood the tiniest, most fragile six year-old ever. The "I'm kind of scared but I won't be afraid" look, complete with crimson coloring, framed her startling blue eyes. I was halfway to her when she focused and recognized me.

"Baby Girl, I am so sorry. I should never have left you alone like that. I'll never do that again." I held her in my arms for the longest time.

"It was kind of scary, Daddy." She sobbed a little into my neck and held on tight.

"What, did you come out these doors?"

"Uh-huh. They were hard to open, but I pushed and pushed."

"You big, strong girl. Did you feel lost?"

"Yes, lost."

"Honey, Daddy's an idiot."

"It's OK. I knew you would come get me."

4. I am not...

an expert on heart disease. As a matter of fact, I'm not an expert on anything. I lack expertise in most areas, as well as the necessary accessories--the hairdo, the glasses, the quirky bowtie, the authoritative voice. Experts come equipped with a very short memory, especially when their expert opinion turns out wrong. My short-term memory is pathetic, but I can't forget the times I was wrong, often dead wrong. Many a night my mistakes keep me wide awake.

During the spring of the American Bicentennial, a professor in a climate class gave me the idea of writing a paper on colonial icehouses in Virginia. These were deep, narrow, cylindrical brick-lined holes in the ground on most of the larger plantations dotting the York, the James, the Rappahannock and the Rivanna rivers during the time of Thomas Jefferson. Ice from frozen rivers was cut into large chunks, loaded onto ships, sailed down the coast and up the rivers to the plantations. The ice was then hauled up from the river, and we are talking UP, courtesy of the local slaves, tossed into the ice pits and covered with sawdust or straw. During that period, most meats were salt-cured or smoked and did not require ice to keep them from spoiling. The ice was used throughout the spring and summer to make chilled desserts, a real treat for those without any other form of refrigeration. Obviously, the cooler the ambient temperature, the more slowly the ice would melt, and the longer into the summer or autumn the ice would last.

Jefferson kept copious records of the temperatures at his home, Monticello, that place on the back of a nickel. His goal was to take the temperature every day at sunrise, noon and sunset. Once in a while he would take a measurement of the level of the ice as well. He and his designees did a remarkably compulsive job of adhering to the plan. In the years since his death, various other residents or caretakers or researchers did their best to continue the tradition. Back then in my Type A days, with the goal of spotting trends and making some predictions, I spent far too many days in the library wading through records laden with temperatures and observations.

In an effort to get up close and personal with the local icehouses, and sick of being cooped up in the library, I fired up my jalopy and headed out to the remnants of the old plantations. At the time, the icehouse was still featured on the tour at Monticello. I spent an afternoon talking with one of the grounds managers there. He was able to add a little to what was published or available. I wasn't satisfied, however, not by a long shot. Like all great explorers, hypnotized by the siren of danger, I felt the urge to venture out into the hinterlands, to engage evil Prince Peril in hand-to-hand combat, to become "embedded" in the story, to discover what became of icehouses that weren't managed by professionals. That sounds courageous and investigative, but all I really wanted to do was pry into people's private lives and see what they were doing with these holes in the ground. I imagined that at least one was being used as a dungeon to house kidnap victims; I'd free them, take a heroic bow, and make off with the most comely of the maidens.

Somewhere in the Jefferson section of the library I found the names of a number of plantations in Virginia where icehouses were at least constructed and used for a few years. I think the list had something to do with sharing the cost of the ice ships. Anyway, on several occasions I travelled down I-64 to York County and the Williamsburg area to investigate. The ice house at the Governor's Palace in Colonial Williamsburg is far and away the best preserved of the bunch; if the Rockefellers are providing your seed money, you are going to have nice digs. I made an appointment with one of the managers there. His family had been in the area for generations, so he knew all about the plantations for miles around. With the help of some very clever hand-drawn maps, he helped me locate a number of the properties, for the most part now divvied up into smaller farms.

In each plantation area I tried to find the oldest residence or the one on the highest hill. The icehouse had to be close to the original owner's home, and that was usually the one with the best view. I'd drive up, knock on the door, and ask if I could take a look at the icehouse on the property. Occasionally I'd get a blank stare, as the hole in the ground had been covered up by previous generations. Once I got a "How'd you know about that thing?" from an old boy who was glad to have someone to talk to and showed me the spot. His was covered up to keep dogs and kids from falling in. Many times it was "Oh, we haven't used that for years", meaning that they were probably embarrassed about employing their icehouse as a septic tank. On a few occasions, feeling adventurous, I drove away, circled around, and, accompanied by my dog Melissa, climbed back up the hill. It was usually pretty easy to find, and indeed, judging by the fragrance, most of the ones I found were being used for waste storage. Pursued one time by an old codger with some sort of long gun, I grabbed the dog by the collar and bolted back down the hill. I felt like an Icehouse Commando, dragging his compadre, making a getaway. Despite my persistent efforts and significant brushes with death, at the end of my explorations there were no dungeons, no prisoners, no rescues and no comely maidens.

By the time I finished my research, I knew more about icehouses in Colonial Virginia than did 99.9% of the world's population. Whoop de doo. Initially very impressed with my wealth of accumulated information, I realized a few months later what 99.9% of the world's population already knew. What is the point of knowing all there is to know about an outdated architectural and culinary artifact now being used to store poop? There was a move afoot to publish my groundbreaking research, a.k.a., my term paper, in the Virginia Climate

Quarterly, a journal with slightly fewer subscribers than National Geographic. I don't know if that ever came to pass. I was feeling pretty darn authoritative. Sleep was difficult for the next year or so. I awakened nightly, imagining a knock on the front door.

"Who is it?"

"It is I, Narvid, from Norway."

"What do you want, Narvid?"

"I bring good news from the House of Nobel."

Icehouses have fallen out of favor, not only as a method of refrigeration but as a point of interest as well. Nowadays, if you take the tour at Monticello, the guide usually doesn't even mention Jefferson's icehouse. H, as in Sally Hemmings, comes before I, as in icehouse. Tourists are much more fascinated by whom Jefferson was doing after dessert than by what he was doing during dessert. Ben and Jerry may be living the dream in Vermont, but at Monticello, sex sells better than Cherry Garcia.

The end of my paper focused on the gradual drop in daily temperatures at Monticello over the previous twenty-five years. I confidently predicted that, within a few decades, icehouses would again be a viable method of chilling food. The earth was obviously cooling off.

Expert.

5. But I am...

(Unsolicited Testimonial)

"Emergency Room, this is Patty speaking. How may I help you?"

"This is Emma Herker. I'm having a migraine. It's the worst migraine ever, and I need a shot."

"I see, Mrs. Herker. Let me ask you a few questions, so that I know how to advise you properly."

"Go ahead, but hurry up. This migraine is killing me, and I might not last much longer."

"On a scale of one to ten, how bad is the pain from the migraine?"

"Oh, Lordy, this one's a twenty at least."

"Oh, I'm so sorry to hear that. Have you spoken with your primary care provider?"

"Oh, he doesn't know anything, that fool. He thinks I should lie down in a dark room, eat some protein, and take some Advil. I've had migraines for thirty years, and I know that doesn't work. And neither do those silly Vicodins. I took a handful of them an hour ago and I still don't feel a thing. My cousin in Tucson gets Dilaudids for hers and she told me to ask my doctor for them, but he won't give 'em to me."

"Well, if you feel this is an emergency, and you don't think you can wait until tomorrow to see your doctor, you are welcome to come in and be evaluated by our emergency physician."

"That's why I called. Who's working there tonight? I hope it's that nice Dr. Holloway. He's such a good doctor. I wish he had his own practice. He takes good care of me."

"I'm afraid not. Dr. Price is here until 10 A.M. tomorrow."

"Lordy, that's no good. I need a shot, and when I need a shot, nothing else helps. I've been to see him before, and all he does is examine me, talk a bunch of nonsense, then give me something to keep me from throwing up. I told him I don't have the flu, you jackass, I'm having a migraine. But he won't give me a shot. I'm not coming in there until he's gone. He's an ASSHOLE!"

6. HOW DID YOU GET HERE?

There are a number of routes you can take to get to the operating table for a Coronary Artery Bypass Graft (CABG) surgical procedure. That statement sounds as if this is something you might choose on a slow day. Only a Munchausen would volunteer to undergo this type of surgery without a very good reason. As a matter of fact, unless you truly need this surgery, it is highly unlikely you could get it done at all. It's not as simple or convenient as renting shoes at a bowling alley.

One of the more common ways to find yourself heading for surgery is through the development of recurrent chest pain. We'll get into the details of cardiac chest pain and its imposters later. Most likely you'd end up seeing your primary care provider, who, wondering whether you might have cardiac disease, refers you to a cardiologist. The cardiologist does one or more tests, which leads to the cath lab, then decides that you have significant coronary disease not amenable to medical therapy or angioplasty and refers you to a cardiac surgeon. The surgeon agrees with the cardiologist, and you are scheduled for elective CABG surgery.

Another pathway to the operating table does not involve chest pain, but somehow you end up on a treadmill for a stress test. Maybe it's for an insurance policy, maybe you have some odd symptom like fatigue or shortness of breath that arouses his suspicion. Maybe it's part of a job application, maybe your physician is concerned about your risk factors, or maybe you just like to take treadmill tests because you want to show off or you are bored. Whatever the case, the treadmill test comes back suspicious for coronary disease, and off you go to the cath lab and subsequently to the operating room (O.R.). If you started out doing the treadmill because you were bored, well, as you are about to discover, there are things far worse than boredom. One of them is postoperative pain.

The third common pathway to the O.R., the least desirable one, goes through the emergency room. It's the least desirable because if there were any prior warning signs that would have landed you on the yellow brick road or the green one, you ignored them and are now on the red one. The horse has left the station. The train has left the barn. That ship has sailed. You awaken in the middle of the night with chest pain or indigestion. After a ride in a car or an ambulance, you end up in the emergency room, surrounded by scary felons handcuffed to their gurneys, meth addicts oozing MRSA from their pustules, screaming hot yard apes (kids with fevers), and equally loud 5-Fs (female, fertile, fair, fat and forty) with gallstones. Your EKG is most likely abnormal, or it may be normal but you have risk factors for coronary disease. Going on the assumption that you are experiencing acute coronary syndrome, which may involve a myocardial infarction (MI or heart attack), you are whisked off to the cath lab pronto, where most likely your blocked coronary artery is opened with meds and/or an angioplasty. Depending on how many other partially blocked coronary arteries they find, you may go to the O.R. for a bypass right away or a few days later.

On the other hand, if your chest pain is controlled in the E.R. and your EKG returns to normal, you may stabilize and end up going to the CVICU overnight and to the cath lab in the morning. In that scenario, waiting for a bed, even one in the CVICU, usually means a longer hang time in your little emergency room nightmare than the fifteen minutes to the cath lab that every heart center brags about nowadays.

As you can see, the final common pathway to CABG surgery is through the cath lab and into the O.R. No matter how you get there, at least two physicians will agree that you require bypass surgery and not some other form of treatment: the guy who does the cath, almost always a cardiologist, and the guy who does the surgery, who had better be a cardiac surgeon. You can walk into a plastic surgeon's office and say you want your northern and southern snot lockers switched or you want a couple of extra nipples, and if you have the dough-re-mi, you might get this done. In this scenario, the plastic surgeon ought to, but doesn't have to, consult with anybody before doing what you want, not even a psychiatrist. He might consult with your banker, however, as health care insurance doesn't usually pay for bizarre elective plastic surgery. You can walk into a general surgeon's office and say you have a really bad stomach ache in the right lower quadrant of your abdomen and he can take you to the O.R., explore your abdomen, and remove your inflamed appendix.

Nowhere in the U.S. will a cardiac surgeon take a new patient to the O.R. for a CABG without someone doing a cath first to identify the anatomy and the pathology. So CABG surgery is much less likely to be performed on you if you don't need it. Although there are undoubtedly doctors in all branches of medicine who in past lives did a brief stint selling used cars, nowadays there is plenty of oversight when it comes to CABG surgery. You won't get sold a procedure you don't need.

About the proboscis transplants? You probably won't be able to get that done, but I like the sound of it. Someone somewhere has gone looking for that procedure, but that's better left for another book. Thank goodness for people. Without them, life might be simpler but so much less interesting.

It is important to bear in mind that every member of the team who has any role in this CABG process desires that you have the best outcome possible. A good outcome means people get to keep their jobs. They sleep better as well.

7. MEDICAL TERMINOLOGY

In the purest form of the language of medicine, you cannot find a single term that is positive. There is "cure" or "remission" or "success", but these are words used by the general public. Even "cure" is a bit dubious, as in "the cure was worse than the disease." Most medical terms refer to something suboptimal, far below normal, or just plain bad.

In virtually every aspect of modern life, the higher the number, the better. Nobody wants to date a 2, but everyone lusts for the 10. Even when it comes to homicide, if you're the perp, you would rather be on trial for Murder 2 than Murder 1, 2nd degree manslaughter rather than Man 1. However, stages of diseases, cancer being the best-known example, are ordered in just the opposite direction, ranging from the best prognosis, Stage 0, to the worst, Stage 4.

The medical profession has come up with a scientific term for just about every conceivable condition. There is even a medical term for "ugly face": "dysmorphic facies". "Nice cans" has a generally positive ring to it, as does "beautiful breasts". Even "huge tracts of land" sounds like a good thing. Excluding the real estate taxes, of course. The medical term "large, pendulous breasts" implies a weighty condition possessed of a guilty conscience.

Medical terminology is also capable of obfuscating fairly simple disease entities. I had a sore red spot on my ear which made me worry about skin cancer. My dermatologist told me I had chondrodermatitis nodularis senilis helicis chronica, presenting only in old men, usually right on the point of their Darwin's tubercle. In terms of causation, it's not exactly a dueling scar. You get them if you sleep on your ear too long. Is that better or worse than basal cell skin cancer? It sure sounds worse, especially the "old men" part. He cut it off, just to be sure. It's never returned, but now, to the investigative eye, I have asymmetrical Darwin's tubercles. How would you like to go through life with that pinned to you?

This concept carries through in the naming of medications as well. Some names, either generic or trade, sound like they can really do the job. Others sound like something you wouldn't give your worst enemy.

Apropos of nothing, in the O.R., you can always tell the pro from the amateur. If, during a procedure, a pro screws something up, rather than cursing himself, the nurses, the world, and especially the patient, he'll usually say, "Oh, very nice." If he's really pissed, between sessions of teeth gritting, he might repeat it a few times, along with a "beautiful" or two. It's a good habit to form. Sometimes, during "twilight sedation", the eighth cranial nerve is still receiving. In other words, the patient can hear what is going on. Some of the other senses work as well. Every so often a patient will awaken after a procedure and ask, "What was that burning smell?" or "I dreamt someone was screaming and throwing metal things."

8. BASIC ANATOMY OF THE HEART

Your heart is nothing more than a pump. Evolved or created over a million years ago, it is an incredibly complex pump, but it is still a pump. Despite all the technology available today, nobody has been able to come up with a permanent replacement that is anywhere near as effective, efficient or long-lasting as the human heart. For your heart to pump blood effectively, all the components of your heart-- coronary arteries, valves, heart muscle cells--must be in good working order. So every single cell in your heart plays a vital role. In the final analysis, however, those components are important only as they affect the ability of your heart to act as a pump.

The simplest way to think about your heart is to compare it to the engine in your automobile. If the engine is defective, it won't run, and all the ancillary support systems--the battery, the starter, the fuel pump, the fuel line, the gas tank--mean nothing. On the other hand, in order for it to run efficiently, all those support systems have to be functioning well.

In an auto, through the use of belts, the engine activates the various pumps--fuel pump for providing an energy source, oil pump for lubrication, water pump for cooling. In the human body, through the transportation of blood, the central pump, your heart, provides the energy source for all the other engines--the brain, internal organs, and skeletal muscles. While the right side of the heart is taking in deoxygented (low oxygen content) blood from the venous system and sending it to the lungs, the left side is taking in oxygenated (high oxygen content) blood from the lungs and pumping it out via the arterial system to all the aforementioned engines throughout the body.

A car has a battery connected to but separate from the engine. Ingeniously, the heart has an internal battery, the sinoatrial (SA) node, located in the right atrium. From the SA node there are specialized bundles of muscle cells which conduct the electrical charge down to the atrioventricular (AV) nodes, which in turn cause the contraction of the two ventricles. When the body is at rest, the SA node, a natural pacemaker, fires somewhere between 60 and 100 times per minute. In runners and others who exercise regularly, the resting heart rate will be significantly lower, anywhere from 40 to 60 beats per minute. During exercise or other forms of stress, a healthy SA node can fire up to 180 times per minute. Over a lifespan of about 80 years with an average heart rate of 80 beats per minute, that battery fires, usually without replacement, over three billion times. Not bad for a design that is over a million years old and powered solely by the flow of ions (electrically charged atoms) back and forth across a cell membrane. Of note, on those relatively rare occasions when the SA node gives out, a "permanent" pacemaker has to be inserted; even with our modern technology, you can't count on that $20,000.00 pacer to last more than ten years.

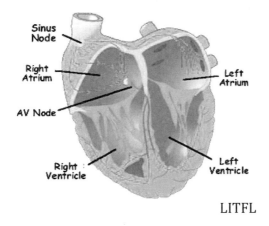

Sinus Node

Right Atrium

Left Atrium

AV Node

Right Ventricle

Left Ventricle

LITFL

When an automobile battery sends out an electrical charge to the engine, the spark causes the combustion of gasoline and air. That combustion causes the individual pistons to move in sequence, turning the crankshaft and causing the car to move. Likewise, in the heart, the electrical charge generated by the SA node and transmitted to the AV nodes causes the myocardium (heart muscle) in the walls of the ventricles to contract. There are two phases to the pumping activity of the heart. Systole (SIS-toh-lee) occurs when the heart muscle contracts, about sixty to eighty times per minute in the normal resting heart. Diastole (di-ASS-toh-lee) is the rest period between each systolic contraction. Both sides of the heart contract more or less at the same time.

The design of the heart pump is a muscle with four interconnected cavities inside. There are two intake chambers, the left atrium and the right atrium, and two outflow chambers, the left ventricle and the right ventricle. An atrium is basically a storage chamber with a small amount of pumping capability, whereas a ventricle is primarily a pumping chamber. Because of pressure in the venous system, deoxygenated blood returning from the body and the brain is constantly flowing into the right atrium. In diastole, between every contraction of the ventricular muscle, the tricuspid valve opens and blood flows from the right atrium into the right ventricle. Then, during systole, the right ventricle contracts, shutting the tricuspid valve and forcing open the pulmonic valve. This allows deoxygenated blood to flow from the right ventricle into the pulmonary arteries. The pulmonary arteries carry the blood into your lungs, where the blood flows into smaller arteries, called arterioles, and then into even smaller vessels, called capillaries. Alongside the capillaries are tiny air pockets known as alveoli. These are the basic building blocks of your lungs. Oxygen diffuses from the alveoli into the capillaries, where the hemoglobin in deoxygenated red blood cells pick up the oxygen; the hemoglobin molecules and red blood cells are now oxygenated. Your blood then enters pulmonary venules, which are tiny veins, and then flows into pulmonary veins which lead to the left side of the heart.

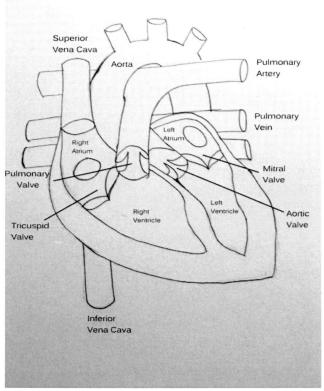

BAC

Chambers of the Heart and Great Vessels

The path of blood through the left side of your heart is similar to that on the right side. Like the tricuspid valve on the right, the mitral valve opens during diastole and allows oxygenated blood to flow from the left atrium into the left ventricle. The left ventricle then contracts at the same time as the right ventricle, shutting the mitral valve and forcing open the aortic valve. With the aortic valve open, blood flows into the aorta. This newly oxygenated blood delivers oxygen to the brain, organs and muscles, allowing them to function aerobically. In summary, the flow of blood through the heart goes as follows.

Systemic veins -> vena cava -> right atrium -> tricuspid valve -> right ventricle -> pulmonic valve -> pulmonary artery -> pulmonary arteriole -> capillary -> pulmonary venule -> pulmonary vein -> left atrium -> mitral valve -> left ventricle -> aortic valve -> aorta-> systemic arteries. Depending on your heart rate, this occurs sixty to eighty times per minute for every minute of your life. If you are stressed or exerting yourself, your muscles, brain, heart and other organs will require more oxygen. Thanks to epinephrine and other catecholamines, your heart will automatically speed up to meet this increased demand.

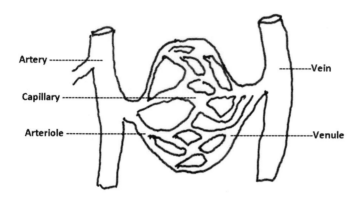

BAC/FMP

Rather than using gasoline and air, the myocardium requires oxygen and glucose in your blood to perform its pumping function. This blood is delivered via the coronary arteries, which act like a fuel line in a car.

There are four major coronary arteries that arise directly or indirectly from the aorta:

1. The left main;
2. The left anterior descending;
3. The circumflex;
4. The right.

The left main, a short stubby, basically splits into the left anterior descending and the circumflex arteries. The right coronary artery is separate from the left main system. In some individuals, one other major coronary artery, the ramus intermedius, also arises from the left main. Each of these major arteries, which are located on the epicardium (outer surface of the heart), also give rise to numerous branches that penetrate into the myocardium.

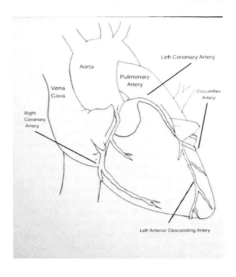

BAC

While the basic layout is similar in most individuals, much like snowflakes, no two coronary artery systems are identical. These coronary arteries direct oxygenated blood to smaller arteries, called arterioles. At the end of each arteriole is a capillary bed, where the myocardial cells extract oxygen and glucose. After the capillary bed comes the venule and then the coronary veins. The coronary veins convey the deoxygenated blood to the right atrium, where it mixes with the blood returning from the rest of your body, and from there it travels through the oxygenating cycle in your lungs.

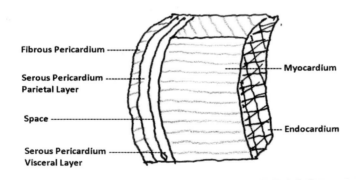

BAC/FMP

Cellular Layers of the Heart

The wall of your heart is composed of three separate layers of cells. Beginning on the inside, in direct contact with the blood flowing through the various chambers of the heart, is a thin layer of cells known as the endocardium. The middle layer, the myocardium, contains the muscle cells that contract to perform the actual pumping function of the heart. The outermost layer of the wall is the epicardium, also known as the visceral layer of the serous pericardium.

Surrounding the wall of your heart is another series of cell layers. Just outside the epicardium is a thin space. This is surrounded by the parietal layer of the serous pericardium, which is in turn surrounded by the outermost layer, the fibrous pericardium. These latter two layers provide protection for the wall of the heart. Disease processes can affect any or all of these layers, but the most important layers in terms of the pump function of your heart are the endocardium and the myocardium. Ironically, these are the two layers most susceptible to damage, especially from lack of blood flow.

There are a few significant differences between your car's engine and your heart. First, when the fuel line is clogged, your car will have trouble climbing hills. That is why your poorly maintained old beater is sluggish or staggers when going uphill. However, despite the various moans and creaks emitted from your vehicle, as far as we know, it does not feel pain. The only pain involved is your pain when you have to pay a mechanic to fix the problem. When you have clogged coronary arteries, you will indeed have trouble climbing hills--in the business, the term is "decreased exercise tolerance"--and you will most likely feel chest pain, also known as angina pectoris.

The most important difference between an engine and your heart shows up when an engine or your heart fails completely. You can rebuild or replace any engine at any time, and the car will run like new again. Once your heart fails to function as a pump or stops for more than a few minutes, all the king's horses and all the king's men and the best heart surgeons in the world can't rebuild it. They can replace it, temporarily with an artificial heart or permanently with a heart transplant, but that heart you were born with is headed for one of the human scrap heaps, either without you to the pathology lab or with you to the morgue.

That's why prevention is so important. From the day you buy it, you perform preventive maintenance on your car on a regular basis, even though you trade it in for a new model every five to ten years. You do that partly because you want to comply with the warranty and partly because you want to protect your investment. However, you take the function of your heart for granted, partly because there is no warranty, and partly because you don't have to invest much money in your healthy heart. Even nowadays, with all the knowledge available, you seek repairs for your heart only when there is a problem. That philosophy often works out just fine, but when it doesn't, oh boy, where do you get another one?

References:

1. Netter, Frank H. "Heart". *The Ciba Collection of Medical Illustrations.* Ed. Fredrick F. Yonkman. Summit, N.J.: Ciba. 1978. 6-21.
2. Libby, Peter. "The Vascular Biology of Atherosclerosis." *Braunwald's Heart Disease.* Ed. Robert O. Bonow, Ed. Douglas L. Mann, Ed. Douglas P. Zipes, Ed. Peter Libby, Ed. Eugene Braunwald. Philadelphia: Elsevier Saunders. 2012. 897-900.
3. Vijayaraman, Pugazhendhi, Ellenbogen, Kenneth A. "Bradyarrhythmias and Pacemakers." *Hurst's The Heart.* Ed. Valentin Fuster, Ed. Robert A. O'Rourke, Ed. Richard A. Walsh, Ed. Philip Poole-Wilson. New York: McGraw-Hill. 2008. 1020-1.
4. Malouf, Joseph E., Edwards, William E., Tajik, A. Jamil, Seward, James B. "Functional Anatomy of the Heart." *Hurst's The Heart.* Ed. Valentin Fuster, Ed. Robert A. O'Rourke, Ed. Richard A. Walsh, Ed. Philip Poole-Wilson. New York: McGraw-Hill. 2008. 51-66. 70-75.

9. CHOLESTEROL AND YOUR CORONARIES

As Americans, we assume our physicians have always been in the forefront of research, particularly when it comes to the big killers: cancer, infections and heart disease. However, until the mid-20th century, most of the important discoveries and advances in medicine came from Europe and Asia.

In 1755, a Swiss physician by the name of Albrecht von Haller first noted aortic deposits during autopsies. He named these deposits *atheromas*, the Greek word for groats or oatmeal. That gives you an idea of the appearance of the innards of a cholesterol plaque. In 1769, Francois de la Salle discovered cholesterol in a solid form in gallstones. In 1815, Michel Chevreul named the compound *cholesterine,* derived from two ancient Greek words, *chole* for bile and *stereos* for solid. While performing autopsies in the late 19th century, the "Father of Pathology" (No, not Quincy), Rudolf Virchow, a Polish-born German physician and researcher, observed that the inner walls of coronary arteries were irregular in contour in patients dying of a heart attack. He subsequently discovered that the irregularities contained cholesterol.

Just before World War I, two Russian histologists (histologists are scientists who spend their lives looking at cells under a microscope, doing various and sundry things to those cells, then looking at them under a microscope again), Nikolay Anichkov and Semen Chalatov, showed that feeding rabbits a diet high in cholesterol rapidly produced atheromatous plaques. Anichkov was also the first to describe foam cells in the walls of coronary arteries. We'll get to foam cells later. Despite their extensive research, not much happened with this information for almost forty years.

In the late 1940s a group of physicians enrolled over five thousand healthy adult males and females between the ages of thirty and sixty-two from the town of Framingham, Massachusetts. The goal was to study cardiovascular risk factors--inheritance, lifestyle and environment--and their effects on the development of high blood pressure and coronary artery disease. The Framingham study was initially expected to last twenty years. Over sixty-five years later, now following the third generation of subjects, it is still running strong. Hundreds of papers based on the findings of the Framingham Heart Study have appeared in the medical literature.

If you pay any attention to advertising, be it in print or on the radio, TV, or internet, you get hammered over the head on an hourly basis by ads informing you about a number of medical conditions--hypercholesterolemia, bipolar disorder, gastroesophageal reflux, and the king of all modern maladies, erectile dysfunction. Before the advent of modern medicine, these things didn't exist, because you were usually dead by the age of forty. These conditions, and a few others like atrial fibrillation, insomnia, and diabetes, have three things in common--they are widespread, they can be treated with highly profitable medications, and, in some cases, the availability of these expensive, easy-to-take medications can lead to overdiagnosis and overtreatment. Just as you are bombarded by media input demanding that you owe it to yourself to pester your physician to prescribe these medications for you, your physician's office manager has to juggle a cavalcade of drug reps wanting to play earwig with the physician and stuff free lunches down the throats of his staff. We'll leave bipolar disease, reflux and E.D. for another day.

As in every single aspect of the minute-by-minute function of the human body, the absorption, synthesis, utilization and breakdown of cholesterol and cholesterol-containing compounds is fascinating and incredibly complex. If you want to learn the entire story of cholesterol, at least the entire story as we believe it to be at this point in time, feel free to pick up *Lehninger Principles of Biochemistry* and read it from cover to cover, just like a first-year medical student. At the time my class was studying biochemistry, a rumor circulated to the effect that the author, Dr. Albert Lehninger, had recently been stabbed at Johns Hopkins University in Baltimore. There was no word as to whether his assailant was a frustrated medical student. Despite the complexity of the subject, in order to maintain acceptable levels of the various components of cholesterol, avoid coronary artery disease, and live long enough to savor the pleasure of soiling your diapers once again, there are just a few things you need to know.

First of all, unlike one of our former vice-presidents, cholesterol is not inherently evil. Cholesterol, a form of lipid, is a necessary ingredient in making normal healthy cells in every part of your body. In the human body, cells are constantly dying and being replaced by new cells. In order to form the walls of cells, you must have cholesterol. If you are a normal, healthy specimen, whatever that is, your liver usually makes all the cholesterol you need for cell synthesis and other functions. When you eat foods that contain cholesterol, that added cholesterol is absorbed from your intestines and circulates in your blood. In addition, your liver will make more cholesterol if you eat foods containing saturated fats or trans fats. Saturated fats are those fats which are completely hydrogenated, or, in other words, saturated with hydrogen atoms. Often solid rather than liquid at room temperature, saturated fats are found in dairy products (cream, ice cream, cheese, butter), lard, red meat, bacon, sausage, even poultry.

Trans fats, which are partially saturated with hydrogen atoms, can be found naturally in small amounts in meats and dairy products. However, most trans fats find their way into our guts and bloodstreams in the form of partially-hydrogenated vegetable oil. That apparently innocuous but ubiquitous liquid is found in shortening, which is used to make cookies, crackers, pie crust, cakes and canned cake frosting. It is used to fry things, like doughnuts, french fries, and chicken. It is found in canned biscuits, cinnamon rolls, and frozen pizza crusts. It is even found in non-dairy coffee creamers and stick margarine. Over the past decade, many food manufacturers have removed (or at least they say they removed) trans fats from their products. Unless you gorge yourself on the above-mentioned foodstuffs, odds are that you are consuming less than half the amount of trans fats that you once did.

Basically, if the American public likes to eat something in large quantities on a regular basis, that something will usually contain saturated fats or trans fats. As damaging as saturated fats are to your heart, researchers currently believe that trans fats are considered to be even more dangerous. In terms of heaters, the current opinion is that saturated fats are Marlboro Lights and trans fats are unfiltered Lucky Strikes. Like everything else in the universe, that belief will probably change in the next twenty years.

Cholesterol is hydrophobic (water-insoluble) and lipophilic (fat-soluble), while your blood is hydrophilic (water-soluble). Normally, the two would not be compatible, and, like oil poured into water, cholesterol would form huge globs in your blood. Fortunately, there are five different compounds, known as lipoproteins, that allow cholesterol to be transported in your bloodstream. Each one of these lipoproteins contains at least three components: cholesterol; a form of fat known as triglyceride; and protein. The amount of each component is different in each type of lipoprotein. We will deal with three of these lipoproteins, LDL, HDL, and VLDL. There are two others, IDL and chylomicrons. We won't get into them, but it is important to know that, like LDL and VLDL, IDL is a bad one. Chylomicrons are the lipoproteins responsible for carrying cholesterol and fats absorbed from your intestines to other parts of your body for storage or use.

Some of the excess cholesterol in your blood is picked up by low-density lipoproteins (LDL) to form LDL-cholesterol (LDL-C, a.k.a. "bad cholesterol") and deposited in the walls of your arteries, between the intimal layer (the inner lining, closest to the blood flowing through the artery), and the medial layer, which contains muscle to make the artery contract. That is a bad thing. It makes you wonder, *Who set up a system that deposits cholesterol in our arteries to kill us more quickly?* Satan? Pharmaceutical companies? Basically, your LDL is placing a badger into your strawberry field, where the badger eats all the fruit, destroys your crop, and drives you into destitution. When John Lennon wrote the lyrics to "Strawberry Fields Forever", clearly he did not take badgers into account.

Monocytes are one of the types of white blood cells circulating in your bloodstream. When they enter the wall of an artery, they convert to macrophages, which are scavengers. These macrophages swallow up the cholesterol that's been deposited by LDL in the wall of your artery. Because the cholesterol inside the macrophage looks like foam, these cells are known as "foam cells". These are the cells first discovered by Anichkov. They will continue to accumulate between the arterial layers to form "fatty streaks". Again, why? Why can't the macrophages go back the way they came with the excess bad cholesterol they picked up? If you send a wiener dog into a hole in a strawberry field in Germany to kill a badger, and the wiener dog gets stuck in the hole with the badger in its mouth, you can pull it out by its specially designed tail. Ditto for a ferret in a London sewer pipe with a rat. Why is there no chemical wiener dog to pull out that macrophage/foam cell?

If nothing happens to reverse this process, the fatty streak eventually grows large enough to form a cholesterol plaque, which is basically a mound. The mound pushes the intimal layer inward into the channel of the artery, narrowing its caliber. As the plaque continues to grow from a mound into a hill and then into a mountain, red blood cells have a harder time getting through the artery. At some point the narrowing becomes severe enough to cause chest pain from lack of blood flow, also known as ischemia. If the plaque ruptures like a dormant volcano going active, a sudden, much more significant narrowing occurs. If the narrowing is 100%, meaning a complete obstruction of the artery, a myocardial infarction (MI) or heart attack usually occurs.

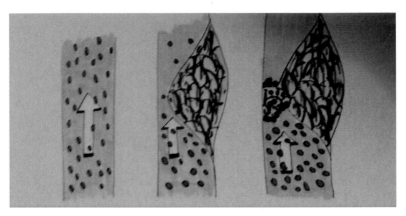

BAC

Normal artery (left). Cholesterol plaque (middle). Ruptured plaque (right).

If you are at risk of coronary artery disease, and let's be honest, who isn't, you would like to have an LDL-C level below 100 mg/dl. If you are at very high risk of coronary disease, meaning you have a scary family history of heart disease or you have other risk factors like smoking or diabetes or high blood pressure, or if you already have coronary disease, ideally you should keep your LDL-C level below 70 mg/dl. The fewer badgers in your strawberry patch the better.

The HDL-cholesterol story makes much more sense from a teleological point of view. Teleology is a philosophy that attempts to explain the reason for something's existence in terms of the result it causes. For instance, take morning sickness. Nobody really knows why it happens, but the teleological reason would be that women puke in the morning to get rid of bacteria-laden food lying in their stomachs and small intestines, bacteria that might kill the mom or her fetus. High-density lipoproteins (HDL) pick up excess cholesterol from your bloodstream, form HDL-cholesterol (HDL-C or "good cholesterol") and transport it back to the liver. Essentially, HDL is in competition with LDL for excess cholesterol floating in your blood. In addition, HDL is believed to help remove cholesterol from macrophages in the walls of your arteries and transport it back to the liver. HDL also carries cholesterol to your adrenal glands and to either your ovaries or testes--one or the other, probably not both--to make steroid hormones. In effect, HDL is the chemical wiener dog with a badger in its mouth. In most people, about a quarter to a third of all circulating cholesterol in the bloodstream is carried as HDL-C. The more HDL you have, the better your chances of removing excess cholesterol from your bloodstream and from foam cells and plaques in the walls of your arteries, thus avoiding coronary artery disease.

A couple of large studies have shown that there is an incremental, inverse relationship between HDL levels and risk of cardiovascular disease and death. The consistent take-home message is that the higher your HDL-C, the lower your risk of coronary disease, and vice versa. Interestingly, some studies have shown that smoking, obesity and diabetes, three independent risk factors for coronary disease, are all associated with low HDL-C levels. So, clearly, a low HDL-C level is bad, and a high level is good. Ideally, you would like to have an HDL-C level of greater than 60 mg/dl. The more wiener dogs patrolling the strawberry patch the better.

Very-low-density lipoprotein (VLDL), the third important lipoprotein, is the body's primary transport system for lipids. VLDL-cholesterol (VLDL-C) is the form of cholesterol that stores the largest amount of triglycerides, which are made in the liver from the carbohydrates, fats and protein you eat. VLDL picks up triglycerides in the liver and takes them into the bloodstream, where they are extracted for storage as fat in adipose cells or for energy production in cardiac and skeletal muscle. As with LDL-C, high levels of VLDL-C or triglycerides will also lead to a greater risk of heart disease. VLDL-C levels tend to be highest in obese people, poorly-controlled diabetics, smokers, heavy drinkers, people who eat a diet that is more than 50% carbohydrates, and those who do not exercise. So, if you are a bad boy with all the bad habits, and some bad genes thrown in for good measure, you will probably end up with high triglyceride levels in your blood. This is probably the only situation where a gambling habit does not add to your risk. On the other hand, if you have all these other bad habits, you are gambling with your health anyway. Although a "normal" triglyceride level is less than 150 mg/dl, the American Heart Association, which, oddly enough, has nothing to do with Valentine's Day, recommends you maintain your triglyceride level below 100 mg/dl. Because your triglyceride level rises after meals, then drops during periods of fasting, it is recommended that you eat nothing and drink nothing but water for eight to sixteen hours before having your blood drawn to check your cholesterol levels.

To calculate your total cholesterol, you add your HDL-cholesterol to your LDL-cholesterol, then add 1/5 of your triglyceride level. In other words:

Total cholesterol = HDL-C + LDL-C + (Triglycerides÷5)

You have to do the triglyceride calculation because there is no simple, direct way to measure your VLDL-C. Ideally, your total cholesterol level should be below 200 mg/dl.

Something you also need to know is that a low-fat diet lowers your total cholesterol, LDL-C, and triglyceride levels, all of which are good things, but it also lowers your HDL-C, which, we now know, is a bad thing. That is where dietary supplementation comes in. We shall get into that in a later chapter.

An important point to remember is that your cholesterol levels are determined mostly by your genes, and a little by your diet. A big fat guy can eat cheeseburgers and fries every day for a year and have a completely normal lipid profile, while skinny runner guy can eat nothing but salads and still have a subterranean HDL-C level and a skyscraper of an LDL-C level. The other point that bears mentioning is that, while people with cholesterol levels above 300 mg/dl. are much more likely to have heart disease than someone with a lower cholesterol level, most heart attacks will occur in people with total cholesterol levels between 200 mg/dl. and 240 mg/dl. That's because there are far more people within that range of cholesterol level than there are at the highest levels.

That is what you need to know about cholesterol. Two hundred years ago, had they even known about cholesterol, nobody would have given a rat's ass about it, because, in all likelihood, you would have died of measles, influenza, strep or some other communicable disease (including the bite of a rabid badger) long before even the worst cholesterol levels could do you in. Fast forward two centuries: you can read nothing but cholesterol drug studies for eight hours a day, five days a week, for twenty years and still not cover all the research devoted to cholesterol, at which point you will have to start over, because by then all the truisms will have been proven to be wrong.

If you take what you've read here, shed all your bad habits, find out what your cholesterol levels are, and treat them appropriately, hopefully you will not end up with a zipper on your chest. Then again, if we all did all of the right things and none of the wrong, I wouldn't have written this, you wouldn't be reading it, and you would never have heard of Viagra, Pepcid, Lipitor or Ambien.

In the 1973 Woody Allen movie, *Sleeper*, Woody plays Miles, a 1970s health food store owner who is cryogenically frozen. He is revived two hundred years later to combat an oppressive government. In one scene, he is being observed by two scientists. One mentions that Miles wants to eat organic health foods, like wheat germ. The other laughs and tells him that, back in the 1970's, people actually thought red meat and hot fudge were bad for you; fortunately, scientists over the next two hundred years determined that they were good for you and all the organic crap was a waste of time.

In 2015 the Dietary Guidelines Advisory Committee (DGAC) reversed its fifty-year-old view on dietary cholesterol. For decades, various experts had recommended lowering your intake of cholesterol because it was believed that eating foods rich in cholesterol would cause your blood levels of cholesterol, particularly LDL-C and VLDL-C, to skyrocket. Now those same experts are saying that only twenty percent of your serum cholesterol comes from your diet. The rest is made by your liver, courtesy of your genes. No longer are there any recommended limits on how much cholesterol you consume, although people with high cholesterol levels or coronary artery disease should restrict their intake of saturated fats and trans-fats. Stay tuned. That view should change in far less than two hundred years.

References:

1. Nelson, David L., Cox, Michael M. *Lehninger Principles of Biochemistry.* New York: W. H. Freeman and Co. 2013. 864-76.
2. Mayes, Peter A. "Lipid Transport and Storage." *Harper's Biochemistry.* Ed. Robert K. Murray, Ed. Daryl K. Granner, Ed. Peter A. Mayes, Ed. Victor W. Rodwell. New York: McGraw-Hill. 2000. 268-84.
3. Mayes, Peter A. "Cholesterol Synthesis, Transport, and Excretion." *Harper's Biochemistry.* Ed. Robert K. Murray, Ed. Daryl K. Granner, Ed. Peter A. Mayes, Ed. Victor W. Rodwell. New York: McGraw-Hill. 2000. 285-97.
4. Bersot, Thomas P. "Drug Therapy for Hypercholesterolemia and Dyslipidemia." *Goodman & Gilman's The Pharmacological Basis of Therapeutics.* Ed. Laurence L. Brunton, Assoc. Ed. Bruce A. Chabner, Assoc. Ed. Bjorn C Knollman. New York: McGraw-Hill. 2011. 877-92.
5. Griendling, Kathy K., Harrison, David G., Alexander, R. Wayne. "Biology of the Vessel Wall." *Hurst's The Heart.* Ed. Valentin Fuster, Ed. Robert A. O'Rourke, Ed. Richard A. Walsh, Ed. Philip Poole-Wilson. New York: McGraw-Hill. 2008. 136-9.

6. Maron, David J., Riker, Paul M., Grundy, Scott M., Pearson, Thomas A. "Preventive Strategies for Coronary Heart Disease." *Hurst's The Heart.* Ed. Valentin Fuster, Ed. Robert A. O'Rourke, Ed. Richard A. Walsh, Ed. Philip Poole-Wilson. New York: McGraw-Hill. 2008. 1203-17.
6. Libby, Peter. "The Vascular Biology of Atherosclerosis." *Braunwald's Heart Disease.* Ed. Robert O. Bonow, Ed. Douglas L. Mann, Ed. Douglas P. Zipes, Ed. Peter Libby, Ed. Eugene Braunwald. Philadelphia: Elsevier Saunders. 2012. 897-912.
7. Ridker, Paul M., Libby, Peter. "Risk Markers for Atherothrombotic Disease." *Braunwald's Heart Disease.* Ed. Robert O. Bonow, Ed. Douglas L. Mann, Ed. Douglas P. Zipes, Ed. Peter Libby, Ed. Eugene Braunwald.

Philadelphia: Elsevier Saunders. 2012. 914-26.
8. Genest, Jacques, Libby, Peter. "Lipoprotein Disorders and Cardiovascular Disease." *Braunwald's Heart Disease*. Ed. Robert O. Bonow, Ed. Douglas L. Mann, Ed. Douglas P. Zipes, Ed. Peter Libby, Ed. Eugene Braunwald. Philadelphia: Elsevier Saunders. 2012. 975-82.
9. Mozzafarian, Dariush. "Nutrition and Cardiovascular Disease." *Braunwald's Heart Disease*. Ed. Robert O. Bonow, Ed. Douglas L. Mann, Ed. Douglas P. Zipes, Ed. Peter Libby, Ed. Eugene Braunwald. Philadelphia: Elsevier Saunders. 2012. 997-1000.
10. Buja LM. "Nikolai N. Anitschkow and the lipid hypothesis of atherosclerosis."*Cardiovasc Path.* 2014. 23(3):183-4.
11. Fye WB. "Albrecht von Haller." *Clinical Cardiol.* 1995. 18(5):291-2.
12. Jarcho S. "Albrecht von Haller on inflammation." *Am J Cardiol.* 1970. 25(6):707-9.
13. Buess H. "Albrecht von Haller and his Elementa Physiologiae as the beginning of pathological physiology." *Med Hist.* 1959. 3(2):123-31.
14. Carmichael EB. "Michel Eugene Chevreul, Experimental chemist and physicist: lipids and dyes." *Ala J Med Sci.* 1973. 10(2):223-32.
15. Barton M. "Mechanisms and therapy of atherosclerosis and its clinical complications." *Curr Opin Pharmacol.* 2013. 13(2):149-53.
Stone, Neil J. "Cholesterol." *World Book Encyclopedia*. Chicago: World Book. 2016. 3:520.

10. INFLAMMATION AND CAD

Inflammation is an essential part of your body's response to irritating stimuli like toxins, dead tissue, and foreign bodies. The process involves immune cells, blood vessels and mediator proteins. Inflammation attacks the cause of injury, removes dead cells, and repairs the damaged tissue. The word inflammation comes from the Latin verb *inflammare*, "to inflame". Big surprise, eh?

The five signs of inflammation are *dolor* (pain), *calor* (heat), *tumor* (swelling), *rubor* (redness), and *functio laesa* (loss of function). Too little inflammation and the insulting agent will continue to kill cells. Too much inflammation that never stops may lead to chronic diseases such as rheumatoid arthritis and other autoimmune processes. Theories abound in the scientific literature as to the initial offending agent--bacteria, viruses, toxins; in many inflammatory diseases, unlike predictable murder mysteries, the villain often remains unidentified.

How do we measure the amount of inflammation in your body? Two of the standard laboratory tests designed for this purpose are the erythrocyte sedimentation rate (ESR or sed rate) and the C-reactive protein (CRP). The ESR is the rate at which red blood cells sediment (fall to the bottom) in one hour. Back in the 1890s, when the test was invented by a Polish pathologist named Edmund Biernacki, anticoagulated blood was placed in an upright tube. The distance the red blood cells fall in one hour is reported in millimeters per hour. When there is inflammation in the blood, a higher than normal concentration of a compound known as fibrinogen (Fibrinogen. Sounds sticky, doesn't it?) causes the red blood cells to stick together. These clumps, or rouleaux, settle faster. The faster the red blood cells fall, the higher the ESR. Nowadays, the sed rate is performed by an automated analyzer. Sed rates can rise or fall in a variety of diseases, particularly those that affect your blood cells, such as anemia or leukemia. Naturally, there is a superb equation to determine the normal sed rate based upon your age and gender--usually 5 mm/hr higher in women than in men--but anything over 20 mm/hr is viewed by suspicious minds as a warning sign of inflammation.

C-reactive protein (CRP) is a protein that, like fibrinogen, falls into the category of acute phase reactants. As the name implies, acute phase reactants are a class of proteins whose concentration in your blood rises (or falls, in the case of some acute phase reactants) as a response to inflammation. In response to injury from toxins, infection or trauma, some of your white blood cells release certain cytokines (molecules released by one type of cell to send messages to another cell type). These messenger boys, adorned in their little flat-top brimless maroon theater usher caps, head straight for your liver, where they deliver marching orders. In response, your tirelessly obedient liver produces acute phase reactants, one of which is CRP. CRP rushes from your liver to the scene of the crime and attaches to dead or dying cells. Once this happens, macrophages, the vultures of the white cell world (Macrophages are like your nephew Stuart. They'll eat anything, especially if it's really disgusting.), actually devour the dead cells. Cytokines and acute phase reactants also attract other cells which begin the healing process. The usual upper limit of normal for a CRP is 10 mg/liter. Once all or part of your body is damaged in some way, CRP levels in your blood rise, as much as 50,000 times normal, within two hours. It will stay up as long as there is ongoing inflammation or injury. It is a more sensitive indicator of inflammation than is the ESR, so in some cases, especially early in the inflammatory process, the CRP can be elevated while the ESR remains normal. The CRP will return to normal much more quickly than the ESR when treatment is instituted. There is a high-sensitivity CRP test (hs-CRP) which can actually predict the risk of a healthy person developing coronary artery disease. While studies are still evaluating its importance, some experts feel that your hs-CRP may one day be as valuable as your cholesterol profile in guiding cardiac counseling and treatment.

Most diseases that are characterized by chronic inflammation involve more than just one organ or body part. In other words, it is a systemic illness. The favored route for nutrients, toxins, or waste products to travel from one organ or body part to another is through the bloodstream. That's why blood tests are so effective in detecting systemic illnesses. If you have rheumatoid arthritis (RA), you suffer from severe inflammation in one or more joints. However, often there is associated inflammation in your muscles, tendons, lungs and pleura (the outer lining of your lungs), brain, peripheral nerves, eyes, skin, spleen, major blood vessels, pericardium (the outer lining of the heart) and coronary arteries. Inflammatory bowel disease, exemplified by ulcerative colitis and Crohn's disease, can also cause inflammation in your skin, eyes, joints and mouth. Many patients with these chronic inflammatory states have elevated sed rates and/or CRPs. In patients with RA, more than 50% of all premature deaths are due to cardiovascular disease. There is some evidence that patients with inflammatory bowel disease may develop coronary artery disease more frequently than their standard cardiac risk factors would predict.

If you get a splinter in your finger and you don't remove it, your body will do its best to wall it off and eventually expel it or break it down into mushy pus. A deer who gets hit with a non-fatal arrow or bullet will surround that foreign body with a dense clump of scar, which will be discovered when some other hunter finally kills and guts it. If you develop a small atheromatous plaque, your body will perceive that plaque as foreign and do its best to isolate or remove it via your immune system, which involves inflammatory cells.

When yours truly was making his way through medical education in the 1970s and '80s, atherosclerosis was considered a bland disease involving the pathological storage of cholesterol in arteries. Nowadays everybody is on board with the inflammation theory.

What is the link between inflammation and coronary artery disease? It starts with LDL. For whatever reason, LDL is preferentially absorbed from the lumen of your coronary arteries through the cells of your endothelium (inner lining) to reside in the space between the layers of your arterial wall. Once inside this extracellular space, LDL is subjected to various enzymes and oxidized. To give you an idea of what happens to LDL, you need only look at one of the commonest examples of oxidation: the oxidation of iron to rust when it is exposed to water and air.

Oxidized LDL, which is much stickier and more irritating than its non-oxidized cousin, stimulates endothelial cells to release various chemicals that attract monocytes, a type of white blood cell circulating in your bloodstream. The monocytes pass through the endothelium and convert to macrophages, which then devour the oxidized LDL, forming a foam cell. Each successive macrophage attracts more macrophages, which cluster and form an atheromatous plaque. Down in the core of the plaque, the oldest foam cells gradually die off, forming a necrotic (dead and rotting, like a corpse or your local cable company) center surrounded by newer macrophages and a fibrous cap. Although the details are sketchy, it appears that one of the functions of HDL is to prevent the oxidation of LDL.

Once an atheromatous plaque grows to a certain size, it inhibits blood flow enough to cause chest pain. In addition, your body senses the plaque as a foreign intruder that must be walled off and/or eliminated. This is when cytokines make their appearance on the scene, attracting even more white blood cells, which are an important component of the inflammatory response. They attempt to devour the plaque. It is a big job, however, and they have to call in reinforcements in the form of antibodies. Now your body has brought in the full weight of your immune system to do the job. If the fibrous cap is fragile, it will eventually break down, releasing the dead foam cells. The dead cells attract even more cells, in the form of platelets and fibroblasts, as well as other acute phase reactants. This causes the formation of a clot, which completely obstructs the lumen of your coronary artery and causes an MI. While this is going on, your heart and blood vessels are working on that plaque as well, stressing it via constriction of the wall of your coronary artery, high blood pressure, and increased rate and contractility of your heart. Given all these stressors going at that innocent little plaque, it's a wonder that more of them don't rupture.

We are a long way from knowing exactly how this inflammatory response affects atherosclerosis. From there, it is an even longer, more circuitous path to figuring out how to prevent or treat it. Then comes the most important step, the treatment itself. Somewhere in there, a brilliant researcher will win a Nobel Prize for turning on the light. It may take decades. Then again, some hapless lab boob brewing the weekly batch of hooch might blow up his moonshine still next week and in the process stumble on the perfect anti-inflammatory for heart disease, once again skipping all the prelims. It happens just like that more often than you think.

References:

1. Falk, Erling, Fuster, Valentin. "Atherothrombosis: Disease Burden, Activity, and Vulnerability." *Hurst's The Heart*. Ed. Valentin Fuster, Ed. Richard A. Walsh, Ed. Robert A. Harrington. New York: McGraw-Hill. 2011. 1215-19.
2. Libby, Peter. "The Vascular Biology of Atherosclerosis." *Braunwald's*

Heart Disease. Ed. Robert O. Bonow, Ed. Douglas L. Mann, Ed. Douglas P. Zipes, Ed. Peter Libby, Ed. Eugene Braunwald. Philadelphia: Elsevier Saunders. 2012. 904-5.

3. Shah, Prediman K., Falk, Erling, Fuster, Valentin. "Atherothrombosis: Role of Inflammation." *Hurst's The Heart.* Ed. Valentin Fuster, Ed. Robert A. O'Rourke, Ed. Richard A. Walsh, Ed. Philip Poole-Wilson. New York: McGraw-Hill. 2008. 1235-41.

4. Ridker, Paul M., Libby, Peter. "Risk Markers for Atherothrombotic Disease." *Braunwald's Heart Disease.* Ed. Robert O. Bonow, Ed. Douglas L. Mann, Ed. Douglas P. Zipes, Ed. Peter Libby, Ed. Eugene Braunwald. Philadelphia: Elsevier Saunders. 2012. 923-6.

11. OLD DRUGS FOR HIGH CHOLESTEROL

In 1987, lovastatin was approved by the Food and Drug Administration for the lowering of cholesterol levels. Compared to many of the older medications approved for this purpose, it was extremely expensive. At the time, I was working as a staff internist at the Phoenix VAMC (Yes, that VA. Motto: If Nixon can get away with it, so can we.). In order to get your patient on lovastatin, even after you had tried all the other meds without success, you had to crawl on your belly to the Cardiology division or the chief of pharmacy and beg for authorization to prescribe it. Not just once, but for every patient. The pharmacy guys especially loved having docs grovel for a signature.

Given the status of the linoleum there, I was going through shirts at an appalling rate. My chief of medicine, hoping to keep me busy and out of trouble, "suggested" I write a review of the currently available hypolipidemic agents, outlining their mechanism of action, indications for usage, and side effects. The idea was to keep physicians from prescribing lovastatin. Not yet in psychoanalysis for my crippling codependency issues, I hopped to it and produced a mini-tome, complete with all sorts of historical gems. Much like this book, it is virtually unreadable. Nevertheless, I find it interesting to know what patients took before the statins came along. Even today, some patients just cannot tolerate the side effects of statins and will end up taking one or more of these medications. If you end up having to take them, as the warden says in the movies just before they throw the switch for Old Sparky, "God help your soul."

NEOMYCIN

Neomycin is one of the oldest members of the aminoglycoside family of antibiotics. Antibiotics work by gaining access to the bloodstream and then traveling to the site of an infection. Some families of antibiotics are well absorbed when taken orally. Aminoglycosides, however, must be given either intravenously or intramuscularly--a SHOT--because they are not well absorbed by the gastrointestinal tract. When injected, like most of the other aminoglycosides, neomycin can cause deafness, neurological disease that stops your breathing, and kidney disease. Except in patients with pre-existing kidney disease, neomycin taken orally stays in your gut and does not cause any problems with hearing or breathing. Neomycin has been used orally to cleanse the intestines, particularly the colon, prior to bowel surgery.

In the late 1950s, researchers serendipitously found that administering neomycin orally would reduce total cholesterol levels by an average of 20%. While it lowered LDL-C levels by up to 25%, it also caused HDL-C levels to fall by 10-15%. Inasmuch as it was observed that neomycin injected intramuscularly had no effect on cholesterol levels, researchers concluded that neomycin worked by preventing the absorption of dietary cholesterol from the intestines. For the first two weeks of treatment, many patients experienced mild nausea and diarrhea. Once people started paying attention to HDL-C levels, this drug fell out of favor.

CHOLESTYRAMINE

Prior to the statins, two bile acid sequestrants, cholestyramine and colestipol, were the most widely studied of all the lipid lowering drugs. These agents bind bile acids in the intestinal tract and aid their removal via the fecal route. The liver then grabs excess cholesterol in the bloodstream to synthesize bile acids to replace the ones you flush down the toilet.

In a study of thousands of men for more than five years, cholestyramine reduced total cholesterol levels by an average of 8% and LDL-C levels by an average of 12%. More importantly, the incidence of coronary disease was reduced by about 20% compared to a placebo group, and coronary deaths were reduced by almost 25%. Other smaller studies found similar decreases in total cholesterol and LDL-C levels, and about a 5% increase in HDL-C levels. VLDL-C levels often rise on this therapy, sometimes strikingly so. Therefore, it was not recommended for patients who already had high VLDL-C levels. The products come in a sandy preparation, have a fairly unpleasant taste and usually require mixing with juices, yogurt or applesauce.

They almost always cause bloating and good luck pooping when you are taking this stuff. In addition, they are not cheap. Owing to their cost and their unpalatable nature, these days they are rarely used to treat hypercholesterolemia. They are still used, however, to treat several types of chronic diarrhea.

GEMFIBROZIL

Gemfibrozil is the best-known member of a group of drugs known as fibrates. Its major effect on lipids is a rise in HDL-C levels and a decrease in VLDL-C levels. This medication increases the breakdown of triglycerides in the body and decreases production of triglycerides by the liver. It also decreases production of LDL-C by the liver.

In two different five-year studies, each involving thousands of men, gemfibrozil caused a reduction in triglyceride levels of more than 30% and a rise in HDL-C levels of 5-15%. Total cholesterol and LDL-C levels fell by 5-10% in one of the studies. Compared to placebo patients, both studies showed a 25% decrease in cardiac events and an equal decrease in cardiac deaths. Oddly, in the Helsinki Heart Study, the gemfibrozil group of patients suffered far more deaths due to accidents and violence. If you've been to Finland, you know that had something to do with booze.

Gemfibrozil is taken in pill form twice daily. Nausea and vomiting can be a problem during the first year of therapy, but tends to lessen thereafter. In other words, it's a good drug to take, especially if you survive the first year of treatment. This medication is still used for patients with high triglyceride levels, both for the cardiovascular benefits and to prevent pancreatitis.

References:

1. Mayes, Peter A. "Cholesterol Synthesis, Transport, and Excretion." Harper's *Biochemistry.* Ed. Robert K. Murray, Ed. Daryl K. Granner, Ed. Peter A. Mayes, Ed. Victor W. Rodwell. New York: McGraw-Hill. 2000. 295.
2. Bersot, Thomas P. "Drug Therapy for Hypercholesterolemia and Dyslipidemia." *Goodman & Gilman's The Pharmacological Basis of Therapeutics.* Ed. Laurence L. Brunton, Assoc. Ed. Bruce A. Chabner, Assoc. Ed. Bjorn C Knollman. New York: McGraw-Hill. 2011. 898-9. 901-3.
3. Genest, Jacques, Libby, Peter. "Lipoprotein Disorders and Cardiovascular Disease." *Braunwald's Heart Disease.* Ed. Robert O. Bonow, Ed. Douglas L. Mann, Ed. Douglas P. Zipes, Ed. Peter Libby, Ed. Eugene Braunwald. Philadelphia: Elsevier Saunders. 2012. 986-7.
4. Price, Frank M. *An Internist's Approach to Hypocholesterolemic Agents.* 1990. 39 p.
5. Frick, MH, Elo, O, et al. "Helsinki Heart Study: Primary-Prevential Trial with Gemfibrozil in Middle-Aged Men with Dyslipidemia." *NEJM.* 1987. 317:1237-45.

12. STATINS

L. Frank Baum was a remarkable writer. In his first draft of *The Wizard of Oz*, he probably didn't pen the couplet:

"All hail statins
Cholesterol is dead."

Eventually, he was persuaded to throw in the Dorothy and Wicked Witch stuff.

Statins, officially known as HMG-CoA reductase inhibitors, were discovered in the 1970s. By then it had been established that the reaction regulated by HMG-CoA reductase was the rate-limiting step in the production of cholesterol. That meant that if you could inhibit that reaction, you could dramatically slow down and perhaps even block the production of cholesterol. In Japan a microbiologist by the name of Akira Endo was searching for compounds that he could use as antibiotics. He discovered compactin, which turned out to be worthless when it came to killing bacteria, but was effective at inhibiting HMG-CoA reductase. In 1978 a group of researchers at Merck Laboratories found another potent inhibitor; eventually, that agent was developed and approved as lovastatin.

After that, the race was on. Every drug company made a bid to have a statin approved. The vast majority of all studies of hypolipidemic drugs published in the last thirty years have centered on statin therapy. You would be hard-pressed to find a study of statins that was not at least partially funded by a drug company, which means two things: there will always be a tendency for the researchers relying on sponsoring drug company money to make the drug look more attractive and effective than its competitors, and, more importantly, as has been shown time and again since the dawn of drug company funding for studies, dangerous adverse effects will be minimized or outright hidden. Sooner or later, though, some doc in the hinterlands, unaware that he's supposed to dispose of bad results, will report said adverse effects to the FDA. That's when the fun begins. Rats scurrying to abandon a sinking ship. The study docs will say they reported those adverse effects to the drug company. The drug company will deny ever receiving those reports. When all else fails, "the dog ate them".

Case in point. After animal safety studies of lovastatin yielded no significant adverse effects, Merck started clinical trials in normal healthy volunteers in 1980. Clinical trials of compactin were proceeding in Japan at the same time, when, suddenly, for reasons NEVER revealed to the general public, Sankyo cancelled all studies in

September 1980. There probably wasn't a conversation like this:

"Hey, Hiroshi!"

"What do you want, Kazuki? I'm busy counting hair follicles on this shih-tzu."

"Come here. You gotta see this."

"Sake bomber! That dog has six eyes. What's he on?"

"Get a load of the extra tail too. Compactin, of course. What else produces shit like this?"

Although the Merck-funded studies of lovastatin showed it to be highly effective in humans in lowering total cholesterol and LDL-C levels with no serious side effects, once compactin was pulled, Merck shut down all research on their product. Since there were significant structural similarities between the two drugs, Merck took a step back and returned to animal safety studies. Eventually they resumed clinical studies, but only in very high risk patients with severe inherited cholesterol disorders. By 1987, lovastatin was approved for use as a cholesterol lowering drug. Its major effects were to significantly reduce total cholesterol and LDL-C levels by as much as 55%. In addition, usually there was a mild reduction in triglyceride levels and an equally mild increase in HDL-C levels.

Between 1987 and 1998, a half-dozen more statins were approved for use. Because of their ease of administration, effectiveness and lack of significant side effects, by the mid-1990s they were considered the one and only pharmacologic step in the treatment of hypercholesterolemia. During its run, revenue for lovastatin peaked at around $1 billion per year.

How exactly do statins do their job? As noted above, they inhibit the action of HMG-CoA reductase, which converts HMG-CoA into mevalonate, which eventually is converted into cholesterol. When you swallow a tablet of statin, it is absorbed from your intestine into your bloodstream. In your blood, it makes its way to your liver. Once in your liver, the statin molecule replaces the molecule of HMG-CoA in the reaction. Cholesterol synthesis by the liver is decreased. When this happens, other liver proteins sense the decrease in circulating cholesterol and respond by increasing the number of receptors for LDL. These receptors attract and attach circulating LDL and VLDL molecules, which are then digested by the liver. The overall result is a decrease in LDL-Cl and VLDL-C. In addition, they raise the level of HDL-C; how this occurs is not clear.

Possibly the most important effect of statins is their ability, at least in high doses, to reduce atheromatous plaque build-up and actually cause plaques to shrink. While the mechanism for this activity remains unexplained, there is some evidence that statins activate a receptor that caused macrophages to be expelled from fatty streaks and plaques. Others think that statins may have a role in reducing the inflammatory response that your body mounts against cholesterol plaques, thus breaking the vicious cycle that results in bigger, more unstable plaques that eventually will rupture and cause an MI. Some researchers specializing in inflammatory bowel disease and rheumatoid arthritis believe that statins hold promise in reducing the inflammation typically seen in those autoimmune diseases.

Ezetimibe is the first of a newer class of drugs known as selective cholesterol absorption inhibitors. Not a very sexy name for that class of drugs. How about SCABS instead? It blocks the uptake of ingested cholesterol by cells in your small intestine. Once your body senses that cholesterol is not being absorbed, it responds by synthesizing more cholesterol. If you are also taking something to block synthesis of cholesterol, then your body is stymied in two ways. That is why ezetimibe is usually combined with a statin. The only one on the market now is a combination with simvastatin, labeled as Vytorin. Any problems with statins? Of course, although compared to other hypolipidemic drugs, they are usually a walk in the park. One of the commonest side effects is myalgia (muscle pain), which can be extremely mild or it can be so debilitating that you can't perform normal activities of daily living. In studies, this occurred in 1-5% of patients taking statins, but it also occurred in a similar percentage of patients taking placebo. Out in the real world, up to 20% of patients over the age of forty taking statins report some sort of myalgia, whereas up to 15% of patients in the same age group who are not taking statins also report sore muscles. The take-home message seems to be that people over the age of forty do a lot of complaining about aches and pains. A more severe muscle complaint, myopathy, which means actual weakness of your muscles, is rare. This will manifest itself as difficulty getting up out of a chair or climbing stairs. If you are taking one or more of the other cholesterol-lowering drugs in combination with a statin, the frequency rises slightly.

The most serious muscular side effect, actual destruction of muscle tissue, is called rhabdomyolysis. It presents as severe muscle pain and weakness, and dark urine caused by the breakdown products of your muscles. If left untreated, it can cause permanent weakness, kidney failure and death. Rhabdomyolysis is dose-dependent, meaning that the higher your dose of statin, the greater your chance of developing the disease. In addition, your chances of developing rhabdomyolysis increase if you have diabetes or you are also taking one of the fibrates to help lower your cholesterol.

As with all drug-related side effects, if you stop your medication immediately and check in with your doctor, you have a much better chance of the side effect resolving completely or causing less severe long-term effects.

The biggest problem with statins is the problem with all high-profit meds in the U.S. For the longest time, drug companies focused on getting physicians to prescribe their products. That involved free lunches hand-delivered by drug reps with short skirts, big hair, bigger boobs, and even bigger expense accounts. The drug booths at medical conventions took on the look of your basic Dallas C&W dance hall on a Friday night. Doctors looking for love in mostly wrong places.

A large portion of the sales strategy involved outrageous "educational" junkets to resorts for golf, sailing, skiing and indulgence in pretty much any vice known to man. "Honoraria" for attendance, to the tune of hundreds or thousands of dollars, were thrown in to sweeten the pot, as were payments for travel, hotel rooms, food and booze out the ass. How do I know about this? As neither a primary care provider in private practice nor a cardiologist, I didn't prescribe statins, so I was not invited to any of this fun stuff. I did hear about it in detail from friends and colleagues who were. Jealous? Bitter? Maybe just a little of both.

This is not unique to statins. It happens with all high-priced medications and medical instruments. However, there are certain classes of medications that make pharmaceutical execs come in their pants. Unlike antibiotics, where you have to wait for someone to get acutely ill and then you can prescribe them for only one to two weeks, when it comes to high cholesterol, you don't have to wait for symptoms to develop, and you can plan on prescribing statins for life. The same is true for meds for high blood pressure, like beta blockers, calcium channel blockers and ACE inhibitors. Speaking of not wanting to wait, Cialis for DAILY use is pure gold. You might want to be ready before an atheromatous plaque forms, but you REALLY want to be ready when the moment is right.

All of this generosity on the part of the big pharmaceutical corporations eventually drew the attention of the IRS, so the drug companies eliminated the middle man, the guy with M.D. after his name, and went directly to the patient. Now, thanks to TV and print ads, the drug companies can tell the patient what he should take, and the patient tells the physician what to write on the script pad. IRS problem solved. In addition, drug companies have gone after health plans. Once their drug is on the formulary and can be prescribed without restrictions, mission accomplished. Just sit back and watch the revenue roll in.

Physicians don't like to be told what to prescribe. Most of that resistance is knowledge; some of it is ego. Problem is, legions of physicians with normal cholesterol panels have been taking statins for years. Even if you have a normal cholesterol profile, you might still have some plaque formation. Any time there is a plaque, there is risk of plaque rupture, the kind that can leave you dead or a cardiac cripple. Low-risk meds to prevent a catastrophic event is a good deal, especially when you get samples on a monthly basis and don't have to shell out for them. With all the advertising, now everyone wants statins for the same reason. It's really not a bad idea. Americans are used to getting what they want in health care, not necessarily what they need.

There is a movement afoot to limit statins to those with a significant risk of developing CAD in the near future. From a cost containment perspective, that is also a good idea. Certainly not everyone taking statins needs them or will benefit from them. The clash will come when Americans want something and their insurance company refuses to pay for them. This is not Great Britain, where the government decides who gets what. It will come down to the drug companies vs. insurance companies, perhaps, and researchers vs. physicians. Of course, physicians will continue to take the statins, no matter what the researchers say.

Had statins been available in the 1970s and early 1980s, Jim Fixx, the ex-smoker and bestselling author who popularized running, would probably still be alive. He died in 1984 at the age of fifty-two. According to experts who researched his risk factors, he had a family history of premature coronary disease and a personal history of smoking and obesity. No mention was made of his cholesterol level. At autopsy he had severe triple-vessel coronary disease. Had he been taking a daily aspirin and a statin, most likely the MI that felled him after his daily run would never have occurred. Of course, had he actually gone to a physician for routine care, his risk factors might have landed him on a treadmill and eventually on the operating table. The take-home message? You can't outrun coronary disease.

Had Mr. Fixx entered the arena of contemporary medical care, then Sonny Jurgensen would never have uttered one of the most tasteless one-liners in history. "All I know about physical fitness is that Richard Burton lived longer than Jim Fixx." Tasteless but true. Burton, a prodigious smoker and drinker from the age of sixteen, died at fifty-eight of a bleed in his brain.

References:

1. Nelson, David L., Cox, Michael M. *Lehninger Principles of Biochemistry*. New York: W. H. Freeman and Co. 2013. 869-70. 872-3.
2. Bersot, Thomas P. "Drug Therapy for Hypercholesterolemia and Dyslipidemia." *Goodman & Gilman's The Pharmacological Basis of Therapeutics*. Ed. Laurence L. Brunton, Assoc. Ed. Bruce A. Chabner, Assoc. Ed. Bjorn C Knollman. New York: McGraw-Hill. 2011. 892-8. 903-4.
3. Genest, Jacques, Libby, Peter. "Lipoprotein Disorders and Cardiovascular Disease." *Braunwald's Heart Disease*. Ed. Robert O. Bonow, Ed. Douglas L. Mann, Ed. Douglas P. Zipes, Ed. Peter Libby, Ed. Eugene Braunwald. Philadelphia: Elsevier Saunders. 2012. 987.

13. Niacin

Niacin, also known as vitamin B3 and nicotinic acid, is clearly beneficial in lowering your LDL-C and triglyceride levels and raising your HDL-C levels. It is absolutely beneficial when used to treat niacin deficiency, also known as pellagra.

Now for the other theoretical indications for niacin. There are anecdotal reports of niacin having a beneficial effect on erectile dysfunction. Some experts recommend taking anywhere from 300 to 1500 mg. daily in three divided doses. The idea is that it dilates your blood vessels everywhere, including your dick. If you surf the net long enough, you will find experts who recommend niacin for age-related macular degeneration, diabetes prevention, osteoarthritis, Altzheimer's, headaches, Hepatitis C, high blood phosphorous levels and "skin conditions". Other than for improving your cholesterol profile and curing pellagra, the evidence for niacin's efficacy is sketchy at best.

Before statins were developed and released for use in the 1980s, there were numerous studies demonstrating that niacin prevented second heart attacks in patients who had suffered a first heart attack and prevented death in those same patients. Seems like a desirable effect, doesn't it? Given that niacin has been available in generic form for about forty years, most likely you will never see a new study showing that niacin alone prevents cardiac events, like heart attacks and death.

Nowadays, any study involving niacin that sees the light of day will probably demonstrate that niacin doesn't help keep people alive but does cause plenty of side effects. Occasionally you can find a study showing that adding niacin to statin therapy will increase HDL-C levels more than statins alone, and that will often correlate to a slight improvement in terms of cardiac events. On the other hand, the aches, pains and muscle damage associated with statins may become more severe or more frequent if you add niacin. In modern medical literature, a generic drug that saves lives is of absolutely no interest. In medicine, as in politics, if you want to find the answer, follow the money.

How does niacin work? There are a number of theoretical mechanisms, some of which have been proven. First, it prevents the breakdown of fats in adipose cells into free fatty acids, which can be used to produce triglycerides, VLDL-C, and LDL-C. In addition, it affects HDL-C levels by preventing the uptake and destruction of HDL-C by the liver. Lastly, it appears to stimulate macrophages and monocytes to encourage removal of cholesterol from arterial plaques.

Almost everyone who takes even a small dose of niacin will experience a flushing sensation, which can be interpreted as burning skin or itching. A fair number of patients will experience headaches. Both of these side effects tend to come on within fifteen minutes of taking a dose and tend to last less than thirty minutes. It is written (It Is Written: sounds very biblical.) that if you take aspirin thirty to sixty minutes prior to a dose of niacin, the flushing will be reduced, sometimes completely prevented. Problem is, you don't really want to be taking aspirin three times a day. Some experts counter that taking one aspirin a day will help as well. Apparently, the long-acting formulations of niacin, which are also significantly more expensive, come with less flushing. Taking niacin on a full stomach tends to lessen the flushing; it is recommended that each dose of niacin be accompanied by twelve ounces of water. Some reports indicate that alcohol tends to worsen the flushing. Why anyone would want niacin's side effects to ruin a perfectly good drink is beyond comprehension. In addition, the combination of niacin and alcohol may be more likely to lead to liver failure. Certain individuals claim that smoking marijuana prior to taking niacin completely prevents flushing and headache. A word of caution here: if you have time to smoke pot three times a day, you have way too much time on your hands. Not only will you most likely forget to take your niacin as well as the rest of your meds, you'll probably forget at lot of other things too, like your family, your dog, and your name, none of which will faze you in the slightest.

When I take niacin, and I take a large dose, within five minutes I get a frontal headache, very mild in severity, and my skin starts tingling and heating up. In other words, niacin gets into your bloodstream faster than asparagus gets into your pee. My headache resolves within ten minutes, and the flushing within fifteen. I take two or three 500 mg. tablets three times a day. Theorizing that spreading out the dose might ameliorate the symptoms, for a few weeks I tried taking one 500 mg. tablet every fifteen minutes rather than 1500 mg. all at once. Instead of one episode of flushing and headache, I got three.

More significant than headache or flushing, niacin also can affect your liver, blood sugar level, and uric acid level, all of which make physicians reluctant to prescribe it. If you have liver problems, niacin will probably make them worse. If you have diabetes, your blood sugars will be harder to control. Your diabetes doc or primary care provider will be on your case to improve your blood sugar control, so unless you get a big kick out of struggling to keep your blood sugar within normal limits, niacin will only complicate your life.

If you tend to have a high uric acid level in your blood, niacin in therapeutic doses will probably cause your serum uric acid level to rise and possibly cause attacks of gout. Acute gouty attacks, characterized by swollen, hot, tender joints, are about as much fun as a hole in a molar. When you have a few minutes and require entertainment, Google "Dialogue between Franklin and the Gout". It is an amusing and informative little essay on gout written by Ben Franklin in the form of a conversation. If you already suffer from gout, niacin may cause more frequent attacks. On the other hand, would you rather die of gout and its complications in thirty years or of coronary artery disease in five? If you have any of these problems, either you have to stop taking niacin or take more medications to control the side effects. The more meds or the higher the doses of meds you take, the more likely you are to encounter side effects. It's a vicious cycle, and the costs, both financial and physical, can become astronomical.

Prescribing niacin is a pain in the ass, which is another reason why physicians don't like to use it. Patients usually feel some headache and flushing with the first couple of doses. Along comes a well-meaning friend who says, "Why are you taking that stuff? It's awful. I know. Years ago I took it for two whole days. Tell your doctor to put you on a statin instead." So then the patient calls his physician and gripes about the side effects, and the physician says, "Screw it, here's a statin. Now go away."

For your best shot at tolerating niacin, you start with a low dose, say 50 to 100 mg. three times a day. Every week you increase the dose by 50 mg. Theoretically, this gradual increase in dosage minimizes the flushing and headaches. Some patients have significant flushing at low doses and don't want to bother with it. If you stick with it, usually you can get to 1500 to 2000 mg. per day with mild flushing. Most experts try to get their patients up to at least 1500 mg. per day and recommend a maximum dose of 4000 mg. per day. Short-acting niacin probably works best when taken three times daily. Again, the long-acting forms of niacin are more expensive, less likely to cause flushing and headache, and can be taken once or twice daily. Any long-acting or extended-release preparations are more likely to build up in your system and cause long-term side effects.

If you have an elevated LDL-C level and you want to lower it, just about all of the hypolipidemics on the market, both new and old, will do the job. However, if you have a very low HDL-C level and you want to raise it significantly, niacin and gemfibrozil are your best bets. I have included my experience taking niacin at the end of the ME section.

References:

1. Bersot, Thomas P. "Drug Therapy for Hypercholesterolemia and Dyslipidemia." *Goodman & Gilman's The Pharmacological Basis of Therapeutics.* Ed. Laurence L. Brunton, Assoc. Ed. Bruce A. Chabner, Assoc. Ed. Bjorn C Knollman. New York: McGraw-Hill. 2011. 899-901.
2. Genest, Jacques, Libby, Peter. "Lipoprotein Disorders and Cardiovascular Disease." *Braunwald's Heart Disease.* Ed. Robert O. Bonow, Ed. Douglas L. Mann, Ed. Douglas P. Zipes, Ed. Peter Libby, Ed. Eugene Braunwald. Philadelphia: Elsevier Saunders. 2012. 988.
3. Shively HL "Correspondence: Ben Franklin's Views" JAMA 2015 313(24):2499
4. Franklin, Benjamin. "III. Dialogue between Franklin and the Gout." *The Oxford Book of American Essays.* Ed. Brander Matthews. New York: Bartleby.com. 2000. Obtained via Google.

14. SUPPLEMENTS TO TREAT HIGH CHOLESTEROL

FIBER

You obtain fiber in your diet when you eat plant-based foods. Fiber is the structural part of vegetables, fruits, and other plants (nuts, whole grains and beans). Unlike animals, you cannot break down fiber with digestive enzymes in your gastrointestinal tract. No digestion, no absorption, so it spends its entire lifespan, as it were, residing in your intestines, making the one-way trip from your mouth to your butthole. There are two types of dietary fiber. The first type, insoluble fiber, found in wheat bran, whole grains, vegetables and the skin of certain fruits, is excreted intact in your feces. It works to speed up the transit of food through the GI tract and helps keep you regular. The second variety, soluble fiber, is found in oats, peas, beans, apples and citrus fruit. This type of fiber dissolves in water to form a gelatinous substance, similar to Steve McQueen's nemesis in *The Blob*. It tends to slow down the transit of food through your intestines.

Soluble fiber is the more important of the two when it comes to lowering your serum cholesterol level. Like cholestyramine, fiber binds bile acids in the intestine so that they can't be absorbed into your bloodstream. When your liver detects low concentrations of bile acids in your blood, it takes up free cholesterol and uses it to make more bile acids. Again, this is a best-guess as to the mechanism of fiber in lowering cholesterol, but it will do for now.

A meta-analysis, the primo scientific example of Mark Twain's comment, "Figures don't lie, but liars figure" is the study of a group of studies, intended to answer a question once and for all. It never does. A meta-analysis done in the late 1990s showed that soluble fiber reduced total cholesterol levels by 2-15%. If you believe that "every little bit helps", then soluble fiber capsules may be just the thing for you. As long as you take them twice daily with a large glass of water, they can't hurt and you will probably live longer than Elvis or Gigi Cestone, both of whom died straining to take a crap.

CHARCOAL

Common charcoal is made from peat, coal, wood or petroleum. Activated charcoal is made by heating common charcoal in the presence of a gas that allows the charcoal to develop internal holes, called "pores", which trap various chemicals. Thankfully, it comes in a pill form, so you don't have to chew on a chunk or swallow a bunch of black granules on a daily basis. In other words, if your teeth are black and you are taking activated charcoal pills, look for another reason for the black teeth. Charcoal is widely used in medication overdoses and toxic ingestions to bind the offending agent before it is absorbed from the GI tract into the bloodstream. Most likely it works to lower cholesterol levels by binding dietary fats, cholesterol and bile acids, again preventing absorption into your bloodstream. Studies have shown that activated charcoal pills can lower total cholesterol and LDL-C levels by as much as 30%. The cholesterol-lowering effect is believed to be dose-dependent, meaning that the more you take, the better it works.

FISH OIL

A tribe of Eskimos in Greenland gave us the first clue that fish oil was beneficial in terms of heart disease. Even though their diet was high in fat content, the fat they ingested was of the fishy variety, with some seal and whale thrown in for blubbery spice (Blubbery Spice: The Spice Girl who can't stop crying.). Their mortality from coronary disease was lower than that of Danes, who live in the same neighborhood, and Americans. A big prevention study, the GISSI-Prevenzione, showed that test subjects who took omega-3 fatty acid supplements had lower rates of death, cardiac death, nonfatal MI and stroke. However, a meta-analysis (remember Mark Twain?) published in 2012 showed that fish oil supplements did not provide a beneficial preventive effect on death, cardiac death, MI or stroke.

In the beginning, before the time of the translucent yellow capsules, experts recommended that, if you wanted to lower your cholesterol, you should eat three ounces of salmon three times a day. While three ounces is not a burdensome amount of salmon, eating it thrice daily would soon have you clapping your flippers and balancing a harlequin soccer ball on the tip of your snout. Or moving to Greenland. Of course, you could change it up by substituting another species of oily fish, like mackerel, sturgeon, tuna, bluefish, anchovies, sardines, herring or trout. Baking or broiling these fish will benefit your heart. Frying them or eating them in a fish sandwich may worsen your chances of heart disease. Approximately 3.5 ounces of any of these fish will provide about one gram of omega-3 fatty acids. In terms of cardiovascular effects, the two most important omega-3's are eicosapentanoic acid (EPA) and docosahexanoic acid (DHA).

Fish oil supplements are usually made from salmon, halibut, mackerel, herring, tuna, cod liver, whale blubber or seal blubber. Yum. They usually contain a tiny amount of vitamin E to prevent spoilage. Fish oil is commonly used to prevent or combat the symptoms of a wide variety of conditions, from psoriasis to Alzheimer's disease. Many of these conditions have been shown in at least one study each to improve with fish oil supplements, but, as is often the case with supplements and health food products, either the study was of questionable quality or subsequent studies were unable to duplicate the results.

Fish oil has its greatest effect on triglyceride levels, which can decrease 10-50%. At least one study has shown that combining fish oil with a standard daily dose of vitamin E will have a greater effect on lowering triglycerides. When you take fish oil supplements, it is especially important to eat a diet low in fat. If you don't, the use of fish oil supplements alone may actually cause a slight increase in levels of LDL-C. Whereas a low-fat diet alone will reduce levels of LDL-C, triglycerides and HDL-C, it has been shown in at least one study that adding one meal of fish each day to a low fat diet will increase HDL-C levels and further reduce triglyceride levels. I'm no expert (remember?), but I think the take away message is to eat a diet low in total fats and eat one meal of fish every day or take fish oil supplements.

It is amazing how vague the experts are when it comes to recommending a daily dosage of fish oil. From what I can gather, unless you have dramatically elevated levels of triglycerides in a fasting specimen, you will want to take at least 300 mg. of DHA twice daily. Given the relative composition of most fish oil supplement capsules, that means you will probably receive 450 mg. of EPA with each dose as well. While you want to limit your intake of fat-soluble vitamins (A, D, E, K) to prevent excessive buildup of those in your liver, a dose of 400 IU of Vitamin E twice daily shouldn't hurt you, and may improve the triglyceride-lowering effect of fish oil. Bear in mind that vitamin E may counteract the lipid-lowering effects of niacin and statins. When it comes to cholesterol, nothing is simple or straightforward.

RED YEAST RICE

Red yeast rice (RYR) is made by fermenting a specific type of red yeast over rice. Initially, the yeast is red, and after fermentation, the rice is red too. RYR has been used in China for centuries to color Peking duck, to enhance flavor in rice wine and fish sauce, and to preserve foods. It has also long been used to treat indigestion, diarrhea and circulatory problems.

RYR contains a number of monocolins, which are believed to be converted in the human body to a substance which inhibits HMG-CoA reductase. In modern medicine, the best known of the monocolins is lovastatin, which was the first statin approved by the FDA. Because of this cholesterol-lowering effect, RYR products containing higher concentrations of monocolins have been developed and are marketed as natural dietary supplements. effective in lowering cholesterol levels.

Ironically, when the FDA realized that RYR contained lovastatin, it banned RYR products containing lovastatin, mainly because of case reports of statin-related muscle damage from the use of RYR. No RYR products containing lovastatin have been available here since around 2007. None of the commercially available RYR preparations in the U.S. make any claims stronger than "supports a healthy cardiovascular system" and "contains beneficial properties that support heart health". None of them even mention monocolins, let alone lovastatin. There is ongoing debate as to whether RYR containing lovastatin should be reclassified as a drug.

For that species known as homo sapiens, nothing is sexier and more desirable than a product banned by a governmental agency, especially when that product is known to contain a regulated drug that ameliorates a serious medical condition. Add to that the fun of circumventing both the medical profession and the pharmaceutical industry, and you have a product that will sell millions. Despite the FDA ban, if you want it badly enough, it is available in dozens of products on Alibaba, both with and without lovastatin.

The recommended dosage of RYR is 1200 mg once or twice daily. Many of the RYR preparations contain CoQ10, which jacks up the price of the product considerably. At least two studies have shown that RYR lowered total cholesterol and LDL cholesterol levels by 15% and 20-25% respectively. Both of these studies were published in well-respected European medical journals.

CoQ10

Coenzyme Q10, an antioxidant synthesized by your body, is required for basic cell function. A coenzyme is a non-protein compound necessary for the function of an enzyme. An enzyme is a substance produced by a living organism that acts as a catalyst to activate a specific biochemical reaction. CoQ10 levels normally decrease with age and are low in a variety of diseases such as cancer, HIV, Parkinson's Disease, Muscular Dystrophy, asthma and heart disease.

Taking CoQ10 may reduce the serious cardiac side effects of daunorubicin and doxorubicin, two chemotherapeutic medications used to treat various forms of cancer. CoQ10 may also improve the effectiveness of certain blood pressure medications, like calcium-channel blockers, beta-blockers, ACE inhibitors, and nitrates, meaning that you might obtain adequate blood pressure control with lower doses of these meds. Lastly, CoQ10 may decrease the blood-thinning effectiveness of warfarin and clopidogrel.

CoQ10 levels are also decreased in patients taking beta-blockers, tricyclic antidepressants, fibric acid derivatives (Gemfibrozil) and statins. When CoQ10 levels drop in patients taking statins, both muscle pain and muscle breakdown increase. While it is not generally recommended that all patients on statins take CoQ10 supplements, some physicians believe it will benefit those with statin-related muscular side effects. There is a possibility that CoQ10 supplements also help lower cholesterol levels, but that theory requires a large study be done before recommending it for that purpose.

References:

1. Genest, Jacques, Libby, Peter. "Lipoprotein Disorders and Cardiovascular Disease." *Braunwald's Heart Disease*. Ed. Robert O. Bonow, Ed. Douglas L. Mann, Ed. Douglas P. Zipes, Ed. Peter Libby, Ed.

Eugene Braunwald. Philadelphia: Elsevier Saunders. 2012. 989.

2. Mozzafarian, Dariush. "Nutrition and Cardiovascular Disease." *Braunwald's Heart Disease*. Ed. Robert O. Bonow, Ed. Douglas L. Mann, Ed. Douglas P. Zipes, Ed. Peter Libby, Ed. Eugene Braunwald. Philadelphia: Elsevier Saunders. 2012. 996-1001.

3. Anderson JW, Tietyen-Clark J. "Dietary fiber: Hyperlipidemia, hypertension, and coronary heart disease." *Am J Gastroenterol.* 1986. 81(10):907-19.

4. Van Horn L, et al. "Serum lipid response to a fat-modified, oatmeal-enhanced diet." *Prev Med.* 1988. 17(3):377-86.

5. Leven EG, et al. "Comparison of psyllium hydrophilic mucilloid and cellulose as adjuncts to a prudent diet in the treatment of mild to moderate hypercholesterolemia." *Arch Intern Med.* 1990. 150:1822-7.

6. Hoekstra JBL, Erkelens DW. "Effect of activated charcoal on hypercholesterolemia." *Lancet.* 1987. 2:455.

7. Kuusisto R, et al. "Effect of activated charcoal on hypercholesterolemia." *Lancet.* 1986. 2:366-7.

8. Haglund O, et al. "The effects of fish oil on triglycerides, cholesterol, fibrinogen and malondialdehyde in humans supplemented with vitamin E." *J Nutr.* 1991. 121:165-9.

9. Blonk MC, et al. "Dose-response effects of fish-oil supplementation in healthy volunteers." *Am J Clin Nutr.* 1990. 52:120-7.

10. Hanaki Y, Sugiyama S, Ozawa T. "Ratio of low-density lipoprotein cholesterol to ubiquinone as a coronary risk factor." *NEJM.* 1991. 325(11):814-5.

11. Burke FM. "Red yeast rice for the treatment of dyslipidemia." *Curr Atheroscler Rep.* 2015. 17(4):495.

12. Chen HH, Neher J, Safranek S. "Clinical inquiry: is red-yeast rice a safe and effective alternative to statins?" *J Fam Pract.* 2015. 64(2):128-35.

15. LOVE

The sign read "Lowest Priced New and Used Appliances in Town". Simmons thought, *"Lowest". God help me.* For the first time in his life, owing to an ill-advised and poorly executed ice-caving adventure, he was going to buy an appliance.

It was all Murphy's fault. The trouble began when his friend stopped by on the way home from a workout at the gym. He grabbed a Coke from the refrigerator and opened the freezer door to get some ice.

"David, your freezer is solid ice!" Simmons, who never cooked and never used ice cubes, hadn't so much as opened the freezer door for months. He looked over Robert Murphy's shoulder. A four-inch wall of white ice, complete with frosty accents, covered every surface in the tiny freezer.

"What's the problem? It's supposed to be cold in there."

Murphy shut the door and popped the top on the Coke can. "Cold enough to keep ice cream from melting and cold enough to freeze ice cubes."

David said, "Well, there you go." He started to walk out of the kitchen.

"Problem is, Dave, there's so much ice built up in there it's blocking the air flow. Pretty soon your fan will burn out, then the condenser motor will burn out, then you'll either have to repair this relic or replace it."

That brought Simmons up short. Money was tight, tight enough that replacing or even repairing that ugly little box of a refrigerator could mean the difference between eating or starving and buying gas or walking everywhere. Until his grant kicked in next semester, a good five months away, he was bare-bonesing everything so that he wouldn't have to go back to part-time night shift jobs, which would send his sleep and his studies in the wrong direction. Any kind of a social life requiring more than spare change was already out of the question. A setback of any magnitude meant double dating out of the dumpster at Dairy Queen.

"Are you fucking with me, Robert?"

"Absolutely not." Simmons was adept at all sorts of car repairs, but Murphy was a genius when it came to any problem around the house, from unclogging a toilet to rewiring an air conditioner. He'd fixed all sorts of appliances for friends free of charge. Despite his goofy exterior, when it came to the homestead, his opinion was not to be doubted.

"What do you think I should do?"

Murphy opened the refrigerator door and looked in at the temperature dials. "Well, you have separate controls for each compartment, so that makes it easier. Turn off the freezer--that's the dial that says "Freezer"--and let the ice melt. Once the compartment fills with melted ice, it'll drip down the front of the fridge, so you'll have to hang out here and mop it up from time to time."

"How long will that take?"

"Four, six, eight hours, something like that."

"I don't have time for that. I'm on call every third night. When I'm home, all I do is sleep, and I'm barely getting five hours a night."

Robert Murphy thought for a minute. "You could use a hair dryer to speed it up. Might take only a couple of hours." He started down the stairs with his Coke. "Either way, make sure you stick around to mop up. That linoleum floor doesn't look too watertight; you don't want to have to pay to repair the ceiling downstairs in what's-his-name's apartment." He descended the steps to the foyer.

"I think I'll give the hair dryer a try. Thanks."

"Just don't try to chop that ice out of there. It'll take forever and you might damage the coils. Damage the coils and there you are, back to replacing the whole unit." Murphy closed the front door behind him.

Within seconds, armed with a table knife and a brick rescued from doorstop duty, David was pounding away at the glacier occupying his freezer. Or rather, the freezer he was renting, along with the apartment, from Oscar Gibson.

At first the chunks of ice broke away in nice thick slabs. *Eight hours, my ass.* Within ten minutes, he could see the row of coils lining the back wall of the compartment. Taking more careful aim, he split off smaller pieces, stopping occasionally to drop them into the sink.

Just this last piece on the bottom and I can let the rest of the back wall melt. I bet it doesn't take more than an hour. He positioned the knife and tapped it ever so slightly with his trusty brick hammer. The ice broke off and slid up against the frosted coils. *Hah. Done.* He laid his excavation tools on the kitchen table and reached to retrieve the last piece of ice. It came out, jagged and cold, without resistance.

After dropping it in the sink, Simmons opened the refrigerator door and turned the freezer section's cooling dial to "Off". He closed the lower door and was just about to throw a dish towel in the freezer when he heard the hiss. Unable to believe his ears, he put his head inside the compartment. Sure enough, there was a high-pitched spitting sound emanating from a tiny dent in the lowest rail of the coils. His first cranial nerve, the olfactory one, picked up the faint scent of ether.

That last piece of ice. Aw, fuck me. He spent a moment wondering why, once again, he had been so stupid, then realized, *Stupid is where I hang out.* He watched the coil until the hissing subsided, then closed the door and picked up the phone to call Oscar Gibson.

The landlord was a busy man. After David bumbled his way through a description of the recent leakage of freon, Oscar got straight to the point.

"Mr. Simmons, did you use an ice pick on that freezer ice?"

"Ah, no sir. It was a table knife." There was muffled swearing in the background. "I'll be glad to help pay for the repair."

"Not worth repairing. Tell you what. First thing tomorrow morning, head down to Thomas Faust's store, at 9th St. and East Main. Tell him you need a used refrigerator and freezer. Tell him I sent you. Have him put it on my bill. I'll add half the price to your rent next month. That way I won't have to dip into your security deposit. How's that sound?"

Good-bye food and gas. "How much do you want me to spend?"

There was a pause. "Seeing as how I'm paying half, as little as possible."

The next morning, Simmons begged Jerry Greenlee to cover admissions for him. His classmate would take the hits from 7 A.M. until noon, then Simmons would be on from noon until 7 A.M. the next morning. He arrived at the Faust storefront at 9 AM.

"Mr. Faust won't be in until 10. You can wait or I can help you." His name tag said Andy Rummel. *A Rummel working for a Faust. Will wonders never cease.* The two families, allegedly descended from Hessian soldiers released from local prison camps at the end of the Revolutionary War, had been feuding for almost two centuries. Every so often, the Daily Crier reported on the latest outbreak of hostilities between the two clans, usually something classy like a shootout at a wedding reception or a drunken fistfight during a baptism. Numerous family members on each side boasted weighty E.R. charts. *Must be married to a Faust, or he wouldn't be working here.*

"Well, Mr. Oscar Gibson sent me to pick out a used refrigerator-freezer. I..."

Andy Rummel's rat face sneered at Simmons. "He called last night. I heard all about your little adventure." He shook his head sympathetically, then added, "That sure was stupid." Simmons kept his mouth shut. *I can get through this without squeezing that little neck of yours until your head pops like a zit.*

After looking at various models in the back room, following Homer's instructions, he selected an old rounded model, repainted in "Approximately Baby Shit". Andy plugged it in, twisted the dials, and it wheezed to life. *Good enough*, David thought. He followed the salesman up to the front counter to fill out the delivery slip.

"Looks like we can drop it off between two and four this afternoon. Will someone be home?"

"No, but I'll leave the front door open. It's apartment number 2, up the stairs."

"Upstairs, huh? The boys will love that. Bet it's a nice wide stairway."

"No, it's pretty tight. Will they take the old one away?"

"You want them to take the old refrigerator too?"

"If it's not too much trouble."

"Well, it will be trouble. It's not like they can just drop it down the stairs or out the window, you know."

"Right. Well, if they can't take it, maybe you can give Mr. Gibson a call and explain how troublesome it would be."

Andy sighed. "Never mind. They'll take it." He glanced over at an RCA console color TV. "Christ Almighty, will you look at that."

It was Simmons' turn to sigh. *Semi-slick TV salesman's trick number 1.* For politeness' sake, he followed the direction of Rummel's pointy little teeth. *Oh my.*

It was a remote broadcast, coming live from Nelson County. Andy reached over and turned up the volume.

"...and the firemen just finished cutting a hole in the side of the single-wide." The camera moved forward slowly and erratically to capture the scene inside. Dozens of flies swirled in the air. Accompanied by the reporter's "Fucking flies", a meaty hand came up and swatted them away from the camera lens.

Another voice from behind the camera whispered, "Fred, you know we're live, right?"

"Oh shit, I mean, look at all those flies."

Through the rough-cut hole in the sheet metal and insulation, a single light bulb could be seen hanging from the ceiling. The camera was now just inside the trailer, angled slightly downward and to the right. More flies flew insanely around the room, occasionally bumping into the lens. A blobby shape on the floor gradually came into focus. At first, Simmons thought it was a bear, but a massive hand and arm, presumably human, came up to wave at the camera. The back of the reporter's head popped into view.

"Well, folks, he's alive. What's that crawling on the floor? Holy shit, there's maggots everywhere."

"Fred!" The reporter's head disappeared; gagging could be heard in the background.

Andy Rummel snorted. "Look at that fat fuck. Bet you anything he's one of those miserable Nelson County Faust bastards."

The cameraman voiced in for Fred, who was indisposed off-screen.

"The firemen are trying to figure out how to get the young man out of the trailer and into their ambulance. This is Fred Afton, live from Nelson County." The camera backed up to show the trailer and a collection of faded shacks. Vomiting sounds emanated from a bent-over figure off to the right. Simmons stared at the screen until regular programming resumed. He said good-bye to his new friend Andy Rummel, then turned to go, wondering, *Where are they going to take him?*

It didn't take long to find out. Right at noon, he received a page from Derek Sylvester, his team's resident.

"David, I have an admission for you. Samuel Faust, age 25." Simmons jotted down the name.

"Room number?"

"Kitchen."

"Excuse me?"

"He's in the kitchen. We don't have a room assignment for him yet. Sandy's probably already down there." Sandy Hillman was one of the two interns on the team.

"If he doesn't have a room, why isn't he in the E.R.?"

Sylvester laughed; Simmons' antennae shot up in alarm. The resident's sense of humor hovered between arcane and repulsive. If something made him laugh, somebody was going to suffer. "When you get to the kitchen, you'll see. Good-bye." He hung up without giving David the fourth part of the admission info package: an admitting diagnosis.

Simmons left the team's office on the fourth floor and headed down to the kitchen. Along the way he stopped in to see Arlen Goodnight. Only sixty-two but looking ninety, the tobacco farmer from down the James River was getting started on dialysis for his multiple myeloma. Simmons had done his first H & P on him three months ago, during Arlen's admission to the hospital for weight loss and bone pain. When he found out he didn't have metastatic lung cancer, his Weyanoke internist's working diagnosis, the old man had laughed ironically.

"Ain't that a bitch, Yankee Boy? Here I been smokin' and chewin' since the age of ten, never ate worth a damn, and now they tell me I don't have lung cancer. I've got too much protein in my blood? Don't that beat all. They tell me I can live another ten years if that son of a bitch," he jerked his thumb toward the ceiling, "is in the mood."

"Yes, Mr. Goodnight. Of course, you have to take medications every day, and your kidneys are in rough shape, so dialysis might be coming down the road."

"The hell with that dialysis nonsense, Sonny. I've heard about that. Doc Turner said it's worse than dying, being hooked up to a machine three times a week. Course, he was wrong about me having lung cancer too. Probably thought he'd be rid of me in a month or two." He'd smiled pensively. "Might be worth the aggravation just to stick around and pester him at that."

As scrawny as Goodnight had been on his first admission, he was now at least twenty pounds lighter. His former bronzed skin had dulled down to merely sallow. Simmons made every effort to avoid talking about the old man's health. They discussed tobacco prices, land swindlers, a.k.a. developers, and the Redskins. After a few minutes, the old man nodded off and David left.

Normally, Simmons ran to pick up his admissions. You never knew when a stable patient would drop down the sinkhole of life within minutes of arriving on the floor; showing up after your new admission had coded and died never sounded good the next day at morning report. From the cryptic details proffered by Derek, he had the idea that this one wasn't going to try to die right away, so he took his time.

He started once again toward the kitchen, then thought, *What the hell,* and took a side door outside. The medical student took a couple of deep breaths, thinking this would be his last taste of fresh air until checkout at 5 P.M. the next day. From there he walked the perimeter of the hospital to the kitchen loading dock. Nestled up against the dock bumpers was a flatbed truck from Rockfish, which David remembered as being located right in the heart of Nelson County. Something nudged at his memory, then disappeared. The big steel loading doors to the kitchen were shut. He climbed the stairs and went in.

Inside there must have been thirty people. All David could see above the crowd was Sandy Hillman's curly black coiffure, up 6 1/2 feet in the air. He made his way past firemen, cooks, nurses and four big men in bib overalls. *Must be the guys from Rockfish.* It wasn't until he reached his intern and the center of attention that he finally put it all together.

Sitting on the floor, wrapped in two layers of heavy canvas, lay the guest of honor. A cook and two firemen were attaching the corners of the canvas slings to a huge hook suspended from a thick steel cable. Lying on its side, forever bent like a broken leg, sat the shiny steel frame of a Hoyer lift, capacity well over five hundred pounds. Simmons remembered the legions of nursing home hefties he'd moved from their beds to gurneys. None of them, mostly in the three-fifty to four-twenty-five pound range, had produced the slightest groan from the Hoyer.

He tapped Sandy on the shoulder. "This is Samuel Faust? This is the guy who was on TV this morning?"

"Right you are. We're admitting a celebrity. That is, we're admitting him once we weigh him and figure out a way to get him off the floor."

"I didn't see the ambulance from Nelson County out there."

Sandy laughed and stroked his beard. "Did you see the flatbed?"

"No kidding, they brought him in that?"

"Him and the fireman who tore his shoulder and threw out his back trying to lift him up onto the flatbed. That guy's in the E.R., getting admitted to Orthopedics."

"How are we going to get him up to the fourth floor? He's huge."

"They're getting a bed ready for him down in the Tazewell wing."

"The TV guy said something about maggots."

"Yeah, he has a bunch of decubitus ulcers on his ass, one or two up near his shoulders. They're all clean though, the maggots did their job." When the corners of the canvas were affixed to the hook, Sandy turned to the head chef. "Ready?"

The chef nodded. He punched a button on the wall. The cable, hook, and canvas-swathed patient rose in the air until his body floated six inches off the ground. Simmons got down on his hands and knees to make sure Samuel Faust was completely levitated. The chef eased around the patient and looked at the arrow on the meat scale.

He called out, "Six hundred forty-one pounds, ten ounces." When Sandy nodded, the chef squeezed back around and hit the button. Down went Samuel Faust to settle softly on the floor.

****

Simmons had often passed the carpenters strolling the halls in a pack, as jocular as a quartet of morticians, pushing a metal cart full of lumber and tools at all hours of the day and night. It had never occurred to him that they actually worked on projects. He just assumed they wandered with the cart for days on end, like Charon, the ferryman of the dead. By the time the assembled volunteers loaded Samuel Faust onto a stout low-lying table and rolled him over to the Tazewell wing, a mere ninety minutes, the carpenters had erected a throne, installed it in a semi-private room, and resumed their endless journey. Simmons couldn't believe his eyes. Constructed of 4 x 4s and 2 x 10s in what looked to be Southern yellow pine, the giant chair had a drop-down back, adjustable foot rest, and an enormous hole in the seat. Nothing about it said "temporary". His new patient wasn't going anywhere soon; David would be rounding on Faust for the remaining six weeks of his internal medicine rotation.

Sandy and David did their workups on the massively obese man together. Other than a few very clean bedsores, overall weakness due to inactivity, and poor hygiene, Faust was in surprisingly good condition. He clearly suffered from a very low IQ, but answered their questions appropriately and did his best to comply with their requests to turn over on his side. Sitting up on his own was an impossibility. He exuded an air of complete passivity and dependency. They ordered up a 1200-calorie diet, fired off consults to Nutrition, Dermatology, Plastic Surgery and Psychiatry, and figured out the daily activity logistics, a.k.a. nursing orders.

When he broke the news about the bedpan situation to the charge nurse, Sandy added, "Look on the bright side. At least your team won't have to lift him or roll him over. It's a straight shot to the ground." She gave him a look that would freeze fire.

Around 6 P.M. they received a call from Samuel's mother. Apparently she worked for a lawyer over in Lovingston, the county seat, and hadn't heard about all the excitement until she returned home. Sandy had David pick up another phone and listen in.

"How's my baby Samuel?" Sandy rolled his eyes, then stroked his beard before replying.

"He's doing just fine, Ma'am."

"Good. When can I bring him home?"

"Well, Ma'am, with his weight problem..."

"I know, he's gotten a little heavy. But it's only been in the last six months." There was a pause in the conversation for a few seconds.

"He also has several deep bedsores, which will need care and possibly skin grafts." David thought, *That guy lying on his stomach for months while the grafts take? Not a chance.*

"I think while he's here we'll start him on a diet, help him shed a few pounds."

"Well, whatever you think, Doctor. I'm sure you know what's best."

"Yes, Ma'am. Will you be able to come over sometime? We'd like to get some more information on Samuel."

"I'll be there late tonight or early tomorrow morning."

"Great. Please bring his immunization records and any of his medical records you might have access to."

"You mean his baby shots? Yes, I have them. But Baby Samuel hasn't been to the doctor in years. After all, he's as healthy as a horse."

"Yes indeed, Mrs. Faust. We'll look for you tomorrow morning. He's in Room 104, Bed 1. Just ask at the front desk and a volunteer will show you the way."

After finishing his workup on Samuel, Simmons admitted one other patient, a thirty-four-year-old mother of three coming in for chemotherapy for an islet cell cancer of the pancreas. She'd burst into tears a half-dozen times during the history and physical; he walked out of her room feeling sad and exhausted. Faust, on the other hand, left him feeling only pitiful numbness. Beginning around 10 P.M., the patient from Nelson County began crying "Mama, Samuel's hungry!" and as of 2 A.M. still hadn't let up. Simmons thought, *I'm taking care of the world's biggest crybaby. Literally.*

During the night more information surfaced, from neighbors and relatives calling in with their two cents. He hadn't left the trailer in almost five years, just he and his mother in there. The last two years he'd been too heavy and weak to stand or even sit up. His Mama had fed him, cleaned him, changed his diapers twice every day. He'd still be out there with his maggots had it not been for the serviceman from the county water department, checking on a low pressure problem in the main running through their yard. All the flies buzzing in and out of a hole in a window screen caught his attention. When nobody answered his knock on the door, he figured there was a dead body inside and had his dispatcher call the fire department.

****

It was 3 A.M., time for the night shift cafeteria feed. Simmons decided to swing by Tazewell 1, make sure Faust was finally settled in for his first night in the hospital. The night shift charge nurse looked up as he walked by, then went back to her charting. He cracked open the door to 104. There were muffled sounds but no more crying, thank God. In bed 2, Mr. Prentice Tazewell III, stroked out to the gills, lay on his back, breathing slowly, still alive. He'd been in the same bed, unresponsive for over five months, but as long as his family kept the donations coming to the medical center, the octogenarian would not be seeing the inside of a nursing home anytime soon. Not wanting the hall lights to awaken Samuel, David squeezed through the opening and peered around the corner toward bed 1.

Mrs. Faust had arrived. A picnic basket of Brobdingnagian dimensions sat on Samuel's lap. The woman was bent over her son, his head elevated at 45 degrees. She was shoving handfuls of mashed potatoes and fried chicken into his mouth, whispering over and over, "Mama loves her Baby Samuel. Baby Samuel is hungry." He chewed and swallowed as fast as she could fill his mouth.

Simmons blushed. Feeling like a witness to an intimate sex act, he backed out of the room and pulled the door to. After considering a heads-up to the charge nurse, he figured, *Fuck it, there's always tomorrow. Everyone should be so lucky.* On his way to meet Sandy in the cafeteria, he tried to make sense of this newly-discovered demonstration of love.

16. OBESITY

Obesity is a condition characterized by the excessive accumulation and storage of fat in the body. If you employ the eyeball test, it is pretty easy to tell who is obese. If your gut hangs down over your belt, or you look down and can't see your throbbing thrill hammer of love without the assistance of a mirror, you are obese. That's not precise enough for scientists. Researchers always need a gold standard when performing studies; for obesity, it is the body mass index (BMI). The BMI is determined by dividing your weight in kilograms by the square of your height in meters. Say you are 6 feet tall and weigh 165 pounds. Your weight in kilograms, 74.8, divided by the square of your height in meters, 3.31 (1.82 x 1.82), equals 22.6. That is your BMI.

A normal BMI runs from 18.5 to 24.9. In order to have a normal BMI, an American man of average height, about 5'10", must weigh between 130 and 174 pounds. An American woman of average height, about 5'5", should weigh between 112 and 150 pounds. As you can see, there is a lot of leeway when it comes to a normal BMI. If your BMI is less than 18.5, you are considered to be underweight. If it's above 24.9, you are considered overweight. While an extremely muscular person can also have a high BMI (muscle weighs quite a bit more than fat), unless you are a very devoted weightlifter, a BMI above 25 usually means you are fat.

A normal BMI does not mean you are fat-free. I am 6 feet tall--okay, 5'11 1/2"--and I weigh about 165 pounds. My BMI is right at 23, well within the normal range, but, thanks to a long and loving relationship with carbs and beer, I sport a significant spare tire up front. If you have the misfortune to eyeball my unclothed physique, I guarantee you that "Greek god" is not what pops into your head. The BMI is great for research studies on large populations and works well as a screening device when looking for people who are overweight, but when it comes to an individual, it is not a good estimate of how much fat you own, nor does it say anything about your overall health.

Nonetheless, BMI is the key number when it comes to determining who is overweight. So, in theory, obese and overweight can be two different things. On the other hand, unless you are a dedicated athlete, or, as your mother used to say, "There there, dear, you're not fat, you just have big bones," overweight usually means obese.

Being overweight is a problem. Usually, but not always, if you are overweight, you are less attractive to the opposite sex. Excess weight is a significant risk factor for diabetes mellitus and hypertension. Although it is clear that the average American is heavier now than at any other time in history, fashion designers and retailers continue to favor underweight or average body shapes in their clothing lines. If you are overweight, it is harder to find clothes that fit, and when you do, you have to pay more for them than for skinny people clothes. Airline seats are too narrow for you. I don't have any special desire to sit next to you if you are obese, but even with you sitting next to me and pushing me over in my seat, the flight is much easier for me than for you. We are rapidly heading for a time when obesity is the single greatest cause of increased health insurance rates. It already impacts life insurance premiums. So, on the one hand we have this recognition that obesity is a massive problem, but on the other, except for a few lines of clothing designed for the "fuller figure gal", American industry acts as if it does not exist. In other countries, especially in men, obesity is perceived as a sign of affluence and success. Not here. In the U.S., for every skinny joke there are ten fat jokes.

In terms of your health, obesity contributes to your risk of heart disease. It increases your risk for high blood pressure and type 2 diabetes, both of which significantly worsen your chances of developing coronary artery disease. In addition, in the early 1980s the Framingham Heart Study showed that obesity was an independent risk factor for heart disease in both men and women. This means that even if you exclude other risk factors such as smoking, older age, diabetes, high blood pressure and high cholesterol, just being overweight increases your chance of having CAD. In addition, obesity is a significant risk factor for the development of high cholesterol, high triglycerides, uterine, breast and colon cancers, stroke, gallbladder and liver disease, and sleep apnea.

Every day the incentives to lose weight become more significant for obese people. In the U.S., the general perception is that every obese person wants to lose weight. That may or may not be true. However, given the amount of money spent every year in the U.S. on weight loss solutions, clearly there are a lot of people who want to move from obese to normal. Losing weight is very difficult. The average American lifestyle does not include physical activity on a daily basis. Portions in restaurants are far larger than what is needed to sustain you until your next meal. It is hard enough to lose weight when you want to and everybody around you is on board with your goal. If your being fat provides a secondary gain for someone else, it is almost impossible.

For some obese people, overeating is truly an addiction. Some research indicates that a small number of overweight people do not get full when they eat, so they eat more food than they require because it still tastes good.

Like any other risk factor, obesity is easier to prevent than to cure. In other words, the best way to treat the overweight condition is to never become overweight. For most of us, gaining weight is much easier than losing weight. To gain weight, all you have to do is sit on your ass and put food in your mouth. The less willpower you employ, the easier it is to gain weight. Losing weight usually requires willpower on two fronts: you have to resist the urge to eat excessively and you have to get up and exercise. Food tastes good. Exercise hurts. In terms of time expenditure, it takes anywhere from ten minutes to a half-hour to eat a 2000-calorie cheeseburger. Say you could run six miles per hour, and you burn off 150 to 200 calories per mile. To burn off 2000 calories, you would have to run between ten and fourteen miles in two hours. Nobody has that kind of time, and not many of us can run at that clip for more than a few minutes, let alone hours.

No matter how much you eat at breakfast and lunch, if you are overweight, you most likely eat too much in the evening, during and after dinner. There are many Americans, overweight or not, who do most of their overeating while watching TV at night. This is probably not an addiction, but watching TV probably is. Why eat while watching TV? Smoking used to be a favorite evening pastime after dinner. In general, the more you smoke, the less you tend to eat. Far fewer Americans smoke than did twenty or thirty years ago. Of those who do smoke, far fewer are willing or permitted to smoke indoors, whether at work, public functions, or home. Perhaps eating has replaced smoking as something you can do with your hands and your mouth indoors at night. In terms of keeping your hands occupied while watching TV, it is probably considered more acceptable than firing a gun.

One of the ways you can lose weight is by not eating anything after dinner. If you do not eat for three hours before you go to bed, you will lose weight, sleep better, and have much less chance of developing acid reflux. As at other times of the day, drinking alcohol at night tends to lead to increased eating. Smoking pot ALWAYS leads to increased eating. In addition to aiding weight loss, a walk around the neighborhood before bed improves digestion, and better digestion leads to better sleep. Please note that riding around with a loaded gun in your pickup truck while "protecting" the neighborhood is not an effective substitute for an after-dinner walk.

I've never met an obese patient who admitted to overeating, but I've heard this one more than a few times. "But Doctor, I don't eat but once or twice a day. I've always had a very slow metabolism. It runs in our family. It's hormonal."

This might be what they teach in medical school on Planet Gullible, but here on earth that really doesn't fly. There are the rare causes of obesity that may not relate to overeating, but for the most part, obesity is simply a matter of taking in (eating) more than you put out (excretion and exercise). Most of what we lose on a daily basis is water weight, from sweating, urinating, and breathing. Losing the fat stuff requires more than just those three bodily functions.

One of the simplest ways to lose weight is to eat half of what you normally eat. If you buy a sandwich and normally eat the whole thing, eat half. Additionally, if you eat a large meal at lunch and forego dinner, you will lose weight and sleep more soundly. Eat SLOWLY— you will be satiated before you finish your meal. No seconds ever. More and more, researchers are finding that fasting for more than twelve hours a day will lead to significant weight loss. Naturally, if you are diabetic, this type of dieting will lead to periods of low blood sugar, which is bad for your brain and a number of other organs as well.

Another effective way to lose weight is to watch what obese people eat and avoid those foods. High on the list would be junk food, fast food, carbohydrates, beer (pretty much any kind of alcohol will do). Nutritionists and those grotesquely thin experts on TV are always harping on processed foods as the root of all evil. Because they are experts, undoubtedly they are correct. Unfortunately, most Americans, especially those who work full-time and are raising families (Do you know anybody like that?) don't have the time, the energy, or the financial wherewithal to make everything from scratch. Personally, I like to make my own meals, and if you cook you are more likely to be selective about what you eat, but a pizza once a month won't kill you. One other thing: No matter how compliant your toddler is with healthy eating habits, keep the bragging to a minimum, because sooner or later peer pressure will kick in and you'll be blowing through the take-out window for a couple of kiddy meals.

Then you have Tom Hanks' alleged comments about losing weight while filming *Castaway*. Something to the effect of, "It's not rocket science. Watch what you eat and climb a few hills." If he's telling the truth, it seems like a pretty simple proposition. Of course, if you throw in the incentive of a movie contract and a watchdog to make sure you don't cheat, maybe a personal chef to keep you full of healthy low-calorie food items, and someone to nag you up those hills, it might be just a tad easier. Then there's the problem of keeping it off once the movie wraps.

There are all sorts of medications on the market that will "help you lose weight". I am talking here about non-prescription substances, most of which you can buy in health food stores and supplement emporia. Depending on the brand and the vendor, they may be safe or unsafe. Substances that are sold only on the internet are more likely to contain some sketchy ingredients. For this reason, avoid those fat-buster products hawked on the tube. Some will contain thyroid extract, probably from dead pigs--yes, pigs--and will cause you all sorts of problems. Taking excessive amounts of thyroid hormone will cause you to lose weight over time, but if you have significant heart disease, you will experience increasing levels of chest pain, unstable angina, possibly a heart attack, possibly death. Some supplements will contain diuretics, so all you lose is water weight and potassium. Get yourself dehydrated enough, or drive your potassium low enough, and you have found yet another way to die. As for amphetamines, also known as speed, just look on the Internet for Frank Zappa's public service announcement regarding speed. A tad on the sarcastic side, but right to the point. If you are interested in other Zappa gems, look up his verbal jousts with Tipper Gore on the subject of music censorship.

If you have diabetes, high blood sugars will lead to rapid weight loss. Excessive sugar in your blood acts like a diuretic, causing you to pee like a racehorse. In addition, sugar doesn't make it into your muscles or fat cells, so they shrink as well. Some diabetic patients understand this and let their blood sugars run around 300-400 mg/dl, usually so they can fit into the special dress or tux for the upcoming wedding. You can drop weight, but you will become extremely dehydrated and probably lose as much muscle as fat. If you survive, after a corrective stay in the hospital, you will regain most of what you lost.

Dieting sucks, and over time it usually fails. Some programs that supply you with healthy food do indeed work, but they can be extremely expensive. In some cases, you have to stay on the program forever if you want to keep the weight off forever. Like a 12-step program, Weight Watchers works through peer pressure, but, again, many working people do not have the time to attend meetings.

Exercise has been shown to be much more effective over time than is simply dieting. If exercise were easy, there would be virtually no obesity. The hardest thing about exercise, like anything else, is that first step, i.e., getting off your ass and getting to it. One other thing about exercise. It doesn't guarantee weight loss if you don't cut back on what you put in your mouth.

Surgeons have been doing procedures to promote weight loss since the 1950s. They started out with the jejuno-ileal bypass, in which a large portion of the small intestine is removed. Along with the weight loss, which is rapid and significant, this particular bypass procedure also leads to incredibly large volumes of yellow, foul-smelling diarrhea. There have been all sorts of manipulations of the stomach, from cutting out a part of it to stapling a part of it shut. If you don't have any direct complications from the surgery, you will indeed lose weight. The theory is that if you have a smaller stomach, you will reach satiety, or the full feeling, with smaller amounts of food. If you are obese, you know you don't necessarily stop eating when you are satiated. If you are determined, you can easily stretch what little stomach is left. In other words, the issues that made you fat in the first place are not going to go away just because of a few staples in your stomach. Ongoing weight counseling is absolutely necessary and effective; if you return to your old habits you will gain back all the weight you have lost, sometimes more.

This is nothing more than a personal observation. I've seen nothing in the way of research to support my theory and, as you well know, I'm no expert. Nonetheless, I believe once-obese people who lose a ton of weight, no matter how, will probably always have to eat significantly fewer calories to keep their weight at a given level than their never-obese peers. I suspect there is a reset of their weight scales.

For the massively obese, there is always a feeder. Often it is the patient's mother, doing what she does best, feeding her child. Sometimes it's a spouse, sometimes an obedient offspring. Sometimes it's simply the angry child locked inside the supersized adult.

References:

1. Maron, David J., Riker, Paul M., Grundy, Scott M., Pearson, Thomas A. "Preventive Strategies for Coronary Heart Disease." *Hurst's The Heart.* Ed. Valentin Fuster, Ed. Robert A. O'Rourke, Ed. Richard A. Walsh, Ed. Philip Poole-Wilson. New York: McGraw-Hill. 2008. 1220-1.
2. Ridker, Paul M., Libby, Peter. "Risk Markers for Atherothrombotic Disease." *Braunwald's Heart Disease.* Ed. Robert O. Bonow, Ed. Douglas L. Mann, Ed. Douglas P. Zipes, Ed. Peter Libby, Ed. Eugene Braunwald. Philadelphia: Elsevier Saunders. 2012. 921-2.

17. EXERCISE

Exercise is any activity that helps to maintain or improve physical fitness. When you exercise, your body burns calories more quickly than at rest. While there are a multitude of goals achievable through exercise, for the purposes of this book, we shall focus on weight loss and cardiovascular conditioning, both of which help to prevent or eliminate diabetes, coronary artery disease, and obesity.
There are three categories of exercise: stretching and flexibility, anaerobic, and aerobic. For your cardiovascular system and overall health, including weight loss, nothing beats aerobic exercise. This includes swimming, brisk walking, hiking, cycling and long- distance running.

Numerous studies have shown the benefits of aerobic exercise. Clearly there is an inverse relationship between the amount of exercise a person undertakes per week and mortality from heart disease as well as all other causes. The greatest reduction in mortality has been documented in sedentary individuals who get up out of the Barcalounger and start walking briskly on a regular basis. If you suffer a heart attack, you can greatly improve your chances of survival simply by taking a brisk walk for thirty minutes three times per week. Obviously, pursuing any aerobic exercise on a daily basis is better than every other day.

While exercise is a wonderful way to maintain or lose weight, it is important to note that diet is equally important. This doesn't mean that starvation plus exercise is an optimal combination. On the contrary, exercise is most beneficial when you eat a diet containing adequate calories and essential vitamins and minerals. In other words, exercising and eating fast food on a regular basis is not a prescription for good cardiac health. Cut down on your total calories per day, cut out as much fast food as possible, and walk briskly on a regular basis. Your exercise tolerance will improve and your weight will go down.

18. DIABETES MELLITUS

Diabetes was first described by the Egyptians around 1500 B.C. as "too great emptying of the urine". About the same time, it was described in India as "honey urine" because it attracted ants. The modern term diabetes mellitus, describing an excess of sugar in the urine, comes from the combination of *diabetes*, meaning "to siphon", and *mellitus*, meaning "sweet". It was coined around 200 B.C. by a Greek physician, Appollonius of Memphis. That would be Memphis, Egypt, not

Tennessee. The great Greek physician Galen described the disease as "diarrhea of the urine". Why all the emphasis on urine? It was something they could observe, collect and play with.

Diabetes mellitus is a disorder in which carbohydrates--sugars and starches--are not metabolized correctly. Let's say you are a normal, non-diabetic person. When you eat a meal, carbohydrates are broken down in your stomach and small intestine, then absorbed as glucose, a simple form of sugar, from your small intestine into your bloodstream. The rise in glucose levels in your bloodstream causes your pancreas to secrete insulin, a hormone. The insulin causes your liver, muscle and adipose (fat) cells to absorb glucose from your bloodstream. In the muscle cells, including your heart muscle, the glucose is used for energy; a small amount is also stored in your muscle cells as fat. In liver cells, the glucose is stored as glycogen, a form of starch. In your adipose cells, glucose is stored as fat. Once all this dietary glucose is stored or used, your blood glucose levels return to normal and your insulin returns to a low, baseline level.

As far back as 400 A.D., physicians in India differentiated type 1 and type 2 diabetes; type 1 was associated with young people, type 2 with overweight adults. If you suffer from Type 1 diabetes, your pancreas cannot secrete insulin into your bloodstream because your pancreatic islet cells, the ones that make insulin, have been destroyed. Although it is not yet clear how the islet cells in your pancreas came to be destroyed, the current theory is that your immune system did the dirty work. Genetics may play a role, as may viruses. Since there is no insulin to facilitate the absorption of glucose into muscle, fat and liver cells, your blood glucose level remains higher than normal. Some of that excess sugar in your blood is filtered through your kidneys into your urine, where it acts like a diuretic, causing you to pee much more than normal.

In the meantime, because there is no insulin to move glucose from your bloodstream to your muscle cells, your muscle cells start crying out for glucose for energy. In response, your liver, which apparently hates the sound of a crying muscle cell, begins to break glycogen back down into glucose, which travels through your bloodstream to your muscle cells to make them stop crying. This is just dandy, as long as your glycogen stores hold up. Once your liver's glycogen stores are all used up and your muscle cells start that goddamned crying again, your adipose cells are tapped to supply energy. Fat is released as fatty acids, which travel in your bloodstream to your liver, where they are broken down into ketones. Initially, the ketones supply energy to your muscle cells, but as the level of ketones, which are acidic, builds up in your bloodstream, it causes your blood to become more acidic. The pH of your blood falls from its normal level, around 7.4, to dangerously low levels, anywhere from 7.0 on down. This results in ketoacidosis, which requires emergency treatment in a hospital and can cause permanent damage to various organs or even death. All of this can be prevented in the Type 1 diabetic with the administration of insulin shots on a regular basis, from one to four times daily.

This is a good time to inject some American history into the diabetes story, particularly type 2, which is far more common than type 1. Prior to modern medicine's first real appearance on the Navajo reservation in the mid-1950s in the form of the Indian Health Service, there was a relative paucity of diabetes. Complications of diabetes, such as MI or chronic kidney disease, were almost unheard of. Part of this was the lack of adequate medical care to diagnose these conditions, and part was due to the economic and social circumstances of the Navajo. They were poor, had no vehicles, and had no access to processed food. They walked or rode horses to get around. They were skinny. By the early 1970s, pickup trucks and processed food were more plentiful. The residents stopped walking so much, ate commercially available processed food, and gained weight; with the weight came type 2 diabetes. Lots of it.

The "Thrifty Gene" theory, set forth by Dr. James V. Neel in the early 1960s, proposed that certain Native American populations, subjected to alternating periods of feast and famine, developed the ability to store energy (food) and use it sparingly. Hunter tribes would kill a woolly mammoth, eat it, cough up a woolly fur ball, then move on and possibly not eat for days or weeks until the next kill. Thanks to high levels of insulin, they stored the food efficiently as fat. During periods without food, insulin levels tumbled and the fat broke down to be used for energy. As long as they were mobile and ate intermittently, they remained skinny. Even though automobiles and greater availability of food supplies made it unnecessary to store energy as fat, their thrifty gene continued to be stingy with energy expenditure, and their weight went up. The only constant in life is change, so who knows? Perhaps a couple thousands of years from now, subjected to adequate availability of food on a regular basis, the thrifty gene will become less thrifty, and much of the type 2 diabetes seen in Native Americans may disappear. In the meantime, southwestern tribes like the Navajo and the Pima will continue to have problems with weight and the attendant diabetic complications.

In Type 2 diabetes, there is sufficient or even excessive insulin production. The problem seems to be that your cells are resistant to insulin. So even though there is plenty of glucose and plenty of insulin, the glucose can't get into muscle cells for energy, or into fat cells for storage. Once again, you have too much glucose in your blood and not enough in your muscles. You get weak and you start spilling glucose through your kidneys into your urine. Treatment for Type 2 diabetes is weight loss, which reduces fat stores and the size of your fat cells, oral hypoglycemic agents, which can help get glucose into cells, or huge doses of insulin to overcome your insulin resistance.

Is diabetes a big problem? You bet, Chet. According to a CDC report released in 2014, twenty-nine million Americans, about 9% of the population, suffered from diabetes. About 1.25 million were type 1; the rest, over twenty-seven million, were type 2. Over 1.5 million new cases of diabetes, mostly type 2, are diagnosed every year. Here's the real stunner. In 2012, it was estimated that eighty-six million Americans aged 20 or older had prediabetes. That's a quarter of the population of the U.S.

Suppose you learn from your doctor or from a screening exam at work that you are "prediabetic". Whenever and wherever that occurred, you were probably given some instructions and a pamphlet or two to read, which, if you are a normal human being, you left in your car or threw in the "to be read" pile at home or work. When most folks hear "pre-" anything, they figure, why worry about something that hasn't happened yet? There's more than enough already happening to occupy the brain's worry lobe. Why worry about a low HDL-C and a high LDL-C if nothing has happened yet? That's how people end up with heart problems. Prediabetes, also known as borderline diabetes or impaired glucose tolerance, means that your body is not doing a perfect job of regulating your blood sugar, but, at least in that respect, it hasn't crapped out entirely. Not yet, anyway. Prediabetes is a diagnosis associated only with type 2 diabetes.

Condition	Hgb A1C	Fasting Glucose	Oral GTT
Diabetes	>= 6.5 %	>=126 mg/dl.	>=200 mg/dl.
Prediabetes	5.7 - 6.4	100 - 125	140 - 199
Normal	About 5.0	<=99	<=139

There are three types of blood testing available to make the diagnosis. The handy dandy chart lists the values of each. The simplest, the Hemoglobin (Hgb) A1C, measures the percentage of the hemoglobin in your blood that is glycosylated. Glycosylation occurs when your hemoglobin is exposed to glucose over a period of time. The higher your average blood glucose over a three-month period, the higher your Hgb A1C. A mildly elevated level means you have prediabetes. A markedly elevated level indicates diabetes. The nice thing about the

HgbA1C measurement is that it involves a single blood draw, it can be done at any time of the day, and does not require fasting.

The classic standard blood test for diabetes is the fasting blood glucose (FBG). This is performed, preferably first thing in the morning, after fasting for at least eight hours. Again, if it is mildly elevated, you probably have prediabetes. A marked elevation usually means diabetes. The drawback is the fasting part, but one nice thing about the FBG is that a finger stick is often the only test required to make the diagnosis. That finger stick can be done in the office and you have the result within seconds. Unless your health care provider is bent on squeezing every dime out of you, it shouldn't cost you much either, certainly no lab fee for drawing blood.

The method with the highest PITA (pain-in-the-ass) score is the postprandial (after eating) blood glucose level. Traditionally, patients with a normal fasting blood glucose level who were suspected of having diabetes would eat a normal meal and then get a blood glucose level drawn two hours later. Even less convenient is the oral glucose tolerance test (OGTT). For that special event, you have to fast for eight hours. Then you get your blood drawn for a fasting blood glucose level. Then you drink a specific amount of glucose within five minutes. Even though you might be starving by now, this stuff rarely tastes good. Then you sit on your ass for two hours. Then you have your blood drawn a second time. If your health care provider really has it in for you, there is even a protocol in which you have your blood drawn at 0, 2, 4 and 6 hours. Nowadays, health care providers with no grudge reserve the OGTT for diagnosing gestational diabetes in pregnant women and prediabetes in non-pregnant individuals when there is high suspicion but the other two tests are normal.

Think of prediabetes as your one last shot at a normal life. This is your chance to shape up. If you don't, most likely you will eventually develop type 2 diabetes, and your life will become much more complicated. Keep it simple.

All very interesting, you might say. However, I am reading this book to learn about heart disease, so how about sticking to the topic? Fair enough. You want to know how diabetes can affect your heart, specifically, what diabetes does to your coronary arteries. High blood glucose levels over a period of time leads to increased fatty deposits in the walls of your coronary arteries, increasing the likelihood of atherosclerotic plaques. If you are diabetic, you are twice as likely to suffer from coronary artery disease (CAD) as your non-diabetic buddies. In addition, diabetic patients tend to develop CAD at an earlier age. If you are middle-aged and have type 2 diabetes, some studies suggest that you have as great a risk of having a heart attack as a non-diabetic who has already had one heart attack. If you are diabetic and have already had one heart attack, your chance of suffering a second heart attack is much higher than in non-diabetics who have had one heart attack. Heart attacks in diabetics tend to be more serious and are more likely to be fatal than in non-diabetics. About two-thirds of all diabetics die of heart disease or stroke. A recent study hot off the presses shows that type 2 diabetes shortens your lifespan by an average of twelve years, more than either smoking or HIV.

All that sounds pretty dark, doesn't it? What can you do about it? Studies consistently show that diabetics, especially type 2 diabetics, with lower, better-controlled blood glucose levels have fewer and milder complications than do their poorly-controlled counterparts. This refers primarily to neurologic complications, such as peripheral neuropathy (numbness and burning in your feet), and microvascular (small vessel) complications in your eyes and kidneys. In addition, if you have type 2 diabetes, you may suffer from cardiac syndrome X, a disorder of tiny vessels in the heart.

Poorly-controlled diabetics also have higher rates of macrovascular (large vessel) disease, such as cerebrovascular disease, which can cause strokes, peripheral arterial disease (PAD), which can lead to leg amputations, and CAD, which eventually will lead to MIs and death. When combined with a little luck, the closer to normal you keep your blood glucose levels, the better the chance you will live a normal lifespan without losing any essential body parts.

If you exercise (get out of the pickup truck and walk), eat right, lose weight and take your medications, your blood glucose levels will almost always come under better control. Good control begets good control, meaning that once you have your blood glucose level under good control, it is much easier to keep it there than it was to get it there in the first place. Doing all the right things is very simple when it comes to tying your shoes, but incredibly difficult when it comes to controlling your diabetes. Then again, if it were easy, anyone could do it.

Diabetes is a fascinating disease to study. From a distance, it is nothing short of shocking that the loss or lack of effect of a single hormone, insulin, can cause so much devastation, both in the short run and over the course of a lifetime. Up close and personal, for you and your physician, it can feel like an endless climb up a steep mountain. If you have hypothyroidism due to a lack of thyroid hormone, you take a pill, check your levels twice a year, and go on with your life. If your testosterone level is low, you take a shot once a month or rub on the clear or the cream, get your PSA checked, and enjoy a gloved urologic finger up your butt every year; every part of your body will feel more energetic and work more effectively, especially your you-know-what. But if your insulin is absent or ineffective, every move you make, every donut you shove through your pie hole has an enormous effect on how you feel and how long you live. Diabetes has a negative impact on virtually every part of your body, from your brain to your toes and everywhere in between. If you are diabetic, two of the seven deadly sins, sloth and gluttony, really can kill you. The treatment of diabetes is not just the treatment of a disease. It is the understanding, acceptance, incentivization and management of human nature. Like the temptation to sit on your ass and overeat, diabetes never goes away. At least not yet it doesn't.

References:

1. Bersot, Thomas P. "Drug Therapy for Hypercholesterolemia and Dyslipidemia." Goodman & Gilman's The Pharmacological Basis of Therapeutics. Ed. Laurence L. Brunton, Assoc. Ed. Bruce A. Chabner, Assoc. Ed. Bjorn C Knollman. New York: McGraw-Hill. 2011. 890-2.
2. Maron, David J., Ridker, Paul M., Grundy, Scott M., Pearson, Thomas A. "Preventive Strategies for Coronary Heart Disease." Hurst's The Heart. Ed. Valentin Fuster, Ed. Robert A. O'Rourke, Ed. Richard A. Walsh, Ed. Philip Poole-Wilson. New York: McGraw-Hill. 2008. 1219-20.
3. Ridker, Paul M., Libby, Peter. "Risk Markers for Atherothrombotic Disease." Braunwald's Heart Disease. Ed. Robert O. Bonow, Ed. Douglas L. Mann, Ed. Douglas P. Zipes, Ed. Peter Libby, Ed. Eugene Braunwald. Philadelphia: Elsevier Saunders. 2012. 919-21.
4. Laios K, Karamanou M, Saridaki Z, Androutsos G. "Aretaeus of Cappadocia and the first description of diabetes." Hormones. 2012. 11(1):109–113.
5. Centers for Disease Control and Prevention. National Diabetes Statistics Report: Estimates of Diabetes and Its Burden in the United States, 2014. Atlanta, GA: U.S. Department of Health and Human Services.

19. HYPERTENSION

Hypertension (HTN) is the medical term for high blood pressure. The word "hypertension" is of mixed Greek and Latin origin, meaning "overstretching". Blood pressure (BP) is the force exerted on your arteries by a wave of blood propelled from your heart. In order to increase your BP, there must be an increase either in your cardiac output (CO), the amount of blood pumped by your heart every minute, or in your systemic vascular resistance (SVR), the degree of tightness in your arteries. The concept of BP was first described by William Harvey in 1628.

Stephen Hales, an English clergyman, recorded the first measurement of blood pressure in 1733. How did he do this back then? He stuck fine tubes into the arteries of animals and measured how high the blood rose in the tubes. In the first three decades of the nineteenth century, several physicians described HTN as a specific disease process. The invention of the cuff-based sphygmomanometer by Scipione Riva-Rocci in 1896 permitted the easy measurement of BP. Ten years later, Nikolai Korotkoff described the sounds heard while measuring BP. These are still referred to as "Korotkoff sounds".

Your BP is recorded as one number over another, as in 120/80. Both numbers refer to the height in millimeters (mmHg.) of a column of mercury on a sphygmomanometer, the device used to measure your BP. First your physician or nurse places an inflatable velcro cuff around your arm just above your elbow. Then he tightens an air valve on the end of a hollow egg-shaped ball of rubber. The greater the pressure exerted by the cuff on your arm, the higher the rise of the column of mercury. By squeezing the ball repeatedly, the cuff is inflated until the column of mercury is high up on the sphygmomanometer, usually above 200 mmHg. but as high as 300 mmHg. At this point, the cuff has completely occluded your artery, preventing any blood flow below your elbow. Then he opens the valve a little, to allow air to slowly escape from the cuff while he listens with his stethoscope over your brachial artery, at the crook of your elbow.

The first number, your systolic blood pressure (SBP), signifies the height of the mercury column when your physician first hears your pulse, the first Korotkoff sound. The second number, your diastolic blood pressure (DBP), represents the height of the column when the sound of your pulse disappears, the fifth Korotkoff sound. Nowadays, most offices and E.R.s use an automated system to measure your BP. These devices do not require listening to your pulse with a stethoscope.

Most BP authorities consider your blood pressure to be normal if your SBP is 120 mmHg. or less AND your DBP is 80 mmHg. or less. Hypertension (HTN) is present when your SBP is 140 mmHg. or higher (systolic HTN) OR your DBP is 90 mmHg. or higher (diastolic HTN). There are all sorts of guidelines available for goals of treatment of HTN based on your age and any coexisting diseases, like diabetes or chronic kidney problems. Although 120/80 is the gold standard for normal, numerous studies have shown that, as long as you don't feel lightheaded or pass out, the lower your blood pressure, even as low as 90/50, the better your odds of living a long and productive life without fear of heart disease or stroke.

When physicians use the word "hypertension", they are usually referring to essential hypertension. This entity, first described in 1925 by Otto Frank, refers to high blood pressure unassociated with any other disease process. A disease that is just there, not because of any other disease process, is usually referred to as "idiopathic". Essential HTN is idiopathic. Prior to Dr. Frank, physicians assumed that HTN was caused by other disease processes, most notably kidney disease. Nowadays we refer to HTN caused by other processes as "secondary hypertension", meaning that another disease had caused changes in the body, resulting in HTN. Essential hypertension is by far the commonest form of HTN.

Our old friend, the Framingham Heart Study, studied the effects of HTN over a thirty-year period. During this time, thanks to it and numerous other studies from many countries around the globe, it was determined that HTN is the leading cause of death in the world.

What does a person with HTN look like? Well, that overweight guy with the beet-red face and steam coming out his ears as he screams at other drivers during rush hour probably has HTN. That would be the "tension" part of the equation. But that pale skinny guy who sits quietly waiting for the light to change could have it too. You can't tell who is hypertensive and who is not just by looking at them. That's why HTN is called "a silent killer". You can't pick the hypertensive guy out of a crowd and you don't know whether you are that guy unless you get your BP checked. By the time you have symptoms related to HTN, a significant amount of damage may have been done to your heart, your blood vessels, your kidneys, your eyes and your brain, damage that is irreversible and permanent.

If you run massive volumes of water through a garden hose, the force exerted on the walls is increased. In response, unless the hose is made of inflexible steel, there will be a mild stretching of the wall of the hose, allowing the diameter of the lumen to increase and accommodate the flow of water. If you continue to run these volumes of water through the hose for years, eventually the inner lining of the hose will erode. In your arteries, HTN causes increased force on the walls of your arteries. Like the garden hose, your arteries will initially stretch a bit, dilating to accommodate the increased flow. Over time, in response to the increased pressure and force, your arteries will build up muscle and elastic tissue, narrowing the lumen. This is a change for the worse.

In addition to the narrow lumen thing, over a period of years, the increased force exerted on the walls of your arteries will cause damage to the inner lining, the endothelium. In the case of arteries, this damage consists of microtears. Once you have a microtear in the wall of your artery, chemical transmitters will initiate the healing process. What results is a scar. Repeated scars from these microtears will build up, further narrowing the lumen of your artery. Scar tissue will not stretch like normal arterial endothelium, so over time, subjected to continued high pressure and forces, the difference in flexibility between the scar tissue and normal endothelial tissue will cause more microtears. More microtears means more scar.

As you age, like elsewhere in your body, it is normal to lose muscle and replace it with less flexible tissue in the walls of your arteries. This leads to hardening of the arteries, a term you probably heard as a kid when someone had a stroke or a heart attack. If you have longstanding high blood pressure, the hardening process is accelerated. By the time your reach sixty years of age, with forty years of untreated HTN in your back pocket, you have the arteries of an eighty-year-old. That doesn't sound any better than being thirty years old and having the complexion of a sixty-five-year-old. And while an aging complexion is indeed a tragedy, it probably won't cause a heart attack.

Even worse, the microtear-related scar, which causes irregularities in the lining of your arterial wall, is an ideal place for cholesterol, fat, platelets and white blood cells to lodge. As we know, whenever those guys get together and hang out in one place in a blood vessel, an atheromatous plaque is sure to follow. So while HTN doesn't cause atherosclerosis, its action on the walls of your arteries provides an ideal setting for incubating and accelerating the process. Means, motive, and opportunity. Guilty as charged.

The hypertension conspiracy doesn't stop there. Your arterioles, those mini-arteries downstream from your arteries, are also affected. In response to high blood pressure, your arterioles develop thicker walls, thus narrowing their lumen. Eventually the lumen becomes so narrow that red blood cells can no longer pass through on their way to your capillaries. No blood to the capillaries means no oxygen or other nutrients making their way to your organs. Eventually, when you lose enough of your arterioles and capillaries, your organs suffer from ischemia and the resistance in your blood vessels rises even higher. Here are just a few consequences of high blood pressure's effects on your blood vessels.

1. Brain-- Long-term cerebrovascular results. Narrowing of arteries and arterioles prevents blood flow, leading to ischemia and stroke. Aneurysms form at the branching points of your arteries. Assailed by the forces associated with high blood pressure, these weak-walled balloons can rupture and cause bleeding inside your brain, leading to paralysis or death.

2. Eye--The usual result of long-term HTN is thickening of the walls of the retinal arterioles. This leads to poor blood flow and loss of nerve fibers, which are responsible for your vision. Additionally, microaneurysms can rupture, causing a retinal bleed, which can result in temporary or permanent blindness.

3. Kidney--Thickening of the wall of your arterioles blocks blood flow to the glomeruli, the unit responsible for filtration. Starved of blood, eventually your glomeruli die off. An absence of glomeruli means no filtration, which means that waste materials in your blood cannot be removed by your kidneys. This leads to kidney failure, for which you must undergo dialysis for years, several times per week in a windowless room full of other sick people, until you luck out and get a kidney transplant. After diabetes, HTN is the second-leading cause of kidney failure in the U.S.

4. Coronary arteries--HTN accelerates the normal age-related hardening of your coronary arteries. In addition, microtears and the resulting scarring allow the accelerated formation of atheromatous plaques. High blood pressure is more damaging to these plaques, making their rupture much more likely. This is one of the leading causes of MI.

5. Heart--How about your heart? The higher your blood pressure, the greater the resistance in your arteries. The greater the resistance, the harder your heart must pump to push out blood into your bloodstream. Years of heavier pumping against higher resistance results in thickening of your heart muscle, especially the most important pumping chamber, your left ventricle. This thickening is known as LVH or left ventricular hypertrophy.

Gee, that sounds like a good thing, a thicker than normal heart muscle. Unfortunately, along with increased muscle mass comes increased demand for blood and nutrients. When those demands aren't met, that big strong thick myocardium begins to scar up, causing the left ventricle to become stiffer and much less efficient at pumping blood. Eventually, all the backed-up blood causes dilation of the other chambers of the heart, especially the left atrium. Eventually the imbalance between oxygen demand and oxygen supply to that thick left ventricle causes it to become flabby, resulting in hypertensive cardiomyopathy and congestive heart failure. In addition, that dilated left atrium no longer pumps or conducts electricity well, and atrial fibrillation results.

What causes HTN? There is no known cause of essential hypertension. It just is. Hypertension is one of the most widely-studied disease processes and, as long as it causes damage to humans and can be treated with expensive medications, it will continue to be so. Researchers have already come up with a myriad of abnormalities associated with HTN, and will undoubtedly come up with more in the future, but sometimes, despite everyone's best efforts to find the unifying, ground-level zero cause, a disease entity remains "idiopathic".

Is salt good or bad for you? As long as there are physicians, nutritionists and research funds, the debate over salt will continue to rage. It is safe to say that the less sodium or salt that you take in, the lower your chances of developing high blood pressure. On the other hand, some individuals can eat all the salt they want and never develop any problems from it. It is difficult to predict whose blood pressure is salt-sensitive and whose is not. When a researcher gets a room full of these salt-insensitive guys together and writes a paper, that's when the salt debate gets up and running again. Don't let anyone tell you that kosher salt or sea salt or any other oddball form of salt is better for you than table salt. They all contain the same amount of sodium, about 40%, and the fact that the most recently-discovered Dead Sea Scroll extols the virtue of green kosher sandy sea salt doesn't mean you should eat the stuff. Remember Lot's wife and the Sodom and Gomorrah deal.

Every few years an editorial appears in the medical literature on the importance of calcium in preventing hypertension. It is well-known that if the level of calcium in your blood is low, your parathyroid glands are stimulated to release higher than normal levels of parathyroid hormone (PTH) into your blood. The increase in PTH causes several things to happen: release of calcium from your bones; increased absorption of calcium from your intestines; decreased excretion of calcium into your urine by your kidneys; a rise in blood pressure. However, unless you are eating a diet extremely deficient in calcium or have some other metabolic problem, your serum calcium levels are usually in the normal range, not low.

Numerous studies have shown that increasing dietary calcium or taking calcium supplements will tend to lower your SBP by about 2 mmHg. and your DBP by 1 mmHg. In subjects, particularly Asians, who follow a diet extremely low in calcium, less than 800 mg/day, the addition of calcium supplements or a change to a diet high in calcium may lower your blood pressure even more. Given that a reduction of DBP by 5 mmHg. will decrease your risks of stroke by as much as 30% and CAD by 20%, if you are eating a diet low in calcium, you might consider adding calcium supplements to get your daily intake of calcium up to 1200 mg/day. If you are already consuming more than 1200 mg. of calcium per day, adding calcium supplementation probably won't help when it comes to your blood pressure.

Magnesium is another element that may affect your blood pressure. In your body's tissues, the concentration of calcium outside your cells is about one thousand times as high as it is inside your cells. The membranes of some types of cells, notably in your arteries, heart, and adrenal glands, contain calcium channels. When these cells receive certain signals, the calcium channels open, allowing calcium to enter the cells in higher concentrations. This influx of calcium causes your arteries to constrict, your heart muscle cells to beat faster and more forcefully, and your adrenal gland to release aldosterone, which causes your kidneys to retain salt and water. All of these actions tend to raise your blood pressure.

Magnesium acts as a calcium channel blocker. This prevents calcium from entering through the channels. Blocking your calcium channels causes your arteries to relax and dilate, which decreases your peripheral resistance, which lowers your blood pressure. Magnesium also stimulates the production of nitric oxide, which dilates your arteries. If you take Viagra, you know that when you get sexually aroused, the nerves in the erectile tissue of your proboscis of procreation release nitric oxide, which dilates the arteries, allowing more blood to flow in and cause an erection. Enough about your dick. That's for another book.

Anyway, low serum magnesium levels have been associated with HTN. From experiments in the lab and from large epidemiological studies we know there is an inverse correlation between blood magnesium and your blood pressure. Low magnesium levels=high blood pressure. What has not been shown yet is whether giving magnesium supplements to patients with low or normal magnesium levels will prevent or treat HTN. As with calcium, if your serum magnesium level is low, you will want to figure out why. In the meantime, you should be taking supplements to get it up to normal. After that, everything is pure speculation.

Isn't it odd that a low calcium level can be associated with high blood pressure, but a low magnesium level, which blocks the effects of calcium, is also associated with high blood pressure? The two minerals are sometimes antagonistic, sometimes cooperative with each other. In pre-eclampsia, a condition in pregnant women that features high blood pressure and hyperactive reflexes, the standard treatment regimen includes IV magnesium. If you give too much magnesium and the woman loses her reflexes--sometimes her ability to breathe, too-- the treatment is IV calcium. On the cooperative side, a low calcium level can be caused by a low magnesium level, and treating the low magnesium level will often correct the low calcium level.

What can you do to prevent or minimize high blood pressure? The usual stuff. Push away from the table and get up to take a walk. In adults and children, although the exact mechanism remains to be determined, there is a clear link between obesity and HTN, meaning that if you are markedly overweight, you have a much higher risk of developing high blood pressure. Cook your own meals without the benefit of a salt shaker. The less salt you ingest, even in cooking, the lower your blood pressure and the lower your chance of developing HTN. Limit your alcohol intake. If you want to prevent HTN or want to bring it under better control, avoid alcohol entirely or drink only in moderation. Alcohol is also a source of excess calories, which lead to weight gain. Lastly, alcohol can limit the effectiveness of some BP meds and worsen the side effects of others. We'll discuss alcohol more in the chapter on alcohol. Make sense?

If your efforts fail to adequately control your blood pressure, your doctor most likely will start you on a medication. Look at this move as a way of saying, "I am concerned about your blood pressure and want to help you avoid a stroke or a heart attack." rather than "You failed. Now it's my turn." Of all the classes of medications, antihypertensives have more diverse indications outside of their intended target disease than any others. That increases their distribution but also tends to increase the number of adverse effects associated with their use.

Four hormones essential to the discussion of blood pressure are renin, angiotensin I, angiotensin II, and aldosterone. If your blood pressure drops, often because of blood loss or dehydration, blood flow to your kidneys is reduced. The decrease in renal (kidney) blood flow triggers certain cells in your kidneys to convert prorenin to renin and release it into your bloodstream. Renin then converts angiotensinogen, which is produced in your liver, into angiotensin I. Angiotensin I is converted to angiotensin II by angiotensin converting enzyme (ACE), which hangs out in your lungs. Angiotensin II causes blood vessels throughout your body to constrict, raising your blood pressure. Angiotensin II also causes your adrenal glands to release aldosterone into your bloodstream. Aldosterone causes your kidneys to retain water and sodium, to raise your blood pressure back to normal. This nicely-orchestrated series of events goes by the catchy moniker "the renin-angiotensin system".

Every protocol for treating HTN lists angiotensin converting enzyme inhibitors, a.k.a. ACE inhibitors or ACEIs. Included in this group are captopril (Capoten), enalapril (Vasotec), benazepril (Lotensin), lisinopril (Zestril), quinapril (Accupril), and ramipril (Altace). There are others as well. As the name implies, ACEIs block the activity of angiotensin converting enzyme. This enzyme converts angiotensin I to angiotensin II, a hormone that constricts blood vessels. The older versions of these meds were taken two to four times per day, the newer ones once or twice per day. Things to watch out for include a dry cough that won't go away, swelling and shortness of breath due to congestive heart failure, high blood potassium levels, lightheadedness from low blood pressure, metallic taste, headache and rash. Much rarer but much more serious side effects include swelling of the lips and face, kidney failure, liver failure, and low white blood cell count. A significant side effect of ACE inhibitors is the "first dose effect". Not infrequently, patients will experience significant orthostatic hypotension (a drop in blood pressure when standing up from a lying position) after their first dose. This side effect also occurs in patients taking their first dose of an alpha-blocker like prazosin (Minipress). Up to 1% of all patients starting either of these classes of medications will experience syncope, a temporary loss of consciousness. To avoid symptoms when you take your first dose, it is advisable to stop any diuretics for twenty-four hours, take the first dose at night when you go to bed, start at a low dose and gradually increase it.

Another group of medications that are prescribed frequently for HTN are the angiotensin II receptor blockers (ARBs). Examples include losartan (Cozaar), valsartan (Diovan), and candesartan (Atacand), among others. These agents block the vasoconstrictive effects of angiotensin II by preventing it from binding with specific receptors on blood vessel walls. This allows arteries to relax and dilate, lowering your blood pressure. Side effects of ARBs include all of the ACEI side effects plus diarrhea.

Introduced in the late 1950s, one of the oldest classes of medications, thiazide diuretics, are still used by millions of patients worldwide. In most countries they are by far the cheapest drugs available to treat HTN. The most popular of the thiazides today are hydrochlorothizide and chlorthalidone. How they work is still not fully explained. Initially they cause you to urinate larger volumes of salt and water than normal. This lowers your blood volume, which tends to lower your cardiac output. With chronic use, they cause your blood vessels to dilate. Common side effects include lightheadedness due to low blood pressure, headache, low potassium, low sodium and worsening of gout. Like any other blood pressure medication, thiazides may cause sexual dysfunction.

The first beta blocker, propanolol (Inderal), was introduced in 1964. Other than propanolol, which is still used for a variety of indications, beta blockers on the market include metoprolol (Toprol XL), atenolol (Tenormin), carvedilol (Coreg), nadolol (Corgard), and sotalol (Betapace). Beta blockers exert their effects through the beta receptors found on myocardial cells and arteries. They prevent the attachment of catecholamines, epinephrine and norepinephrine, which tend to speed up your heart rate and cause your blood vessels to constrict. While many of the older preparations are available in generic form for pennies per day, the newer formulations tend to be longer-acting and are easier to take. Side effects include lightheadedness from low BP, worsening of asthma, nausea, diarrhea, nightmares, fatigue and erectile dysfunction.

Calcium channel blockers have been available since the 1970s. Popular brands include diltiazem (Cardizem), nifedipine (Procardia), nicardipine (Cardene), verapamil (Calan) and amlodipine (Norvasc). They block calcium channels (really?) on arterial, myocardial and adrenal gland cells. In the arteries, this leads to dilation and decreased resistance. In myocardial cells, this leads to a slowing of the conduction of electrical activity, thus slowing the heart rate. In addition, they decrease the force of contraction of myocardial cells. In your adrenal gland, they block the production of aldosterone, so you don't retain salt. All three of these effects tend to lower your blood pressure. Side effects may include low blood pressure, congestive heart failure, constipation, headache, rashes and bradycardia.

A couple of other things about hypertension. The first one tells you something about interpreting the results of research studies. In the late 1970's, a much-heralded study came out about hypertension. Based on their experience at a major medical center, the authors concluded that up to 10% of patients with high blood pressure had a pheochromocytoma. A pheo is a small tumor found in the adrenal gland. It secretes massive amounts of two catecholamines, epinephrine and norepinephrine, causing wild fluctuations in blood pressure, palpitations and headaches. This was shocking news, because, prior to the report, pheos were considered to be extremely rare, as in less than one in one thousand patients with HTN. Many academic institutions went directly to sheep mode and fervently followed the leader. This was, after all, a lead article in the New England Journal of Medicine. Anyone who came in with high blood pressure that was difficult to control was put through the pheochromocytoma workup, which entailed expensive blood tests, twenty-four-hour urine collections, arteriograms and numerous other time-consuming exercises in search of a zebra. Meanwhile, the average doc in the community, obviously not interested enough in staying up to date to read the NEJM, was just trying different meds to keep his patients normotensive. After much time, more money, and a lot of patients full of needle holes, it became clear that pheochromocytomas were indeed as rare as hen's teeth, at least in the general population.

A patient came to the study institution, the local Mecca (the hospital where the really tough cases end up), only if every other attempt to control his blood pressure failed, so the group of patients the authors wrote about were a very select few compared to all patients with HTN. When you hear that a study proves one thing or another, it is very important to determine whom the researchers included in their study, just your average Joe off the street or a pre-screened special Joe who's been referred up the ladder. What is common as dirt at the Mecca is exceedingly rare at St. Elsewhere.

The other thing to note about high blood pressure is the "white coat syndrome". When you are being seen at your doctor's office for high blood pressure, the gold standard is to let you sit quietly for a few minutes before your blood pressure is measured. That's because when you walk around, your blood pressure and your heart rate increase, and it takes a while for them to return to normal. Owing to the need to see the most patients in the shortest time possible, many offices and clinics do not strictly adhere to that recommendation. In addition, for some patients, the anxiety of going to the doctor's office is so great that they just can't unwind around medical personnel, the ones in the white coats, no matter how long they sit and "relax". Their catecholamine levels get jacked up just thinking about going to the doctor. You might not even be aware of that anxiety, but your blood pressure sure is. That's why it is so important to measure your blood pressure at home, record it, and bring it to the office for your visit. The goal is to control your blood pressure during your normal daily life, not during your stressful appointment.

References:

1. Hoyt, Brian D., Walsh, Richard A. "Normal Physiology of the Cardiovascular System." *Hurst's The Heart*. Ed. Valentin Fuster, Ed. Robert A. O'Rourke, Ed. Richard A. Walsh, Ed. Philip Poole-Wilson. New York: McGraw-Hill. 2008. 83-6. 100-1. 105-6.
2. Samarel, Allen M., Walsh, Richard A. "Molecular and Cellular Biology of the Normal, Hypertrophied, and Failing Heart." *Hurst's The Heart*.

Ed. Valentin Fuster, Ed. Robert A. O'Rourke, Ed. Richard A. Walsh, Ed. Philip Poole-Wilson. New York: McGraw-Hill. 2008. 124-33.

3. O'Rourke, Robert A., Shaver, James A., Silverman, Mark E. "The History, Physical Examination, and Cardiac Auscultation." *Hurst's The Heart.* Ed. Valentin Fuster, Ed. Robert A. O'Rourke, Ed. Richard A. Walsh, Ed. Philip Poole-Wilson. New York: McGraw-Hill. 2008. 239-41.

4. Hilal-Dandan, Randa. "Renin and Angiotensin." *Goodman & Gilman's The Pharmacological Basis of Therapeutics.* Ed. Laurence L. Brunton, Assoc. Ed. Bruce A. Chabner, Assoc. Ed. Bjorn C Knollman. New York: McGraw-Hill. 2011. 721-41.

5. Michel, Thomas, Hoffman, Brian B. "Treatment of Myocardial Ischemia and Hypertension." *Goodman & Gilman's The Pharmacological Basis of Therapeutics.* Ed. Laurence L. Brunton, Assoc. Ed. Bruce A. Chabner, Assoc. Ed. Bjorn C Knollman. New York: McGraw-Hill. 2011. 765-83.

6. Westfall, Thomas C., Westfall, David P. "Adrenergic Agonists and Antagonists." *Goodman & Gilman's The Pharmacological Basis of Therapeutics.* Ed. Laurence L. Brunton, Assoc. Ed. Bruce A. Chabner, Assoc. Ed. Bjorn C Knollman. New York: McGraw-Hill. 2011. 304-30.

7. Reilly, Robert F., Jackson, Edwin K. "Regulation of Renal Function and Vascular Volume." G*oodman & Gilman's The Pharmacological Basis of Therapeutics.* Ed. Laurence L. Brunton, Assoc. Ed. Bruce A. Chabner, Assoc. Ed. Bjorn C Knollman. New York: McGraw-Hill. 2011. 671-701.

8. Pickering, Thomas G., Ogedegbe, Gbenga, "Epidemiology of Hypertension." *Hurst's The Heart.* Ed. Valentin Fuster, Ed. Robert A. O'Rourke, Ed. Richard A. Walsh, Ed. Philip Poole-Wilson. New York: McGraw-Hill. 2008. 1551-63.

9. Hall, John E., Granger, Joey P., Hall, Michael E., Jones, Daniel W."Pathophysiology of Hypertension." *Hurst's The Heart.* Ed. Valentin Fuster, Ed. Robert A. O'Rourke, Ed. Richard A. Walsh, Ed. Philip Poole-Wilson. New York: McGraw-Hill. 2008. 1580-1605.

9. Rashidi, Arash, Rahman, Mahboob, Wright, Jackson T., Jr."Diagnosis and Treatment of Hypertension." *Hurst's The Heart.* Ed. Valentin Fuster, Ed. Robert A. O'Rourke, Ed. Richard A. Walsh, Ed. Philip Poole-Wilson. New York: McGraw-Hill. 2008. 1610-19.

10. Victor, Ronald G. "Systemic Hypertension: Mechanisms and Diagnosis." *Braunwald's Heart Disease*. Ed. Robert O. Bonow, Ed. Douglas L. Mann, Ed. Douglas P. Zipes, Ed. Peter Libby, Ed. Eugene Braunwald. Philadelphia: Elsevier Saunders. 2012. 935-44. 961-8.

20. SUGAR AND CORONARY DISEASE

Sugar is the name given to sweet-tasting, soluble, short chain carbohydrates, which are substances composed solely of carbon, hydrogen and oxygen. Sugars are found in most plants, but only sugar beets and sugar cane contain enough sugar to allow practical refinement. Sugar cane has been cultivated in tropical climates in southeast Asia for centuries. There is evidence of its growth by South Pacific islanders 8,000 years ago. It became a valuable trade commodity when, in the 5th century A.D., growers on the Indian subcontinent figured out how to turn sugarcane juice into granulated crystals, making its transport much easier. It first arrived in Europe in the mid-seventh century A.D. By the early 1400s, Europeans were growing sugar cane in north Africa and in the Canaries and other islands in the Atlantic Ocean. On his way to the New World, Christopher Columbus stopped off in the Canaries and from there brought sugar to the Americas for the first time. Thanks to the establishment of sugar plantations in the New World by European countries, sugar became available to the common man in the eighteenth century. Prior to that, just plain folks had to rely on honey for sweetness. Since then, the sugar industry has played a hand in wars, slavery, industrialization of third-world colonies, and, most recently here in the U.S., massive subsidies to sugar kings in Louisiana, Florida, Hawaii and Texas.

According to nutritionists, the world of sweetness is divided into two categories: good carbohydrates and bad carbohydrates. All carbohydrates eventually break down into glucose. The difference between the good and the bad is the rate at which they break down as well as their nutritional content. Generally speaking, the good ones are complex carbohydrates, like oatmeal, which tend to contain large quantities of fiber. Other sources of complex carbohydrates include low-fat yogurt, lentils and other beans, whole grain breads and pastas, and most fruits and vegetables. The fiber content slows digestion of carbs into glucose, preventing spikes in your blood sugar and leaving you feeling full for a longer period of time. Simple carbohydrates include sucrose (table sugar), brown sugar, and foods with added sugars, which are sugars or syrups added to foods during preparation or processing. Common examples of foods containing added sugars are sweetened beverages, like soft drinks and fruit drinks, sweetened cereals, candy, and dairy desserts. These are digested very quickly, cause a bump in your blood glucose level, and thus may cause inflammation throughout your body, especially inside your blood vessels.

It is estimated that the average American adult consumes twenty-two teaspoons of added sugar every day. Over 70% of Americans obtain at least 10% of their daily calories from added sugar. Research has shown that the higher the percentage of sugar in your total daily caloric intake, the higher your risk of cardiovascular disease. If you consume more than 20% of your calories in the form of sugar, you double your risk.

The American Heart Association recommends no more than six teaspoons (100 calories) of sugar per day for women and nine tsp. (150 cal.) for men. Sugar-sweetened beverages are the largest contributors to added sugar in the American diet. The AHA recommends limiting these beverages to thirty-six ounces per week.

What is the link between dietary sugar and CAD? Studies have shown that limiting sucrose in the diet will result in a significant decrease in your levels of total cholesterol, LDL-C and triglycerides. Now that experts are backing off their attack on dietary cholesterol, sugar is the new whipping boy. Oddly enough, given all the media focus on sugar, there is a dearth of good research available. It's not even clear that eating sugar leads to diabetes. There is a ton of "information" available, much of which relies on the author's favorite theory or poorly-designed studies.

One possible connection to CAD is the stimulation of your immune system when you ingest added sugar. To combat trauma, infection and poisons, certain types of white blood cells, notably B lymphocytes, T lymphocytes and macrophages, release cytokines, which are potent mediators of your immune response. It is postulated that these cytokines treat added sugar as an invader, triggering an inflammatory response. Of course, you get cytokine release whenever you eat anything, be it protein, carbohydrate, fat or any combination thereof. Leading members of the anti-sugar crowd, those terminally thin talking heads doling out dietary advice so that you can end up resembling them or their first cousin, the praying mantis, insist that added sugar prompts a much greater release of cytokines than do other food groups. Perhaps they do, perhaps not.

Inflammatory responses are all the rage now; If you are selling potions and elixirs, a.k.a. antioxidants, to fight inflammation, you have to postulate that inflammation is everywhere and, left untreated, invariably leads to hideous disfigurement, painful death, or, worst of all, aging. If you don't want to get old, stay away from sugar and keep those cytokines on the shelf.

It is fair to say that nobody has a clear understanding of how added sugar contributes to CAD, but it probably does. If that's the case, it would behoove you to eat as little added sugar as possible, and, when you eat carbs, stick to the complex ones. You know, the ones that aren't as much fun.

Now that cholesterol, no longer the Grand Poobah of dietary cardiac risk factors, has folded its tent and slunk off, expect an ass full of studies looking at sugar and its role in the development of CAD. Eventually, the market will be overrun with drugs designed solely to inactivate dietary sugar before it triggers the inflammatory response that sends you down that spiral ending up in the CVICU. Consider this: According to the sugar-is-the-root-of-all-evil crowd, the ingredient in a BLT that hurts you the most isn't the bacon or the mayo. It's the bread. Perhaps someday you'll receive a low dose of ibuprofen in each slice of Wonder Bread. On the other hand, in a decade or two we might be receiving continuous conks on the noggin by reports of the dangers of tomatoes and lettuce.

References:

1.Wyse, Roger E. "Sugar." *World Book Encyclopedia*. Chicago: World Book. 2016. 18:959-62.
2. Abbott, Elizabeth. *Sugar: A Bittersweet History*. London: Duckworth Overlook. 2009. 1-269.
3. Mozzafarian, Dariush. "Nutrition and Cardiovascular Disease." *Braunwald's Heart Disease*. Ed. Robert O. Bonow, Ed. Douglas L. Mann, Ed. Douglas P. Zipes, Ed. Peter Libby, Ed. Eugene Braunwald. Philadelphia: Elsevier Saunders. 2012. 1003.
4. Werbach, *Melvin R. Nutritional Influence on Illness*. Tarzana, CA: Third Line Press. 1996. 66-7.
5. Kushi, LH, Lew RA, Stare FJ, Ellison CR, el Lozy M, et al. "Diet and 20-year mortality from coronary heart disease. The Ireland-Boston Diet-Heart Study." *NEJM*. 1985. 312(13):811-8.
6. Mensiunk R, et al. "Effects of monounsaturated fatty acids versus complex carbohydrates on serum lipoprotein and apolipoproteins in healthy men and women." *Metabolism*. 1989. 38:172-8.
7. Temple NJ. "Coronary heart disease: Dietary lipids or refined carbohydrates?" *Med Hypothesis*. 1983. 10(4):425-35.
8. Yudkin J. "Metabolic changes induced by sugar in relation to coronary heart disease and diabetes." *Nutr Health*. 1987.5(1/2):5-8.
9. Cohen AM, Bavly S, Poznanski R. "Change of diet of Yemenite Jews in relation to diabetes and ischaemic heart-disease." *Lancet*. 1961. 2:1399-1401.
10. Reiser S, Hallfrisch J, Michaelis OE 4th, Lazar FL., Martin RE, Prather ES. "Isocaloric exchange of dietary starch and sucrose in humans 1. Effects on levels of fasting blood lipids." *Am J Clin Nutr*. 1979. 32(8):1659-69.
11. Yudkin J, "Effects of high dietary sugar." *Brit Med J*. 1980. 281:1396.

12. Winitz M, Seedman DA, Graff J. "Studies in metabolic nutrition employing chemically defined diets 1. Extended feeding of normal human adult males." *Am J Clin Nutr.* 1970. 23:525-45.

21. CAFFEINE AND CORONARY DISEASE

Coffee is a drink made by brewing roasted coffee beans, the seeds of the Coffea plant berry. Coffee plants are raised in dozens of countries concentrated around the equator, mostly in Latin America, India, Southeast Asia and Africa. After coffee beans are picked, they are processed and dried. They are then sold as green coffee beans, one of the world's most widely traded commodities. Once roasted and ground, they can be used to make coffee.

The effects of coffee were first noted in Ethiopia. Goatherds observed that their flocks stayed up all night after feeding on coffee berries and leaves. Coffee cultivation first took place in southern Arabia, probably in the thirteenth century A.D. It served as a food, a wine, and a medication before it became popular as a drink. It was often used for religious services, and in the intervening years, coffee has been banned for various reasons by churches and governments. The first coffee houses in Europe appeared in the middle of the seventeenth century, and the plant was introduced to the Americas, initially in Brazil, during the eighteenth century.

If you ask the average Joe on the street about coffee and its effects, he will most likely focus on caffeine. Caffeine is found in coffee, tea, soft drinks, chocolate and some nuts. It stimulates your central nervous system (CNS), promotes the release of free fatty acids from fats, and is a potent diuretic, capable of making you pee until you are dehydrated. If you are caffeine-naive (That's a sexy way of describing people who don't drink coffee or other caffeine-containing drinks.), starting a regular intake of caffeine will cause decreased sensitivity to insulin, leading to higher postprandial (after meals) blood glucose levels. In addition, as a caffeine neophyte, you will experience significantly higher epinephrine (adrenaline) levels in your blood and a higher blood pressure. After a week or so of continuing caffeine intake, your blood pressure will fall towards but not completely back to normal, as will your circulating epinephrine levels.

Studies show that caffeine increases LDL-C levels, but only if the coffee is boiled, not filtered. The active cholesterol-raising component is cafestol, which is removed by paper filters but not by boiling or using a French press. Given that an increase in LDL-C is a bad thing, it is reasonable to ask whether drinking coffee is bad for your heart.

A meta-analysis of twenty-one studies showed some conflicting results. In subjects who drank four to six cups of coffee and in those who drank more than six cups of coffee per day, two studies showed a positive correlation between coffee drinking and coronary artery disease (CAD), while two others showed a negative correlation. Overall, there was a slight increase in CAD associated with coffee intake. Other recent studies, each following more than thirty-five thousand subjects for nine to thirteen years, also produced conflicting results. One showed that subjects who drank two to three cups of coffee per day had a lower risk of CAD than those who drank more or less coffee. The second showed a definite benefit to women who drank coffee, but not to men. The third study showed no relationship between coffee consumption and heart failure, not even for those who drank more than five cups per day. So we are left with the understanding that caffeine does some bad things that you would expect to cause a significant increase in CAD, but coffee use has only a mild effect on heart disease, if any.

There is a tendency to extrapolate results of caffeine studies onto coffee drinking, but some research indicates that the effect of coffee on blood pressure, epinephrine levels, exercise performance and blood glucose levels are not as profound as those of similar doses of straight caffeine. There are hundreds of chemical compounds in coffee, some of which may lessen the effects of caffeine on your heart. In fact, caffeinated non-coffee drinks (energy drinks, some soft drinks) have an effect on blood pressure similar to that of pure caffeine, while caffeinated coffee has almost none. Interestingly, whereas caffeine significantly elevates blood glucose levels, caffeinated coffee causes an insignificant rise and decaffeinated coffee causes a drop.

Most experts now believe that coffee has little or no effect on your chances of developing CAD when consumed in moderate quantities. Conversely, overuse of caffeine can be disastrous. A seventeen-year-old male drank near-lethal doses of caffeine, developed angina and had an MI, all due to coronary artery spasm. Even if you are a moderate coffee drinker, habituated to caffeine, you can experience caffeine withdrawal within twelve to twenty-four hours after your last cup of coffee. Headache is the commonest symptom, but you can also experience anxiety, fatigue, drowsiness and depression.

One of the strangest connections between coffee and illness came to light in a 1981 New England Journal of Medicine article. Researchers focused on a group of several hundred patients who developed cancer of the pancreas, to see if there was a common thread when it came to risk factors. While there was a weak link between cigarettes (but not cigars or pipes) and pancreatic cancer, there was no increase in risk from drinking alcohol or tea. However, in both men and women, there was a strong link between coffee and pancreatic cancer. Drinking one or two cups of coffee per day almost doubled the risk of developing pancreatic cancer, and drinking three or more cups almost tripled the risk.

As you may imagine, the coffee industry sat up and took notice. A flurry of studies and editorials surfaced within the next few years. One study discovered that only decaffeinated coffee posed a risk of pancreatic cancer. That finding produced even more studies, purportedly showing that only certain types of decaffeination processes were risky. There was even a case report of a husband and wife who routinely poured coffee syrup into their coffee. Both developed pancreatic cancer. Recently, however, studies have shown absolutely no increase in the risk of pancreatic cancer in coffee drinkers, decaffeinated or otherwise. Go figure.

More than anything else about coffee, I want to know what is it about Starbucks coffee that makes it so addictive. It certainly isn't the flavor.

References:

1. Clark, JCD. "Coffee". *World Book Encyclopedia*. Chicago: World Book. 2016. 4:754-5.
2. Hoffman, James. *The World Atlas of Coffee: From Beans to Brewing-- Coffees Explored, Explained and Enjoyed*. Buffalo, NY: Firefly Books. 2014. 247 p.
3. Illy, Elisabetta. *Aroma of the World: A Journey into the Mysteries and Delights of Coffee*. Vercelli, Italy: Whitestar Publishers. 2012. 15-69.
4. O'Brien, Charles P. "Drug Addiction." *Goodman & Gilman's The Pharmacological Basis of Therapeutics*. Ed. Laurence L. Brunton, Assoc. Ed. Bruce A. Chabner, Assoc. Ed. Bjorn C Knollman. New York: McGraw-Hill. 2011. 663.
5. Mozzafarian, Dariush. "Nutrition and Cardiovascular Disease." *Braunwald's Heart Disease*. Ed. Robert O. Bonow, Ed. Douglas L. Mann, Ed. Douglas P. Zipes, Ed. Peter Libby, Ed. Eugene Braunwald. Philadelphia: Elsevier Saunders. 2012. 1003.
6. Klatsky AL, Friedman GD, Armstrong MA. "Coffee use prior to myocardial infarction restudied: heavier intake may increase the risk." *Am J Epidemiol*. 1990. 132:479-88.
7. Grobbee DE, Rimm EB, Giovannucci E, Colditz G, Stampfer M, Willett W. "Coffee, caffeine, and cardiovascular disease in men." *NEJM*. 1990. 323:1026-32.
8. Thelle DS. "Coffee, cholesterol, and coronary heart disease: The secret is in the brewing." *Brit Med J*. 1991. 302:804.

9. Forde OH, Knutsen SF, Arnesen E, Thelle DS. "The Tromso heart study: Coffee consumption and serum lipid concentrations in men with hypercholesterolemia: A randomised intervention study." *Brit Med J.* 1985. 290:893-5.

10. Wu J, Ho SC, Zhou, C, Ling W, Chen W, Wang C, Chen Y. "Coffee consumption and risk of coronary heart diseases: A meta-analysis of 21 prospective cohort studies." *Internat J Cardiol.* 2009. 137(3):216–5.

11. Mostofsky E, Rice MS, Levitan EB, Mittleman MA. "Habitual Coffee Consumption and Risk of Heart Failure: A Dose-Response Meta-Analysis." *Circulation: Heart Failure.* 2012. 5(4):401–5.

12. Siasos G, Tousoulis D, Stefanadis C. (2013). "Effects of Habitual Coffee Consumption on Vascular Function." *J Amer Coll Cardiol.* 2013. 63(6):606–7.

22. THE GIVER

Simmons waited silently while the skinny old man wiped the blood from his lips and put his handkerchief away. When the coughing started, he'd put his hand up to his ribs, under his left armpit. He took a slow breath, then looked up.

"So now, Mr. Halsey, I am going to ask you about your habits. Smoking, drinking, exercise, drugs, that sort of thing." Halsey crossed his arms and set his jaw.

"I don't use drugs. Never did, never will. Don't have much use for exercise either."

"Okay. How much do you drink in an average day?"

"Never drink during the day." He curled his upper lip back, pushed his upper denture plate out a good inch, sucked it back in, and clacked it against his lower plate. Simmons couldn't tell whether this was a longstanding habit when he cut up or a recent addition to his repertoire associated with the weight loss, but he liked it. It fit the old codger like his sporty Sam Snead snap-brim.

"How about in an average night?"

"Don't drink any more. Used to have a couple of bourbon and branches at old Joe's Buddy Buddy every day after work. That was Joe's house, you know. Joe and his cousin Buddy and his other buddy, me. Maybe a few on the weekends. Quit drinking when I retired, oh, nine years ago."

"So you don't drink anymore?"

"Nope."

"Nothing? Really?" David gave him his most sincere look.

"No siree. Just beer."

"Mm-hmm. How many beers in a day? Make that how many in a night?"

"Six-pack a night. Budweiser."

"Oh? Always Bud?"

"Yeah Boy. Got a brother over to the Busch Gardens. He'd set me on fire with my own Zippo I drank something else." This time he didn't do the clacker thing. *Guess he isn't kidding about that part.*

"Okay. Ever had any problems when you stopped drinking?"

"Well, along about eleven or so my wife tells me to take that ankle-biter of hers out back to piss. I hate that dog. So I guess that's the main problem when I stop drinking." That brought a clack.

"Excuse me?"

"When I finish my six-pack, she tells me to throw away the cans and take that rat terrier out back to take a piss. I go out there and drain the old dragon too. Never did like taking a leak in a toilet when there was some perfectly good yard available." He clacked. David felt like he was listening to a lecture in an obscure foreign dialect, not knowing if the speaker were a bona-fide genius or the village idiot. Either way, he knew he was getting worked but good.

"So that's the only time you quit drinking, when you to go to bed?"

"Course. Can't drink beer all night."

"Got it." *Oh, well,* he thought, *he's not here in Pulmonary clinic for alcohol-related problems.*

"Tell me about your cigarette habit."

"Ain't a habit. Not exactly."

"Oh, so you're not a daily smoker?"

"Course I am. It's not a habit, though."

"It's not?" Simmons waited for the next punch line. Halsey gave him a look, resolved something in his head, and moved on.

"Nope. It's a, what they call a 'condition of employment."

"How's that?" This guy was starting to grow on him.

"I worked for RJR."

"RJ Reynolds?"

"Is there any other RJR in Petersburg?"

"Petersburg? You live in Petersburg?"

"All my life, 'cept for a couple of months in Richmond. The wife wanted a change in scenery. Too big-city for me, so I told her I was moving back home, with or without her."

"Oh. How far a move was that?"

"Six and one-half miles, not a inch less."

"Okay. So you worked for RJR all your adult life, right?"

"Yup."

"And how many packs of cigarettes did you smoke a day?" Halsey stared at Simmons with such an odd look, he wondered if the guy was seizing from a brain met. After a long period, the patient stopped staring.

"One."

"Okay. A pack a day for how many years?"

"Going on forty-four years next month. June 18th."

"Ever smoke more than a pack a day?" Halsey reddened up like a zit on the verge of eruption.

"Doc, where exactly are you from?"

"Delaware."

"Delaware. Border state. They grow any tobacco up in Delaware?"

"A little in the southern part of the state."

"Mm-hmm. And are you from the north or south part of Delaware?"

"South." Actually, about seven miles south of Wilmington, which was about as far north as you could go in Delaware and not be in Pennsylvania. A meaningless white lie, but it might lessen his Yankeeness in the patient's eyes. Holding his rib cage, Halsey coughed into his handkerchief, examined it, then put it back in his pocket. No blood this time. Too weak for satisfaction, he looked up with distracted curiosity.

"Doc, when you work for a tobacco company, at least one that's not in Delaware, you get a pack of cigarettes a day. Now, excepting fellas that had a family field and cut their own, I never met a man at RJR who smoked more'n one pack a day. Period."

"How about the weekend?"

"Friday you get three packs stead'a one. One for Friday, one for Saturday, one for Sunday. Period."

"Holidays like Christmas you get a pack a day too?"

"Christmas, New Year's, Thanksgiving, two weeks of vacation. Yeah Boy."

"When you retire?"

"I can go down to the factory store, show my tag, and get a carton a week. Too far, though, so I buy 'em myself." *Yeah, too far, what with a twenty-pound weight loss and that cough and maybe some godawful rib pain from the crab spreading out from its perfect little sphere into his lung like bamboo roots invading a pipe.*

"Mr. Halsey, can I ask you a personal question?" Halsey sat back a little, looking a little defensive. "If I get too personal, you can tell me to go piss up a rope." Halsey clacked his dentures and nodded.

"You have a bad cough, maybe some blood in it, you've lost weight, you lived and worked with lifelong smokers for decades. Ever seen any of your buddies go through what you're going through?"

"Maybe a couple over the years."

"Any of them still alive?" The patient seemed to ponder this for a moment, then looked down at the floor.

"Mr. Halsey, are you by any chance related to the Halseys at MCV?"

"Dr. Stringfellow Halsey's my second cousin. Called him Slap when we were kids. Can't exactly remember why anymore. My middle name's Stringfellow. Named after his daddy, also a surgeon."

"And there's been a Stringfellow Halsey at MCV for a long time, right?"

"There's been a Stringfellow Halsey operating at the medical college since the turn of the century," he said with a touch of familial pride.

"Can I ask you why you came all the way to Charlottesville when you drove right by MCV on your way here?" Simmons figured he was going to get a really interesting answer or he was going to watch Halsey get up and march out.

"Slap sends me a card every Christmas. Twenty-five years now. He always writes, 'Homer, please stop smoking.' Before that, his daddy sent me one for about five or so." Simmons was surprised. Twenty-five years ago, nobody thought to urge patients to quit smoking, especially in Richmond, Virginia. That'd be like telling a guy in Detroit to go buy a Datsun.

"Whenever I'd see them, I'd say, 'Don't worry about me. If I get cancer, I'll just up and die.'"

"Yes." *That's what every smoker says.* "What'd they say to that?"

"They said cigarettes don't let you just up and die. You cough for years, you lug around an oxygen tank, you lose a leg, you have a heart attack or two, you shrivel up like a prune, like an idiot you roll around on the ground having fits and pissing your pants, then they let you die."

"Didn't leave much to the imagination, eh?"

"Folks in my family see a job through, Doc."

"You quit yet?" Every smoker quit once they got the news that they were actually dying of lung cancer. Simmons wondered, *When the thing that you needed most in life has done its job, satisfying your craving day in and day out, why do you cast it away when it finally can't hurt you anymore. Remorse? Hope?*

"Not a chance, Doc. I reckon I knew they were telling me the truth, but I guess deep down I figured I could decide what happened to me and when."

"Were you unwilling to go see them because they were right?"

"I feel like a dumb shit. Here I had these famous doctors coming to family weddings and funerals and telling me what I should do and I thought I was smarter than them. Homer S. Halsey, the smart guy working at the factory, thinking I was getting away with something. A free pack a day and three on Fridays."

"We all do stupid stuff, Sir. Even doctors." *If he only knew.* "When I started out by asking you what brought you in today, you said, 'My wife in our car.' Are you really here because you want a diagnosis?"

"I know what's wrong with me. Don't need a medical diploma to know I got cancer."

"Okay. If you know what's wrong, and you don't want surgery, radiation or chemo, what can we do for you?"

"Doc from Delaware, it should be pretty plain to see. I want to donate my body to science."

That brought Simmons up short. After a few seconds, he said, "Why here, Mr. Halsey? Why not to MCV?"

"Too much RJR around MCV. They already got forty-four years out of me and now they got my health too. I don't owe them my corpse."

"I hadn't thought of it that way. No, Sir, I guess you don't."

"Yeah Boy, you got that right." He clacked his teeth. "I guess we should talk about what you're gonna do with me."

"I'm no expert, and I've never known anyone who donated their body, but my guess is that once you pass away, your local funeral home will embalm your body. After your wake and funeral, the funeral company would transport your body here. For intact bodies, the medical school assigns four students to dissect you."

Halsey winced when he heard "dissect". "How long does that take?"

"They'll study you for their entire first year in anatomy class. One or all of them will be working on you five days a week. The lab is open 24/7, so they can come in at night or on weekends to work on you. I did that myself my first year, almost every weeknight." Simmons thought for a moment. "We even named ours. Chet, after Chet Huntley. At the end of class each day, we'd all say, 'Good night, Chet. Good night, David.' Kind of wishing him a decent sleep." It suddenly occurred to Simmons that Chet Huntley had died of lung cancer too.

"I don't want any old name, and I'm tired of being called 'Homer'." He clacked his teeth once. "How about 'Mr. President'?"

"Shouldn't be a problem, Sir. 'Good Morning, Mr. President. Good Night, Mr. President.' Something like that?"

Halsey began to cough. He pulled out his handkerchief, coughed into it a couple of times, then wiped the blood from his mouth. "That sounds about right, Doc." He looked out the window for a minute.

"Something on your mind, Mr. President?" At that, Halsey smiled and turned to look at David.

"I heard a story a few years back. Cousin of my next door neighbor, fella by the name of Thomas Jefferson Bailey, worked as a housekeeper in the labs here. Said a dog got into the dissecting lab one Sunday morning. Said the dog ended up on the front steps of St. Paul's, right across the street on University Avenue, chewing on a corpse's innards. Said it happened just as the 9 o'clock service was getting out. Created a ruckus. A rich lady fainted. Anything to that?"

"Yes, Mr. Halsey, I heard that story too. We got a lecture on dos and don'ts the very first day from the Dean of Students. Two sources, so it's probably true." Even three and a half years later, Simmons could remember the lecture verbatim.

"On the way over this morning, my wife, she's dead set against this by the way, thinks I'm crazy, thinks I should go see Slap and get treated, well she told me a medical student got caught jump roping with a corpse's intestines in the lab one night."

"Mm-hmm, that was right at the top of the dos and don'ts list too. I also heard that fellow got tossed out of school permanently. I can't vouch for the students, but as far as the dog goes, we have a combination lock on the door, so, unless it's one smart dog, you won't end up on the steps of St. Paul's for breakfast." Halsey thought about this.

"So, once they're done with me at the end of the year, what do they do with me, just throw me into a dumpster out back?" The vision of someone tossing Homer Halsey, still clacking his dentures, into a dumpster almost made Simmons laugh, then he felt a chill go down his spine. The whole conversation was getting a little distant, a little smug, a little too objectified.

"No, nothing like that. If you wanted to be buried, we would make sure you got back to the funeral home."

"That sounds good. I got a couple of plots for me and the missus at the First Baptist Church of Petersburg. Right next to my Mama and Daddy and my brother Billy. That'll leave one when me and her are gone. Bought them lots my first year at Reynolds. They had a six-pack deal worked out with the church. Guess they knew something, even back then, eh?"

"Yes, Sir, I'm afraid so."

Halsey nodded his head. "They stuff all my innards back in and sew me up?"

"Yes. Unless you want us to save some of your organs for a pot case."

"A what?"

"A pot case. We study anatomy the first year, then pathology the second. These pot cases, they're plastic buckets full of formaldehyde. Lids comes included. If you wanted them to, they'd put your lung into the formaldehyde. If the cancer spread to your ribs, they'd put a rib or two in as well. Same for your liver and adrenal glands, as well as any other organ or body tissue that had metastases. That way, more students can see what you died from."

"And how long would I hang around in the bucket?"

"I know of at least one pot case they've been using for ten years or so."

Homer tried to whistle, but his dentures got in the way. "Ten years? God Almighty." He pondered this last bit. "Could I have my name on the bucket? 'Mr. President'? And how about, 'Courtesy of RJ Reynolds'?"

"I don't see why not. Of course, you'd have a number on the bucket too, so they could find you when they want to. Sure." The two sat thinking.

"You know, Mr. Halsey, some radiation might help that sore spot you keep holding. It wouldn't be anything long-term, just a week or so. That way, coughing might not be so painful."

"That's alright, Doc. It ain't that bad. I got some APCs at home. Between them and the Bud, I'm doing okay. But I'll let you know if it gets too bad."

"And you plan to continue smoking?"

"Of course, Doc. Always enjoyed a good smoke. Takes my mind off of everything for a little while. Besides, if I was gonna quit smoking, I shoulda done it forty-four years ago, right?"

"Very true, Mr. Halsey. Very true."

"Listen, Doc, I'm gonna pass on the physical exam and get along. Me and the Missus are going downtown for lunch. Thought we'd check out the new walking mall. Then we'll head back. Okay if I drop by in a few weeks?"

"Sure, that would be great. Do you want to sign the papers today or think on it a bit?"

"I'll think on it. Like I said, the Missus is dead set against this. We'll pray on it together, then I'll get back to you."

"That would be fine. If we can help in any way, please just say the word. I'll be done with my rotation here in the Pulmonary Clinic in ten days. After that, if you want to find me, just ask the lady at the front desk to page me, okay? I'd like to visit with you if you get back this way."

Halsey nodded, then stood up. "Will do. Ya know, Doc? For a Yankee you're not half bad. But that southern Delaware stuff? What a pile of crap. You didn't fool me one bit."

"Glad to hear it, Sir. Nothing wrong with your brain."

"That's what you think. You better write your name down for me. Starting to lose my memory."

Simmons jotted his name on a sheet of paper and handed it to the old man.

As he walked to the door, Halsey turned. "Speakin' a brains. Do me a favor, Doc?"

"Absolutely."

"If you ever see me rolling around on the ground like an idiot having fits and pissing my pants, just drop a blanket over me. Skip all that other stuff and throw me in the dumpster." On the way out, he clacked once more.

Following behind him, Simmons said, "Good Night, Mr. President."

23. SMOKE 'EM IF YOU GOT 'EM

The patch came in at 6:30 A.M. Tina, the night charge nurse, answered the call on the radio phone.

"I need a doc for a cardiac patch." Only a month ago, after a spate of cardiac patients dying en route in ambulances, the powers that be decided that anytime an ambulance transported a patient with chest pain or an arrhythmia, they had to call in a report to be recorded by a physician rather than a nurse. To Simmons' way of thinking, by the time the patch was done, the ambulance was usually pulling up at the door, so nothing he said was going to make much difference.

"This is Dr. Simmons. Whatcha got?"

"Hi, Doc, this is Greg Alexander on Engine 40." E-40 was based about fifteen miles south, and they would be passing at least four major hospitals on their way to him. Either all the ERs along the way were closed to ambulances because they were full or the patient had convinced the paramedics to take him to Simmons' hospital. Didn't matter either way to Simmons. "We are bringing you John Walcott, a fifty-one-year-old male with chest pain. He woke up about 5 A.M. with substernal chest pain, radiating to his left arm, shortness of breath, and sweats. He was sitting on his front porch smoking a cigarette when we got there. His BP is 160/95, pulse 88 and regular, respirations 20. His oxygen saturation is 100% on a non-rebreather. Monitor shows sinus rhythm with occasional unifocal PVC's and ST elevations in a few of the leads. We gave him four baby aspirins to chew and four of MS. His pain's still about three on a scale of ten, so we're going to give him the other six of MS. We should be to you in about ten minutes."

"Sounds like he's doing pretty well overall." *For an acute MI*, Simmons thought. "Do you need any orders?"

"Naw, Doc, just following the chest pain protocol, you know."

"Right. How come you're coming this far up north?" Simmons knew the paramedics weren't any happier about the long ride than he was. After the drop off, they'd have to drive back down to South Phoenix, clean up the ambulance and restock before they could go home from their twenty-four-hour shift.

"Doc, he's seeing a pulmonary doc up your way for a cough, and three of the four closest facilities are closed to ambulances, two don't even have any CCU or ICU beds open. The only one that's open is Lutheran, and you're only two minutes further than them."

"Got it. Who's the doc?"

"Schreiner."

"Okay, see you when you get here. Give me a call back if you need anything."

"Engine 40, over and out."

While waiting for the chest pain to arrive, Simmons discharged two patients he'd sutured up and admitted a ninety-five-year-old with diverticulitis. Twenty minutes passed, and still no ambulance. No day shift replacement for Simmons either. Mike Williams was supposed to be here at 7. He lived down in Chandler, a good thirty miles south. Depending on traffic, the drive could take thirty minutes or over an hour. Mike usually showed up fifteen minutes early, and despite the iffy traffic conditions, had never been late for a shift. Simmons thought about asking the unit secretary to call, just in case he'd overslept, but he didn't have anything pressing today and was off for the next four days, so he just sat down at his desk, dictated a few old charts and waited. An hour or two of overtime always looked good on the paycheck.

"I need a doc for a patch." The other guy working the day shift, Ray Epstein, was already sewing up a screaming three-year-old's chin laceration, so Simmons went over to the patch phone.

"This is Dr. Simmons, go ahead."

"Doc, this is Greg Alexander on Engine 40 again. Doc, we're going to have to upgrade Mr. Walcott."

Simmons thought, *Upgrade him to what, a DOA?* "What exactly do you mean, upgrade him?"

"Doc, he's now a Level I trauma." *Well*, thought Simmons, *we are a Level I trauma center.*

"How did that happen?"

"Well, Doc, you remember I told you the patient was smoking a cigarette on the porch when we arrived?"

"Yeah?" Simmons thought, *Please don't tell me you stopped at a Circle K to get him a pack of heaters for the ride. With the 100% oxygen mask, no less.*

"Well, it turns out he smokes about three packs a day. We gave him the other six of MS and his pain went down to a one. While I was charting, all of a sudden he sits up, rips off his O2 mask, opens the back door of the ambo, and jumps out onto Seventh Street, right in the middle of traffic. I don't know how, but he must have unbuckled the gurney straps earlier. His IV was out too. He hits the ground, rolls a few times, by this time we're fifty yards up the road, then he stands up and pulls out a pack of cigarettes and a lighter. We stop, start to back up, when a blue Hummer goes to pass on the left and clobbers him. He flew a good twenty feet in the air before he landed." Simmons thought, *Hummer. That must have hurt.* Tina, who was standing next to Simmons, checking off each of the log book entries from her shift, gave him an odd look.

"Patient Walcott is back in the ambulance, looks like he has a tension pneumothorax on the left, so we needled that, got a new IV established, and got him back on O2. The driver of the Hummer is a Level 2; I'll give you his information when we get there. He jammed his right ankle into the floorboard, looks like a dislocation, and a few facial burns from the airbag deployment, but otherwise OK. We'll be to you in ten."

"So is Walcott a trauma code or just a Level I?"

"No, Doc, actually he looks pretty good. He's having a hard time breathing, because of the pain and all, but he's still talking, wants to get out and have a cigarette." Simmons could hear gasping and yelling in the background.

"So his vitals are good?"

"Yes. BP 140/86, pulse 96, respirations 24. We have his sats back up to 94%."

"Okay, thanks. If you have time, stick an IV in the driver. See you when you get here."

Ten minutes later, the ambulance pulled up. The guy with two kinds of chest pain was wheeled in. Sorkin the trauma surgeon introduced himself. The patient gasped, coughed, and tried to say something. Sorkin bent down while the x-ray tech wheeled in his machine for a chest x-ray. He pulled the non-rebreather mask a little to the side and bent closer. Walcott promptly coughed up a couple tablespoons of blood that covered Sorkin's face and scrub top.

"Beautiful." He looked up to see Escobedo the trauma anesthesiologist walk in. "Arturo, he's going to need to be intubated. ASAP." Simmons listened to Walcott's breath sounds. He definitely had a tension pneumothorax. Still. He pulled at the catheter the paramedics had placed to relieve the tension. It came out without a sound, which told Simmons it had never made it to the pleural space.

David asked, "Okay if I put a chest tube in once he's paralyzed and sedated?" Sorkin, wiping himself off, nodded. "I'll stick a subclavian in on the pneumo side once I have the chest tube in." Lauren, Tina's dayshift replacement, came up to Simmons.

"I have the driver in Trauma 2. He has a dislocation of the ankle. They're doing a chest x-ray, two views of the ankle, and a C-spine series."

"Sounds good. Is the ankle open?"

"No."

"You want to call the orthopod on call to come see him?"

"He wants you to reduce it." Simmons looked up from his chest tube set-up. "You'll see. I'll have him sign a consent before I give him any MS."

"Okay. I'll need about twenty minutes here." Lauren started to walk away. "Hey, has anyone heard from Mike yet?"

"Yes."

"Is he here yet?"

"Sort of." She left the trauma room.

It all went smooth as silk. Escobedo had the guy down and out and intubated in minutes. Simmons punched in a chest tube and felt the gratifying gush of air as the tension pneumothorax was reduced. Once the lung was back up, the left-sided thoracic architecture was stabilized, and he hit the subclavian vein on the second stick. He was done within fifteen minutes, Walcott's vitals were relatively stable, and except for the need to suction bright red blood out of his ET tube every couple of minutes, things calmed down. His EKG showed an acute anterior MI, the chest x-ray showed a massive density of the left upper lobe. His hemoglobin was down to 8, so Sorkin ordered a bunch of packed cells. Harry Chong, the TCV surgeon on call, arrived just as Simmons, wondering where Mike Williams was, went next door.

As he walked in to Trauma 2, the x-ray tech rushed past him with a pile of film cassettes. He walked over to the patient on the backboard, still wearing the hard C-spine collar.

Without looking down, he stuck out his right hand. "Hi, I'm Dr. Simmons."

"Hi, Dave." Simmons twisted around to look at his face.

"Oh, shit. Hi, Mike." He had found Williams. *That's why Tina had the funny look on her face when she heard about the blue Hummer. Apparently she has knowledge of Mike's vehicle.* "You

okay?" "Yeah, good. Lauren gave me a little MS."

"Does your neck hurt?"

"Nah, it's fine. Just the ankle and my face."

"Okay, let's get you out of the collar and off the board." Simmons removed the hard collar, felt Mike's neck for any point tenderness. When that went well, he had him lift his head off the gurney, again with no pain or tenderness.

"Why don't you leave me on the board until you straighten out my ankle. I'd rather not move if that's okay with you."

"Sure. How come you don't want me to call the orthopod?"

"Number one, it's Lance Keller, who hates me with a passion. Number two, he sucks. Number three, with all the shit going on with my divorce, it'll be two weeks before my new health insurance kicks in." The x-ray tech came in with the films. Simmons walked over to the view box and took a look. C-spine okay, chest okay. The ankle was a jumble of broken bones and a dislocation.

"No matter what I do here, you're gonna need a bunch of screws and plates."

"If you reduce it and put me in a splint, I can go down to the VA today and they can schedule me for an elective repair. Won't cost me anything."

"How about I just reduce it and transfer you there today?"

"They won't take me in transfer. I'm not service connected. If I go through the walk-in clinic, they'll take me." Simmons pondered the logic of that, shook his head, and cut the ankle free of the dressings and cardboard splint. He asked Lauren to set Mike up for conscious sedation, and walked across the way to let the ladies in the office know that Mike would be out for a while and they'd need to round someone up to cover today's shift. When he got back, Mike was set up. Lauren pumped the MS and Versed, and soon Mike was snoring.

Lauren asked, "Why don't you just splint him like that?"

"Come here. See that pale spot there?" He pointed to a triangular area of skin that was ghost-white on the lateral aspect of the ankle. She nodded.

"If I don't reduce that promptly, that skin will necrose and he'll most likely need a skin graft. Skin grafts on lower extremities have a habit of getting infected."

"MRSA?"

He shook his head. "Shit bugs. From his butt. They tend to wend their way south." Lauren looked at him to see if he was kidding, saw that he wasn't, and returned to the head of the bed to check Mike's vitals.

During his training in Portland, Simmons did a month with an orthopod named Fenstermacher. He let David reduce a dislocated ankle in the O.R.

"Do you have any special advice before I do this, Bob?"

"Yes I do. Don't be a pussy."

Simmons grabbed Mike's ankle and yanked for all he was worth. The crunch startled Lauren and made Mike groan, more like a yodel, but everything was back in alignment. He checked for pulses, saw that the pale spot had disappeared, and loosely wrapped the ankle with an ace. He walked out, asked the unit secretary to call for a post-reduction x-ray. When he returned to Trauma 2, he told Lauren, "Okay to let him wake up."

"Reverse it?" When there was a need for prompt reversal of the Versed, an IV injection of Romazicon did the trick in seconds. Otherwise, it would wear off of its own accord in anywhere from ten minutes to an hour.

"No, let him enjoy the buzz while I finish up his paperwork." He walked next door to Trauma I. Sorkin was dictating, and Chong was talking on the phone. The respiratory therapy student was learning how to suction through Walcott's ET tube. There was about 300 cc of bright red blood in the suction canister on the wall. Packed cells were dripping through the peripheral IV and one of the ports of the subclavian. Chong hung up and smiled. When he wasn't doing bypasses or thoracotomies here, he taught the TCV fellows at County. He was reputed to have a warped sense of humor.

Simmons asked, "O.R.?"

Chong smiled. "By way of the cath lab, yes."

"Seriously?"

"Yeah, something about this guy's bleeding isn't right. Dunhill's going to shoot his coronaries, then do a pulmonary angio and an aortogram, then we're going to the O.R. Other than the blood loss, he's looking surprisingly good. So far, we have two legs of the TCV tripod." Simmons looked at him. "He has an MI, so if there's a single vessel, I'll bypass that. Maybe I'll do two. And, he needs an exploratory thoracotomy to look at his left upper lobe. I have a perfusionist available, so either way, he's going on the bypass machine. What I don't want is some surprise bizarre vascular surprise, which would be the third leg, and a most unfortunate one at that."

"He's supposed to be a patient of Schreiner's. For the cough."

"I talked to Sol. He hasn't seen this guy yet, so that opacity in his left upper lobe may not be just traumatic. Too bad I don't have a surgery resident or TCV fellow here. This is a great case." He punched Simmons in the arm, laughed, and walked out. The Trauma crew packed up the pumps, the monitor, all the IV's, and wheeled Mr. Walcott out the door to the elevator.

Over the next hour, David checked Mike's post-reduction films, splinted him up, and dictated him and Walcott. Tina showed up to take Mike to the VA--when Simmons gave Lauren a look, she shook her head--and David and the tech wheeled him out to her SUV, then cradled him up into the back seat to lie down. Getting the seat belts around him took some doing. By the time she drove away, Ted Segall was seeing patients in the E.R. David went to lie down in the call room for a few hours. With all the excitement gone, his catecholamines did their disappearing act. He was exhausted and didn't feel like running over a crossing guard or a handful of school kids on his way home.

At 10:30 Simmons woke up to an overhead announcement about an incoming trauma patient. He grabbed his backpack, checked his phone, and walked back to the E.R. All of his dictations were done, so he signed his time sheet and said good-bye to Lauren. In the parking lot, he ran into Harry Chong.

"The guy make it?"

"Huh? Oh, hi. Yeah, he's fine." He started to get into his pickup. "Oh, yeah, that's right, you didn't hear." He stood back up. "He had a complete occlusion of his LAD, so I bypassed that with his LIMA. Only about 200 cc. of blood came out of that chest tube you placed, and the seventh and eighth ribs were fractured and indented on the left, so I straightened them out." He smiled wickedly. "That 'contusion' in his left upper lobe turned out to be a giant A-V malformation. He had almost no lung tissue up there, just a bronchus."

"So that's where the hemoptysis was coming from?"

"Yeah, but here's the best part. I found a one centimeter tumor, probably a squamous cell, connecting the bronchus and the AVM. It was basically growing into both, and blood just started leaking out of the AVM this morning. I talked to his wife. She said when he took a drag on his cigarette on the porch this morning, he coughed up a little blood for the first time ever. Another day or two, or maybe just one bad cough, and that guy would have exsanguinated and died."

Simmons said, "So the MI saved his life."

Harry Chong nodded, "And the car-pedestrian accident." He climbed into his truck.

"But what really saved him was the cigarette."

Before he closed his door, Chong laughed and said, "That and the fact that it obviously wasn't his day to die."

24. CIGARETTES AND CAD

Tobacco has been grown around the world, mostly in warmer climates, for centuries. The word *tobacco* most likely derives from *tobaca,* a hollow Y-shaped tube used by Native American tribes to inhale tobacco smoke. Varieties of tobacco thrive in Syria, Turkey, Cyprus, Greece, Bulgaria and Iran. There is evidence of its cultivation and use in Mexico as far back as 1400 B.C. Several islands in the Caribbean, most notably Cuba, have grown tobacco since the time of Columbus.

Early settlers in Connecticut and Massachusetts learned to smoke tobacco in peace pipes from local Indian tribes, who used it for sacred ceremonies or to seal a deal. Tobacco hit the big time when some seeds were taken from the New World and grown in Spain. Prior to being decapitated, Sir Walter Raleigh popularized its use in Elizabethan England. Cigarettes took off in the U.S. when James Bonsack invented the first automated cigarette rolling machine in 1880. Until then, even the most skillful cigarette roller could manage only four per minute. Bonsack's machine could roll fifty times that many.

The American medical establishment had a torrid fling with tobacco for decades. From the 1930s well into the 1960s, advertisements abounded in magazines depicting doctors (in their Floyd of Mayberry jackets and official head mirrors) endorsing various brands, the smoke curling seductively around their heads. Just imagine the photo shoots:

"Professionally speaking, I recommend Salems, because the menthol soothes your throat." Just one more toxic chemical to send, as hot as the fires of hell, into your lungs.

"I love Luckies. You will too. Smoke one. Light one up and smoke it right now. I'm your doctor and I know what the hell I'm talking about. Smoke it, goddammit."

No doubt you've come across a cute little guy by the name of Dr. Kool, holding a black medical bag emblazoned with his name. Somewhere I have a porcelain figurine of the gent. By far the most frequently photographed penguin of his time, you often find him smoking a mentholated heater, nattily attired in a bow tie, accessorized with cane, stethoscope, and, of course, the obligatory head mirror, presumably to detect the throat cancers caused by his product. In one ad, decked out in a dapper little top hat, he's looking refreshed and ready to paint the town. In another, he's bushed after a long day in the office, so his comely penguin nurse lights one up for him. In my favorite, he's lying back on a chair, his penguin nurse once again preparing his cigarette. You don't have to be the suspicious type to wonder whether this is merely a soothing follow-up to a world-class penguin beak job. Okay, maybe you do. Just what the doctor ordered.

In the early 1980s, after twenty years of publicity focused on the dangers of tobacco, the love affair ground to a tawdry halt; the American Medical Association (AMA) got caught with its investor pants down around its ankles. The largest group of American doctors had been the proud possessor of large chunks of tobacco company stocks for years. By December of 1981, it had sold more than thirty thousand shares of R.J Reynolds and Phillip Morris stock for more than $1 million, netting a profit of over $500,000. At this point in time, the medical community is firmly in the corner of condemning all nicotine-containing tobacco products as dangerous to our health. However, they are still pushing nicotine in the form of Nicorette gum and Nicoderm patches.

What's so bad about tobacco? After all, even lifelong smokers have only a 20-30% chance of developing COPD (emphysema or chronic bronchitis) severe enough to cause symptoms and require medications. Not to mention that fewer than 10% of all smokers will get lung cancer, and even fewer will get one of the other cancers linked to tobacco, such as cancers of the mouth, throat, larynx, esophagus, stomach, pancreas, liver, kidney, bladder, cervix, colon and rectum. Of course, smoking does account for 30% of all cancer deaths, and 87% of all deaths from lung cancer. The risk of developing lung cancer is twenty times as great for males who smoke than for non-smokers. And the life expectancy for an American smoker is sixty-four years, almost fifteen years less than for non-smokers.

Besides the lung issues, the biggest effect of cigarette smoke is on your vascular system--your heart and your arteries. How does that happen? Thousands of studies on smoking have identified many of the pieces of that particular puzzle. However, the completed puzzle, the way in which they all fit together, remains to be seen. While nicotine is the most widely studied of the toxins in cigarette smoke, when it comes to the relationship between smoking and heart disease, some of the other chemicals may eventually turn out to be just as dangerous.

Many of cigarette smoke's ill effects on your heart are related to the stimulation of your sympathetic nervous system when you smoke a cigarette. Nicotine appears to be the major bad actor. Smoking a single cigarette causes an increase in the amount of catecholamines (adrenaline), specifically epinephrine and norepinephrine, in your bloodstream. These hormones, which are released during any physical or emotional stress, increase your heart rate, constrict your blood vessels, and raise your blood pressure. This happens every time you smoke a cigarette. If you are a daily smoker, nicotine persists in your bloodstream twenty-four hours a day. Ironically, the agents often prescribed to help you quit smoking, i.e. nicotine gum and patches, do the same thing to your heart and blood vessels as cigarettes.

We already know that the chore of delivering blood to your myocardial cells falls on your coronary arteries, right? Right? When you are stimulated, by fear or exercise or lust, your myocardial cells work harder, so they require more blood and oxygen. There are two ways that this increased need can be accommodated. One is that the pump--your heart--works harder and faster. The other is that the blood vessel, in this case your coronary artery, relaxes and dilates (opens up). Cigarette smoke causes your heart to work harder, but it prevents dilation of your coronary arteries. In fact, cigarette smoke causes your arteries to constrict (tighten up), which makes it harder for blood to get where it is going. So, given your heart rate and blood pressure and the amount of work your myocardial cells are performing, the increase in coronary blood flow is not as great as it should be. Even early in your smoking career, long before your teeth start to brown, before your fingertips turn to a lovely shade of burnt sienna, before your voice acquires that sexy gravelly timbre, even before your face takes on that chronic wrinkly stench, a single cigarette decreases your heart's ability to respond to increased demand for blood and oxygen. So if you are smoking while running, climbing uphill, riding a bicycle or swimming laps (backstroke, unless you want a soggy smoke), your heart is not getting all the oxygen it needs. Once you develop even mild cholesterol plaques in your coronary arteries, it becomes that much harder for your myocardial cells to obtain enough oxygen to do their job.

In addition to the vascular issues, cigarette smoke changes LDL-C so that it is more easily deposited into the walls of your coronary arteries, forming foam cells. Cigarette smoke causes cholesterol plaques to become less stable, and thus more likely to rupture. Cigarette smoke also affects your clotting cascade, making blood clots more likely. In addition, it causes inflammation of the lining of your arteries, and that's never good. All of these factors put cigarette smokers at much higher risk for angina, MI, and sudden cardiac death.

These days, smoking makes about as much sense as letting your pet chimp play with your loaded handgun. On the one hand, as a devoted member of the NRA, you've been living in Denial World, where handguns are not inherently dangerous, so it's okay to let Bobo handle the "safe" gun. On the other hand, deep in the common sense lobes of your primitive brain, the lobes you should be listening to, the ones otherwise known as "your gut", you know it is stupid to let anyone play with a loaded gun, so when he pops you once or twice in the chest and belly, as you lie bleeding out on the living room dirty mustard shag, just before you lose consciousness, you feel stupid and angry. It's destructive to feel anger toward yourself, so you blame Bobo. Once complications like COPD, vascular disease, bladder or lung cancer show up, the denial that keeps smokers on the nicotine highway often gets replaced by resentment. It's hard to continue to deny when you have a BKA (below-the-knee amputation) stump or an MI staring you in the face.

If you don't already have a BKA stump or an MI staring you in the face, or even if you do, the only thing about smoking that is important is quitting. There isn't much you can do about the damage already done, but you can prevent future damage. For the sake of argument, let's assume you don't already have lung cancer. Once you quit, your risk of developing lung cancer drops every non-smoking year you survive. After ten non-smoking years your risk will be significantly lower than it is now. After twenty-five non-smoking years, your chances are almost as low as a never-smoker. In addition, the levels of carbon monoxide in your blood will drop to normal in less than a day. The long-term effects of chronic carbon monoxide poisoning are still being elucidated, but I'll hazard a guess that there aren't any good ones. In terms of COPD, your lung function will improve, sometimes dramatically, within the first six months after quitting.

What happens to your risk of MI, stroke or amputation when you quit? In the first hour of quitting, your heart rate and blood pressure will begin to fall. Your risk of MI will drop within the first day. Within three months, your peripheral circulation will improve, and you may notice that walking will be easier. Inside your vessels there will be less inflammation, a decrease in foam cell formation and growth, and less likelihood of any of your atheromatous plaques rupturing and causing a potentially fatal MI.

Why are cigarettes so addictive? The current theory is that nicotine attaches to certain receptors in your brain. Once these receptors are activated, your brain releases dopamine, which makes you feel good. After you are finished your heater, dopamine levels drop, making you want another cigarette. From there, it's Go Time.

How do you quit? Like any other addictive substance that you eat, drink or smoke for a long time, if you stop using it, your body and your brain will crave it. Stop it long enough and you will experience physical and psychological withdrawal symptoms. For nicotine, the common symptoms are headache, nausea, fatigue, drowsiness, insomnia, constipation, irritability, anxiety, depression, and difficulty concentrating. Sounds pretty daunting, eh? You have to really want to get off cigarettes to be willing to endure all those symptoms. Fortunately, there are a number of medications on the market to help you.

Nicotine replacement therapy (NRT) substitutes pure nicotine for smoking cigarettes. It comes in gum, lozenge, and patch, all of which are available over the counter, or nasal spray and oral inhaler, both of which require a prescription. The idea is to gradually reduce the amount of nicotine you put into your body while minimizing the severity of your withdrawal symptoms. The milder your withdrawal symptoms, the easier it will be for you to quit. The other major benefit of NRT is that, although you are still using nicotine, you are not being exposed to the other toxic chemicals and side effects associated with smoking.

Besides nicotine withdrawal, there are other difficulties associated with smoking cessation. For some smokers, the oral fixation that is satisfied by sticking a fag into your mouth is as important as the nicotine craving. For other smokers, holding a cig in your hand is equally addictive. If you are interested in battling one or more of these habits or cravings, the American Cancer Society website has plenty of suggestions. Attending a counseling program will improve your chances of quitting permanently. If you are worried about putting on the pounds when you quit, NRT has been shown to prevent weight gain, but you may gain weight when you stop NRT.

The single most important point regarding NRT is that it doesn't work if you cheat (smoke). According to the experts, if you don't cheat on the first day of NRT, you are ten times as likely to quit permanently as if you do cheat. From a physical as well as a psychological perspective, it is worse to smoke while using NRT than it is to do one or the other. If you use NRT and continue to smoke, it is possible to develop nicotine poisoning, which can cause restlessness, agitation, muscular twitching, abdominal cramps, high blood pressure, rapid heartbeat, excessive drooling, confusion, seizures, coma and death.

I vividly remember a photo from thirty years ago. A large man with a big shit-eating grin sits in a hot tub between two women. His arms are draped across their shoulders. On his chest is a nitroglycerine patch. His right arm features a Nicoderm patch. His right hand holds a beer can. Positioned between his left index and middle fingers is a freshly-lit cigarette. Poster boy for the combo nicotine regimen and the good life, he's ready for anything, including sudden death.

Bupropion started its life as an antidepressant, marketed in this country as Welbutrin in 1985. Doesn't that sound nice and soothing, Welbutrin? In 1997 it started its second life as Zyban. Zyban sounds edgier, makes you think it can really kill something off, like giant cockroaches or pit vipers. It was the first non-nicotine medication approved for smoking cessation and the first medication available in tablet form. Interestingly, Zyban was approved for use in smoking cessation even though nobody knows how it works.

Most smoking cessation studies run about four weeks. Occasionally, if the manufacturer is extremely confident, it will support longer studies. According to studies of Zyban vs. NRT, either one produces about the same results. Using both in combination yields a slightly better result. In terms of withdrawal symptoms, users of Zyban reported decreases in restlessness, irritability, frustration, difficulty concentrating and depression. Nobody knows whether this is due to its overall anti-depressant effect or to an effect directly linked to smoking. Side effects, which improve with time, include dry mouth and insomnia. If you take more than the recommended dose of Zyban, you run the risk of seizures. On the plus side, unlike many other anti-depressants, Zyban does not cause weight gain, drowsiness or sexual dysfunction. That means you can take it, maintain your Charles Atlas physique, and stay awake long enough to get it up.

Varenicline tartrate--doesn't sound like something you want to put in your mouth, does it--was approved for use as Chantix in 2006. It works by attaching to nicotine receptors in the brain, thus blocking access for nicotine molecules. Since there is no nicotine attachment, there is a much smaller release of dopamine. That means you don't get the buzz from Chantix that you do from a cigarette. That also means there is less of a subsequent drop in dopamine levels, so you don't get as much of a craving for the next cigarette. If you do start smoking again while on Chantix, you won't get your usual cigarette buzz.

There are two ways to use Chantix. In the first method, you set a date to quit smoking and start taking Chantix one week before that date. The other is to start taking the medication before you set a quit date and once you are on Chantix, you set a date between eight and thirty-five days after beginning treatment. The most important point is to actually quit on the date you select. You start out at a low dose and gradually increase until you are at the maximum by the end of the first week. If at the end of your twelve-week course you have remained cigarette-free, the manufacturer recommends another twelve-week course, I guess just to seal the deal. Counseling is recommended in addition to Chantix treatment. The most common side effects include vivid dreams, nausea, vomiting, flatulence and constipation. In addition, the manufacturer recommends you stop the drug immediately for changes in behavior or suicidal thoughts. Seizures have been reported, as has aggressive behavior and blackouts if you drink alcohol while taking Chantix. Although overall mortality is lower with Chantix than with other forms of smoking-cessation medications, some studies have shown an increase in cardiovascular events on Chantix. Nobody knows how Chantix and NRTs would interact, so they recommend you not mix the two.

According to several experts, no matter which medication you try to help you quit smoking, the cost will be less than the cost of the cigarettes you would have smoked during the treatment period. Obviously that applies only if you actually quit smoking.

When I first started seeing patients, I decided I would ask every one of them if they were a smoker. Usually you can tell anyway, by the finger stains, the tobacco breath, smelly clothes or the gravelly voice. Women's faces take on a certain coarseness after years of smoking. Occasionally a patient who reeked of tobacco would lie, but for the most part, everyone was open about their smoking, much more so than about drinking alcohol. If the patient told me he didn't smoke, I'd then ask him if he ever did. From my personal survey, about ten per cent of current nonsmokers smoked at one time but quit permanently. So then I'd ask them when they quit. Even if it had been fifty years or more, well over ninety per cent remembered the exact date that they last smoked a cigarette or cigar.

Why did they quit? For many ex-smokers, there was a signature event, often related to family. Many quit when they became parents, some when they became grandparents. A surprising number quit for financial reasons. The year I heard most commonly was 1964, when the price of a pack of cigarettes went from twenty-five cents to thirty cents. Ironically, that was right around the time Marlboro began its heavy advertising campaigns. Somewhere in there the percentage of

American adults who smoked rose to over 40%, its all-time high. It is worth noting that the vast majority of Americans who successfully quit smoking do so without the benefit of counseling or medications. Either they quit cold turkey or they cut down and then quit. On the other hand, over 90% of those who try to quit without a program fail.

While NRT reportedly increases your chances of quitting permanently, I have never met a patient who used NRT to get off cigarettes and then stopped using NRT. I've met dozens who tried NRT but stopped because it was expensive and unsuccessful. Many patients tried NRT, successfully quit cigarettes, but were never able to quit NRT. There are a shocking number of patients who have used NRT for years, and continue to use it now, but were never able to completely quit smoking. While this sounds like the worst of all worlds, most of them are pretty proud that they were able to cut their daily cigarette intake by 50% or more. In the long term, this is probably a better outcome than to continue smoking cigarettes at a higher frequency.

Whether it's at the birth of a child, in a hospital bed, or in a casket, eventually everybody quits smoking. It's up to you to decide whether you want to wait for your first stroke, your first MI, or your first amputation to quit. Once you hit the funeral home, the decision has been made for you. The most devout quitters I've ever encountered are the guys who have been diagnosed with terminal lung cancer. At that point, with only weeks or months left on earth, these lifelong cigarette smokers have absolutely no problem putting them down for good.

Most times, before I could even ask them the last question, "Why?", the ex-smoker would offer up the reason for quitting. Why does anyone do anything? In medical training, especially psychiatry, you are told never to ask a "why" question. The official reason for that dictum is that "why" sounds judgmental and tends to put the patient on the defensive. Over the years, I have come to realize the real reason. The answer to any "why" question, the reason at the root of their behavior, is always the same. "Because I wanted to."

Why did you stop smoking?
Why did you eat that candy bar?
Why do you drink every night?
Why have you tried to kill yourself 21 times?

Because I wanted to.

When it comes to smoking, I have never met a patient who didn't want to quit but was able to quit anyway. If you don't want to quit, you won't. In your mind, there will be one good reason to keep smoking, maybe a couple. That's all well and good. The only reason to quit is because you want to. Don't torture yourself with trying. "Trying" to do anything is a waste of time for everyone. If all the scientific data doesn't make you want to quit, no patch or gum or Smokers Anonymous is going to either.

One other tidbit about smoking. When I went down to Roanoke, more or less the northern edge of the Southern Virginia coal region, I met an internist at the Salem VA. Back when coal mining was king, pretty much all the physicians in the small towns of Coal Country would work the monthly Black Lung clinics. He did it for a number of years. He said he'd never met a miner with Black Lung who didn't smoke. I don't know if he was right, but it was his personal observation. Of course, he once said to me, "Nothing slow about you, eh?" Obviously he got that one wrong.

When it comes to cigarettes and a CABG, the longer you abstain from smoking prior to surgery, the faster you will get off the ventilator. For most folks, every minute on the vent seems like an hour. Every tobacco-free day counts.

References:

1. Hibbs, Ryan E., Zambon, Alexander C. "Agents Acting at the Neuromuscular Junction and Autonomic Ganglia." *Goodman & Gilman's The Pharmacological Basis of Therapeutics.* Ed. Laurence L. Brunton, Assoc. Ed. Bruce A. Chabner, Assoc. Ed. Bjorn C Knollman. New York: McGraw-Hill. 2011. 270-2.
2. O'Brien, Charles P. "Drug Addiction." *Goodman & Gilman's The Pharmacological Basis of Therapeutics.* Ed. Laurence L. Brunton, Assoc. Ed. Bruce A. Chabner, Assoc. Ed. Bjorn C Knollman. New York: McGraw-Hill. 2011. 657-8.
3. Maron, David J., Riker, Paul M., Grundy, Scott M., Pearson, Thomas A. "Preventive Strategies for Coronary Heart Disease." *Hurst's The Heart.* Ed. Valentin Fuster, Ed. Robert A. O'Rourke, Ed. Richard A. Walsh, Ed. Philip Poole-Wilson. New York: McGraw-Hill. 2008. 1217-8. 1222.
4. Ridker, Paul M., Libby, Peter. "Risk Markers for Atherothrombotic Disease." *Braunwald's Heart Disease.* Ed. Robert O. Bonow, Ed. Douglas L. Mann, Ed. Douglas P. Zipes, Ed. Peter Libby, Ed. Eugene Braunwald. Philadelphia: Elsevier Saunders. 2012. 914-15.
5. Smith, W. David. "Tobacco." *World Book Encyclopedia.* Chicago: World Book. 2016. 305-8.
6. Oropeza, Ruben. *Between Puffs: Two Thousand Years of Tobacco Use.* Orlando, FL: Rivercross. 2005. 19-91.

25. ALCOHOL AND CAD

When you use the word "alcohol", especially when you blather on about drinking the stuff, you are talking about ethyl alcohol, also known as ethanol, EtOH, 2-carbon fragments, or booze. As a group, alcohols are chemical compounds with at least one hyroxyl (-OH) group. There are two other very common forms of alcohol, methanol and isopropanol. The first one will cause you to go blind, the second is great for taking the itch out of mosquito bites but not so great in a margarita. Ethanol is made through the fermentation of sugars by yeast.

There is evidence that ethanol was consumed at least nine thousand years ago. Mesopotamian pottery from about 4000 B.C. depicts scenes of wine fermentation. Sumerians, who dominated the area now occupied by Iraq, brewed over a dozen different types of beer, had designated drinking places and celebrated alcohol with official drinking events. They even conjured up a goddess of brewing. Spirits, so named because it was believed that they contained the spirit of the liquid product of fermentation, were produced initially in Europe. Distillation of brandy, the oldest distilled spirit, began around 100 A.D. Whisky was distilled by the Scots and Irish as far back as the fifteenth century A.D. Gin was first made by the Dutch around 1600 A.D. The successful cultivation of sugar cane in Barbados led to the production of rum in the mid-seventeenth century. Bourbon was first distilled in the late eighteenth century in Kentucky. Since man began keeping records of his activities, virtually every society has produced and consumed alcohol, making it one of the oldest and most widely used psychoactive substances.

Given the right environment, ethanol can be produced from almost every species of plant, from juniper berries (gin) to rye (whiskey) to grapes (wine) to barley (beer) to agave (te-kill-ya). While alcohol can be associated with much fun when used in moderation, when used to excess it comes in second only to tobacco in terms of short-term and long term mortality (death) and morbidity (illness), everything from acute alcohol intoxication in teenagers to GI bleeding, dementia, liver failure and nerve damage in chronic heavy drinkers. Not to mention the nice bulbous nose and manly liver you grow when you imbibe excessively for decades.

Most of mankind's vices are not nice to your blood vessels or heart. Tobacco, cocaine, meth, obesity, they all treat your cardiovascular system like a toilet, dumping their adverse effects in on a regular basis. You would be hard-pressed to come up with a scientific study lauding the benefits of smoking crack, and most physicians have given up on the idea that menthol cigarettes are better for you than regulars. Alcohol occupies a niche that no other vice can claim. It can be bad for you and it can be good for you too!

What's alcohol got to do with heart disease? Alcohol increases HDL and triglyceride levels. Increased HDL means a reduction in the risk of coronary artery disease (CAD), while increased triglyceride levels favor an increase in the risk of CAD. Overall, according to some experts, the rise in HDL is more significant than the rise in triglycerides, meaning that the net result of moderate ingestion of alcohol favors a reduction in CAD. Other equally prominent voices would disagree.

Alcohol also causes a reduction in serum fibrinogen levels. Fibrinogen is converted to fibrin during the formation of a blood clot. Less fibrinogen means fewer blood clots, and fewer blood clots means fewer MIs. Alcohol also tends to inhibit platelet aggregation. Again, less active platelet aggregation means fewer blood clots and, theoretically, fewer MIs. More potential for bleeding to death too.

On the other hand, consumption of three or more drinks per day will raise your blood pressure, and the higher your blood pressure, the greater the chance for damage to your coronary arteries and your heart. It has been demonstrated that if a heavy drinker cuts back to moderate drinking, he can lower his systolic blood pressure by 2-4 mmHg. and his diastolic by 1-2 mmHg. That doesn't sound like much, but in the world of hypertension, every little bit helps.

When it comes to quantifying your alcohol consumption, the standard drink consists of twelve ounces of beer, five ounces of wine, or 1 1/2 ounces of 80-proof liquor. Moderate drinking, which is the kind most researchers recommend, consists of two drinks per day for men under sixty-five years old, one drink per day for men aged sixty-five and older, and one drink per day for women of any age. Binge drinking is drinking to the point where your blood alcohol level reaches 0.08 g/dl., a common threshold for DUIs. That level can be reached within two hours by the consumption of four drinks by an average-sized woman or five drinks by her male drinking buddy. Binge drinking on a regular basis will result in an increased blood pressure as well.

For the past several decades, the rumor has been that a couple of glasses of red wine will decrease your chances of developing coronary artery disease and suffering an MI. This belief was triggered by the French Paradox. Despite consuming a diet high in saturated fats and smoking like chimneys, the French have a low incidence of CAD. Some studies have shown a definite reduction in coronary artery disease for individuals who have one or two drinks on a regular basis. Those in the non-drinking corner (Motto: Why have fun doing something that's good for you?) will counter that drinking grape juice is as beneficial as those two glasses of wine. Resveratrol and flavinoids, two antioxidants, are found in stems, leaves, skin and seeds of red and purple grapes; experts theorize that they are responsible for the benefit in terms of heart disease. Lovers of the fermented grape then argue that to get the benefits of two daily glasses of red wine, you would have to consume a couple gallons of grape juice every day. That's a lot of calories to consume on a daily basis, even if it is good for you.

When you make wine from grapes, the first step after picking is the destemming process, where the bunches of grapes are dropped into a bin with a rotating coil inside it. This smashes the grapes into a pulpy juice and removes the seeds, stems and leaves. To make red or rose wine, you then put the semisolid must, consisting of skins, juice and pulp, into tanks to begin the fermenting process. To make white wine, you first press the grapes, toss the skins and pulp, then put the juice into tanks. If the beneficial compounds are contained only in a grape's stem, seeds, leaves and skin, then white wine, which contains none of these, shouldn't help at all.

Does it matter what form of alcohol you drink? Some large studies have seen a bigger reduction in risk of heart disease in wine drinkers than in their fellow beerflies, but almost every study demonstrating a benefit from moderate wine drinking also shows benefits from other varieties of alcohol.

So, in the end, is the consumption of a couple of drinks daily good or bad for your heart? Most cardiologists will say it's okay. However, if you find yourself imbibing more than two per day on a regular basis, you run the risk of losing the benefit and doing some damage. If you get into trouble because of excessive drinking, it's time to board the H.M.S. Rehab, where mental health professionals and substance abuse counselors man the helm; at this point, the recommendation will be for you to get off the sauce completely. When it comes to booze, there's a very fine line between fun and done.

References:

1. Schuckit, Marc A. "Ethanol and Methanol." *Goodman & Gilman's The Pharmacological Basis of Therapeutics.* Ed. Laurence L. Brunton, Assoc. Ed. Bruce A. Chabner, Assoc. Ed. Bjorn C Knollman. New York: McGraw-Hill. 2011. 629-36.

2. Mozzafarian, Dariush. "Nutrition and Cardiovascular Disease." *Braunwald's Heart Disease.* Ed. Robert O. Bonow, Ed. Douglas L. Mann, Ed. Douglas P. Zipes, Ed. Peter Libby, Ed. Eugene Braunwald. Philadelphia: Elsevier Saunders. 2012. 1003.
3. Busch, Marianna A. "Alcohol." *World Book Encyclopedia.* Chicago: World Book. 2016. 1:335.
4. Claus, Michael J. "Alcoholic Beverages." *World Book Encyclopedia.* Chicago: World Book. 2016. 1:336-7.
5. Gately, Iain. *Drink: A Cultural History of Alcohol.* New York: Gotham Books. 2008. 546 p.
6. Rimm EB, Giovannucci EL, et al. "Prospective study of alcohol consumption and risk of coronary disease in men" *Lancet.* 1991. 338:464-8.
7. Moore RD, Pearson TA. "Moderate alcohol consumption and coronary artery disease: A review." *Medicine.* 1986. 65(4):242-67.
8. Davidson DM. "Cardiovascular effects of alcohol." *West J Med.* 1989. 151(4):430–9.
9. Rimm EB, Klatsky A, Grobbee D, Stampfer MJ. "Review of moderate alcohol consumption and reduced risk of coronary heart disease: is the effect due to beer, wine or spirits." Brit Med J. 1996. 312:(7033):731–6.
10. Simini B. "Serge Renaud: from French paradox to Cretan miracle.". *Lancet.* 2000. 355(9197): 48.

26. THE MCGUIRE

A Labor Day weekend Saturday in Flagstaff. Most of the docs from Kayenta and Inscription House were on the Green River, headed down to the confluence with the Colorado, through Cataract Canyon, to eventually land at Hite Marina at the far north end of Lake Powell. It was a weeklong trip, and someone had to stay behind and man the clinic; more importantly, the E.R. had to be covered on nights and weekends. David had alternated call with Tom Reynolds, every other night for the past week. Friday night call had been surprisingly light, probably because many Navajo families went out of town to visit family in Gallup, Cortez or Flagstaff and do some weekend shopping. After signing out to Tom, David lit out first thing Saturday morning, stopping in Tuba to pick up cash and booze orders. He declined $200.00 from one of the new nurses over there, who wanted him to pick up some expensive wine from the Seller. In less than two months, the guy was already known as something of a snob and a world-class whiner. Simmons wasn't taking a chance on wine that might have turned. He stuck to small quantities of beer and a few bottles of hard liquor--less chance of a bad batch. It was a pain in the ass to hide the stuff in the back of his pickup. If stopped by the tribal police on the reservation, they could pour any alcohol out, confiscate it, or impound his truck. On a bad day, it would be all three.

The 150-mile trip went smoothly, and he was in Flag by noon. Marie Kent, an Anglo married to one of the environmental guys in the PHS, had told him stories about making the trip back in the '60s over a washboard dirt road before the mine was fully operational. Brutal on the teeth and the suspension. At the Elephant Feet, Simmons picked up a quartet of hitchhikers, an old lady and her two daughters, each sporting at least four velvet skirts and the aroma of dusty mutton, and a grandson. He had the kid sit up front with him so they could chat on the ride in. The little guy turned out to be a good storyteller. Simmons added a few new words to his Navajo vocabulary. Once in town, he cruised down Santa Fe until one of the daughters rapped on the back window. He pulled over and opened the back of the camper top; they scrambled out onto Santa Fe and, with a nod and an ahéhee', headed up Elden. He turned right at San Francisco and parked in the lot at the Casa Royale.

It took a couple of hours to round up the booze orders and most of the supplies he needed. The perishables he'd pick up Monday morning on the way out of town. That was one of the best things about border towns--the stores were open seven days a week, even holidays, to take advantage of the reservation folks coming in to shop on the weekend. He walked around town, had some pizza and a beer at the Alpine, and took a snooze.

Around six-thirty, after losing a few games of nine-ball downstairs, Simmons headed over to the McGuire Hotel. A placard on the front window advertised Sven Lindstrom, a blues guitarist up from Phoenix. It was an early show, already in progress. David had caught his act a few weeks prior up in Telluride; he hoped to finish up his business with Jorge and still see some of Sven's set. Afterwards, a collection of local bluegrass players planned a jam. Nice way to end the evening.

Terry and a teacher named Paul Finley had asked him to buy $400.00 worth of weed from a supplier named Jorge. At first, David balked. These two were constantly in debt, and he didn't want to get stuck with a bunch of grass. Word would get around and pretty soon he'd be the mooch crowd's best new friend. Terry, who was currently finishing up at Hite, promised that he would take it off his hands first thing Monday morning, give him $400.00 and throw in a quarter ounce for his trouble. Simmons upped the resale price to $425.00. Terry agreed and called Finley to set it up. David still had misgivings about any business arrangement that involved those two knuckleheads, but the way he figured it, once he was out of Jorge's hotel room, he'd have control of the situation and the risk would be minimal.

After he worked his way around the crowd in the lobby of the old hotel, David climbed the stairs to the third floor. The balcony that looked out on Aspen and Leroux was overflowing with people gawking and drinking. He could hear the band two stories below; the windows in the bar were open. Just to his left, an enormous guy who looked like he could handle himself was standing in front of the door to room 39. His black t-shirt had TANK across the front. Beside him was an umbrella stand with a few old bumbershoots and the stock of a long gun. *Probably a shotgun,* he thought. *Really? Kind of messy for a crowded place.* Simmons felt a knot in his gut and thought about turning around and heading back where he came from, but the bald guy was giving him the evil eye, so he thought, *Fuck it* and walked right up to him.

"What do you want?" David literally could not see either side of the doorway around this guy.

"I'm supposed to give Jorge some money."

"You can give it to me."

"Yeah. Probably not. Tell him I'm here."

"He's busy. Go wait in 35 and I'll come get you when he's done. A few minutes."

Again, Simmons considered leaving, grabbing a beer downstairs and sitting on a barstool, ogling girls and enjoying live music. Every component of that plan was non-existent on the res. But he ignored his gut. He was curious about what was going on in 39. Room 35 was two doors down to his left. The door was closed but unlocked. He looked back at the big guy, who nodded and pointed, so he went in.

Clearly this was the waiting room. The single bed was shoved up against the wall under an open window. A half-dozen empty folding chairs were arranged more or less in a circle around an old brass ashtray standing in the middle of the room. David walked over to the other window and looked out. There was no balcony this far west. Two stories below, four guys were standing outside the side door of the bar smoking and laughing. He turned around and headed out the door.

"Where you going?" The fat guy moved to block him from the stairway. Simmons feinted right, darted left and slid between the door of Room 39 and the enforcer, then completely around him and down the first two steps. He turned around to face him.

"This whole setup is ridiculous. I'm leaving." He jumped down two more steps, well out of the big man's reach, then turned to look up the steps again.

Tank stared down at him, then said, "Okay. Wait a minute." He knocked twice on the door and went in. After about ten seconds, he came back into the hallway. "He's ready for you." Simmons climbed back up the stairs and walked into the room. *Oh, fuck.*

The last time he'd seen Jorge, his name wasn't Jorge. It was Chico, or Chaco, or something like that. An old Army buddy of Murphy's, he'd come back to Portland to squeeze five grand out of Robert; that didn't go well, so he pulled a knife. Murphy drop-kicked him down thirty-five steps until he came to rest at David's feet. The two of them hauled him across the street and dumped him unconscious in the employee parking lot of the Duck Flat Inn, then Murphy went inside and called the fire department to report an injured drunk out back.

An ambulance took him to Saint Titus, where he underwent surgery for a broken femur and a depressed skull fracture. In his journey down the steps, the knife had slit his forearm, severing his radial nerve. The last he'd heard, Chico ended up being transferred over to the Rehab Institute, alive and extremely pissed off. From what Murphy told him later, David surmised Chico was a true sociopath, all smiles and smoothness until he didn't get what he wanted. Then the anger surfaced and violence usually followed. One evening a few weeks later in the Duck Flat, David wondered aloud why Saint Titus hadn't shipped him up the hill to the VA.

"He's using an alias. Has some unresolved issues with law enforcement in California. Besides, a general discharge does not earn you VA bennies."

He looked pretty much the same, except he'd grown a goatee. Still had the shiny black hair, the bright blue eyes that seemed out of place. His left hand had some atrophy. David had a moment of panic, then realized that this guy had never met him, at least not while he was conscious. In addition, David had since grown his hair longer and now had a rather full beard.

"What do you want?" Cocky. He thought, *I'm doing a follow-up visit to check on your injuries. How about a couple more?*

Instead, he said, "I'm picking up some reefer for Finley."

"Oh, yeah. What's your name? David or something?" He waited for Simmons to confirm. That wasn't going to happen. No reason to get him in a conversation. For the first time, he noticed they were not alone. A guy who looked to be about fifty in dog years was passed out in a tattered stuffed leather chair over to David's right. On the floor next to his chair was a bottle of cheap Reposado. Someone had taken a tiny red plastic sombrero, probably the bottle cap, and tied it to the top of his head with a shoelace. He wasn't breathing much.

"What happened to him?"

Chico/Jorge looked over at the pale form in the recliner and laughed. "Shorty? Just a little too much tequila. He'll be fine." David walked over and stood watching. Not breathing much was actually not breathing at all. He felt the guy's face. Ice cold.

"How long's he been out?"

"Couple hours. You got the money?" He pulled a leather briefcase up on the card table. Out of the corner of his eye, David could see his left hand wasn't working very smoothly, and it dangled uselessly when he wasn't holding something. Guess the radial nerve repair didn't go too well. He visualized the scene in the parking lot, thought the left thigh was the one with the deformity. He turned back toward the table.

"Yeah. Four hundred. Where's the weed from?"

"No weed. Couldn't get any on short notice. Finley said it'd be okay to give you coke instead."

God-DAMN it. That slippery bastard. He wondered if Terry was in on this. Didn't matter. To give himself time to think, David walked back toward Shorty and picked up the bottle.

"Oh, coke. Did this guy do a bunch of coke today?"

"Naw, just his usual line. Shorty has it all under control. Does a line every morning before work. Keeps him sharp, driving a grader for the state highway department for eighteen years." He punched in some numbers on a small calculator. "Eighteen times three sixty-five.

Counting weekends and holidays, six thousand five hundred seventy. That's a shitloada lines. Let's see the money."

"I don't want the coke." He turned back toward the guy at the table.

"You're taking the coke and I'm taking the money. That was the deal once you walked in the door." He looked at the bottle in David's hand, then stood up, reaching behind him for something. David heard the snick of a switchblade. *Again with the knife,* he thought. Simmons stepped forward and kicked him as hard as he could in the left thigh. Low-middle kick with *kihap.*

"Mother fucker!" Jorge twisted in pain, falling onto and crushing the flimsy card table. As he hit the floor, the knife stuck at an angle into the weathered pine floor. David stomped on it, snapping the blade. The briefcase lay on the floor, dozens of clear plastic packets of cocaine and twenties strewn around Jorge's body. Simmons threw the bottle through the nearest window. Broken glass showered down on Jorge. A second later he heard the bottle shatter in the street. He considered kicking Jorge just for fun, thought better of it, and turned to the door.

Tank was coming in. David said to him, "You got about two minutes before someone calls the cops, maybe another five before they come busting in here. Shorty's dead. If I were you, I'd get the coke and the money and your buddy Jorge and get out of here."

Jorge rolled over onto his back, holding his left thigh. He stopped moaning long enough to say, "I know where to find you, you fuck." Tank looked over at Shorty crumpled in the leather chair, then down at Jorge, then at David.

"Fuck him. He's not my buddy. Shorty is. Was." He stepped over Jorge. As Simmons started down the steps, he looked back. Tank was piling some of the coke packets and all the money into the briefcase. Walking slowly down Aspen, thinking about what Jorge had said, David almost bumped into the phone booth. He pulled out a quarter, dialed 0, and waited.

"Hello, I'd like to report a crime. There's a guy being held against his will by a drug dealer with a knife. Room thirty-nine in the McGuire Hotel. Third floor. Better send an ambulance as well. He looks sick." He wrote off Sven and the bluegrassers and wondered who was playing in the basement bar at the Casa Royale.

27. DRUGS AND CAD

Cocaine is the drug of delusion. Even for someone like Mr. Shorty, who has it all under control, chronic low-dose cocaine use can have devastating effects on the heart. Believe it or not, there are more than a few guys like him out there, dosing themselves with coke the way most of us rev up in the morning with coffee.

In the short term, smoking, snorting or injecting cocaine causes an increase in the level of circulating epinephrine. This causes increased heart rate, a rise in blood pressure, and an increase in the contractility of the heart muscle. These all lead to a marked increase in the demand for oxygen and blood by the heart muscle. At the same time, other catecholamines cause coronary artery constriction and a greater tendency for blood clots to form, so there is less blood flow through the coronary arteries. These two opposing effects can cause ischemia or infarction. In addition, cocaine alters the function of the sodium channels in individual cardiac muscle cells. Much like screwing around with your boss's wife, screwing around with the sodium channels never leads to anything good. In the case of cocaine, this interference with sodium channels causes a decrease in left ventricular contractility and an increase in the tendency toward arrhythmias.

Looking back on this paragraph, I don't see anything that sounds remotely good. So, even in the short term, cocaine can kill you by triggering abnormal heart rhythms or a heart attack.

When used on a long-term basis, cocaine can cause aneurysms in your coronary arteries. In addition, cocaine can cause inflammation in the walls of the coronary arteries. Any time you have long-term inflammation, scarring usually develops. Fibrous plaques are the result in this situation. In addition, chronic use and the resulting inflammation can lead to accelerated deposit of cholesterol plaques or atherosclerosis. Chronic use will also lead to cardiomyopathy, a heart which doesn't pump well, which can develop into congestive heart failure. Again, nothing that anyone would go to K-Mart to buy.

Meth users can suffer pretty much all the complications that cocaine users experience. In addition, given their predisposition to picking at their skin, meth addicts can also develop MRSA infections, including endocarditis, a blood-borne infection of one or more heart valves.

When you check into the hospital for your heart surgery, it is wise to tell the truth about all your bad habits. Other than the occasional well-meaning zealot who will sneak into your room at night and pray for your lost soul, nobody at the hospital really cares what you put into your body. If you are a chronic user of any type of drug, be it alcohol, heroin, prescription narcotics, cocaine, meth, or benzodiazepines like Ambien, Valium, and Librium, it is better to fess up to your nurse or doctor than to run the risk of seizing, dying, stroking out, or just having to stay in the hospital for four or five more days because you suffered withdrawal from not having your fix.

References:

1. O'Brien, Charles P. "Drug Addiction." *Goodman & Gilman's The Pharmacological Basis of Therapeutics.* Ed. Laurence L. Brunton, Assoc. Ed. Bruce A. Chabner, Assoc. Ed. Bjorn C Knollman. New York: McGraw-Hill. 2011. 661-3.

28. NICE NORMAL EKG

Many of the steps in the development of the EKG took place in experiments on frogs. Some discoveries were made on recently-hung criminals. In 1773, a member of the British Parliament, John Walsh, demonstrated a visible spark of electricity from an electric eel and communicated his findings in a letter to Benjamin Franklin, who was fascinated by all things electric. This was over twenty years after the kite-and-key experiment in a lightning storm. Between then and the end of the nineteenth century, a multitude of brilliant, inquisitive men made significant discoveries in the fields of physics and physiology that led to the modern EKG.

Willem Einthoven of the Netherlands is considered the father of the EKG. In 1893 he introduced the term "electrocardiogram" at a meeting of the Dutch Medical Association. Two years later he described five deflections in the tracing of the heart's electrical activity, which he named P, Q, R, S, and T. His first EKG machine, produced in 1901, weighed over six hundred pounds. In 1905, in what was undoubtedly the first telemedicine event in history, he began transmitting EKG's over telephone cables from the hospital to his laboratory about a mile away. Common sense dictates that the abbreviation for "electrocardiogram" is "ECG" rather than "EKG". In 1912, Einthoven referred to the electrocardiogram as EKG. And that is why EKG is still used today. Tradition.

An EKG is basically a tracing of the electrical activity of your heart. That's all. A purist would prefer to put needles into various portions of the heart muscle to obtain an EKG; a fair number of researchers have done just that. Given the nature of inventors and researcher, it stands to reason that at least one of them did it to his own heart muscle, but information in that area is scant, perhaps because he didn't live to tell about it. However, the standard EKG setup, with sensing electrodes attached to skin on each of your arms and legs and across your chest, does very nicely without the need for cutting open your chest. It is a much faster, cheaper and safer alternative. Less invasive.

There are basic laws of physics and electricity that explain how an EKG works. I have replaced plenty of electrical outlets and switches, sometimes successfully, and I aced physics in both high school and college. I've read the explanations of the theory of the EKG at least a dozen times, most recently while preparing to write this chapter, but I still can't explain it to you. I could say that it's too complicated for the scope of this book (That's what experts usually say when they are talking down to you.), but that's just another way of saying I don't understand it; therefore, I'm not going to waste your time by trying to bullshit my way through it. If you are an electrician or a physicist, this is elementary stuff, and you can figure it out on your own. If you are neither, my explanation will provide absolutely nothing in terms of comprehending the underlying concepts. If you want to know everything about EKG's, pick up a copy of *Practical Electrocardiography* by Henry J.L. Marriott, M.D.

When your doctor looks at your resting EKG, which means an EKG done when you are comfortable and lying down, he looks for several things. First he looks to see whether your heart rate is normal or abnormal. Officially, a normal heart beats between sixty and one hundred times per minute. Anything below sixty bpm (beats per minute) is termed bradycardia (pronounced "Tom Brady-cardia"). Anything above one hundred bpm is termed tachycardia (pronounced "Ooh, that's so tacky-cardia").

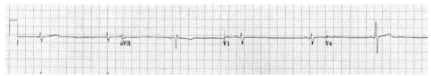

Bradycardia

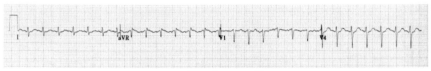

Tachycardia

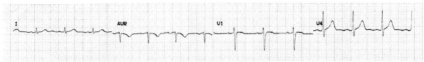

Normal Sinus Rhythm

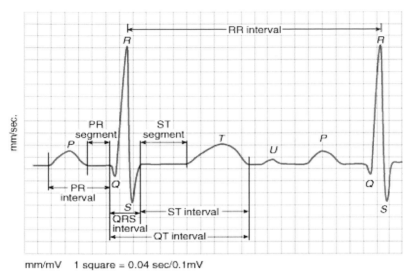

mm/mV   1 square = 0.04 sec/0.1mV

Normal QRS Complex

The next thing to look at is the rhythm. Is it regular or irregular? Regular means the R-R interval, the space between each QRS complex, is the same. If there is a P wave before each QRS complex, your heart rate is between sixty and one hundred bpm, and the rhythm is regular, you are in normal sinus rhythm, the most common type of rhythm. A slower regular rhythm, again with a P wave before each QRS complex, is termed sinus bradycardia, and a faster one sinus tachycardia. Sinus bradycardia is common in healthy runners. The more we learn about the effects of long-term, long-distance running on the human body, the more the terms "healthy" and "runner" seem mutually exclusive. Their heart rates will often be between forty and sixty bpm. Patients on beta-blockers for high blood pressure or heart disease often have rates below sixty bpm.

The important squiggles on your EKG are the P, Q, R, S, and T waves. There are also U waves, but they are relatively rare. Each of these waves is a tracing of the depolarization (electrical firing) or repolarization (recovery or reloading of electrical potential) of a portion of your heart. The P wave represents depolarization of your left and right atria. The Q, R, and S waves, which are usually described together as the "QRS complex" represent the depolarization of the left and right ventricles, the big pumpers in your heart. This is by far the most important complex of the bunch, and, to make things easier, it is almost always the tallest collection of waves. In the QRS complex, if the first wave points downward, it is called a Q wave. Q waves can be normal or abnormal, present or absent. The first upward-pointing wave, whether or not it is preceded by a Q wave, is the R wave. The downward-pointing wave after the R wave is the S wave. The T wave represents the repolarization of the ventricles. Once repolarization occurs, the ventricles are ready to fire and cause the next heartbeat.

There are well-known patterns for each of these waves. P waves, for instance, are usually upright in some leads and inverted in others. Likewise for T waves. P or T waves that are upright or inverted where they shouldn't be may indicate coronary artery disease. Q waves in some leads are considered to be normal. However, Q waves in other leads, or exceptionally large Q waves in any lead, are often a sign of a recent or old MI.

Equally important to the discussion of coronary disease and its manifestations is the ST segment. This is the part of your EKG that spans the space between your QRS complex and your T wave. It should be smooth, somewhat rounded, and at the same level as the segment between the T wave and the next P wave. Elevation or depression below that baseline can indicate potential or actual damage to your heart.

A standard EKG is commonly referred to in the business as a "12 lead". That's because there are twelve different areas of your heart that are evaluated on your EKG. Leads 2, 3, and aVF represent the inferior portion of your heart; the muscle there is often supplied by the right coronary artery. Leads V1 through V4 represent the anterior portion of your heart, often supplied by your left anterior descending coronary artery. Leads aVL, V5 and V6 display the electrical activity of the anterolateral and lateral aspects of your heart. This segment is usually supplied by either the left anterior descending or circumflex or both.

Although there are dozens of interesting variations upon what you've just read, when it comes to diagnosing coronary artery disease, ischemia and injury (MI), that is pretty much all you will need to know. Axis, hypertrophy, bundle branch block are all important aspects of the EKG as well, but usually don't figure much into the diagnosis of ischemia or infarction. As we go through the various manifestations of coronary artery disease, I will point out the typical changes in your EKG. Again, if my explanations are too simplistic, feel free to read further on any subject in Dr. Marriott's book.

The most important thing to know is that a resting EKG, one that is performed while you are lying down and pain-free, tells you almost nothing about the state of your coronary arteries. That's why we have treadmill stress tests and cardiac catheterizations.

References:

1. De Luna, Antonio Bayes, Goldwasser, Diego, Fiol, Miquel, Bayes-Genis, Antoni. "Surface Electrocardiography." *Hurst's The Heart.* Ed. Valentin Fuster, Ed. Richard A. Walsh, Ed. Robert A. Harrington. New York: McGraw-Hill. 2011. 307-19.
2. Wagner, Galen S. "Interpretation of the Normal Electrocardiogram." *Marriott's Practical Electrocardiography.* Philadelphia: Lippincott Williams & Wilkins. 2001. 44-67.
3. Mirvis, David M., Goldberger, Ary L. "Electrocardiography." *Braunwald's Heart Disease.* Ed. Robert O. Bonow, Ed. Douglas L. Mann, Ed. Douglas P. Zipes, Ed. Peter Libby, Ed. Eugene Braunwald. Philadelphia: Elsevier Saunders. 2012. 126-37.

29. NOT SO NORMAL EKG

One of the great things about an EKG is that it can give you clues as to the cause of your chest pain. While there are dozens of subtle EKG signs that indicate you are suffering from ischemia or infarction, there are a few that provide more evidence of ischemia or injury than all the others combined. Specifically, this chapter will look at Q waves, ST segments, and T waves in the setting of coronary artery disease. If you come into your doctor's office or the E.R. with chest pain and your EKG shows abnormal Q waves or abnormalities of the ST segments and T waves, odds are your chest pain is due to ischemia or infarction. If you come in with active chest pain and your EKG is completely normal, there is still a chance that you have heart disease and your symptoms are related to that. Remember that a normal EKG when you are lying down with no discomfort tells you nothing at all about the status of your coronary arteries. And, as low-tech and antiquated as it sounds, there is no substitute for a good history and physical to diagnose any disease, especially coronary artery disease. The EKG is designed to complement the H & P, not replace it. The focus is on ST segment and T wave abnormalities because that's where the action is.

As you may remember, on your normal EKG, the ST segment is the area between your QRS complex and your T wave. It represents the time between depolarization (electrical firing) and repolarization (electrical recovery) of the ventricles. The ST segment should be smooth, slightly rounded, and isoelectric (at the same level as the preceding PR segment and the following TP segment). Minor elevations (less than 1-2 mm) or depressions (less than 0.5 mm) of the ST segment may be normal variants. In healthy young black men who haven't been shot by white cops it is not uncommon to see ST segment elevations of as much as 4 mm in one or more leads. While it looks ominous, this may also represent a normal variant, known as "early repolarization". In general, however, significant ST segment elevations or depressions in the right clinical setting represent infarction or ischemia until proven otherwise.

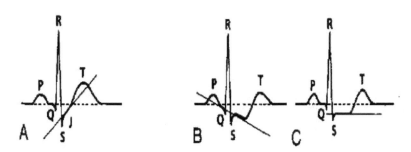

Ischemia with ST depression: upsloping (A), downsloping (B), horizontal (C)

The hallmark of ischemia on an EKG is ST segment depression. If you must get down to the nits and grits, during ischemia there is an increase in the resting potential of ischemic myocardial cells. Because the ST segment represents the period of time when myocardial cells are depolarized, it is less elevated than the rest of the EKG tracing, so it comes out looking depressed. If you are the normal dog in a pack of hyperactive Jack Russell terriers, you will look depressed by comparison. Suffice to say, if your ST segments are depressed, and you are having chest pain, you are probably suffering from coronary ischemia. There is a rare form of ischemia known as Prinzmetal's angina, caused by muscular spasm of the coronary artery, in which the ST segments will be elevated rather than depressed. Other causes of ST segment depression include low blood potassium levels, digitalis, hyperventilation, mitral valve prolapse, left ventricular hypertrophy (thickening of the wall of the left ventricle, usually due to longstanding high blood pressure), bundle branch blocks (conduction abnormalities between the right and left ventricles), hypothermia, tachycardia, and diseases of the central nervous system. While hyperventilation and mitral valve prolapse can cause chest pain, once again, a good history and physical exam will usually differentiate these entities from angina or MI.

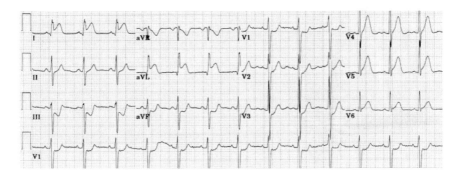

Lateral infarction with ST segment elevation in leads I and aVL; reciprocal ST segment depression in leads III, aVF and V1-V3

Infarction can show up on an EKG in two different patterns. In a transmural MI, involving the entire thickness of the wall of the heart, you will see ST segment elevation. A transmural MI is also known as an ST elevation MI (STEMI) or a Q wave MI. The ST elevation results from early repolarization of the damaged myocardium. Don't ask me to explain it, but please take my word for it. It came to me in a vision.

When a major coronary artery is partially blocked or a smaller branch is completely blocked, you will have a non-ST elevation MI (NSTEMI). Because only a portion of the full thickness of the ventricular wall is involved, your EKG will show ST segment depression rather than elevation. In this scenario, the duration and intensity of the pain may help to distinguish ischemia (angina) from an MI, but usually blood levels of CPK-MB and Troponin I, elevated in an MI but normal or minimally elevated in ischemia, will make the diagnosis.

T waves represent the repolarization phase of the ventricles. This is the recovery period, when they recover their spent electrical energy through the flow of ions back and forth across the cell membrane. The important characteristics of your T wave are its amplitude (height), its shape and its direction. Changes from their normal characteristics in these three categories can indicate ischemia or infarction, often before any other EKG signs develop.

Normally your T waves are upright in leads 1, 2 and V3 - V6. They should always be inverted in lead aVR. They can vary in all the other leads. Whether upright or inverted, your T waves are normally a little asymmetrical. If you are suffering from partial coronary blockage causing ischemia, often your T waves in the corresponding area of the EKG will point in the opposite direction of normal. Normally upright T waves will be inverted and may be of greater amplitude than normal. Likewise, normally inverted T waves will now point upward.

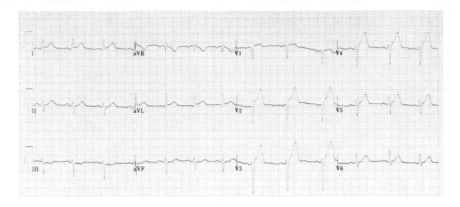

Early infarction: Hyperacute T waves in leads V2-V4

If you are experiencing a STEMI, often the first EKG sign will be "hyperacute" T waves. These are tall, symmetrical, and peaked. After anywhere from a few hours to a few days, if the infarction is not treated, your T waves will invert deeply. On the other hand, in ischemia and NSTEMI, T wave inversion usually accompanies the ST segment depression

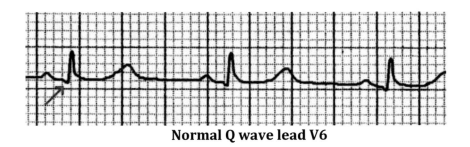

Normal Q wave lead V6

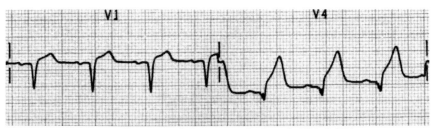

Abnormal Q waves in leads V1 & V4

Small Q waves can be present normally in leads, 1, aVL, aVF, V5 and V6. Moderately sized Q waves can be seen in leads 3, V1 and V2. A very deep Q wave is the norm in aVR. Q waves do not develop during or after ischemia, nor are they seen during or after a NSTEMI. They appear only after a STEMI. While Q waves usually show up within hours or days of an infarct, it is not uncommon for a patient to have a

STEMI and never develop Q waves. The key to determining whether a Q wave is indicative of a STEMI is the clinical setting, i.e., the presence of chest pain, the depth and width of the Q wave, and the leads in which the Q waves appear. The deeper and wider the Q wave, the greater the likelihood it is abnormal.

References:

1. De Luna, Antonio Bayes, Goldwasser, Diego, Fiol, Miquel, Bayes-Genis, Antoni. "Surface Electrocardiography." *Hurst's The Heart.* Ed. Valentin Fuster, Ed. Richard A. Walsh, Ed. Robert A. Harrington. New York: McGraw-Hill. 2011. 333-41. 344-7.
2. Wagner, Galen S. " Myocardial Ischemia and Infarction." *Marriott's Practical Electrocardiography.* Philadelphia: Lippincott Williams & Wilkins. 2001. 140-4.
3. Wagner, Galen S. "Ischemia and Injury Due to Insufficient Blood Supply." *Marriott's Practical Electrocardiography.* Philadelphia: Lippincott Williams & Wilkins. 2001. 164-77.
4. Wagner, Galen S. "Myocardial Infarction." *Marriott's Practical Electrocardiography.* Philadelphia: Lippincott Williams & Wilkins. 2001. 180-94.
5. Mirvis, David M., Goldberger, Ary L. "Electrocardiography." *Braunwald's Heart Disease.* Ed. Robert O. Bonow, Ed. Douglas L. Mann, Ed. Douglas P. Zipes, Ed. Peter Libby, Ed. Eugene Braunwald. Philadelphia: Elsevier Saunders. 2012. 149-59.

30. ARRHYTHMIAS

Technically speaking, an arrhythmia is any rhythm other than normal sinus. You can divide them up into fast, slow and irregular, or you can categorize them the same way you do brain tumors. Like a benign brain tumor, most of the time benign arrhythmias don't cause problems, and they don't end up killing you. Malignant arrhythmias, like malignant brain tumors, definitely cause problems and they can kill you. Unlike a malignant astrocytoma, a malignant arrhythmia can usually be treated and cured. While there are dozens of arrhythmias, both benign and malignant, we'll be dealing only with the ones commonly associated with MI or CABG.

The benign arrhythmias occur commonly. Sometimes they are temporary and sometimes they stick around despite everyone's best efforts. Occasionally they will cause symptoms, which often resolve with little or no treatment. Let's start with the benign ones, then move on to the really bad ones.

Bradyarrhythmias are those that involve a rate less than sixty beats per minute (bpm). Tachyarrhythmias require a rate above one hundred bpm. Irregular rhythms can be associated with fast, slow, or normal rates.

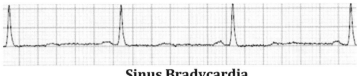

Sinus Bradycardia

The commonest bradyarrhythmia is sinus bradycardia. It consists of a sinus rhythm, usually with a rate between fifty and sixty bpm. It is very common in runners and other aerobic athletes. It is also commonly seen in normal people who are asleep. Beta blockers and calcium-channel blockers for angina or high blood pressure are common causes. It can also occur in patients taking digoxin (digitalis) to slow down a tachyarrhythmia or to improve heart muscle function in congestive heart failure. Other oddball causes of sinus bradycardia include severe anorexia nervosa, increased intracranial pressure (swelling of the brain), glaucoma (increased pressure in the eyeball) or pushing on someone's eyeball or carotid artery with your thumb just for laughs. Because the right coronary artery supplies blood to both the SA node and the inferior portion of the heart, a fair number of patients who suffer an inferior MI will experience sinus bradycardia.

Very few people have symptoms from sinus bradycardia if the rate is above fifty bpm, so this arrhythmia rarely requires treatment. In those rare cases where the rate is below fifty bpm and your blood pressure drops, you may experience symptoms like lightheadedness, weakness or loss of consciousness. When these situations develop while taking a medication known to cause sinus bradycardia, the usual treatment is to decrease the dosage of the medication or stop it altogether. In dramatic cases where the slow rate causes a significant fall in blood pressure, the administration of IV atropine usually affords prompt, temporary relief, and external temporary pacemakers can be used until the drug is out of your system. If it's not due to medications, it almost never causes symptoms.

The commonest tachyarrhythmia is sinus tachycardia. It is a normal response to exercising and emotional upset. Abnormal causes include severe blood loss, dehydration, fever, infections, MI, congestive heart failure, and thyrotoxicosis (overactive thyroid gland). In sufficient doses, caffeine can cause sinus tachycardia. And of course there are the not-quite-organic causes: nicotine, cocaine, methamphetamine, and amyl nitrate (poppers). The treatment regimen for persistent sinus tachycardia usually consists of finding the cause and making it go away. Nicotine, coke and meth addicts tend not to stick to the treatment regimen.

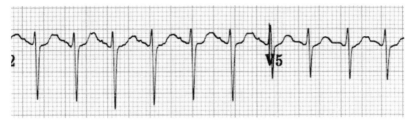

Sinus Tachycardia

Irregular arrhythmias will have varying R-R intervals. In other words, on an EKG, the distance between R waves varies. The commonest irregular rhythm, sinus arrhythmia, occurs so frequently that it is often referred to as a "normal variant", rather than an abnormality. It is a sinus rhythm, meaning each QRS complex is preceded by a P wave. It is neither fast nor slow; usually the rate is between sixty and one hundred bpm. When you take a deep breath, your heart rate increases. When you exhale, your heart rate slows. On your EKG, sinus arrhythmia can be so subtle as to appear regular, and is detectable only by measuring the R-R interval. While this virtually never leads to any symptoms or damage, it is often misdiagnosed as a more serious arrhythmia.

In the grey zone are bradyarrhythmias that are usually benign, but often cause symptoms and almost always require treatment. These usually involve some form of electrical conduction blockage between the atria and the ventricles. Sometimes there will be no P waves, and the QRS complexes fire at a rate in the thirty bpm range. Sometimes there will be P waves at a normal rate, with incomplete conduction to the ventricles. Sometimes the P waves will be seen at a much higher rate than normal, but the conduction to the ventricles is so bad that the ventricular rate is dangerously slow. These conduction abnormalities can be caused by congenital defects, seen in newborns; coronary disease, fibrosis (scarring) and calcifications, especially in the elderly; inflammation of the heart muscle, known as myocarditis; or medications, usually beta blockers, calcium-channel blockers, digitalis or other anti-arrhythmics. When medications are the culprits, decreasing the dosage or stopping the offending agent will often return things to normal. Otherwise, a permanent pacemaker may be required.

If there is one arrhythmia you've heard of, most likely it is atrial fibrillation (AFib). Contrary to what the pharmaceutical companies and their advertising agencies would have you believe, AFib is not merely an excuse to sell you new anticoagulants (blood thinners). You know, those commercials where the overly concerned and persistently intrusive daughter with too much time on her hands toadies her way into her father's medical issues. Not content to allow him to enjoy his retirement and prick his finger once a month to check his ProTime, take his rat poison (Warfarin, a.k.a. Coumadin: Ricky the Forager picks up the yummy-looking warfarin, and, being a co-dependent and dutiful rat, brings it back to share with the rest of the pack, whereupon they enjoy a group gorge and eventually all bleed to death.), and do what his doctor tells him to do, like he's happily done for the past two decades, she invites herself over, shoves his face into the laptop and browbeats him into scheduling an appointment with his cardiologist. When the doctor sees her walk into the waiting room, he thinks, *Oh, God, here she comes. Must have been surfing the internet again.* As her father, who would rather be back in his greenhouse singing to his orchids, asks about Xarelto or Eliquis or Pradaxa, she stares daggers of death at the beleaguered cardiologist. Next week it's off to see the lady ophthalmologist with the eerily luminous eyes. Dad's eyeballs are looking a little dry; he would definitely benefit from some Restasis.

No, AFib is a real disease. Its original name, *delirium cordis*, which translates from Latin to English as "madness of the heart", gives you some idea of its chaotic nature. It comes in two varieties: lone atrial fibrillation, which is not associated with any other heart diseases; and secondary AFib, caused by other diseases, usually rheumatic heart disease (RHD), coronary artery disease (CAD), high blood pressure, aging, CABG surgery or an overactive thyroid gland. In secondary AFib, especially when it is associated with RHD or CAD, there is often marked dilation of the atria. Many of these diseases occur with greater frequency in the elderly; now that people are living longer, AFib is much more common. In 2010 there were more than five million patients in the U.S. with AFib. There are estimates that by 2030, that number will grow to between ten and fifteen million.

In the normal heart, every time the SA node in the right atrium fires on a regular basis, anywhere from sixty to one hundred bpm, the nice obedient atria contract. In atrial fibrillation, instead of the SA node firing regularly and the atria pulsating once for each discharge, the atria quiver (fibrillate) irregularly, up to three hundred sixty bpm. The AV node will conduct only some of these discharges on a seemingly random basis. The ventricles respond to these random conductions by contracting irregularly. In a healthy, untreated heart, the ventricles can contract up to one hundred fifty bpm or more. This results in "AFib with rapid ventricular response". In an unhealthy heart or one subjected to medications (beta blockers, digitalis, calcium blockers), the ventricular response will be significantly slower.

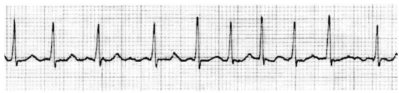

Atrial Fibrillation

In new-onset AFib, the primary goal is to slow the ventricular response to 110 bpm or less. This is fairly easily accomplished with digitalis, beta blockers or calcium channel blockers. Once the ventricular rate is controlled, the secondary goal is to return the heart to normal sinus rhythm. This can be accomplished with a variety of antiarrhythmics like sotalol, flecanide, or amiodarone, with electrical cardioversion (a series of shocks to your chest), or both. If the atria are dilated, the chances of conversion back to normal sinus rhythm are a little better than the chance of being struck by lightning, but not by much. Especially in secondary AFib, where dilated atria are fairly common, many patients will have the arrhythmia the rest of their lives.

In your quivering atria, there is not much contraction or pumping going on. Blood may pool in there and eventually form a blood clot. One of the biggest risks from AFib is embolization of the clot to your peripheral arteries, brain, lungs or kidneys. In the brain, this will cause a stroke (a cerebrovascular accident, or CVA). If this traveling clot makes it to your lungs, you will experience a pulmonary embolus (PE). In your peripheral arteries, the clot may interrupt blood flow and cause the loss of a limb. In your kidneys, you may experience kidney infarcts leading to kidney failure. This is where the money comes in. With more than five million patients currently carrying the diagnosis of AFib and between 100,000 and 200,000 new cases each year in the U.S. alone, there is an enormous, endless market for anticoagulants. Hence all the new meds entering the market in the past couple of years.

The new anticoagulants have been studied head-to-head with warfarin in tens of thousands of patients. In these studies, the new guys, when compared to warfarin, are touted as cutting by half the relative risk of intracranial hemorrhage (ICH = bleeding inside your skull), about the worst possible complication of anticoagulant therapy. While that sounds like a big decrease, the actual numbers are not as impressive. One smart feller concluded that of all the patients in the studies, ICH occurred in less than two per cent of patients on warfarin and in less than one per cent of patients on the newer medications. Obviously, if you are one of the folks who suffers an ICH on warfarin, you and your loved ones will always wonder if you'd have fared better on one of the newer medications. However, these drugs tend to cost forty to fifty times as much as generic warfarin. Even if you have good health insurance, your co-pay will undoubtedly be much higher as well. That's a lot to pay for cutting your chance of a brain bleed from 2% to 1%.

Premature ventricular contractions (PVC's) are abnormal beats that, rather than arising from a discharge in the SA node, originate in one of your ventricles. Often they occur right after a normal beat, preventing the next normal beat from occurring. They disrupt the normal rhythm of your heart, and often can be felt as a skipped beat in your chest. On an EKG or a rhythm strip, a PVC is easily recognizable. It is out of rhythm with the normal beats that precede and follow it. Additionally, it is wider than the other beats and shaped differently as well.

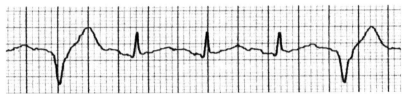

Premature Ventricular Contractions

At some point, PVCs occur in almost everyone. They often arise spontaneously, or they can be associated with caffeine, alcohol, or nicotine use. Abnormally low blood levels of magnesium or potassium can cause PVC's. Benign PVC's tend to disappear with exertion, as your heart rate increases. Malignant PVCs, which can be a sign of ischemia, will often increase in frequency during exercise. It is not unusual to see PVCs after an MI or heart surgery. Unless you've suffered serious damage, eventually they go away.

A single PVC normally does not lead to disastrous consequences. Even a pair of them can be tolerated by most people and will not require treatment. If you have three in a row, however, technically you are experiencing ventricular tachycardia (VT). Treatment of PVC's is usually reserved for patients having unbearable symptoms or sustained runs of VT. Beta blockers and calcium channel blockers have both been used for years to successfully treat PVCs.

Ventricular tachycardia (VT) consists of a series of at least three consecutive PVCs. It is a wide-complex tachycardia, meaning the QRS complexes are wider than normal, and the rate will almost always be greater than one hundred bpm. While in rare instances it can occur in young, healthy individuals and pose almost no risk of sudden cardiac death, VT usually requires prompt treatment with meds or electrical shock (defibrillation). Left untreated, VT can degenerate into ventricular fibrillation, asystole, and cardiac arrest.

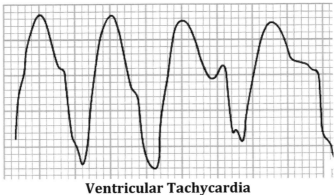

Ventricular Tachycardia

Especially when runs of VT are brief and cardiac output is maintained, you may have no symptoms. Longer runs will usually cause lightheadedness and a pounding sensation in your chest. In most cases, if VT does not cease spontaneously or with the help of medications or shock, you will become pulseless. At this point, there is no perfusion of your coronary arteries, so ischemia will develop. If you are already suffering from ischemia, it will worsen. In your brain, lack of perfusion usually results in loss of consciousness. If circulation is not restored, seizures, stroke and brain death may follow within minutes.

The initial treatment of pulseless VT is electrical defibrillation. IV lidocaine without shock will help to resolve some cases of VT, and is effective in preventing recurrences. For patients with persistent VT, a number of medications are available for long-term use. Some cases will require ablation--destruction of abnormal portions of the heart with radiofrequency electricity. That involves running a catheter from your groin up into your heart, locating the area of irritability, and frying it with radio frequency waves.

Just as in AFib, ventricular fibrillation (VF) involves quivering of one or more chambers of the heart in response to chaotic electrical discharges. While in AFib some of these discharges make it through the conduction system and produce ventricular contractions, in VF the chaos originates in the ventricles themselves. No effective ventricular contractions are produced. Your heart is quivering like jelly. This means no pumping of blood by the heart, no perfusion through the coronary arteries or the brain, no pulse and no blood pressure. When you listen with a stethoscope to the heart of a patient in VF, there are no heart sounds. On an EKG or rhythm strip, you will usually see a wide-complex, very low amplitude sawtooth pattern. In cases of "fine VF", there may be almost no perceptible electrical activity, just a choppy baseline.

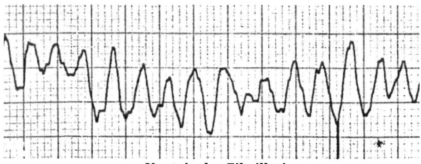

Ventricular Fibrillation

Like VT, VF may occur anytime one or both ventricles are irritated. It usually occurs in chronically diseased hearts or in the setting of acute ischemia or MI. Occasionally it will occur in otherwise normal hearts. Unlike VT, VF does not resolve on its own; it will always result in cardiac arrest if not treated immediately. Time is of the essence. If left untreated, VF can degenerate into asystole in as little as thirty seconds. Treatment is immediate electrical defibrillation. As far back as 1887, John A. MacWilliam of the University of Aberdeen in Scotland demonstrated that VF could be terminated with a series of electrical shocks. If defibrillation is unavailable or unsuccessful, CPR should be started immediately and continued until the patient is transported to an emergency facility. Even after more than thirty minutes of CPR, patients have been known to survive and walk out of the hospital under their own power.

The final rhythm in cardiac arrest is asystole. Also known as "flatline", it occurs when your heart demonstrates no electrical activity. A lack of electric discharges means no contraction of the heart muscle, no pulse, no blood pressure, no nothing. It can occur for any number of reasons besides an MI: very low or very high blood potassium levels, chest trauma, drowning, hypothermia, pulmonary embolus, low blood sugar, excessive blood loss. Treatment consists of correcting the underlying cause, if possible. It does not respond to electrical defibrillation. Patients can be maintained for a while using CPR, IV epinephrine, or external or internal pacemakers.

BTW--Many patients experiencing an MI present to the ER in sinus tachycardia. Once things stabilize, your pain goes away, and you undergo some sort of intervention to limit the damage to your heart, your heart rate should fall once again below one hundred bpm. However, if you leave the hospital in ST, your prognosis is much worse than if you experience VT or VF once or twice in the hospital. Why? Stroke volume (SV) is the amount of blood your heart pumps with each beat. If you have a badly damaged ventricle with a decreased SV, your heart will have to pump at a faster rate (HR) to maintain an adequate cardiac output (CO), the amount of blood your heart pumps every minute. In other words, CO=SV x HR. A damaged ventricle increases the likelihood of congestive heart failure or malignant arrhythmias.

Likewise, if at any time during your hospitalization for an MI you develop AFib, either transiently or permanently, your prognosis both in the hospital and after discharge is significantly worse than a run or two of VT or VF.

References:

1. Sampson, Kevin J., Kass, Robert S. "Anti-Arrhythmic Drugs." *Goodman & Gilman's The Pharmacological Basis of Therapeutics.* Ed. Laurence L. Brunton, Assoc. Ed. Bruce A. Chabner, Assoc. Ed. Bjorn C Knollman. New York: McGraw-Hill. 2011. 815-42.
2. Antzelevitch, Charles. "Mechanisms of Cardiac Arrhythmias and Conduction Disturbances." *Hurst's The Heart.* Ed. Valentin Fuster, Ed. Robert A. O'Rourke, Ed. Richard A. Walsh, Ed. Philip Poole-Wilson. New York: McGraw-Hill. 2008. 913-5.
3. Prystowski, Eric N., Fogel, Richard I. "Approach to the Patient with Cardiac Arrhythmias." *Hurst's The Heart.* Ed. Valentin Fuster, Ed. Robert A. O'Rourke, Ed. Richard A. Walsh, Ed. Philip Poole-Wilson. New York: McGraw-Hill. 2008. 946-9.
4. Prystowski, Eric N., Waldo, Albert L. "Atrial Fibrillation, Atrial Flutter, and Atrial Tachycardia." *Hurst's The Heart.* Ed. Valentin Fuster, Ed. Robert A. O'Rourke, Ed. Richard A. Walsh, Ed. Philip Poole-Wilson. New York: McGraw-Hill. 2008. 953-71.
5. Rho, Robert W., Page, Richard L. "Ventricular Arrhythmias." *Hurst's The Heart.* Ed. Valentin Fuster, Ed. Robert A. O'Rourke, Ed. Richard A. Walsh, Ed. Philip Poole-Wilson. New York: McGraw-Hill. 2008. 1003-16.
6. Vijayaraman, Pugazhedhi, Ellenbogen, Kenneth A. "Bradyarrhythmias and Pacemakers." *Hurst's The Heart.* Ed. Valentin Fuster, Ed. Robert A. O'Rourke, Ed. Richard A. Walsh, Ed. Philip Poole-Wilson. New York: McGraw-Hill. 2008. 1020-5.
7. Olgin, Jeffrey, Zipes, Douglas P. "Specific Arrhythmias: Diagnosis and Treatment." *Braunwald's Heart Disease.* Ed. Robert O. Bonow, Ed. Douglas L. Mann, Ed. Douglas P. Zipes, Ed. Peter Libby, Ed. Eugene Braunwald. Philadelphia: Elsevier Saunders. 2012. 771-4. 798-803. 812-16.

8. Morady, Fred, Zipes, Douglas P. "Atrial Fibrillation: Clinical Features, Mechanisms, and Management." *Braunwald's Heart Disease*. Ed. Robert O. Bonow, Ed. Douglas L. Mann, Ed. Douglas P. Zipes, Ed. Peter Libby, Ed. Eugene Braunwald. Philadelphia: Elsevier Saunders. 2012. 825-30.

31. ANGINA PECTORIS

Angina pectoris is that chest discomfort you have been experiencing during sex. The Latin word *angina* means "infection of the throat", but its precursor, the Greek word *ankhone* means "strangling". The Latin word *pectoris* means "of the chest". Thus, *angina pectoris* has come to mean "strangling of the chest". The concept was first described by Sushruta, a famous surgeon in India, in the sixth century B.C. He called it *Hritshoola* which means "heart pain". His description, developed without the benefit of lab tests, EKG's or x-rays, matches the modern description almost perfectly.

William Heberden, a famous eighteenth century English physician, was the first to use the term *angina pectoris*. A brilliant man, he described numerous disease processes without the benefit of any modern testing or technology. He was also big on coining Latin terms for the medical conditions he described, most of which are still in use today.

Angina pectoris, or angina, is a dull, heavy pain, usually located over the lower half of your sternum (breastbone). Although people with heart attacks or angina are often depicted holding the left side of their chest with an open right palm, ischemic chest pain is best depicted by a clenched fist dead center, neither right nor left. Angina is not the sort of sharp, tearing chest pain that makes you scream in agony. That would be a dissection of the thoracic aorta, or, more commonly, a nipple piercing. Angina drains you of energy. All you want to do is clutch your chest, sometimes push on your sternum with a fist in an effort to relieve the heavy discomfort. Some patients will feel more of a burning sensation, and complain of indigestion or heartburn. It is not unusual to have a patient deny they are having pain; many will describe it as discomfort or soreness. Usually brought on by exertion, sometimes by emotionally upsetting situations, it will last from five to thirty minutes. You might feel the pain spreading to your shoulder or your jaw. That is known as radiation of the pain. Sometimes you can feel it radiate all the way down your arm. While the common perception is that it radiates only to the left arm, it can be felt in the right arm or both arms as well. Sometimes it will radiate straight through to your upper back or shoulder blades.

The pain should not be pleuritic, meaning it should not hurt to breathe, and should not get worse with a deep breath or cough. It should not be caused by or altered in any way by a change in position. In other words, bending forward or twisting your torso shouldn't make it better or worse. Angina is often associated with shortness of breath, sweating, nausea, sometimes lightheadedness or a feeling of fatigue. As with snowflakes and your coronary arterial tree, when it comes to angina, everyone is unique. No two patients describe the pain and associated symptoms exactly the same way. So, despite all the characterizations, all the descriptions of what angina is and what it isn't, what it should do and what it shouldn't, if you see a large number of patients with chest pain, you will eventually come across someone with pleuritic chest pain which gets worse with a deep breath who is indeed experiencing angina.

Besides narrowing of your coronary arteries, there are two other causes of angina. The first, Prinzmetal's angina, is caused by spasm in the muscular layer of one or more coronary arteries. Sometimes there is underlying atherosclerotic CAD, sometimes there is not. The changes seen on EKG will usually differ from those seen with typical angina. Treatment can be different as well but nitroglycerine usually works well in the short term. The other situation, cardiac syndrome X, refers to angina occurring in patients with normal coronary arteries on cardiac cath. These patients are more likely to have angina at rest, more severe pain, and longer lasting episodes. The theory is that narrowing of arterioles, tiny vessels too small to be seen on cardiac catheterization, causes the pain and the EKG changes. Nuclear imaging of the heart and MRI will usually detect the decreased blood flow to the heart muscle.

Any time you are curious about the effects your assorted diseases or vices are having on a particular organ in your body, trot on down to your local library and locate the Ciba Collection of Medical Illustrations. The drawings were created by Frank Netter M.D., an artist who graduated from medical school and trained as a surgeon. While, had he practiced, Dr. Netter might have turned out to be a great surgeon, he is undoubtedly the greatest medical illustrator of modern times. If you are wondering how your lungs will look after thirty years of smoking a pack a day, if you have a hankering to see your scarred and shrunken liver after treating it to a pint of whiskey on a daily basis for a score of years, if you have a need to know what diseases could be the cause of the blood dripping out of your butt, you can see a graphic and completely accurate depiction in his collection of illustrations.

There is a classic Frank Netter illustration of a guy having an attack of angina. Standing at the top of a short set of stairs that lead from a restaurant, he is clutching his chest with his right hand. His heavy briefcase has fallen from his left hand; the cigarette he was holding in his right hand is lying in the snow. The caption lists the usual triggers of angina pectoris: a heavy meal, exertion, cold weather, smoking. Surprisingly, he is not obese. Nor do we know if he's diabetic, since he is not wearing a sign. Inasmuch as Netter lived most of his adult life in the Big Apple and drew from observations on the street, presumably this traveling salesman is standing in Manhattan, having this strange pain in his chest, thinking to himself, *I wish I were back home in Sheboygan.*

Angina occurs when the heart muscle is not receiving enough blood flow through the coronary arteries. At rest, the normal heart beats sixty to eighty times per minute. The heart muscle is consuming a certain amount of oxygen delivered by the hemoglobin in the red cells in your blood. In a normal person or even a patient with angina, the amount of oxygen being delivered at rest is adequate and you feel fine. When you exert yourself by walking, smoking a heater, climbing stairs, having sex, lifting a heavy grocery bag, running a marathon, or attending a family reunion and bumping into creepy old Uncle Dick in an awkward situation, your heart beats faster and harder. Like an automobile climbing a hill, for the heart muscle to work harder, it requires more fuel in the form of oxygenated blood. If there is an area of significant narrowing in a coronary artery, the flow of blood will be restricted and will not be great enough to satisfy the needs of the heart muscle.

At this point your heart muscle cramps and you experience angina. If the angina predictably occurs with the same level of exertion and resolves completely when you stop exerting yourself and/or put a nitroglycerine tablet under your tongue, you are said to have stable angina. If you are walking, stop walking. If you are having sex, take a break but don't light up. If you are carrying a heavy grocery bag, put it down gently. Back slowly out of the guest bathroom and advise Uncle Dick to pull up his pants and put away the Playboy. Some patients walk around in a circle or pace back and forth waiting for the pain to go away. That is known as "walking through angina". I call it "wandering for relief." Even without nitroglycerine, the pain of stable angina will almost always subside within thirty minutes. Nitroglycerine should make it go away more quickly.

Somewhere along the line, unless you are extremely tight-lipped, you will tell your physician, who will tell his favorite cardiologist, who will put you on a treadmill for a stress test. If you are truly having angina, your stress test will be abnormal and you will end up having a cardiac cath. Often in patients with stable angina, the cath will show moderate

CAD with no critical areas of narrowing. Your cardiologist may decide that your disease requires nothing more than medications. No angioplasty, no surgery. He'll put you on a long-acting nitrate, or one of two types of medications also used for hypertension--beta-blockers or calcium channel blockers. When it comes to angina, we think the major effect of these meds is the same: to keep catecholamines like epinephrine from making your heart work so hard at a given level of stress or exertion. If your heart doesn't work as hard, you won't need as much blood flowing through your narrowed coronary arteries and you'll be less likely to develop angina. In addition, beta-blockers prevent catecholamines from constricting your coronary arteries, and we know constricted arteries are very bad. As long as your angina doesn't worsen or become unstable, you may live long and prosper on meds alone. Obviously, eliminating or treating other risk factors for coronary disease such as tobacco, high blood pressure, diabetes, high cholesterol, excessive booze and obesity will allow you to live longer and prosper even more. Count on having a nuclear stress test or stress echocardiogram on a regular basis, say every two years or so, "just to keep an eye on things".

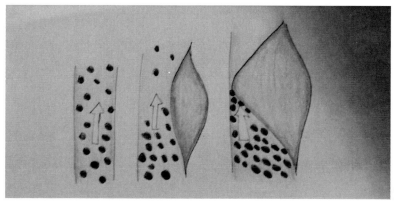
BAC

Normal coronary artery blood flow (Left)
Partially arterial occlusion with mild restriction of blood flow (Middle)
Subtotal arterial occlusion with severe restriction (Right)

As in the case of high-rise window washer platforms, when it comes to angina, stable is better than unstable. Unstable angina is not predictable. The very first time you experience angina pectoris, since you have never had it before and therefore have no set pattern, technically you have unstable angina. If you don't die on the spot and that episode resolves within the thirty-minute time frame, you may settle into a routine with predictability to your anginal episodes. Now you have stable angina. You learn that walking for a block or lifting heavy items and carrying them upstairs or having sex after a heavy meal will cause that pain to return. You casually mention it to your family doctor and he refers you to a cardiologist.

Most commonly the term unstable angina denotes a change in your usual stable anginal pattern. You do something for a shorter period of time or with less effort than is normally required for your stable angina to occur. Instead of developing angina after walking a block, you experience it after walking half a block. Instead of doing the big icky for ten minutes before you get chest pain, now you get it after five minutes. Instead of developing angina after smoking ten cigarettes in a row, it comes on after smoking two cigarettes. Or you wake up out of a sound sleep in the middle of the night and you are having chest pain. These are all common presentations of unstable angina. The pain will usually be more severe and may last longer than stable anginal attacks. The characteristics of the pain, the location, the associated symptoms, may be identical to those of your typical attack or they may be completely different.

Unstable angina is a big deal, a major medical emergency. When your stable angina goes unstable, it usually means something significant has happened in one of your coronary arteries. Perhaps the narrowing that has been causing your stable angina has worsened, to the point that even at rest there is not enough blood flowing to the heart muscle. Alternatively, somewhere in your coronary arterial system a small cholesterol plaque has ruptured, causing a blood clot to completely or almost completely obstruct the artery. Both come under the heading of ACS, "acute coronary syndrome". If it's the former situation, where the narrowing has increased without rupture, you have unstable angina. In the latter, you are heading for an MI, a.k.a. myocardial infarction, coronary thrombosis, heart attack. Either way, it's something different.

When your significant other asks you, "Do you notice anything different, Darling?", in a panic you stall with, "Yes. Yes, I do. You look lovelier than normal." It could be her hair color, her hair style, her new dress, her new tan, her new shoes, new earrings, a tooth whitening, a total body Botox. You scramble to evade her attempt to pin you down. Sometimes it works, sometimes it does not work. In terms of unstable angina, you may not know exactly what happened, but you'd better get to the hospital to find out. And chew an aspirin while you are calling 911.

Say you have a rattlesnake living in a deep pit in the middle of your living room. As long as you don't fall into the pit, the snake doesn't climb out, and you have an adequate supply of rats to toss in on a regular basis, the two of you can coexist in a perfectly amicable relationship for quite some time. So it is with stable angina.

If, however, you do fall into the rattlesnake pit, or you forget to feed your reptilian roommate and he decides to climb out of said pit to find something else to gnaw on, your peaceful coexistence will most assuredly change for the worse. Likewise, if you don't pay attention to and work on your other risk factors, or if you stop taking your meds, which is a huge cardiologic no-no, life will become much less fun and much more complicated. Do what you are told and stay away from the snake.

References:

1. Netter, Frank H. "Heart". *The Ciba Collection of Medical Illustrations.* Ed. Fredrick F. Yonkman. Summit, N.J.: Ciba. 1978. 223.
2. O'Rourke, Robert A., Shaver, James A., Silverman, Mark E. "The History, Physical Examination, and Cardiac Auscultation." *Hurst's The Heart.* Ed. Valentin Fuster, Ed. Robert A. O'Rourke, Ed. Richard A. Walsh, Ed. Philip Poole-Wilson. New York: McGraw-Hill. 2008. 217-22.
3. Michel, Thomas, Hoffman, Brian B. "Treatment of Myocardial Ischemia and Hypertension." *Goodman & Gilman's The Pharmacological Basis of Therapeutics.* Ed. Laurence L. Brunton, Assoc. Ed. Bruce A. Chabner, Assoc. Ed. Bjorn C Knollman. New York: McGraw-Hill. 2011. 745-64.
4. Depre, Christophe, Vatner, Stephen F., Gross, Garrett J. "Coronary Blood Flow and Myocardial Ischemia." *Hurst's The Heart.* Ed. Valentin Fuster, Ed. Robert A. O'Rourke, Ed. Richard A. Walsh, Ed. Philip Poole-Wilson. New York: McGraw-Hill. 2008. 1259-74.
5. Canty, John M., Jr. "Coronary Blood Flow and Myocardial Ischemia." *Braunwald's Heart Disease.* Ed. Robert O. Bonow, Ed. Douglas L. Mann, Ed. Douglas P. Zipes, Ed. Peter Libby, Ed. Eugene Braunwald. Philadelphia: Elsevier Saunders. 2012. 1049-50.
6. Sabatine, Marc S., Cannon, Christopher P. "Approach to the Patient with Chest Pain." *Braunwald's Heart Disease.* Ed. Robert O. Bonow, Ed. Douglas L. Mann, Ed. Douglas P. Zipes, Ed. Peter Libby, Ed. Eugene Braunwald. Philadelphia: Elsevier Saunders. 2012. 1076-9.
7. Morrow, David A., Boden, William E. "Stable Ischemic Heart Disease." *Braunwald's Heart Disease.* Ed. Robert O. Bonow, Ed. Douglas L. Mann, Ed. Douglas P. Zipes, Ed. Peter Libby, Ed. Eugene Braunwald. Philadelphia: Elsevier Saunders. 2012. 1210-14.

32. ATYPICAL CHEST PAIN

Cardiology joke:

Q: What's the worst kind of atypical chest pain?
A: The kind that kills you.

Atypical chest pain is any pain in the chest or upper abdomen that doesn't fit the description of angina pectoris. Atypical chest pain is a daily cause of patients presenting to the E.R. Perhaps when you bend forward or twist to the right or left or lift something heavy, you feel pain in the front or side of your chest. This is usually musculoskeletal pain, resulting from excessive or unusual physical activity, like digging all day to put in a new garden or beginning a new weightlifting regimen. You might experience a squeezing pain in the center of your chest, perhaps associated with difficulty swallowing, the feeling of something stuck in your throat, or regurgitation of food or liquids. Often that will represent esophageal spasm due to reflux.

You may have sharp, penetrating chest pain that worsens when you breathe, cough or sneeze. This is known as pleuritic chest pain, a symptom of pleurisy; you are feeling "The Devil's Grippe", often caused by Coxsackie B virus. More importantly, sometimes pleuritic chest pain results from a pulmonary embolus, a blood clot that has traveled from your leg vein to your lung, infarcted (killed off) a segment of your lung, and might kill you. An agonizing, unrelenting burning pain anywhere in your chest, usually on one side or the other, may represent the early stages of shingles, before the blisters appear.

A particularly common form of atypical chest pain is often associated with pain down one or both arms, lightheadedness, and shortness of breath. Unlike many other causes of atypical chest pain, this one can be associated with EKG changes. On the discharge sheet, it is known as Hyperventilation Syndrome. You wake up in the middle of the night with shallow, rapid respirations because you can't catch your breath. Your chest aches. The aching gets worse every time you inhale. The pain goes into your arms. Your fingers are tingly. You are lightheaded and feel like you are going to pass out. Ironic, isn't it? You wake up feeling like you're going to pass out.

You go to the E.R., where your blood pressure is noted to be elevated and your heart rate is up around one hundred twenty beats per minute. Your EKG shows sinus tachycardia with inverted T waves in leads V3 through V5. Your cardiac enzymes are normal, as is your chest x-ray. If you are given a sublingual nitroglycerine tablet, it does nothing to alleviate your symptoms. In fact, it adds a new one, a bitch of a headache. The nurse comes over and puts an oxygen mask over your face and nose, but doesn't turn on the oxygen. Or she puts a brown paper bag over your nose and mouth. She tells you to breathe deeply in and out. You feel like you are suffocating, but she is stronger than you are, so the mask or bag stays on. Eventually all your symptoms disappear. You go home with a prescription for Ativan and a recommendation to see your doctor.

Each of these examples of disease processes causing atypical chest pain are interesting and may cause severe discomfort and serious illness, even death. Occasionally, however, atypical chest pain may be caused by coronary artery disease. Virtually every physician who has cared for patients with chest pain can remember thinking, *This guy has pleurisy or a chest wall muscle strain,* only to find that his EKG is wildly abnormal, because he is experiencing unstable angina or an MI. Far and away, however, the commonest scenario in which coronary artery disease masquerades as atypical chest pain is the onset of "heartburn" in the middle of the night.

The Labor Day cookout at your home came off as a big success. Planting the new blue spruce tree was hard, sweaty work, and you felt tired all day after that, but you finished up by 2 P.M., then got the food on the grill. Hamburgers, hot dogs, pizza, wings. Everyone went home fat and happy. Because of all that hard work earlier in the day, around 9 P.M. you're hungry again, so you grab a few wings, a piece of pizza, and head out back to watch the stars. After a round of gratifying burps, you fall asleep by 11 P.M. Around 4 A.M. you awaken with burning in your mid-chest. It feels like heartburn, so you try some Maalox. Your wife wants you to take some Alka-Seltzer, but you blow her off. What does she know about indigestion?

The burning isn't any better, and you keep whining about it, so your wife drives you to the hospital, but not before she lets you know what she thinks of you and your heartburn. "You big baby." You think, *Oh yeah, well I wasn't a baby when I dug that hole for your blue spruce tree this morning.* Then, while you're getting checked into a bed in the E.R., she has to go and complain to the nurse. Implies that you are a pig; you always have to eat and drink more than anyone else. Looks you right in the eye and tells you it's time to go on a diet. Then you find out she counted everything you ate and drank. Five beers, two hot dogs, three pieces of pizza, fourteen wings and two hamburgers. Everybody on the night shift is looking forward to a little bit of a lull; clean up the lingering patients and coast downhill to change of shift at 7 A.M. Instead they get to be entertained by your wife going off about your dietary indiscretions.

The E.R. doctor is tired, he's been up all night, but he goes through your entire history. After examining you from head to toe, he describes his findings as "unremarkable". When your EKG comes back normal, he orders a GI cocktail, a.k.a. "grasshopper", with Mylanta, viscous lidocaine to numb up your esophagus, and donnatal to relieve spasms in your esophagus and intestines. The nurse also injects Pepcid intravenously, to reduce the amount of acid in your stomach. Voilà, your pain goes away. About an hour later, the doc returns to tell you your chest x-ray and blood tests, including something called "cardiac enzymes", which can detect a heart attack, are all within normal limits. He says that even though your pain went away with the GI cocktail, you still might have something going on with your heart. He thinks you should be admitted for twenty-four hours, to get a couple more sets of cardiac enzymes, see a cardiologist, maybe get on a treadmill for a stress test. Your pain is gone, so you don't want to stay. Your wife is fed up and wants to get home and get the kids up for school, so off you go with a diagnosis of esophageal reflux and discharge instructions recommending you follow up with your family doctor later in the day.

On the way home, your wife is so tired she doesn't even bother to get on your case. Thank God for small favors. With any luck, she'll forget all that talk about a diet. After all the hard work with the blue spruce, doing grill duty, and spending three hours in the E.R., you're beat too. You crawl into bed for a brief snooze. Unfortunately, you never wake up. Only thing left is to call the local mortician. If it's any consolation, nobody at your funeral will use the terms "big baby" or "fat slob". You'll be remembered as the loving husband and father who spent his last day on earth planting a tree and slaving away over a hot grill. On the other hand, your wife was right. You should have taken the Alka-Seltzer. The 325 mg. of aspirin in each one of those effervescent wafers might have prevented or dissolved the clot in your coronary artery and saved your life. The blue spruce thrives for decades, eventually dwarfing your house.

The take-away lesson here is that heartburn might keep you up at 11 P.M., but any kind of chest, upper abdominal, upper back, jaw or arm discomfort that comes on in your sleep, especially after 4 A.M. or during the morning hours, is a heart attack until proven otherwise. Not a giant burp that's stuck in your tummy. Not stable angina that will resolve in five to thirty minutes. It might be unstable angina, caused by a non-obstructive clot irritating one of your coronary arteries. Most likely it's a heart attack. Normal EKG's, chest x-rays and a single set of cardiac enzymes mean nothing. The only way to prove it's not an MI is a cardiac catheterization. If the E.R. doc wants to admit you to rule out an MI, let him. If he doesn't want to admit you, well, nobody's perfect, especially at the end of a night shift. You might want to stick around anyway, despite the fact that staying in the hospital sucks and if you call in sick the day after a holiday weekend, your boss will assume you are hung over.

However, consider this. Every year a little over a million people in the U.S. suffer an MI. Almost half are fatal, meaning they kill you. Almost half the patients who suffer a fatal MI will die before they reach the hospital. Once you've made it there, you might as well benefit from the odds. Pat yourself on the back for your good fortune and stick around. You don't want one of your kids to find you dead in your bed, and you don't want your friends saying, "I can't believe he left the hospital while he was having a heart attack."

The early morning time frame may have something to do with increased cortisol secretion just before sunrise. Cortisol is secreted by the adrenal glands in anticipation of stress. For most working people, it's probably the stress of getting up for work. If you awaken in the middle of the night or even first thing in the morning with discomfort in any of the aforementioned areas, chew an aspirin immediately and call 911. It might be a false alarm, but if it's not, you might save your life.

One other thing. The scenario depicted above is as common as the mulch you so lovingly shoveled around the blue spruce. Ask any medical malpractice attorney or hospital risk management director. One loves it, one hates it.

References:

1. O'Rourke, Robert A., Shaver, James D., Silverman, Mark E. "The History, Physical Examination, and Cardiac Auscultation." *Hurst's The Heart.* Ed. Valentin Fuster, Ed. Robert A. O'Rourke, Ed. Richard A. Walsh, Ed. Philip Poole-Wilson. New York: McGraw-Hill. 2008. 224.
2. Sabatine, Marc S., Cannon, Christopher P. "Approach to the Patient with Chest Pain." *Braunwald's Heart Disease.* Ed. Robert O. Bonow, Ed. Douglas L. Mann, Ed. Douglas P. Zipes, Ed. Peter Libby, Ed. Eugene Braunwald. Philadelphia: Elsevier Saunders. 2012. 1077.

33. ACUTE CORONARY SYNDROME

Acute coronary syndrome (ACS) is an umbrella term for any situation in which there is a sudden complete or partial blockage of blood flow in one or more of your coronary arteries. The two processes covered by the term ACS are unstable angina and non ST-segment elevation MI.

ACS is something you will hear or see under these circumstances:

1) You come to the E.R. with chest pain, usually in the middle of the night. It may be your admitting diagnosis to the cath lab or the CVICU;
2) You happen to read medical journals for fun;
3) You learn of a new study reported on the internet or on television;
4) You read your bill from the hospital. Be aware that a hospital bill in and of itself can bring on chest pain. In some situations, ACS may be reimbursed by insurance companies or Medicare at a higher rate than unstable angina or even MI.

The current thinking is that the mechanisms of both unstable angina and NSTEMI are similar. The theory is that when a plaque ruptures, a platelet clot forms to prevent further bleeding from that rupture. If the body's natural thrombolytic (clot busting) defenses act sufficiently to break up the clot, the pain will go away. However, the clot formation/clot thrombolysis cascade is a dynamic one, so theoretically, as long as the ruptured plaque remains as an irritant, clots will continue to form and then break up. This causes unstable angina, where the pain comes on acutely but then comes and goes. If, however, your body can not break up the clot on its own, the coronary artery remains completely blocked. If the clot is not removed, a portion of your heart muscle dies and you suffer an MI.

Initially, before balloon angioplasty was employed in an emergent situation, the treatment for an acute MI was the use of thrombolytics, mainly streptokinase and urokinase. At first, they were administered systemically, which meant you just injected them into a peripheral vein, and they worked throughout your body. Someone got the idea to drip them through a coronary artery catheter into a blocked coronary artery. Obviously, this required smaller doses, and theoretically would lead to fewer bleeding complications, especially in the brain. For unstable angina, intravenous heparin was employed. An anticoagulant, heparin thinned the blood and prevented new clots from forming, but it rarely affected clots that had already formed.

What really got the term ACS into the conversation was the development of much more expensive, more profitable thrombolytics like tPA and rPA. Several studies yielded conflicting results on their use in unstable angina and MI. Given that in the middle of the night, an E.R. doctor or a cardiologist might not be able to distinguish between unstable angina and MI, someone came up with the term ACS. Thereafter, most studies of thrombolytics utilized the umbrella term

ACS rather than unstable angina or MI. In addition, Glycoprotein IIB/IIIA inhibitors, which prevent platelets from clotting, also were investigated in studies focusing on ACS. Both thrombolytics and GpIIB/IIIA inhibitors will be discussed extensively in the exciting upcoming chapter on thrombolytics.

Balloon angioplasty was first employed in cases of stable angina in the late 1970s. By the mid-1990s, Percutaneous Coronary Intervention (PCI = balloon angioplasty + stent, roto-rooter, laser, or brachytherapy) was being used for patients with acute MI. At the turn of the century, most major medical centers were performing PCI on patients with ACS. Now it is the standard of care for patients with ACS to undergo PCI within one hour of presentation to the E.R. If you present with ACS at a facility that does not perform emergent PCI, there is a good chance you will be offered the option of being transferred to one that does. If you choose not to be transferred, you will most likely receive thrombolytic therapy and then have a cardiac cath done later to identify the extent of your disease. It is important to note that, depending on your coronary anatomy, PCI may be a temporary solution or a permanent one. Patients with ACS who are shown to have multiple severe coronary lesions may be referred for a CABG soon after the emergent PCI is performed. Those with single vessel disease who have no further symptoms after PCI may need no further interventional therapy.

References:

1. 1. Weitz, Jeffrey I., "Blood Coagulation and Anticoagulant, Fibrinolytic, and Antiplatelet Drugs." *Goodman & Gilman's The Pharmacological Basis of Therapeutics.* Ed. Laurence L. Brunton, Assoc. Ed. Bruce A. Chabner, Assoc. Ed. Bjorn C Knollman. New York: McGraw-Hill. 2011. 849-71.
2. Kim, Michael C., Kini, Annapoorna S., Fuster, Valentin. "Definitions of Acute Coronary Syndromes." *Hurst's The Heart.* Ed. Valentin Fuster, Ed. Robert A. O'Rourke, Ed. Richard A. Walsh, Ed. Philip Poole-Wilson. New York: McGraw-Hill. 2008. 1311-8.
3. De Lemos, James A., O'Rourke, Robert A. "Unstable Angina and Non - ST-Segment Elevation Myocardial Infarction." *Hurst's The Heart.* Ed. Valentin Fuster, Ed. Robert A. O'Rourke, Ed. Richard A. Walsh, Ed. Philip Poole-Wilson. New York: McGraw-Hill. 2008. 1351-70.
4. Cannon, Christopher P., Braunwald, Eugene. "Unstable Angina and Non-ST Elevation Myocardial Infarction." *Braunwald's Heart Disease.* Ed. Robert O. Bonow, Ed. Douglas L. Mann, Ed. Douglas P. Zipes, Ed. Peter Libby, Ed. Eugene Braunwald. Philadelphia: Elsevier Saunders. 2012. 1178-9.

34. MYOCARDIAL INFARCTION

Let's not spend too much time on this topic, as the goal of this tome and of most research into coronary artery disease is to prevent myocardial infarction (MI) and death. We'll just go over the basics so that if you continue to be a bad boy and do bad things, you will know what you can expect. If you do the right things and have any kind of good luck, you will not end up with the diagnosis of acute MI.

Myocardial infarction is the medical term for a heart attack. It occurs when a coronary artery is completely occluded (blocked). Usually this is caused by the rupture of a cholesterol plaque inside the artery. This attracts platelets, the cells in the bloodstream whose function is to stop bleeding. They form a clump, a coronary thrombus, around the ruptured plaque to prevent any bleeding inside the wall of the artery. This thrombus blocks the artery. Blood can't flow to a certain area of the heart muscle, and, if nothing is done to open the artery, or it doesn't open on its own, that portion of the heart muscle deprived of blood will infarct, or die.

In 1912, a Chicago physician by the name of James B. Herrick wrote an article describing myocardial infarction. He theorized that a thrombosis in a coronary artery was the cause. Although every patient is unique and their myocardial infarction is as well, you can pretty well predict what portion of the myocardium will die off if you know which coronary artery is involved. A patient may have severe cholesterol plaque deposition in several arteries, but almost always, only one artery infarcts at a time. Obviously, knowing what we do about how the left main coronary artery gives rise to two coronary arteries, the circumflex and the left anterior descending, an infarct of the left main will often involve the muscle supplied by both of those major branches.

There have been reports of MIs caused by spasm in an otherwise normal coronary artery with no sign of cholesterol plaques, but these are rare.

There are two types of MI. Each has at least three names attributed to it and one or two abbreviations. The type of MI most people associate with the term heart attack is known as a transmural MI or Q-wave MI or ST segment elevation myocardial infarction (STEMI). This is caused by blockage of one of the major coronary arteries or one of its large branches. This type of infarction is known as transmural because it involves the entire thickness of the myocardial wall, from the epicardium to the endocarium. It tends to leave a permanent calling card on your EKG, an abnormal Q-wave. When your doctor refers to "a massive heart attack", he is usually talking about a transmural MI, often involving the left anterior descending coronary artery.

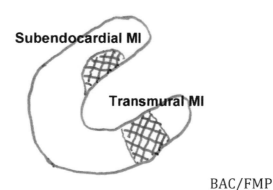

BAC/FMP

Depending on the coronary artery involved, transmural MI's tend to cause necrosis (muscle death) in a predictable area of the heart. If a million beavers congregated in a single spot in a river and chewed up millions of trees with those big buck teeth of theirs, pretty soon the river would be dammed. The water level behind the dam would rise, and eventually the backed-up water would flow off to the sides. Beyond the dam, the river bed would soon be dry. After a while, all vegetation downstream in the river valley would dry up and die. When blood flow is blocked in a coronary artery, within a few hours you will be able to detect on nuclear scan, echocardiogram, or autopsy, muscle cell necrosis and loss of muscular contraction in the area of the muscle downstream from the blockage. In other words, that part of the heart muscle, deprived of oxygenated blood, literally turns to jelly and eventually to scar tissue. Instead of contracting like muscle, it just sits there and does nothing. Depending on the size of the scar, this can have a profoundly bad effect on the pump function of your heart.

The EKG in a transmural MI initially shows ST segment elevation, probably some T wave inversion. Eventually, if the coronary thrombus is not removed or does not break up spontaneously, abnormal Q waves will appear. After healing, the ST segment elevation usually goes away, but the Q wave stays.

The use of blood tests to help diagnose a transmural MI has evolved over the past six decades. Initially, nonspecific blood tests were available. SGOT levels in your blood will rise after an MI, but they can also rise during acute liver damage, as in hepatitis, or after skeletal muscle injury or inflammation. The same is true for LDH levels. CPK levels will rise when there is injury or inflammation of any muscle in your body.

However, the MB band percentage of CPK (CPK-MB) rises only when there is injury to the heart muscle. If your loan shark, the aptly-named Carmine the Crusher, puts your leg through a wringer because you didn't come up with the vig in a timely fashion, your CPK will go through the roof, but your CPK-MB band percentage will remain normal. However, if Carmine is sick and tired of your excuses as to why you repeatedly can't come up with the vig and says, *To hell with it, I'm done with this deadbeat,* and puts your HEART through his beloved pink Home Queen wringer, your total CPK level and your CPK-MB band percentage will both go into orbit. More recently, researchers discovered that an elevation in the Troponin I level in your blood is the earliest and usually the most reliable blood test to detect acute MI. Between the CPK-MB and the Troponin I levels, most MIs won't go undetected.

So, if you arrive at the ER with chest pain, your EKG shows ST elevations in one or more leads, and your Troponin I level is elevated, you are having a transmural MI. Hopefully you have already had an aspirin. With any luck, you should be in the cath lab and have the occluded vessel opened during PCI .

The other type of infarct, a subendocardial (SEMI) or non-Q-wave MI or non-ST segment elevation myocardial infarction (NSTEMI), is caused by blockage of a much smaller branch of a coronary artery or a partial blockage of a major artery. It is called subendocardial because it involves only the portion of the heart muscle closest to the endocardium, which lines the chambers on the inside of the heart. It does not cause the appearance of an abnormal Q-wave on your EKG. As one of its names (NSTEMI) would indicate, a subendocardial MI does not feature ST segment elevations in the acute phase. Instead, as in the case of acute angina, you tend to see ST segment depression with T wave inversion. A week or so after a NSTEMI, your EKG may have returned to normal. In addition to blockage by a blood clot, some cardiologists subscribe to the theory that spasm of a small artery or arteriole can also cause this type of MI. In the past, a subendocardial MI has been referred to as a "minor heart attack", but more recently, physicians have come to realize that these can be minor or major, and the prognosis can often be much worse than that of a transmural MI.

Unlike their transmural kinfolk, subendocardial MIs tend to have a more diffuse, less well-defined area of damage, probably because of the interdependence of the smaller arteries to supply the subendocardium. Rather than a dammed river, a subendocardial MI is more like the sudden disappearance of an underground aquifer that you cannot see. From above ground, it is unclear how much farmland will be deprived of water. Eventually, however, you will find that a small or very large area has been involved.

The majority of MIs occur early in the morning, between 6 A.M. and noon. You dig a hole for a tree, you have a stressful day with the family or the job, and you awaken at 6 A.M. with chest pain. Researchers have long suggested that the timing probably has something to do with cortisol levels being at their peak in the early morning. A growing area of interest is the role of inflammatory mediators in MIs and whether their levels in your blood rise at that time of the day.

The symptoms of an MI are similar to those of angina. Chest pain behind your breastbone is common. Some patients who have had angina in the past say the onset of pain with an MI is more sudden, more severe, and, obviously, lasts longer. Others say it comes on more gradually than angina. The chest discomfort is often accompanied by radiation of the pain to the jaw or one or both arms, shortness of breath, sweating, nausea and vomiting. Patients often have a feeling of anxiety, and irregular heartbeat is not uncommon. Unlike typical angina, when you suffer an MI, the pain will not resolve within thirty minutes, and nitroglycerine will relieve the pain only temporarily or not at all.

If you have a "Silent MI", you do not experience chest pain or the associated symptoms. Some experts estimate that 40-60% of MI's are silent. Patients who suffer a silent MI say they had a flu-like illness for a couple of days, feeling fatigued, perhaps nauseated, perhaps a little sweaty. These are usually detected at autopsy or at a later time on an EKG or during a cardiac workup.

Risk factors for an MI are pretty much the same as those for CAD: previous CAD, high LDL-C, low HDL-C, high blood pressure, obesity, smoking, diabetes, sedentary life style, alcohol abuse, and cocaine and amphetamine abuse. As you can see, most of the risk factors can be addressed and prevented or improved through lifestyle changes and/or meds.

Anywhere from one-half to two-thirds of the deaths associated with an MI occur before the patient reaches the hospital. If you are having a heart attack, do not try to drive to the hospital. Call 911. Chew a standard 325 mg. aspirin tablet or four baby aspirin tablets. Regular aspirin tastes terrible, but it works faster if you chew. Do not chew tobacco. A nitroglycerine tablet under the tongue may help. If you have an oxygen tank, use it. If you have morphine lying around the house, inject 5-10 mg. into your thigh or upper arm, but not into a vein or artery. Although heroin is in the same category of medications as morphine sulfate, it is not an acceptable substitute in this situation. This next caveat should be obvious, but bears mentioning anyway: do not light up a cigarette while you are waiting for the ambulance. The toxins in the tobacco could cause spasm of your coronary artery and may worsen the damage or just plain kill you on the spot. A shot of whiskey, even for "purely medicinal purposes", is also ill-advised.

References:

1. Yazdani, Saami K., Ladich, Elena, Virmani, Renu. "Pathology of Myocardial Ischemia, Infarction, Reperfusion, and Sudden Death." *Hurst's The Heart.* Ed. Valentin Fuster, Ed. Richard A. Walsh, Ed. Robert A. Harrington. New York: McGraw-Hill. 2011. 1296-1305.
2. Badimon, Juan Jose, Ibanez, Borja, Fuster, Valentin, Badimon, Lina. "Coronary Thrombosis: Systemic and Local Factors." *Hurst's The Heart.* Ed. Valentin Fuster, Ed. Robert A. O'Rourke, Ed. Richard A. Walsh, Ed. Philip Poole-Wilson. New York: McGraw-Hill. 2008. 1245-53.
3. Yang, Eric H., Gersh, Bernard J., O'Rourke, Robert A. "ST-Segment Elevation Myocardial Infarction." *Hurst's The Heart.* Ed. Valentin Fuster, Ed. Robert A. O'Rourke, Ed. Richard A. Walsh, Ed. Philip Poole-Wilson. New York: McGraw-Hill. 2008. 1375-90.
4. Antman, Elliott M. "ST-Segment Elevation Myocardial Infarction: Pathology, Pathophysiology, and Clinical Features." *Braunwald's Heart Disease*. Ed. Robert O. Bonow, Ed. Douglas L. Mann, Ed. Douglas P. Zipes, Ed. Peter Libby, Ed. Eugene Braunwald. Philadelphia: Elsevier Saunders. 2012. 1087-1107.
5. Antman, Elliott M., Morrow, David A., "ST-Segment Elevation Myocardial Infarction: Management." *Braunwald's Heart Disease*. Ed. Robert O. Bonow, Ed. Douglas L. Mann, Ed. Douglas P. Zipes, Ed. Peter Libby, Ed. Eugene Braunwald. Philadelphia: Elsevier Saunders. 2012. 1118-35.

35. COLLATERALS

Collaterals are naturally-occurring vessels that can save your life. While there are three or four major coronary arteries supplying blood to your myocardium, there are hundreds or thousands of microscopic vessels which form connections between the major arteries and between each of their branches. Normally these vessels are so small that they cannot be visualized on a cardiac cath. If a blockage gradually develops in a major coronary artery, the worsening ischemia triggers the transformation of these tiny vessels. The wall of the collateral vessel thins out, allowing the lumen to enlarge. At this point, the collateral can transport enough blood to be visualized on a cath. These collateral vessels then supply blood to the major coronary artery downstream from the blockage.

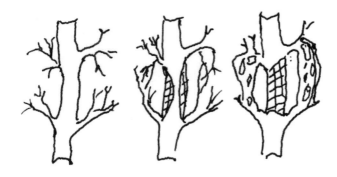

Normal coronary artery (left)
Partially occluded artery with collaterals beginning to form (middle)
Completely occluded artery with collaterals providing bypass around occlusion (right)

If a ruptured plaque or blood clot suddenly completely obstructs a coronary artery, collaterals will begin the transformation process. Unfortunately, there is not enough time for collaterals to provide adequate blood flow, so in most cases an MI occurs downstream from the blockage. If, however, an incomplete blockage occurs, the transformation process can begin in less than two minutes. In order to stimulate transformation, most researchers believe the blockage has to be at least 90%. Maximum enlargement of these collaterals occurs within about four weeks, though some theorize that changes conducive to increased blood flow can continue for up to six months.

Some cath studies have shown completely occluded coronary arteries in patients with no evidence of a heart attack. Usually these patients have excellent collateral flow. The theory is that they had enough ischemia prior to the complete occlusion that collaterals were transformed and were able to supply adequate blood flow downstream from the blockage. Patients with gradually worsening angina probably have cholesterol plaques that are slowly growing. These patients are the ones who most likely will develop extensive collateral systems.

Coronary collateral vessels were first described by Dr. Richard Lower in England in 1669. Of note, he is also the first to transfuse blood from animals to man. The 1960s saw research begin in earnest on collaterals. Several growth factors, proteins which stimulate the development of new vessels, have been isolated; experimental trials utilizing some of these factors have yielded mixed results. The ultimate goal of these investigations is to develop a drug or gene therapy agent that can be injected and cause the growth of collateral vessels which will deliver blood to ischemic areas of the heart, preventing angina and infarction. Thus far, nobody has come up with a workable plan to grow collaterals through diet or exercise.

References:

1. Malouf, J., Edwards, W., Tajik, A., Seward, J.. "Functional Anatomy of the Heart." *Hurst's The Heart*. Ed. Valentin Fuster, Ed. Robert A. O'Rourke, Ed. Richard A. Walsh, Ed. Philip Poole-Wilson. New York: McGraw-Hill, 2008. 75.
2. Kern, M., King, S. III, "Cardiac Catheterization, Cardiac Angiography, and Coronary Blood Flow and Pressure Measurements." *Hurst's The Heart*. Ed. Valentin Fuster, Ed. Robert A. O'Rourke, Ed. Richard A. Walsh, Ed. Philip Poole-Wilson. New York: McGraw-Hill, 2008. 485.
3. Davidson, C., Bonow, R. "Cardiac Catheterization." *Braunwald's Heart Disease*. Ed. Robert O Bonow, Ed. Douglas L. Mann, Ed. Douglas P. Zipes, Ed. Peter Libby, Ed. Eugene Braunwald. Philadelphia: Elsevier Saunders. 2012. 428-9.
4. Canty, J. M., Jr.. "Coronary Blood Flow and Myocardial Ischemia." *Braunwald's Heart Disease*. Ed. Robert O Bonow, Ed. Douglas L. Mann, Ed. Douglas P. Zipes, Ed. Peter Libby, Ed. Eugene Braunwald. Philadelphia: Elsevier Saunders. 2012. 1064-6.
5. Seiler C, Meier P "Historical aspects and relevance of the human coronary collateral circulation" Curr Cardiol Rev 2014 10(1):2-16.

36. NOSEPICKER ALERT

The term "blood thinners" encompasses several groups of medications, including anticoagulants, platelet poisons, direct thrombin inhibitors and thrombolytics. None of these actually thin your blood, they just make it less likely to clot, or, in the case of thrombolytics, they break up clots and prevent new ones.

If you are an inveterate nose pickin' fool, be very careful around any of these medications. That includes warfarin (Coumadin), aspirin, heparin, enoxaparin (Lovenox) and any other medication prescribed to prevent clots. Some of these are prescribed only while in the hospital, and most folks tend to pick their noses less often if there is a chance that someone is watching over a closed circuit TV system. The ones you take at home will get you into trouble. If mining gold from your snot locker is a favorite pastime, do yourself a favor and wrap those prospecting digits in bulky cotton gauze until they look like baseball bats and are too fat to fit into your nasal cavity. Otherwise, should you scrape the mucosal lining inside your favorite mother lode, be prepared for a red river that won't stop for days. Inevitably you will end up in the E.R. or in an ear, nose and throat specialist's office, getting all sorts of chemicals and instruments jammed halfway up the nasal route to your brainpan. That's more than enough unpleasantness for one day, but not the end of your misery.

After you've been treated, you'll have to walk around for a few days with one side of your nose twice the size of the other, your nostril filled with vaseline gauze, a nasal tampon, or an inflated balloon, all of which label you as a booger-picking moron. Good luck preventing your significant other, your kids, or your grandkids from snapping a pic or two on the ever-present smart phone to preserve the moment for all eternity.

37. ANTICOAGULANTS

Anticoagulants are medications administered to prevent blood clots. For the most part, they do not break up pre-existing clots, but they are effective in preventing small clots from getting bigger. That's important because the bigger the clot, the more likely it is to break off and travel somewhere to do major damage. Thrombolytics, which do indeed dissolve clots, are a separate category of medications and are discussed in another chapter.

In order to thoroughly understand how and where each anticoagulant works, it is necessary to study and memorize the coagulation cascade. Coagulation is the process by which the body halts bleeding, as from a cut. That's a good thing. Unfortunately, the coagulation cascade also entails thrombosis, the process in which your body forms blood clots inside blood vessels or organs, particularly your heart. That is a bad thing. If you get the coagulation bug, you can find a diagram and explanation of the cascade in any internal medicine or hematology text. We'll keep this discussion of anticoagulants simple.

Heparin sodium, more appropriately called unfractionated heparin (UH) because it has not been fractionated to separate out the low molecular weight molecules, is usually given intravenously in the hospital. It may also be given subcutaneously (SQ=under your skin) in the hospital or at home.

Heparin was first isolated around the end of World War I at Johns Hopkins University. It is a naturally-occurring substance, produced by certain types of white blood cells. Your body releases it only at the site of an injury, where it may prevent clots but also may prevent further damage by bacteria and other foreign invaders. Nowadays it is isolated in large quantities from pig intestines and cow lungs.

Heparin is used in a variety of situations:

1. Atrial fibrillation (AF)--UH prevents clots in your atrium from breaking off and travelling through your arteries to wreak havoc in your lungs (pulmonary embolus), brain (stroke), coronary arteries (MI), extremities or other organs.
2. Acute coronary syndrome, specifically unstable angina or NSTEMI--UH prevents further clotting in your coronary arteries.
3. Deep vein thrombosis (DVT)--UH prevents existing clots in your legs or pelvis from growing larger and breaking off to travel to your lungs.
4. Pulmonary Embolus (PE)--UH prevents recurrence of blood clots travelling to your lungs.
5. Coronary artery bypass surgery (CABG)--prevents clots in your blood while you are on the bypass machine.
6. Indwelling central or peripheral IV catheters--prevents them from clotting off.
7. Hemofiltration--prevents clots from forming while your blood is running through a cleansing machine.
8. Cryonics--Prevents clots from forming while some weirdo sci-fi company keeps you frozen until they figure out how to bring you back to life. Ted Williams tried this route and ended up getting his dead head smashed with a monkey wrench in an effort to dislodge a cat food tuna can used as a pedestal. Allegedly.

If you actually read the stuff above, you don't have to be a genius to figure out that heparin is used almost exclusively to prevent blood clots in patients who find themselves in high-risk situations.

Heparin is not well absorbed from your gut, so administering it by mouth (enterally) does not work; it has to be given via a needle (parenterally). It has a short half-life (doesn't last long in your bloodstream), so when it is used IV, either you receive an injection every four hours or you are on a continuous infusion, which means an IV bag and a pump on a pole. It's not a good idea to administer it by giving shots deep into your muscle (IM = intramuscularly) because it will cause bleeding and lead to big fat painful blood clots inside your muscles, which can become infected. It can be given every 12 hours SQ in low doses to prevent blood clots in bedridden patients, and in larger doses to treat existing blood clots. The low-dose SQ regimen will cause black and blues, but otherwise doesn't do much damage. The high-dose SQ regimen, rarely used to treat DVT or PE, can cause more significant bruising.

One of the few nice things about using heparin is the ease with which you can tell whether your blood is thin enough to prevent blood clots. A simple blood test, the partial thromboplastin time (PTT), will tell you what you need to know. Depending on the laboratory, in a healthy person who is not taking any blood thinners, the PTT should be less than seventy seconds. A newer test, the activated PTT (aPTT), has a normal range of less than fifty seconds. When you are started on heparin to treat a clot, you want to prolong your aPTT by 1.5 to 2.5 times. So if your normal baseline aPTT is forty seconds, the goal of heparin therapy is an aPTT of sixty to one hundred seconds. While testing is easy, the concentration of heparin in your blood can fluctuate significantly, so, while you are being treated for a DVT or PE, frequent monitoring of your PTT is necessary.

One other nice thing about heparin is that if you receive too much, your blood gets too thin, and somebody figures it out in time, the whole heparin experience can be reversed by injecting protamine sulfate. That may prevent the commonest side effect of heparin, bleeding (nose, gums, GI tract, brain). If not detected early, blood loss can be significant enough to require blood transfusions. Other serious complications include thrombocytopenia (low platelet count) due to an immune response, and hyperkalemia (high blood potassium level) caused by suppression of aldosterone.

Because of the relative unpredictability of UH, researchers started looking at low molecular weight heparin (LMWH) in the 1980s. LMWH is produced by chemically chopping off small fractions of the heparin molecule and discarding the big chunk. It has advantages over UH in terms of safety and ease of use.

Unlike UH, the blood-thinning effect of LMWH cannot be monitored by the aPTT. Instead, you must use the anti-factor Xa assay. At the present time, this test is more expensive to perform and not available in some labs 24/7. However, it may turn out to be a better test, and the cost should come down as more physicians order it and testing companies streamline the process. The good news is that you rarely have to monitor LMWH therapy. You inject it SQ once or twice daily, and that is that, unless you are markedly overweight or have significant kidney disease, in which case you have to run the assay and adjust the dose. Patients with DVT or PE who normally would have to stay in the hospital on IV heparin for five to seven days can be sent home within a day or two to self-administer LMWH or have home health come in once daily for the injections.

Depending on where you cleave the big heparin molecule, you can come up with different species of LMWH. There are about ten of them. The most widely-used in the U.S. is enoxaparin (Lovenox); its use should increase now that there is a generic available, which will cut the cost considerably.

LMWHs are used primarily in the prevention of DVT in bedridden patients and the treatment of existing DVT and PE. They may have some role in the treatment of acute coronary syndrome when PCI is performed, to prevent clots at the site of stent placement.

If you have a DVT or PE, you may treat with SQ heparin or LMWH for an extended period of time, but most likely you will complete your treatment with an oral agent. The oldest one, warfarin, a vitamin K antagonist, has been in use for over sixty years as an anticoagulant. The warfarin story started in the early 1920s. Rather than dying of embarrassment after dehorning or castration, cattle began bleeding to death. Veterinary researchers in the northern U.S. and Canada determined that they were prone to hemorrhage because they were eating moldy silage made from sweet clover. It was one of those "Oh, look at that!" moments in science. Taking it one step further, they fed clean clover to one rabbit and moldy clover to another. Mr. Moldy bled to death, while Mr. Clean did just fine. By 1929, veterinarians determined that the bleeding was due to a lack of functioning prothrombin. Just goes to show you that when the stock market crashes, you don't have to jump out of a tenth-story window. There are other options. You can do research on bleeding cattle.

It took another ten years for researchers at the University of Wisconsin to identify, isolate and synthesize the compound causing all the bleeding. They eventually named it dicoumeral. It is a derivative of coumarin, a naturally-occurring chemical that gives clover its sweet smell. Various fungi commonly found in hay can convert coumarin to dicoumerol, which is why the bleeding disorder was associated only with spoiled sweet clover.

Over the next few years, the Wisconsin researchers worked with dicoumerol to develop a more potent rat poison, and eventually came up with warfarin, named for the Wisconsin Alumni Research Foundation, which financially supported the project and obtained the patent. It was registered for use in 1948 and was an immediate hit among rat killing aficionados. By the early 1950s it was determined that warfarin could be used on humans, and in 1955, President Eisenhower was prescribed warfarin after a heart attack.

Where in your coagulation cascade does warfarin work? It took unti 1978 for researchers to figure out that it inhibits an enzyme, epoxide reductase, thus interfering with the activity of Vitamin K, a specific antidote for warfarin overdose. How well does it work? It is theorized that Khrushchev and his Commie cohorts poisoned Joseph Stalin with warfarin, causing a fatal cerebral hemorrhage (bleeding in his brain). Up against the almighty warfarin, even Uncle Joe, the Man of Steel, fared no better than a rat.

The indications for warfarin use include:

1. Outpatient treatment of DVT;
2. Outpatient treatment of PE;
3. Outpatient treatment of AFib;
4. Outpatient treatment after an MI.

In each of these indications, heparin or a LMWH is started in the hospital, and after a day or two, warfarin is added. Upon discharge from the hospital, heparin or LMWH is discontinued and warfarin is continued for anywhere from three months to indefinitely, depending on circumstances.

Because you can bleed like a stuck pig if you take too much warfarin, yet risk a stroke, MI, or PE if you don't take enough, you must make sure on a regular basis that you are getting the right amount. The old perfect test is the prothrombin time (PT or Protime). In a healthy person who is not taking any blood thinners, the normal PT is 12-13 seconds. In most cases, the goal of warfarin treatment is a PT anywhere from 1.5 to 2.5 times normal. Because of differences in labs, in the 1980s the new perfect test, the International Normalized Ratio (INR) was developed. The INR is basically the ratio of the patient's PT divided by the control PT, which is derived by measuring the PT of 20 local normal adults in the same lab and taking the average. In a healthy person who is not taking blood thinners, the INR runs between 0.8 and 1.2. The goal of warfarin therapy (therapeutic range) is an INR of 2.0 - 3.0. When you are first started on warfarin, plan on checking your INR at least once a week, either at home on your own or in your doctor's office. After the first month, assuming it stabilizes in the therapeutic range, you will probably have to check your INR once a month.

Plenty of diseases and medications can mess with your PT and INR, but the biggest problem is dietary. Eating green leafy vegetables or other sources of Vitamin K will counteract the effects of warfarin; that makes your blood more coagulable (yes, it really is a word) and lowers the values of both your PT and INR, exposing you to the risk of blood clots. Unless you plan on eating absolutely no leafy vegetables ever again, the simplest way around this is to eat the same amount every day and adjust your warfarin dose accordingly. One solution is to eat a salad every day. It's good for you. If you substantially change your diet or add or subtract meds from your regimen, be sure to keep a close eye on your INR and notify your doctor if it goes too high or too low. Interestingly, patients in Germany who take warfarin often are permitted to adjust their dosage themselves, based on home monitoring of their INR.

If your INR consistently runs too high but you aren't bleeding anywhere, your health care provider will have you hold your warfarin for a day or two until your INR gets back to the therapeutic range. He may also decrease your dose. If your INR gets above 10, you will probably have to take vitamin K orally for a day or two, hold your warfarin until it returns to the therapeutic range, and then restart at a lower dose. If your INR is too high and you have major bleeding, you will probably require some IV vitamin K and either PCC (prothrombin complex concentrate) or FFP (fresh frozen plasma). The latter two will correct your PT and INR more quickly, but don't hang around very long, so you will need the vitamin K to continue to counteract the excess of warfarin in your bloodstream.

As we learned in the chapter on arrhythmias, there are several new anticoagulants on the market. Each one has a generic and a trade name that is a mouthful, and none of the names make sense like warfarin. Dabigatran (Pradaxa) is a direct thrombin inhibitor (DTI) approved to prevent strokes in patients with atrial fibrillation not associated with valvular heart disease. Rivaroxaban (Xarelto) and apixaban (Eliquis) are Factor Xa inhibitors that are also approved for use in AFib and in certain situations to prevent or treat DVT and PE. For each of these agents, their upside is also their downside. In patients without access to frequent PT and INR testing, these three medications might be preferable to warfarin, which requires monthly testing. On the flip side, you can't tell how "thin" your blood is on these meds like you can with warfarin. Studies show that there is less chance of a brain bleed on the newer meds than on the old rat poison, but GI bleeds may be more frequent. There is no specific antidote to these medications, although a report or two indicates that reversal treatment may be coming down the pike in the near future.

There's an old medical adage (Is there such a thing as a new adage?):

Be not the first by which the new is tried,
Nor the last to lay the old aside.

As with all new medications, expect the research dirt swept under the rug by their manufacturers to surface in the coming years. The longer a medication is on the market and the more widely it is prescribed, the more likely side effects will pop up.

References:

1. Weitz, Jeffrey I., "Blood Coagulation and Anticoagulant, Fibrinolytic, and Antiplatelet Drugs." *Goodman & Gilman's The Pharmacological Basis of Therapeutics.* Ed. Laurence L. Brunton, Assoc. Ed. Bruce A. Chabner, Assoc. Ed. Bjorn C Knollman. New York: McGraw-Hill. 2011. 849-66. 872-4.
2. Mohler, Emile R. III, Schafer, Andrew I. "Atherothrombosis: Disease initiation, progression, and treatment." *Williams Hematology.* Ed. Kenneth Kaushansky, Ed. Marshall A. Lichtman, Ed. Ernest Beutler, Ed. Thomas J. Kipps, Ed. Uri Seligsohn, Ed. Josef T. Prchal. New York: McGraw-Hill. 2011. 2210-12.
3. Francis, Charles W., Crowther, Mark. "Principles of antithrombotic therapy." *Williams Hematology.* Ed. Kenneth Kaushansky, Ed. Marshall A. Lichtman, Ed. Ernest Beutler, Ed. Thomas J. Kipps, Ed. Uri Seligsohn, Ed. Josef T. Prchal. New York: McGraw-Hill. 2011. 353-61.
4. Deitcher, Steven R., Rodgers, George M. "Thrombosis and antithrombotic activity." *Wintrobe's Clinical Hematology.* Ed. John P. Greer, Ed. John Foerster, Ed. John M. Lukens, Ed. George M. Rodgers, Ed. Frixos Paraskevas, Ed. Bertil Glader. Philadelphia: Lippincott Williams & Wilkins. 2004. 1729-39.

38. ASPIRIN

Aspirin, a.k.a. acetylsalicylic acid (ASA), made from the bark of the willow tree, is the oldest pain reliever still in use. At least as far back as 2000 B.C., Egyptians were drinking tea from the willow and other plants rich in salicylates to reduce fevers. They probably also used it to help their hangovers from wine and mead. Willow bark extract was prescribed for fevers and the pain of childbirth by Hippocrates as far back as 400 B.C. Before and during the Middle Ages, Western medicine relied on willow bark for relief of inflammation, pain and fever. During their expedition in the early 1800s, Lewis and Clark allegedly used willow bark tea to reduce fevers.

Edward Stone, a rector in the Church of England, is credited with isolating the active ingredient in aspirin. In 1758, while walking through a meadow in a place called Chipping Norton, he stopped to pull a piece of bark from a willow tree. Rector Stone found it to be very bitter, and, instead of spitting it out like any normal person, after working through a series of arcane assumptions and deductions, he ended up drying out a pound of bark which he made into a powder.

Now, if you are a church rector in 18th century England, and you want to test out a hypothesis, how do you go about recruiting a large number of test subjects? Although there is no record of this, most likely he compressed the powder into wafers and distributed them at communion. In a time when raves were non-existent, what options would you have for getting a bunch of arthritic middle-aged guys to knock back a non-alcoholic homemade potion? Lo and behold, after a few doses of the Body of Bark, all of the Chipping Norton willow junkies were up dancing a jig in the aisles of St. Mary's Church. Stone sent a letter to the head of the Royal Society describing his findings. He had discovered salicylic acid, the basic ingredient in aspirin. His Rectorness was roundly praised for his research. As a matter of fact, his letter is still on file at the Royal Society HQ. Nowadays he'd be hauled up before an institutional review board and most likely be sued by a flotilla of personal injury lawyers right after he finished up his two-month stint in the stocks.

In 1853, ninety years after Stone's discovery, a French chemist by the name of Charles Gerhardt combined acetyl chloride with sodium salicylate to form an impure and unstable form of acetylsalicylic acid, the active ingredient in modern aspirin. In 1856, two days shy of his fortieth birthday, Gerhardt died after being poisoned in his laboratory. There is no mention of whether ASA was the culprit.

In 1897, chemists at Bayer AG in Germany began experimenting with a pure form of ASA. By 1899, Bayer was marketing their product under the name aspirin. Although the chemical and its name were protected by patent, their rights were lost or sold in countless countries throughout the world; now any preparation of ASA can be sold as aspirin. During World War I, Germany cut off supplies of aspirin to the Allies, so after the war the victorious Allies forced Bayer to give up their patent.

During the Spanish flu epidemic of 1918, aspirin was the best option for reducing the fevers and aches associated with influenza. Adhering to the wrongheaded logic of the "If a little bit is good, then more is better" school of medicine, aspirin was given in much higher doses and much more frequently than is now recommended. It stands to reason that some of the deaths during that period were caused not by influenza but by aspirin overdose.

With the development of acetaminophen and ibuprofen in the late 1950s and early 1960s, aspirin use declined. Interestingly, in the 1940s, doctors noted that children given aspirin-containing gum for pain after tonsillectomy bled more than other children. The authors of some of these reports theorized that since aspirin caused more bleeding, it might also prevent blood clotting. As is so often true in research, a bit of wisdom lies dormant until someone stumbles upon it serendipitously and cries, "Ah-HA"! It was more than two decades before anyone looked closely at that possibility. By the 1980s, after twenty years of research in that direction, aspirin was established as an effective anti-coagulant.

When a cholesterol plaque ruptures in the wall of an artery, platelets, the clotting agents in your blood, adhere to the tear in the wall and form a clot. While this is beneficial in halting further bleeding, if the clot becomes too large, it may obstruct the artery completely and prevent normal blood flow. In a carotid artery, this will lead to a stroke. In a coronary artery, this will lead to an MI. Aspirin prevents the formation of thromboxane A2, which helps to bind platelets together to form the clot. When it comes to heart disease, its main benefit is the prevention of blood clots. In most of the population, no thromboxane means no clot. No clot means no MI.

In 1978, the Canadian Cooperative Study Group (Doesn't "cooperative" sound so Canadian?) published the findings of a trial of aspirin in patients with "threatened stroke". This high-risk group consisted of over five hundred patients who had experienced TIAs or non-disabling strokes in the past. A TIA, transient ischemic attack, is a temporary loss of feeling and/or function in one side of your face and/or body. By definition, a TIA must resolve completely within twenty-four hours or it is called a CVA (cerebrovascular accident) or stroke. In this high-risk group of patients who'd experienced TIAs, aspirin was shown to reduce by almost half the risk of stroke or death in men. Oddly, little or no benefit was seen in women. From this study, it was recommended that patients with a history of TIA or stroke take aspirin on a daily basis.

Large studies have shown that eighty mg per day of uncoated aspirin--one baby aspirin--can prevent second heart attacks in patients who have already had one. So it is reasonable to take a baby aspirin every day to prevent a heart attack if you have already had one. This is known as secondary prevention. Studies to determine whether a daily aspirin will prevent a first heart attack in healthy adults--primary prevention--have been much less conclusive. Some experts argue that those studies tended to use coated aspirin, which was developed to prevent upset stomach and ulcers, and the coating tends to block the release of one of the active ingredients in aspirin, thus rendering the study findings useless.

A large literature review published in 2009 by the Agency for Healthcare Research and Quality, a division of the U.S. Department of Health and Human Services, evaluated the risks and rewards of daily aspirin use for the primary prevention of MI and strokes. They looked at all the studies published between 2001 and 2008. They found that aspirin in healthy adults reduced the incidence of MI in men and strokes in women. Aspirin use did not have any effect on death due to cardiovascular disease or death from all causes. Aspirin caused an increase in hemorrhagic strokes (bleeding in the brain) in men and an increase in GI bleeds (bleeding ulcers and gastritis) in both men and women.

Many experts say that, because of all its side effects, mostly related to bleeding, if aspirin were a new drug seeking approval from the FDA today, most likely it would be rejected. This despite the fact that no other drug has the spectrum of activity in common diseases that aspirin has. Aspirin has antipyretic (fever reducing), analgesic (pain relieving), anti-inflammatory and anti-platelet effects. Acetaminophen (Tylenol) has antipyretic and analgesic activity, but has no anti-inflammatory or anti-platelet effect. Ibuprofen has antipyretic, analgesic, and anti-inflammatory effects but possesses no activity when it comes to preventing blood clots. Clopidogrel (Plavix), the other major anti-platelet drug besides aspirin, has no anti-inflammatory, analgesic or antipyretic effect.

Here are some of the uses for aspirin, past and present. It has a benefit in the treatment of tension headaches. In adults, it is an excellent treatment for fever of any cause. Because of the risk of Reye's syndrome, it should not be used in children when treating fever due to viral infections like the flu or the common cold, or in bacterial infections. There are rare case reports of Reye's syndrome in adults as well. In general, when it comes to infections, acetaminophen and ibuprofen have largely supplanted aspirin for the treatment of fever. For years, aspirin was a first-line treatment for rheumatoid arthritis and other inflammatory conditions. Aspirin is combined with clopidogrel after the placement of coronary stents for twelve months, then aspirin alone is recommended for lifetime treatment. ASA is a first-line treatment for acute rheumatic fever. There is evidence that aspirin reduces the risk of developing colon cancer and of dying from it. There are studies suggesting that ASA can prevent sunburn and skin cancer. While low-dose ASA (two 325 mg. tablets every four hours) can cause a rise in serum uric acid levels, thus causing an attack of gout, treatment with much higher doses will usually lower uric acid levels and prevent attacks of gout.

Because of the risk of bleeding, in both your stomach and your brain, the FDA no longer recommends the use of a daily dose of aspirin to prevent heart attack or stroke in healthy people. Probably what is needed is a large-scale study of normal adults using uncoated baby aspirin. Until then, you and your doctor get to decide: nosebleeds, shaving nicks that won't stop bleeding, massive GI bleeds, the rare hemorrhage into your brainpan, versus a massive heart attack that cripples or kills you or a stroke that leaves you paralyzed on one side of your body. Speaking from personal experience, into which I shall delve later in the "Me" section, were it not for daily aspirin use, doubtless I would not be here, and this book would never have been written. I'll leave it to you to decide the pros and cons of that one.

References:

1. Grosser, Tilo, Smyth, Emer, FitzGerald, Garret A., "Anti-Inflammatory, Antipyretic, and Analgesic Agents: Pharmacotherapy of Gout." *Goodman & Gilman's The Pharmacological Basis of Therapeutics.* Ed. Laurence L. Brunton, Assoc. Ed. Bruce A. Chabner, Assoc. Ed. Bjorn C Knollman. New York: McGraw-Hill. 2011. 959-82.
2. Francis, Charles W., Crowther, Mark, "Principles of Antithrombotic Therapy." *Williams Hematology.* Ed. Kenneth Kaushansky, Ed. Marshall A. Lichtman,Ed. Ernest Beutler, Ed. Thomas J. Kipps, Ed. Uri Seligsohn, Ed. Josef T. Prchal. New York: McGraw-Hill. 2011. 362-4.
3. Mohler, Emile R. III, Schafer, Andrew J., "Atherothrombosis: Disease Initiation, Progression, and Treatment." *Williams Hematology.* Ed. Kenneth Kaushansky, Ed. Marshall A. Lichtman,Ed. Ernest Beutler, Ed. Thomas J. Kipps, Ed. Uri Seligsohn, Ed. Josef T. Prchal. New York: McGraw-Hill. 2011. 2211-2.
4. Wood JN "From plant extract to molecular panacea: a commentary on Stone (1763) 'An account of the success f the bark of the willow in the cure of the agues'." Philos Trans R Soc Lond B Biol Sci. 2015. 370.
5. Pierpoint WS, " Samuel James (c 1763-1831) of Hoddeson and the medicinal use of willow bark" J Med Biogr.2007. 15(1):23-30.
6. The Canadian Cooperative Study Group. "A randomized trial of aspirin and sulfinpyrazone in threatened stroke. The Canadian Cooperative Study Group" NEJM. 1978. 299(2):53-9.
7. Wolff T, Miller T, Ko S "Aspirin for the primary prevention of cardiovascular events: an update of the evidence for the U.S. Preventive Services Task Force." Ann Intern Med 2009. 150(6):405-10.

39. OTHER ANTI-PLATELET MEDICATIONS

Outside of aspirin, clopidogrel (Plavix) is the most commonly used medication to prevent platelets from clotting in your arteries. Before the expiration of its patent, Plavix was the second-largest grossing prescription medication in the world. Clopidogrel works by inhibiting receptors on the surface of platelets, preventing platelets from binding together to form a clot. If you have one or more stents placed for coronary artery disease, most likely you will be on clopidogrel for a year or more. This gets you through the risky period for the stent to become obstructed by clot. After the first year, the risk falls significantly.

Either alone or in combination with aspirin, clopidogrel is often prescribed to prevent heart attacks and strokes in patients who are at high risk for either of these. That would include anyone who has already had a heart attack, stroke, peripheral arterial disease or acute coronary syndrome. If you are allergic to aspirin, you can substitute clopidogrel in any situation where aspirin would be used as an anti-platelet medication. Prior to 2012, when its patent expired, that was a financially painful substitution. Now that a generic form is available, your wallet won't scream anywhere near as much.

As with any other blood thinner, the downside to using clopidogrel is the risk of bleeding and bruising. In a large study looking at the risk of major bleeding, clopidogrel plus aspirin caused major bleeding in 3.7% of patients as compared to 2.7% with placebo plus aspirin. So while there was an almost 60% increase in major bleeding, the risk was still pretty low. In a head-to-head study of aspirin vs. clopidogrel in patients with a recent MI, the rates of GI bleeding and bleeding inside the brain were about the same.

Some studies suggest that certain proton-pump inhibitors (Prilosec or Nexium) which are prescribed for acid reflux or to prevent GI bleeding, may decrease the effectiveness of clopidogrel, worsening your chances of a bad cardiac outcome, i.e., a heart attack or death. Other studies show no effect of Prilosec or Nexium on clopidogrel's function. Once again, who knows?

There is no doubt that any combination of clopidogrel with another blood thinner, either IV or oral, increases your risk of bleeding. If you take clopidogrel on a daily basis, count on bleeding longer from any cut, even if you nick yourself shaving, and huge bruises from even a mild bump against your skin. A patient who suffers significant trauma, such as a car accident, fall, laceration, stabbing or gunshot wound while on clopidogrel will require transfusions of red blood cells and platelets far more often than a similarly-injured patient who is not taking clopidogrel. There is a collective groan in the trauma room whenever the paramedics list clopidogrel as one of the meds the guy on the backboard is taking.

Glycoprotein IIb/IIIa inhibitors (GPI) are the other major class of anti-platelet medications in use for cardiac disease. This group includes abciximab (ReoPro), eptifibatide (Integrilin), and tirofiban (Aggrastat). These medications block the receptor known as glycoprotein IIb/IIIa (You were wondering where they came up with that terrific name, weren't you? Now you know.) on the surface of platelets. If this receptor is blocked, fibrinogen cannot bind to platelets, and platelets cannot bind together to form clots. When it comes to platelets, it's all about teamwork--forming the clot.

The discovery of the GpIIb/IIIa receptor and its function came about through the study of a bleeding disorder called Glanzmann's Thrombasthenia. Quite a mouthful. Fortunately, it is extremely rare, occurring in about one in a million people, so, unless you are a hematologist, you almost never have to use the term. It was first described in 1918 by a Swiss pediatrician named Eduard Glanzmann. He observed it in a little girl with extensive bruising all over her body. He found other children with the same symptoms; the disease tended to occur in families, which led him to conclude it was inherited. He called the disorder hereditary hemorrhagic thrombasthenia. The word "thrombasthenia" means "weak platelets". Later on, somebody named the disease after him. Eventually, researchers figured out that a defective or low level of glycoprotein IIb/IIIa on platelets was the underlying cause of Glanzmann's Thrombasthenia. From there, it was a race to discover compounds that would block the glycoprotein receptor.

Patients with this disease, whose platelets contain defective or low levels of glycoprotein IIb/IIIa, tend to bleed at the drop of a hat. Women with the disorder tend to bleed excessively during their periods and after childbirth, while both sexes can suffer from heavy nosebleeds, easy bruising, bleeding from their gums, gastrointestinal bleeding, and excessive bleeding after surgery. It can be inherited or acquired as an autoimmune disease.

Initially, GpIIb/IIIa inhibitors (It sure would be nice if someone could come up with an easier name to type, like "Glibitors" or even "Glypibitors") were once used in STEMI, NSTEMI, unstable angina, and during PCI procedures. Currently they are employed for patients undergoing PCI, either for stable angina, unstable angina, or NSTEMI.

So if you find yourself in one of these situations, you will probably be given a Glibitor (There, that's much better.) at the beginning of your balloon angioplasty and stent placement. Since all of these agents are only given intravenously, you won't be taking them once you leave the hospital and go home. Then you'll be on clopidogrel, aspirin, or both.

References:

1.Weitz, Jeffrey I., "Blood Coagulation and Anticoagulant, Fibrinolytic, and Antiplatelet Drugs." *Goodman & Gilman's The Pharmacological Basis of Therapeutics.* Ed. Laurence L. Brunton, Assoc. Ed. Bruce A. Chabner, Assoc. Ed. Bjorn C Knollman. New York: McGraw-Hill. 2011. 868-72.
2. Mohler, Emile R. III, Schafer, Andrew J., "Atherothrombosis: Disease Initiation, Progression, and Treatment." *Williams Hematology.* Ed. Kenneth Kaushansky, Ed. Marshall A. Lichtman, Ed. Ernest Beutler, Ed. Thomas J. Kipps, Ed. Uri Seligsohn, Ed. Josef T. Prchal. New York: McGraw-Hill. 2011. 2211-2.
3. Deitcher, Steven R., Rodgers, George M., "Thrombosis and Antithrombotic Activity." *Wintrobe's Clinical Hematology.* Ed. John P. Greer, Ed. John Foerster, Ed. John M. Lukens, Ed. George M. Rodgers, Ed. Frixos Paraskevas, Ed. Bertil Glader. Philadelphia: Lippincott Williams & Wilkins. 2004. 1731-2.
4. Weitz, Jeffrey I., "Antithrombotic Drugs." *Hematology: Basic Principles and Practice.* Ed. Ronald Hoffman, Ed. Edward J. Benz, Jr., Ed. Sanford J. Shattil, Ed. Bruce Furie, Ed. Leslie E. Silberstein, Ed. Philip McGlave, Ed. Helen E. Heslop, Ed. John Anastasi. Philadelphia: Churchill Livingstone Elsevier. 2009. 2067-70.
5. Stevens RF, Meyer S. "Fanconi and Glanzmann: the men and their works." *Brit J Haem. 2002.* 119(4):901-4.

40. TAKE GOOD CARE

Gus Van der Berg followed the driveway up from the EMERGENCY sign on the highway. There were no tire tracks to follow, but in the blowing snow he could just make out the yellow reflectors every few feet. The visibility had to be down to less than ten yards. He looked over at his wife in the dark.

"Honey, we're gonna stop here for a little bit and get you checked out. Maybe they can call a doctor in to see you tonight." Gus doubted it. There was a good five inches of snow on the ground here. When they'd come down from the pass into town, the city snow plow passed them heading up, thick heavy flakes blasting straight south in its headlights.

"Donh stah. I'nh okay."

"I know, Honey. I know. Snow's pretty bad, though, and seeing as it's coming from where we're going, that next pass'll probably be closed for a while." A thought occurred to him. "Besides, you don't want to meet Wade's parents for the first time until we fix that problem with your mouth."

"Fhees fhunny, mhy mhouh."

"And the way your arm's all stiff, you won't be able to help the women set up for the party." He drove the big GMC past a bright AMBULANCES ONLY sign and parked in the lot.

"Nhoh stih. Ihs nuunh."

"Right, Honey. Numb." Gus got out of the truck and walked around to her side. As he opened her door and grabbed his wife to keep her from falling out, a gust of wind blew his hat into the bed of the truck next to his.

When Janelle looked up, the tall man in the cowboy hat was standing right in front of the nursing station desk. She hadn't heard him come in, and thought for a second, *He must have taken his shoes off.*

"Yes, Sir, how may I help you?" When she stood up, Janelle realized he must be six-six or more, a good eight inches taller than her husband Fred, and quite a bit leaner too. Maybe forty-five years old. The Marlboro Man, from when she was a kid. Before the oxygen tank and the nasal prongs.

"My wife," he turned slightly to his left, jerking his thumb slightly up toward his shoulder, "is having some trouble with her mouth. Her arm too." He wore a helpless smile. Janelle looked past him, saw a bundled figure on the gurney in Bay 4. The overhead fluorescents were on, both side rails up.

"Oh. I didn't hear her get in the bed."

"I carried her in. She's not walking real well either, I guess from being dizzy."

Janelle picked up a clipboard and hurried around the desk. As she passed Gus, she looked down and saw his work boots. *A rancher*, she thought. He didn't move, so she asked over her shoulder, "Would you please come in here with me? I need to get a little history from you."

She looked down at the figure on the gurney, then across at the tall man.

"My name's Janelle. I'll be the nurse taking care of your wife tonight. May I have your name, please?"

"Van der Berg." When she asked, he spelled it for her. "Gus Van der Berg." Instinctively he stuck out his hand. As they shook across the gurney, he smiled; Janelle noticed the lines around his eyes. Either he was closer to sixty or, like her Grandpa down in Cochise County, he'd spent most of his life squinting in the sun. Maybe both. *Men like him don't sport Wayfarers astride their palominos.*

"That's something," Janelle smiled.

"What's that?"

"My grandfather and grandmother Merrill had a cattle ranch down on Van der Berg Road when I was a kid. Near that abandoned mine town, um..."

"You mean Pearce?"

"That's it. The Commonwealth mine."

"Right. Your grandpa's ranch was on Van der Berg Cutoff Road. That goes down to what used to be the north end of my family's ranch. There's a small road at the end, Van der Berg Ranch Road, that led east to our gates. My place, what's left of the old ranch, starts about eight miles south of there. I remember your grandpa's place all right. Had a stream ran right through."

"Yes. I loved that creek. So cold, deep and fast in the summer."

"When we were kids, probably a good fifteen years before you were born, everybody went up to his place for the Fourth of July, big cookout in the yard and little kids' rodeo in his corral there. We'd spend all year making little canoes out of throwaway pieces of leather, then, just before supper, we'd let them run down that creek toward the road. Every year I carved a new wooden Chokonen brave to sit in mine.

"Chokonen?"

"Real Chiricahua. Cochise's band."

Janelle snapped out of her reverie and looked down at the patient. "Hi, Mrs. Van der Berg. My name is Janelle. Can you tell me your first name?" Kind, patient hazel eyes looked up at her.

"Merabeh."

"Maribel. Nice to meet you." She put down her right hand to shake. The patient shrugged her shoulder. The rest of her right arm lay flaccid on the gurney. Janelle picked up her pen and began writing the first name on the chart.

"If you're like most folks, it's not what you think."

She looked up at Gus. "What's not?"

"Her name. Not Maribel. Mary Belle." He spelled it for Janelle. "Mary after her mother's sister, and Belle after her daddy's favorite mare. When she was little, while Belle was still alive, she called herself Mare Belle. She liked thinking she was part horse. That way she could run faster. Ran all the way to first place in the state for the 880." He looked down at his wife. "Didn't you, Belle?" He smiled and rubbed the back of his hand down her cheek. She smiled with the left side of her face; the right side stayed in place, oblivious to her lifelong affection for him.

"Mr. Van der Berg..."

"Gus. Mr. Van der Berg was my Grandpa." He smiled.

"Gus, my tech is down with his wife in Phoenix having their first baby tonight, an emergency C-section, so we're a little short-staffed. Would you mind helping me get your wife's coat off? We can roll her towards me, then back towards you." Janelle started to roll the woman her way, but the tall man put his hands softly on her forearms. She looked up.

"Let's try something else." Without bending, he slid both hands under his wife, at her shoulders and thighs, like a forklift. He slowly lifted her straight up and held her chest-high, a good two feet above the gurney. Stunned for a second, Janelle quickly removed the patient's jacket from her right arm, which promptly fell straight down. Janelle looked at Mary Belle, ready to apologize. The woman's eyes were locked onto her husband's face. The nurse hurried around to the other side of the gurney and pulled the jacket off of her left shoulder, then slid it down and off.

"Okay, we're good. Thank you." Gus lowered his wife back down to the gurney. "How did you do that?"

"I don't know. Just did it."

Janelle reached over and pressed the intercom button. Her words echoed overhead. "Dr. Smith, we have a new patient in Bay 4." She turned back to the cowboy, who was holding his hat in his hands. Just below his sandy salt and pepper hairline, a pale white band ran across his forehead. "Mr. Van...Gus, why don't you have a seat out there by the nursing station. Gloria from registration will get some more information from you there. Dr. Smith will be here in just a minute and will want to talk with you. I'm going to help your wife into a gown so he can examine her."

Van der Berg turned to leave. "I don't mean to push, but we'd sure appreciate it if you could fix her up and we could be on our way. We still have to drive to St. Joseph tonight."

Janelle didn't know what to say to that. "Yes, Sir, we'll do our best."

She followed him to the hallway, then pulled the curtain across the bay and went back to her patient.

Gus sat at the low counter on a stool with a wicker back to it and calculated in his head. Normally the trip to St. Joseph, about three hundred miles, took five, maybe five and one-half hours without pushing it. They were already six hours into it, and still had one thirty or so to go. It was going to be a long night. Nice hospital, though, and the Merrill lady seemed friendly enough. He hoped they could get Mary Belle fixed up and maybe they'd make it to the motel before midnight.

The young girl, Gloria, came and took down some more information, then went off to make a copy of his insurance card. When she came back with the card and a cup of coffee, he signed a bunch of forms and she smiled and went back out front somewhere.

"Mr. Van der Berg?" Gus swiveled on his stool and stuck out his hand.

"Gus Van der Berg." He shook hands with a young doctor in one of those outfits doctors wore, like on the TV shows. This one was bright turquoise with pink around the edges. The fella looked to be about thirty-five, longish dark hair and a full beard, just a tinge of gray in his sideburns. He had a stethoscope around his neck with two black tubes instead of one like the Elfrida vet's.

"My name's Smith. I'm the physician on call here tonight. I took a quick look at your wife. She's stable. While we're getting her workup started, I want to ask you a few questions if I may."

"Sure, Dr. Smith. I want to say I'm real sorry they had to call you at night to come see Mary Belle." Smith thought he was kidding, then revamped his perspective on the Van der Bergs.

"I appreciate that, but I stay here all night, 9 P.M. to 9 A.M. There's always a doc here to see patients." When he said this, Van der Berg looked genuinely surprised. "And it's Joe. Fewer syllables than Dr. Smith." He smiled.

"Oh, okay, Joe. What can I tell you?"

"I understand this problem your wife is having started earlier today. Why don't you begin by telling me about her day. While you're going through it, it's very important to let me know times, because the timing in this sort of problem is critical. I'm going to be writing while you talk. I may interrupt you from time to time to ask a question. Please go ahead." Smith pulled up a stool and lay a clipboard on the counter.

"Well, we got up usual time, 4:30. Coffee first, then Mary Belle made breakfast for me and her and Deron. He's our hand, lives out in the old bunkhouse. Around 5:30 we went out to tend the horses..."

"You have a farm?"

"Used to. Not anymore. Only farming we do now is Mary Belle's." he looked over at the drawn curtain, "summer vegetables." I break and train horses. Racers and a few trotters. Mostly Californians shipping their two-year-olds over to me for a few months. Now and then we get a four-year-old cutter from Montana or British Columbia. Five acre spread is all."

"Where do you live, Sir?"

"Cochise County." The young doctor looked up at him. "We're halfway between Willcox and Bisbee. You heard of them?"

"Yes, thanks." Smith nodded.

"Yup. Seeing as we were going to be up north for a few days, I had to go over a few things with Deron..."

"Where are you headed, Mr.... Is it okay if I call you Gus?"

"That would be just fine, Joe." Gus smiled. "Our daughter Sophie teaches up in St. Joseph. Kindergarten." Smith nodded and smiled. "She met a local fella about a year ago. Looks like they're gonna get hitched."

"Congratulations. So the wedding is this weekend?"

"No, not until the fall. That'll be down at our spread. This is an engagement party, chance for us to meet one another. We're having it up there because Wade's, Wade Young is his name, Wade's grandma is too weak to travel. They say she had a stroke a few months back." Smith nodded.

"We planned to leave around ten, but Mary Belle has been having this headache the past couple of days, so she slept until almost two. Slept through her yoga thing on T.V. and all. I made lunch for me and Deron. When she woke up, her headache was better, so we got moving by three."

"Was she acting normally then?"

"Yes she was, but still a little sleepy from her nap. Fell asleep as soon as we got in the truck. Normally she's a talker, especially in the truck, and it was kind of lonely with Mary Belle sleeping, so I just listened to crop reports, stuff like that, on the radio. I stopped around 4, 4:15, and got some new wipers put on at the NAPA in Benson, then grabbed a cup of coffee before we headed for Tucson."

"Mrs. Van der Berg was asleep the whole time?"

"Yes. I think all the excitement about our trip wore her out. You can call her Mary Belle."

"Okay, thanks. Please go on."

"It was getting on to rush hour when we got to Tucson. We don't usually go into the city unless we have to, because of all the traffic and such. Normally we like to take the Cascabel around the city to the San Pedro, then up to catch 77 just outside of San Manuel. That can be a rough ride, and I didn't want to wake Mary Belle up. So instead I drove a little further into town, got off at Houghton, wound around Sabino Canyon and got on 77 before Oro Valley."

"Did you stop anywhere else?"

"Yup. There's a little barbecue place near there, we like it, so we stopped to eat. Mary Belle was still sleeping, so I carried her in."

"Did she wake up then?"

"Oh, sure. We got a booth. She was starting to have more trouble with her mouth, and she still couldn't use her arm, so I propped her up in the booth so she could lean up against the wall."

"Wait a minute, Gus. She was having trouble with her mouth and her arm before that?"

"Yes indeed. Didn't I mention that?" Joe Smith shook his head. "Yeah, around three, when we were getting started, after I carried her from the bathroom to the truck, it was a little hard to understand what she was saying." Smith sat with his mouth agape like a bass, then realized it and shut it, biting the inside of his cheek.

"You carried her from the bathroom at your home?"

"Of course. She was a little unsteady on her feet."

"Gus, can I ask you a question?"

"Sure, Doc. I mean Joe."

"Did you think about stopping in Benson or Tucson to have your, to have Mary Belle evaluated at a hospital?"

"Sure did. Asked Mary Belle what she thought about the idea, but I knew what she'd say. She's scared to death of hospitals, doctors too, so of course she said no. As a matter of fact, Joe, she didn't even want to stop here. No offense. Me, I'm glad we stopped here. You and Janelle seem like real nice folks."

"Thanks. Did your wife eat anything?"

"She wasn't hungry, and she still had a headache. I asked the waitress for some ibuprofen, but all they had was aspirin, and Mary Belle's allergic..."

"She's allergic to aspirin?"

"All her life. The nurse at our clinic wanted her to take a baby aspirin every day, but Mary Belle told her about her allergy, guess she has a hard time breathing, so that was the end of that."

Gus continued, "So I sat next to her and fed her some potatoes and a little barbecue. She had a hard time, because of her problem with her mouth. Some of it went down, but she kept letting it fall out of her mouth or choking on it, so I quit after a while." Behind them, the drape was pulled back abruptly. Janelle emerged walking backwards, pulling the gurney. Gus looked over, then back at Smith. "Where are they going?"

Smith looked over and smiled at Janelle as she switched to pushing the gurney. "CT." Gus waited for clarification. "Cat scan." No response. "We are going to take pictures of her brain."

"Something's wrong with her brain?" For the first time, Gus looked worried.

"Gus, let me ask you something. What do people in your and your wife's families die of?"

Van der Berg thought for a moment. "Farm accidents." He paused. "That or old age." Another pause. "Sometimes the old age causes the farm accident."

****

After he looked at the C.T., Smith called a neurologist in Phoenix.

"How long's it been?" His accent was pure Brooklyn.

"At least six hours." Joe recounted the essentials of the story.

"That's incredible. He's been carrying her places for six hours and went right past all those hospitals in Tucson? What's with this guy?"

"I don't think medicine's his thing. Would you know a horse emergency if you saw one?"

"True. All right, I'd go ahead and give her the tPA anyway."

"You think it'll help this far out?" The standard was three hours or less after a stroke. Beyond that, the risks of bleeding, especially in the brain, outweighed the benefits.

"Probably won't do much for the acute infarct, but some of the guys down here have seen it help with rehab. Their recovery might be more complete, and it'll definitely happen sooner. And unless you have a neurosurgeon up there, you should fly her down here ASAP. Just in case there's a complication."

"Okay, thanks. I'll talk it over with her husband and let you know."

"Don't wait too long. Whether you give her the tPA or not, she's not going to get better anytime soon. If she gets worse, I don't think you want to be dealing with it up there."

Gus was sitting by his wife's gurney, holding her left hand. She was sleeping.

"Gus, I talked with the neurologist down in Phoenix. We both agree Mary Belle has had a stroke."

"She had a stroke? Where?"

"There's a blood clot in a small vessel in her brain. That's what a stroke is. That's why she is having trouble with her mouth and her arm and leg." Joe waited for that to sink in. After a bit, Gus nodded.

"This is a serious one. We both feel she might benefit from giving her some medicine to break up the blood clot."

"Sure, Joe, that would be fine. Can we get the prescription filled here in town before we head out? We have to be in St. Joseph by 10 A.M."

"Gus, drug stores here don't carry this. It has to be given in a hospital and the patient has to be watched very closely for a while."

"Well, we could go to the hospital in St. Joseph and get it."

"Gus, I don't know anything about the medical facilities up in St. Joseph, but I do know that's not the direction we want to be sending Mary Belle. I was thinking Phoenix would be more appropriate."

"Phoenix? That's a long drive, Joe."

"Gus, we're talking about a helicopter ride."

"God in de hemel!"

"Exactly."

"Joe, I don't want to sound ungrateful, but this isn't what we had planned for today."

"That's why I have a job, Gus. If you come in here, it means your day isn't going as expected. Don't worry, we'll take good care of Mary Belle."

****

It took a while, but Gus finally seemed to grasp what was going on. He signed the consent for the tPA and Janelle administered it. Now that the storm was winding down to a few flurries and almost no wind, the pilot figured he'd be able to take off in about a half-hour. Joe Smith crossed his fingers and attended to the brave souls who made it in to the E.R. despite the snow on the ground. A three-year-old with the usual chin laceration, a high school wrestler with a broken wrist and an old miner with a COPD exacerbation. Around 10:30, Janelle wheeled an Apache girl past him on her way to the OB-GYN exam room.

"Dr. Smith, quick. This girl's thirty-five weeks pregnant. She broke her water about four hours ago and now she's contracting every sixty seconds." Smith followed her in and helped lift the girl onto the exam table and put her feet up in the stirrups. She looked to be about sixteen. Joe put on a pair of sterile gloves and took a look.

"How did she get here? There must be close to six inches on the ground."

"She walked. She and her mother and her younger sister are all staying down the street at the Casa Mia. About a quarter-mile or so."

"Any prenatal care?" He felt around inside. Massively dilated, effaced cervix. This was going to happen soon.

"Not in the past four months. She had the ultrasound for dates around eighteen weeks, had another one at twenty-four weeks, and was supposed to go back for a procedure two weeks after that, but she didn't follow up."

"Wonder what the procedure was. Okay, we'll get through it." Just as the girl began a new contraction, the code arrest bell went off.

"Code 99, ICU. Code 99, ICU."

Janelle looked at him. "It must be that baby with RSV. A six month-old from Weaver that was admitted this morning. They've been giving her breathing treatments all day. I think she's going to need to be intubated."

"Perfect. I gotta go. Janelle, sit here and catch whatever comes out. I hope it's an easy one. I'll be back as soon as I can. If one of the family docs comes through, grab him."

"Tonight? Nobody's wandering around in the snow looking for work."

Smith smiled. "I know, but you can hope."

He shot off his gloves into the trashcan, stood up and turned. Gus was standing there, his face aglow with a smile.

"She's all better, Joe. Hungry and sitting up, talking like her usual self, brushing her hair. She wants to get back on the road."

"Who, Gus?" Joe had no idea what he was talking about.

"Mary Belle, of course. Boy, you really know what you're doing, don't you now."

"Gus, I have a delivery here and a baby that's trying to die right around the corner. I have to go. I'll be back as soon as I can and we'll talk."

Gus looked around him and nodded. "Go ahead, Doc. I got this covered."

Again, Smith had no idea what Gus was talking about. A he started running toward the ICU, he heard Gus say to Janelle, "You and I, Janelle, we can take care of her."

****

Three helicopter lift-offs later, Joe and Gus were sitting drinking fresh coffee at the nursing station counter. First to go was the baby on a ventilator to St. Mortimer's Childrens, then the new mother and her baby to Wakefield, then Mary Belle to Meadows. Janelle sat at her desk, sipping tea and charting.

"So my Belle's all better. I sure am glad we ended up here with you folks."

"Gus, I'll be honest with you. Nobody would ever have expected your wife to recover the way she did that quickly. That just doesn't happen. So I can't tell you that she won't relapse. But the fact that she's back to normal, at least for now, is a real good sign."

"Joe, I believe we ended up here for a reason, and I know she's gonna be just fine. You think the pass is open yet? I want to get started."

"They'll call us on the patch phone just as soon as they're done plowing. We're lucky there weren't any wrecks up there."

Janelle looked up. "I wrote down that you delivered the baby boy, Dr. Smith. I can't really list Mr. Van der Berg..." Gus smiled at her and shook his head. She smiled back. "...can't list Gus, as the attending physician."

"Well, it means I'm on the hook for the next eighteen years if that kid goes bad, maybe twenty-one, but whatever. Hope you knew what you were doing, Gus."

Van der Berg smiled at him. "That's gotta be somewhere around two hundred fifty deliveries, Joe. After about the fiftieth or so, you sort of feel like you know what you're doing."

"Two hundred fifty?" Smith coughed a little on his coffee. Then he thought, *Gus is pulling my leg.*

"Oh, at least. Cats, dogs, horses, cows, a few sheep, a couple deer. Even delivered a few humans along the way. This was my first human breech, though." He looked over at Janelle. "How'd I do?" She smiled.

Joe sat stunned. "It was a breech? You delivered a breech baby?"

Janelle looked up, tapping her pen against her chin. "Once Gus told me, I thought the procedure she missed probably had something to do with the baby being a breech."

The patch phone rang. Janelle answered it, hung up, and announced, "The pass is clear." Gus stood up, turned toward Smith, and extended his hand.

"No big deal, Joe. Down at my place, that's all I do. Just like people, animals know how to deliver a head-first baby on their own."

"Gus, thank you. You saved a life or two tonight. Take care driving down. Be careful going through Superior. Good luck to you and Mary Belle."

"Thanks, Joe. You take good care too."

41. THROMBOLYTICS AND FIBRINOLYTICS

Thrombolytics, or fibrinolytics, also known as clot busters, are medications that are used to break up blood clots that have decided to form in bad places. Bad places include deep veins in your legs (DVT or deep vein thrombosis), pulmonary arteries (PE or pulmonary embolism), arteries in your arms or legs (peripheral arterial occlusion), arteries in your neck or brain (CVA or cerebrovascular accident), and, of course, our new best friend, coronary arteries in your heart (MI). The first four are still treated on a regular basis with thrombolytics. For a while, thrombolytics were all the rage when it came to acute MI. Now that most major medical centers have PCI (Percutaneous coronary intervention--balloon angioplasty + stent, laser, roto-rooter or brachytherapy) available 24/7, thrombolytics play less of a role in the management of acute MI. However, if you live in an area where PCI is not available, you will most likely receive thrombolytics and be shipped (That would be via ambulance or helicopter, not UPS or FedEx.) somewhere for PCI. In the earliest stages of thrombolytics, you had three choices of where to get it: streptococcal bacteria, human urine, or poisonous snakes.

The clot-busting characteristic of streptococcal bacteria was first discovered by Dr. Tillett at Johns Hopkins in 1933. As usual, it was almost completely serendipitous. By 1945 the specific enzyme had been isolated and was officially named streptokinase (SK). It was found to activate plasminogen to produce more plasmin. Plasmin breaks down fibrin, a major constituent of blood clots, after the clot has stopped the bleeding. The more plasmin in the area of the clot, the faster the clot will dissolve. Within four days of use, antibodies are formed to SK, so it is not recommended for use in a second MI or PE.

During the 1950s, streptokinase was used primarily to improve drainage of fluid around the lungs and to prevent scarring in meningitis caused by tuberculosis. Also during this time reports surfaced regarding the use of streptokinase to dissolve blood clots in arteries. From the mid-1960s, for about two decades, studies showed that in patients with MI treated as quickly as possible with streptokinase, there was less damage to heart muscle and better survival. The take-home message was, the sooner it was given through the veins, the better the result. Numerous cardiologists tried dripping it directly onto a clot in a coronary artery through a cardiac catheter, but in the end, it appeared that intravenous administration could be started much more quickly and produced equally impressive results.

The ability of urine to dissolve blood clots was first discovered in 1947 in Great Britain by a British hematologist named McFarlane. Like streptokinase, urokinase activates plasminogen to form plasmin, which breaks up fibrin clots. In the past it has been used to improve drainage of pleural effusions (collections of fluid around the lungs) and for years it was the drug of choice to open clotted dialysis cannulas and permanent central venous catheters. While it has been shown to be effective in DVT, PE, and MI, currently it is indicated only for use in DVT.

Studies of these two oldest fibrinolytics in the late 1960s showed for the first time that these agents were more effective in treating PE than standard anticoagulants like heparin and warfarin. Basically, it was better for you to be treated with products from strep bacteria and urine than with rat poison.

In the 1960s, a British physician isolated ancrod, a component of pit viper venom that prevented blood from clotting. While similar thrombolytics are found in many vipers, including cobras, the Malayan pit viper produces the largest quantity of ancrod. Pit viper farms were not uncommon in Germany, as the drug was marketed for decades there and in Austria. Eventually, in the 1980s it was withdrawn from the market in favor of other thrombolytics. Interestingly, it was also used quite successfully to treat priapism, that thing they warn you about in the Viagra commercials. You know, the side effect where you have to call your doctor after four hours of a continuous hard-on. In 2005, the FDA gave approval for clinical trials of ancrod, under the name Viprinex (Nice sinister name.), for the treatment of acute strokes.

Tissue plasminogen activator (tPA) is an enzyme found in humans that dissolves blood clots. There are two major commercially available forms, alteplase and reteplase. Both are manufactured using recombinant DNA. Marketed respectively as Activase and Retavase, tPA is the most commonly used thrombolytic in the treatment of acute MI and acute CVA. Retavase is extremely easy to administer, a couple of IV pushes thirty minutes apart rather than the prolonged IV infusion required for SK. Its ease of administration comes at a hefty price, about ten times the cost of SK. Despite decades of studies involving over ten thousand patients, it has not been proven to work better than SK in MI, and may cause a higher risk of bleeding in your brain. Most E.R. docs and nurses would much rather use Retavase, which is why it has become so popular.

In many European countries, there is more centralization of specialty services. When it comes to cardiac care, you are less likely to have a cath lab and cardiac surgery available in your home town. We in the U.S. are used to having our medical services determined more by free market economics than by central governmental policy. Even back in the 1970s, an American city of moderate size would have several hospitals or medical centers with cardiac surgery capability, whereas a city of the same size in Europe, partly because of the socialization of medicine there, might have none. Our standard in the U.S. for patients with an MI was to travel less than ten miles to a cardiac center, where they were then admitted and started on SK. Europeans suffering an MI would travel about the same distance to their local hospital; there they would be put in an ambulance ASAP and transported to a regional cardiac center. Along the way, ambulance personnel would start the infusion of SK.

As far back as the 1980s, when DRGs were first introduced, the cry was that we were heading for socialization of medicine. While a single-payer system is inevitable, our way of life in the U.S., everything from getting what we want to the tort system, dictates that we will not end up with the centralization of services that prevails in Europe, and, to a lesser extent, in Canada. Here, if you have an MI near a major medical center, you will receive the option of emergency PCI because, as a cardiologist once told me, "That's what I would want."

It would be a shame to omit bivalirudin here, because, even though it is not technically a thrombolytic, it is commonly used in the cath lab, and has a couple of characteristics worth mentioning. Bivalirudin is the most prominent of a group of medications called direct thrombin inhibitors, which bind to thrombin, a protein that plays a key role in blood clot formation. It is easier and safer to use than heparin, the most popular intravenous blood thinner, an indirect thrombin inhibitor. It prevents the formation of clots in the area of angioplasty and stent placement in your coronary artery.

 Bivalirudin is given intravenously at the beginning of an angioplasty procedure, usually in combination with aspirin and often with other anti-platelet medications, to prevent clotting in your coronary artery. The first thing to like about the drug is one of its trade names. Angiomax. If ever there was a reassuring name for a medication, it is Angiomax. *Angio* is a Greco-Latin prefix which refers to blood vessels. As for *max*, well, can it get any better than Max? The other great thing about bivalirudin is that it is a synthetic drug designed to resemble and work like a naturally occurring chemical compound known as hirudin. Where does hirudin come from? The saliva of leeches. That's why a leech can keep on sucking your blood out. Its saliva has an anticoagulant that prevents your blood from clotting and can actually liquefy clotted blood.

Leeches were originally used for bloodletting--sucking the bad humors out of sick patients. Instead of cutting open one of your veins, the physician merely attached a couple of leeches and then presumably went out to the local tavern for a few hours while the leeches sucked away. Leeches have been used since the time of the ancient Egyptians to treat everything from headaches to hemorrhoids; they reached their peak popularity in the mid-1800s in Europe. It is estimated that, from the 1830s on, French physicians alone were using up to one hundred million leeches for bloodletting every year. A lecturer at the Royal College of Physicians said in 1840, "Blood letting is a remedy which, when judiciously employed, is hardly possible to estimate too highly."

Over two hundred years ago, Wales was known as the leech farming capital of Europe. Recently that UK country has returned to leech prominence. Russia and Germany never gave up the use of leeches. If you are truly interested in leeches, there is an organization that would be glad to number you among its membership, the American Hirudotherapy Association. Nowadays in the U.S. leeches are used primarily to suck clotted blood (Remember that leech saliva!) from skin flaps rotated during reconstructive plastic surgery and from reattached limbs.

Instead of sticking a leech on your chest au naturel and hoping it sucks in the right place, your cardiologist will give you a dose of bivalirudin in your vein, knowing that it will eventually make its way to the action zone, your coronary arteries.

References:

1. Weitz, Jeffrey I., "Blood Coagulation and Anticoagulant, Fibrinolytic, and Antiplatelet Drugs." *Goodman & Gilman's The Pharmacological Basis of Therapeutics.* Ed. Laurence L. Brunton, Assoc. Ed. Bruce A. Chabner, Assoc. Ed. Bjorn C Knollman. New York: McGraw-Hill. 2011. 849-71.
2. De Lemos, James A., O'Rourke, Robert A. "Unstable Angina and Non - ST-Segment Elevation Myocardial Infarction." *Hurst's The Heart.* Ed. Valentin Fuster, Ed. Robert A. O'Rourke, Ed. Richard A. Walsh, Ed. Philip Poole-Wilson. New York: McGraw-Hill. 2008. 1367.
3. Iqbal Z, Cohen M. "Emerging antithrombotic agents: what does the intensivist need to know?" *Curr Opin Crit Care.* 2010. 16(5):419-25.
4. Thearle MJ. "Leeches in medicine." *Aust N Z J Surg.* 1998. 68(4):292-5.

42. FLYING HIGH

Gladys Anthony, delicate as a flower, sat with hands clasped in her lap, the picture of late middle-aged Catholic schoolgirl propriety, thinking it would be nice to go home and take a long hot bath. It was late afternoon, and the waiting room for the CCU was empty. A tall man in nicely creased black pants and a short-sleeved white linen shirt walked purposefully toward her, extending his hand. Instinctively, Gladys responded in like fashion. She started to stand.

"Mrs. Anthony? Hi, I'm Michael Wolff. Please don't get up." He handed her a business card. She laid it carefully on her lap without reading it, and looked back up at him.

"Nice to meet you, Mr. Wolff." Although he wasn't dressed in one of those operating room outfits, she couldn't remember the term, she expected him to give her information, an update on Dick's condition. "Are you with the hospital?"

Michael Wolff laughed. "No, Ma'am, I'm not. I'm with the NTSB." He paused and waited for her to respond, see if she knew what the initials stood for. Let her take her time, not rush her.

"Oh, yes, you're the ones I see on TV now and then, whenever there's a plane crash or train wreck. Let me see, National Transportation Something Something."

Something Something. I'll have to remember that. "National Transportation Safety Board, yes Ma'am." Again he let her move at her own pace, keep things nice and friendly.

After thinking for a moment, Gladys said, "Well, we didn't, that is, Dick and I, we didn't crash."

Wolff took the seat to her right. "Yes, that's true. But you did radio in a Mayday, your pilot friend lost consciousness, and you were about to land a plane, possibly for the first time. Then your pilot loses consciousness again coming out of the plane. That warrants what we call an informal interview. It's on the record, but it's purely a matter of gathering information."

"While it is true that Dick lost consciousness twice, and I did call in a Mayday, it was not the first time I've landed a plane."

"Do you have an active pilot's license?"

"No, I've never had a pilot's license." She sat still, now letting him come to her.

Wolff hadn't expected this. Feistier than she looks. Good. He smiled. "So you're taking flying lessons from Mr. Withnin?"

"Oh, no, we were just out for a ride."

"Mrs. Anthony, you've piqued my curiosity. When and where were you flying and landing a plane without the appropriate license?"

"I grew up in Northern Nebraska, Mr. Wolff. All the ranchers in Cherry County had their own planes, for dusting and getting around. The first time I landed a plane with my father, I was twelve years old." She smiled proudly.

Not as fragile as she looks, this Nebraska farm girl. "Ah, yes. Mrs. Anthony, I thought I could save you the trouble of a drive downtown in the next few days by interviewing you here while you are waiting to see Mr. Withnin."

"Of course. And please call me Gladys, Mr. Wolff."

"It's Michael. Good. How long have you known Mr. Withnin, Gladys?"

"We met over coffee a week ago last Saturday. That would be eleven days."

"Oh, a first date?"

"Yes. We were both registered on Active Seniors." She blushed. "That's a website for ladies and gentlemen over the age of sixty-five. I listed flying as an interest and so did he." She lifted her hands from her lap, palms up, for just a second, then let them fall back together, clasped.

"I take it coffee went well?"

"Very. We've met every day since. This was our maiden flight together. Dick wanted to take me up sooner but he had to wait for a part for his plane. He's very careful, Michael, does all his own maintenance on his planes."

"He only has one registered with the FAA. Where's the other one?"

"Oh, he keeps it up at a friend's wheat ranch near Winnipeg. A beautiful banana yellow Piper J-3 Cub, from World War II. I've seen pictures of it."

"He's still crop dusting? At his age?"

"Not here in the States, only in Canada, occasionally down in Mexico, and only for friends. It's in his blood, you know."

"By the way, Gladys, how old is Mr. Withnin?"

"You wouldn't know it to look at Dick, but he'll be seventy-eight in November. He could easily pass for sixty-eight. I've always been partial to older men. My husband Sam, God rest his soul, he was thirty-two when we married. I was just out of high school, barely eighteen." She gave just the hint of a shy smile.

Wolff made a mental note to alert the Canadians. *The old guy probably had no license to dust, maybe no license at all up there. Seventy-seven. Jesus.* "Do you have a phone number for Mr. Withnin? I'll need to talk to him, but the nurse says he should be home in a few days, so I won't bother him here in the hospital."

"Yes, of course. He gave me his card on our first date. Isn't that funny, I haven't called him yet, nor has he called me. We had such fun each time we were together that we'd simply make plans for the next day." She put Michael Wolff's card into her clutch purse and pulled out an oatmeal-colored business card. Wolff took out his cell phone and typed in the phone number on the card. Then he handed the card back to Gladys.

"Oh, you may keep it, Michael. Dick gave me a dozen or more and said I was to give out his card freely to anyone at all."

"Thank you, Gladys." He put the card in his breast pocket of his shirt. Gladys could read the red lettering through the linen. "Before we start, I'd like your permission to tape our conversation. As I said earlier, it's only an informal interview, but I'd like to have a tape for reference when I write my report. After the report is finished, I promise to erase the entire interview."

"Oh, I don't mind at all." She waited while he started a portable tape recorder. "Where would you like me to start?"

"I'm assuming he picked you up this morning. Why don't you start there?"

"Actually, Michael, I rode my bicycle out to P & R Field. I arrived there by 6 A.M. It took me a little over an hour."

"That's quite a ride so early in the morning."

"Oh, heavens, I'm up every day at 4:30. Yoga first, then breakfast, then a bike ride. Keeps me limber." Wolff thought he caught the slightest trace of a smile. "I had to skip my yoga this morning. By the time I arrived, Dick had already loaded up his toolbox and inspected his Cessna. We pushed it out of the hangar together."

"What was the toolbox for?"

"Our plan for the day included a ride up to Jackson Hole. A friend needed a part for his plane, so Dick offered to pick up the part and install it for him. The owner lives in Southern California and does all his own maintenance, but he won't be able to get up there for a month. Dick was flattered that his friend trusted him enough to let him work on the plane."

"So you were flying to Jackson and then coming back the same day?"

"Yes. I packed us a picnic lunch. Dick thought the repair would take about an hour, after which we would eat, then fly back."

"How was Mr. Withnin on the flight to Jackson?"

"Oh, he was his usual charming self. We have so much to talk about whenever we're together, the time just flew by. Next thing we knew, we were landing at a small airport south of town. It was just lovely there. During our approach, we'd spotted a creek near the airport, so I walked over and made myself comfortable while Dick completed his repairs. He told me his friend is a well-known actor. He appeared in several of those Star Something movies." She raised her hands from her lap again, then let them fall back into their clasp.

"Star Wars?"

"Yes, I believe that was the name. His last name had something to do with automobiles. What was it now?"

"Harrison Ford?"

"Yes. How did you know?" She seemed genuinely amazed.

"Dick was working on Harrison Ford's plane?" *Mother of God.* He made a mental note to notify someone up in Jackson. *That plane bears looking at before it goes up again.*

"Yes."

"Isn't that something. Please go on."

"After he finished his repairs, Dick walked over to the creek. We sat and enjoyed the view, ate our lunch..." She stopped, blinked a couple of times, then turned to Wolff with a look of disbelief.

"Yes, Gladys?"

"And then Dick proposed to me."

Wolff jaw dropped. He hadn't been expecting that one. *One surprise after another. I can't wait to meet this old coot.* After he closed his mouth, he realized that she was waiting for him to say something.

"Con-congratulations, Gladys!" It came out more of a choke than a salutation.

"Thank you."

"Wasn't that kind of sudden?"

"You know, Michael, it was and it wasn't. When I woke up this morning, I had an inkling that something special would happen today, and, don't you know, getting proposed to qualifies as something special, at least in my book." She looked at him without saying anything more.

"Oh, mine too. Definitely." She nodded at each of his words.

"Gladys, after your picnic lunch and proposal...By the way, did you accept?"

"Of course. I think we both knew from the moment we met that we were kindred souls. After all, I grew up only twelve years and twenty-three miles from Dick."

"Oh, that's terrific. So, after lunch and proposal, what happened next?"

"We walked back to the airport, got in the Cessna, and headed back here."

"All right. When did you notice that Mr. Withnin was not feeling well?"

"We were about thirty miles outside of Boise, talking back and forth, of course. Dick wants to get married up at Coeur d'Alene, on the lake at a friend's cabin. Such a planner, Michael. He said he had something to show me; he reached behind his seat but couldn't find what he was looking for, so he turned his head around to his right and looked down at the floor. All of a sudden, he went limp. His head hung down toward me, and he turned this awful blue grey color. I thought, oh my goodness, he's had a stroke or a heart attack. That's when I called in the Mayday. Then I pushed his head back up and took over the controls. I thought about giving him CPR, but I decided the best thing was to land the plane and get him to the hospital as quickly as I could."

"His Cessna, you pretty much have to be sitting in the pilot's seat to land it."

"Michael, remember I told you about my daily yoga sessions?"

"Yes, Ma'am, I do."

"Well, as a result I am extremely limber. Flexible."

"Still pretty dangerous to try and land that plane from the passenger's seat."

"That's how I learned to fly, Michael."

"From the passenger seat?"

"Of course. You don't think my father would let me sit in the pilot's seat, now do you? After all, I was only twelve. That would have been irresponsible." Wolff thought, *Of course. Silly me.*

"I reached over him with my hands and my feet to take control. By the time I started my descent, Dick woke up. At first he seemed confused, but after a little bit, he realized where he was and started flying again. I sat back in my seat and buckled up. Next thing I knew, we were coming out of the descent and heading back up."

"Did he say why he didn't want to land, Gladys?"

"Yes, of course he did."

"Could you tell me?"

She smiled demurely. "I'd rather not say, Michael." She looked down at her hands, still clasped in her lap.

"How about a hint?"

Gladys Anthony thought for a moment, then looked at Wolff. "Dick said he wanted to take us up to eight thousand feet above sea level." She looked back down, smiling.

"Why eight thousand...?" He stopped. *Boise is twenty-seven hundred feet above sea level. Eight thousand minus twenty-seven hundred came to fifty-three hundred feet.* "Oh." He blushed.

"May I ask you something, Gladys?"

"Yes?"

"Did you give your consent?"

"Oh, yes. Dick wanted our first time to be special. I was a bit shocked at first, but you see, Michael, my dear husband Sam, well, he became extremely agoraphobic. As a matter of fact, for the last eighteen years of our marriage, he never left our house, not even to do business. We never went anywhere, never did anything out of the ordinary. I'd never imagined it was possible, but when Dick said we could join the mile-high club right then and there, I was so excited."

"And how did it go, Gladys?"

"It was superb. As I said, my dedication to yoga has left me very flexible. This doesn't have to go into your report, does it?"

"No, Ma'am, it does not. Again, congratulations."

A few minutes later, Dr. Holden came out to talk to them. "Mrs. Anthony, I understand you are Mr. Withnin's fiancée?"

"Yes, Doctor."

"Well, he's given his consent to discuss his condition with you, but only with you." He looked at Michael Wolff.

"Oh, Michael is a dear friend. I'm sure Dick wouldn't mind your discussing anything in front of him. And I'm sure Michael will keep everything confidential." She reached over and gave Wolff's hand a squeeze. *Nicely done, Gladys.*

"Well, to be honest with you, he's very lucky to be alive. Either one of his syncopal episodes today could have been his last."

"Oh dear. When Dick told me he had them all the time, I assumed they weren't serious."

"Very serious. Mr. Withnin has two major heart problems. First, he has severe aortic stenosis. His aortic valve barely opens at all, so even on his best days, his heart is barely pumping adequate amounts of blood to his brain. Anything that compromises his heart rate causes his blood flow to drop even further. In addition, he has a very sensitive carotid sinus, especially on the right side of his neck." The cardiologist pointed to a spot just below his right ear. "Any time he turns his head down and to the right, his heart rate slows dramatically. When I first examined him, I just palpated his right carotid pulse ever so lightly. His heart rate dropped from eighty beats per minute to twenty and he passed out."

Oh, dear. Yes, that must be what happened in the plane."

Michael Wolff asked, "What about after you deplaned?"

"Oh, he's such a gentleman, Michael. I was carrying the picnic basket. When he noticed, he reached down to carry it for me. That's when he had another of those spells. I held him up, but thank goodness those nice young men in the ambulance arrived just then." She turned back to the doctor. "Dr. Holden, what can we do about all this?"

"Well, I've already inserted a temporary pacemaker. We'll put in a permanent one tomorrow. That should take care of his heart's tendency to slow down. In terms of his aortic stenosis, I'll consult with Dr. Akers, the cardiac surgeon tonight. I'm afraid Mr. Withnin is going to require a replacement of his aortic valve, probably later tomorrow or Friday first thing." Just then his pager rang. He looked at the number. "I'm due in the cath lab. Excuse me."

Michael turned to Gladys. "If you two are going to fly again, you might think about getting a pilot's license, Gladys. Mr. Withnin is going to be out of commission for a few months. If he gets a mechanical valve replacement, he'll be on Coumadin to thin his blood, and his flying days are over, period. Even if he gets a pig or cow valve replacement, he'll need to be retested for his license."

"Goodness, Michael, how do you know all that? Don't tell me you have to have a medical background to investigate crashes."

"It doesn't hurt, but no. My dad spent twenty years as a flight surgeon in the Air Force." He turned off his tape recorder and stood up. "Thank you for talking with me, Gladys. It looks like I won't be able to interview Mr. Withnin for quite a while. I'll be in touch." He turned to go, then turned back. "Gladys, promise me. No more mile-high business, okay?"

She smiled. "I promise. Good-bye, Michael."

Out in the parking lot, Wolff felt the card in his shirt pocket. For the first time he noticed the red block lettering above the phone number. The second line read, "Aerial Adventures and Crop Dusting". He thought, *That's over and done with.* The top line made him smile. "Dick Withnin(e) Lives". *He just used two of them.*

43. SYNCOPE

Syncope (SINK-oh-pee) is a sudden temporary loss of consciousness and posture, meaning you black out and fall down. If you are standing, you fall to the ground in a heap. If you are sitting, you slump in your chair. I've never heard of anyone having a syncopal episode while lying down, but in theory it is possible. The cause is almost always the interruption of the flow of blood and oxygen to the brain. There are numerous causes for this interruption. In the setting of syncope, the causes can be grouped into three categories: neural (relating to the nervous system), cardiac, and orthostatic hypotension.

Perhaps the commonest cause of syncope, vasovagal syncope, falls in the neurally-induced category. It is mediated by the vagus nerve, which, among its many duties, is responsible for slowing your heart rate. At the end of a hard day, you walk in the door to find your wife crying her eyes out. When you ask her what's wrong, she tells you that Slimey, your favorite pet sea slug, just died. Overcome with emotion, your brain sends a signal to your vagus nerve, which fires, causing your heart to slow down. We are talking SLOW, as in thirty or fewer beats per minute. As a result, your blood pressure drops, and voilà, so do you. One minute you are standing up, the next you are on the ground. For some people, all it takes to cause a syncopal episode is getting their blood drawn. If you've ever seen a woman faint on screen, that's vasovagal syncope. Of course, the non-Hollywood variety does not involve putting the back of your hand to your forehead or falling into Clark Gable's conveniently available arms.

Once you hit the ground, the spell is usually broken; because you are now more or less horizontal, blood doesn't have to climb vertically to as high a level. After an episode of vasovagal syncope, your blood pressure returns to normal, you awaken almost immediately and you can stand up. Unless, of course, the fall has broken your hip or your neck. Other neurologic causes of syncope include strokes and seizures. People have been known to experience syncope from coughing, swallowing, vomiting and urinating.

Orthostatic hypotension is defined as a significant fall in blood pressure when you change position. Normally when you stand up, gravity causes blood to pool in your legs and feet; up where it's measured in your arm, your blood pressure will fall a bit. At that point, your heart will start beating faster and your blood vessels will tighten up to restore your blood pressure to its previous normal level. If your heart or blood vessels don't do their jobs, the drop in your blood pressure will be steeper and longer-lasting. Eventually, your brain will be starved of blood and down you go. Some people are born with orthostatic hypotension owing to a lack of overall regulation of blood pressure. Previously normal individuals who are severely dehydrated or suffer significant blood loss will experience orthostatic hypotension and syncope because the volume of circulating blood has been depleted. Serious systemic infections tend to dilate your blood vessels throughout your body, so blood pools in your lower extremities when you stand up. Once again, down you go.

A variety of conditions can cause cardiac syncope. Every so often a high school or college athlete falls down and blacks out either during or right after strenuous exercise. The cause is usually cardiac in nature. When caused by an arrhythmia, V Tach (Ventricular tachycardia, remember?) is frequently the culprit. In addition to the arrhythmia, there is often a congenital heart valve or heart muscle malformation which hinders the outflow of blood from the heart to the brain. Some of these presumably healthy young people suffer cardiac arrest and die on the spot.

Anyone of any age can experience syncope due to pulmonary embolus, a blood clot which travels from your leg through your heart to your lung. In older individuals, i.e., guys like you, syncope is often caused by arrhythmias; until proven otherwise, the safe route is to assume the underlying culprit is coronary artery disease or valvular heart disease. So if you or someone you know passes out for no reason, it's off to the doctor to find out why. Lots of people survive their first episode of syncope. Consider it a warning. Those who choose to ignore that warning may or may not have a second episode, and they may or may not survive that one. Of all patients seeking medical attention for syncope, 10% will have an underlying cardiac problem, usually treatable and often life-threatening. Of all patients experiencing an episode of syncope, 4%, one out of every twenty-five, will die within thirty days. Syncope during exercise is much more likely to have a cardiac cause than syncope at rest.

Old farts tend to have interesting causes for their syncopal episodes. A guy in his seventies or eighties who has a large, obstructive prostate gland may not have fallen into the clutches of the local urologist yet. Because of that big old prostate gland, which may be three or four times normal size, he has to strain to empty his bladder. That straining stimulates his vagus nerve, causing his heart rate to drop; like an obedient lap dog, his blood pressure follows suit. The resulting lack of blood flow to his brain leaves him draped across the toilet or on the floor. At that point, his urine flows like Niagara Falls, leaving his pants and other articles of clothing soaked. Very embarrassing, but, again, better than a broken hip or neck. Other than getting his prostate whittled down, the simplest remedy to prevent further syncopal episodes is to sit to pee. Not only is it safer in terms of distance he will fall if he blacks out, it is also easier to empty one's bladder while sitting. Ask any female.

Another odd and interesting syndrome that causes old guys to fall down unconscious is necktie syncope. A tight necktie will compress the carotid sinus, which is located on the side of your neck below your ear. This pressure will stimulate your vagus nerve and cause your heart to slow down. A variation of necktie syncope can also be seen in old guys who wear high, tight collars. The only case of necktie syncope I ever saw was a guy in his eighties who would have syncopal episodes only on Sundays. The answer to the puzzle was the high collar he wore to church.

Like many other medical phenomena, the worst kind of syncope is the kind that eventually kills you. Just as in those healthy young athletes, when an arrhythmia is involved, it is very often V Tach. Occasionally, just to keep things interesting, a patient like Dickie Nine Lives will suffer a syncopal episode due to severe bradycardia (slow heart beat) or a brief run of asystole (no heart beat). If left undetected and untreated, any of these can eventually result in cardiac arrest. The take-home message is that when you have an episode of syncope associated with an arrhythmia, it is vitally important to look behind the rhythm disturbance marionette and find the evil horned puppet master lurking there, pulling all your strings in the wrong direction.

References:

1. Carlson, Mark D., Grubb, Blair P. "Diagnosis and Management of Syncope." *Hurst's The Heart.* Ed. Valentin Fuster, Ed. Richard A. Walsh, Ed. Robert A. Harrington. New York: McGraw-Hill. 2011. 1125-30.
2. Calkins, Hugh, Zipes, Douglas P. "Hypotension and Syncope." *Braunwald's Heart Disease.* Ed. Robert O. Bonow, Ed. Douglas L. Mann,

Ed. Douglas P. Zipes, Ed. Peter Libby, Ed. Eugene Braunwald. Philadelphia: Elsevier Saunders. 2012. 885-6.

44. CODES AND CARDIAC ARREST

In July of 1774, a Mr. Squires of London applied electrical shocks to a three-year-old girl who had fallen out of a first-story window and was pulseless. He started administering the shocks at least twenty minutes after she was pronounced dead. There was no response until he applied shocks to her chest, after which she was noted to have a pulse. She sighed, vomited, and within a week was back to normal.

The word "Code" is short for Code Arrest, Code Blue, Code 99, or Code 1. All of these commonly used terms mean the same thing: someone in the hospital is trying to die, usually because their heart has stopped beating effectively. These events are classified as cardiac arrest. Every year in the U.S., approximately 200,000 patients suffer cardiac arrest in the hospital. Around 20% of adults and 30-40% of children survive long enough to be discharged from the hospital.

"Code" can be used in a number of ways. It can be a passive verb, as in "When I got there, he was coding", meaning trying to die. It can also be an active verb, as in, "We coded him for an hour", which means the code team attempted to resuscitate the dying patient. It can be a noun, representing the procedure, as in "I ran my first code today." It can also be used as a noun to represent the patient's code status, as in "Are you telling me that old gomer is a code?" In this situation, you can also use the phrase "full code", to mean that no futile effort or monetary expense should be spared in attempting to resuscitate said gomer.

Every patient should have a "code status" determined upon admission to the hospital. Most patients will be what is called a "full code". That means that, no matter what happens to you, no matter how hopeless your situation becomes, your health care team will do everything possible to keep you alive. That includes meds, shocks, intubation and ventilator life support. Most patients, particularly the young and healthy ones, will fall into this category. Even patients with serious chronic illnesses, like early-stage cancer or mild congestive heart failure or mild COPD, will be full codes. If you are admitted to the hospital for a cath or bypass surgery, most assuredly you will be a full code. Lots of patients undergoing either will have at least a transient episode where their heart unexpectedly stops beating.

"No Code" means the same as DNR--Do Not Resuscitate. If you sign a form, you can (almost) rest assured that if you try to die, nobody will stop you. This designation is usually reserved for the chronically ill (terminal stages of cancer, severe heart disease, severe COPD), the extremely old, or anyone who doesn't want to end up with a tracheostomy on a ventilator with multiple tubes sticking out of natural and man-made holes in his body, slowly losing an unwinnable battle against MRSA and other opportunistic bacteria and fungi. Many patients who are designated as a no code have either signed a living will which outlines their wishes or made their preference known to their physician before or at the time of admission.

There is also a term known as "mini-code" or "Baby Blue" which will be discussed in more detail later on. Generally speaking, the mini-code status allows for IV meds and fluids, which are sometimes successful in resuscitations, but no intubation, no CPR, and no shock.

Although a code can be called for anything from an irregular, potentially life-threatening arrhythmia to a severe asthma attack to an extremely low blood pressure, usually there is a cardiac arrest--loss of consciousness associated with ventricular tachycardia (V Tach), ventricular fibrillation (V Fib) or asystole. On the monitor, V Tach is a series of wide-complex R and S waves at 100 per minute or more. V Fib is nothing more than a choppy saw tooth pattern with no discernible P waves or QRS complexes. Asystole is a flat line.

As opposed to adult codes, pediatric codes often start with respiratory distress. If you get to the infant or toddler quickly enough and correct the breathing problem, either by dislodging the hot dog with a Heimlich maneuver, like Burt Lancaster in *Field of Dreams,* or by intubating the child and putting him on a ventilator, you may avoid having to deal with any cardiac arrhythmias.

A code starts with a nurse walking into a room, then running out into the hallway and yelling, "Call a code. Room 432 Bed 1". Some hospitals have a special button at each bed. Rather than run out into the hallway, the nurse can push the button to notify the nurse at the desk, who then calls the hospital operator and tells her to call a code. Then you hear it over the loudspeaker. That's when all the fun begins. In teaching hospitals, especially university hospitals with med students, interns and residents, everyone runs at breakneck speed to the scene of the code. That's because they think they are going to save a life. That also because some of the smoking hot ICU nurses will arrive to help out. Mostly it's because they're young and have all this unexpended energy. As you age, the running gives way to walking purposefully; after a few dozen codes, you realize there is no reason to run, because:

A. A lead from the patient's chest to the monitor is disconnected and the patient is fine;

B. Someone, either the housekeeper or the nurse, bumped the code button accidentally;

C. The patient's nephew, Little Dickbrain, pushed the button to see what would happen;

D. The patient, 95 years old, is rotting away slowly and painfully from lung cancer, but nobody bothered to put a DNR order on the chart;

E. It is change of shift, and the code is on a ward without cardiac monitors. That means the patient has most likely been dead for hours and was just discovered by the oncoming nursing staff.

In addition, as you age, running entails the risk of spraining an ankle, spilling your coffee, or falling down.

According to *The House of God*, the first thing to do at a cardiac arrest is to take your own pulse. Probably a better first step is to make sure all the EKG leads are connected to the patient at one end and to the monitor at the other. Plenty of guys, sleeping peacefully and minding their own business in a hospital bed, have been rudely awakened by a fist to the chest or, worse, by three-hundred joules of electricity from a defibrillator. It's not as hard as you think to break someone's ribs or breastbone with a good solid thump from on high, even easier when performing vigorous CPR. If a shock administered in error doesn't convert your normal rhythm to a lethally abnormal one, at the very least it'll make you sit up and take notice. In the movies, a defibrillator is the shocky thing that zaps the dead guy right after they yell "Clear". That's immediately before they say, "Live, damn it!" while performing piss-poor CPR, then stop, shake their collective heads and walk out of the room.

Most hospitals have a protocol for a "code team". The members of the team usually change on a daily basis. Back when pagers were all the rage, each member of the code team carried a separate pager that went off only when a code was called. You've seen one. Dr. Beeper wore a code pager in *Caddyshack*. Although spot-on most of the time, that classic movie contained one glaring error. In most hospitals, the code team does not include a proctologist. Nowadays the code team members probably carry special cell phones or iPads. Maybe you get called to a code via your Zuckerface page. Don't forget to update your status. "Running to a code."

The code team usually includes an anesthesiologist to intubate you. A respiratory therapist will be there to manage the airway before and after you are intubated. There's usually an intensivist, which is a physician who specializes in critical care, or at least an internist who is working in the ICU, to run the code. An EKG tech will be there to run 12-lead EKG if you survive. A nurse or two from the ICU or CVICU will be there to administer meds. The patient's nurse or the charge nurse usually takes notes to keep track of the progress of the code. A cavalcade of rubberneckers will also crowd your room, spouting off "helpful" suggestions. Eventually the doc in charge will have had enough of the second-guessers; at that point he'll direct everyone not on the code team to leave. Once that happens, the average IQ in the room rises dramatically.

In-hospital codes on a monitored ward--that would be telemetry or a step-down unit--are initially a little rougher than in the units, but after a minute or two, everything should be running smoothly. On unmonitored wards (medical or surgical floors), expect a dash of what the old timey wrestling announcers called "organized mayhem". Many times the patient doesn't have an IV in place. The patient's code status may be unclear. The staff may be unfamiliar with the layout of the code cart, which contains cardiac meds, IV fluids, and endotracheal tubes. Although the use of the defibrillator is supposed to be reviewed on a regular basis on each ward, in the heat of the moment it can be challenging to operate it correctly. If a code is called on you on an unmonitored unit, most likely you will be just fine, mainly because you weren't coding in the first place and the code was called in error. Otherwise, it might be a tough go. If you survive a real code, expect to spend a day or two in the CVICU. If you've come in for a cath or bypass surgery, there's no good reason for you to be languishing on an unmonitored unit anyway.

For the better part of two decades it has been all the rage to have your family stay in the room during a code. It's supposed to allow them to see how hard the code team is working to save your life. This is a great idea when the code occurs in the ICU, everyone on the code team is already there, and you wake up after the first shock from the defibrillator. On a general medical ward, a code often starts out as a giant cluster fuck; occasionally it ends up better than it started. Nowadays, count on a family member to film the whole thing on an iPhone, so that the malpractice lawyer has some hard data on hand.

Over one thousand people suffer a cardiac arrest outside the hospital in the U.S. every day. If you suffer a cardiac arrest "in the field", which means anywhere other than a hospital or a very well-equipped outpatient facility or ambulance, your chances of survival--being discharged from the hospital alive--are at best about 10%. There are certain subsets who do much better. If witnesses see you fall down and immediately start CPR (chest compressions only; no mouth-to-mouth, thank God.), your chance of survival rises to about 30%. Out in the field, children fare worse than adults. Even if you do survive a cardiac arrest outside the hospital, there is a fair chance your brain won't be working as well as it did before.

When discussing the cost of medical care in the U.S., it is important to remember that $125 billion, 25% of all Medicare funds, are spent on 5% of the Medicare population in the last year of life. That means that far too many terminally ill elderly patients are treated far too aggressively, usually in ICU's. Cardiac arrest is often the inciting factor in those end-of-the-line attempts to repel the Reaper. Everybody wants to die at home, but most Americans die in a hospital, nursing home, or extended care facility. The solution? Make your wishes known to your physician and your family, and sign one of those sheets detailing specifically your code status, so that the paramedics will know that you're not keen on a ride down Code Road. Stick it on your refrigerator door. That's where they'll look first.

References:

1. Kerber, Richard E. "Indications and Techniques of Electrical Defibrillation and Cardioversion." *Hurst's The Heart.* Ed. Valentin Fuster, Ed. Robert A. O'Rourke, Ed. Richard A. Walsh, Ed. Philip Poole-Wilson. New York: McGraw-Hill. 2008. 1102-3.
2. Reynolds, Matthew R., Pinto, Duane S., Josephson, Mark E. "Sudden Cardiac Death." *Hurst's The Heart.* Ed. Valentin Fuster, Ed. Robert A. O'Rourke, Ed. Richard A. Walsh, Ed. Philip Poole-Wilson. New York: McGraw-Hill. 2008. 1161-74.
3. Myerburg, Robert J., Castellanos, Agustin. "Cardiac Arrest and Sudden Cardiac Death." *Braunwald's Heart Disease.* Ed. Robert O. Bonow, Ed. Douglas L. Mann, Ed. Douglas P. Zipes, Ed. Peter Libby, Ed. Eugene Braunwald. Philadelphia: Elsevier Saunders. 2012. 845-6. 860-1.

45. GOING FOR THE GOLD

It was Wednesday afternoon, David's time to do treadmill stress tests. From a purely aesthetic perspective, this ranked far and away as the best of the specialty clinics. There was none of the patient moaning associated with the Friday morning straight sigmoidoscopy clinic. Whether you were on-call for the weekend or not, that session left a dark brown taste in your mouth through to Monday. The Tuesday morning diabetic foot care clinic was sure to produce at least one whiff of wet gangrene. There was a column on the flow sheet for the examiner to indicate the number of attached toes. Occasionally a lump in a sock turned out to be a newly-shed black peanut, and the number decreased once more.

Usually three or four stress tests were scheduled per afternoon session. Most lasted only five to ten minutes, as the patient population tended to be at least twenty pounds overweight with a fair number of smokers and the occasional patient with arthritis, vascular disease or nerve damage, sometimes all three. He got to the treadmill room right at 1:00 P.M. The first patient was all hooked up with the leads on his arms and legs; the vest-like contraption sprouted wires all over his chest. Marcy was doing the grunt work today, attaching all the EKG leads, running the tracings, and filling in the vital signs every few minutes.

The first three went off without a blip. Two of the three tired out before they got to their goal heart rate, so their tests were inconclusive. The third, a wiry old WWII vet with legs bowed in a perfect circle from years in the saddle, hung in there like a trooper and got through the whole protocol with no chest pain and no EKG changes. David told him he was a tough guy, shook his hand, and advised him that the chest pain was probably due to esophageal reflux. Realizing the stupidity of that statement, he added, "Be sure to follow up with your doctor. He might want to do some further tests."

Simmons filled out the report, closed the chart and walked back to the treadmill room. A guy with a crew cut and glasses by the name of Larsen, about forty or so, was bouncing up and down in his expensive new running shoes. He looked surprisingly fit for a patient.

Maybe it was a pre-employment or insurance thing. David had been shocked by the number of blond-haired, blue-eyed Indians in Oklahoma, and had learned not to ask, but something about this guy didn't seem to fit. He asked Marcy to follow him into the office.

"Shut the door, will you, Marce." She gave him a look and complied.

"What's up with this guy?"

"Whatever do you mean?" Innocent brown eyes. *Something's up.*

"This fellow does not in the least resemble one of our folks. What's he doing here?"

"Oh, so he doesn't look native enough for our Navajo expert?" She smirked. On Navajo, everyone was at least half Native American, and most were full-bloods. Normally Simmons would play along, but something about this guy bugged him, so he got pushier than normal.

"Is he a patient of this service unit or not? I haven't seen too many of our folks bouncing around in brand-new $200 running shoes."

She laughed. "He's a friend of Tacconelli's from Area Office. Runs one of the departments up there, maybe pharmacy or procurement, I can't remember. The two of them have been friends for years. Couple of drinking and whoring buddies, those two." Marcy had family all over the state. Nothing was beyond her reach when it came to scandalous info.

"If he's from Area Office, then he's got insurance. What's he doing here?"

"I think you'd better hear it from the horse's mouth." She picked up the phone, punched in three numbers and waited. "Hi, Esther, it's Marcy. Is Mr. T. available? Dr. Simmons has a question for him." She handed the receiver to David.

"Hi, Sam, it's David. I am trying to solve the riddle of the hyperactive guy who's here for a stress test. Yeah, the one from Area. Seriously? A bet? You know there's a four-month backup for routine stress tests, right? Yeah, I know, one more won't make a difference. Unless some guy got bumped for this and has a heart attack tonight and dies because we didn't diagnose him in time. Oh, okay, as long as it's that serious. Yeah, sure. Thanks. Bye." He looked at Marcy, shook his head, and put the receiver down. "What the fuck. Sorry, Marce."

"Relax, Doc."

"This idiot's here because he bet Tacconelli he could break the hospital record for endurance. Tacconelli said he had to do it here so the guy couldn't cheat. You make sure your tribal council hears about this, understand? Matter of fact, make sure the chief knows."

Marcy saluted and grinned. "Aye-aye, Sir!" She had no problem sticking a pin in Tacconelli's ass whenever she could. The feeling among the tribes was that, as good as he was at running the service unit and the hospital, Indian health care should be administered by Indians. Period. Tacconelli had kept his job longer than anyone else in IHS because this service unit provided for nineteen tribes. Nineteen chiefs, nineteen councils. It was like juggling nineteen ice picks at once. His thespian skills kept him on top.

As they went out to the treadmill room, David whispered in her ear, "This is just plain wrong."

"Things have a way of working themselves out." Marcy's dad was two years out from a quadruple bypass and was having some weird chest pains. When she brought it up to Simmons yesterday, he expected to see him on the schedule for today. Maybe Tacconelli had bumped him in favor of Larsen. David made sure Larsen signed both the informed consent for the procedure and a non-beneficiary release of liability. Larsen put up a fuss when Marcy handed him the latter.

"What's this?"

David said, "Unless you have a direct blood relative on the Dawes Rolls, you have to sign that or we can't treat you."

"Sam never said anything about this."

"If you were in a patient care position, you'd have seen this before."

"I don't know."

"Sign it or get out." Marcy stared at Simmons, who looked at Larsen with mild disinterest.

The guy turned out to be even more of a dick than Simmons had imagined. Instead of just walking on the treadmill, he babbled on about himself through the first twelve minutes. Simmons had to admit he was in great shape. As they started Stage 5, the guy switched from a brisk walk to a run.

"What's the record here for this thing, twenty minutes or something?"

Marcy looked up. "Twenty-two minutes, forty seconds." There was the slightest edge to her voice. David imagined the absurdity of the situation was finally getting to her.

"Hah. Whoever that dumb bastard was, if he'd gone twenty-four minutes, he'd have been in Alberto Salazar territory." That surprised David. He had no idea that Salazar had ever performed one of these things, but it made some sense. "Some time I'd like to run a marathon he's entered in, see how I do against him." *Oh, please*, Simmons thought. When he'd worked in Portland, in exchange for a free membership, he'd done stress tests at the YMCA. Watching one of the greats run, even on a treadmill, was unlike any running he'd ever seen. They didn't really run, they bounced on invisible springs. He'd worked the Cascade Runoff and the Portland Marathon a couple of times as well. When Salazar ran, he floated above the pavement. This guy could run a long time, but there was no comparison.

At around twenty minutes, the guy still had enough gas to chatter away about his boat up on Grand Lake, his drinking parties up there with Tacconelli, and how David should join them for one of their weekend orgies. Marcy rolled her eyes when he brought up his mistress. She walked to the office door, then turned to Simmons.

"I have to make a call. You okay here?"

"Sure, Marce. We're fine." He picked up the clipboard as she walked into the office and closed the door.

At twenty-one minutes he was still going, his mouth as much as his legs. Talking about the diamond bracelet he'd bought for "Princess". Marcy came out of the office and took back the clipboard. She looked at the timer and called out "Ready." Simmons put the earpieces in and was about to take Larsen's blood pressure.

The room went black. There was a shout from Larsen, then a thud from below. Immediately the lights came back on. Larsen was lying on his left side on the treadmill, moaning, clutching his right knee. David saw a little blood on the treadmill up by Larsen's face. Marcy was staring down at the fallen runner, her mouth agape, her eyes wide as saucers. It was a weak attempt at horror.

"Goddamn this hurts!" Larsen was rocking back and forth, holding his knee. They helped him up into a chair, then called x-ray to come get him for a knee film, after which he would be heading to the ER or home. When he was gone, David turned to Marcy.

"How in the world did you do that?"

"Timmy Leo in engineering. My dad taught him how to night fish for croppies when he was a kid. They are very close. Timmy was concerned about my dad's chest pains."

"I hope the ventilators in the ICU are still running."

"Just this room. He promised." Simmons shouldered his backpack and they headed out into the hall together.

"Guess he doesn't break our record or Salazar's."

"I don't know who this Salazar is, but there was no way that guy was breaking our service unit record."

"Oh?"

"It was set by Robert Bible, a tribal police officer from over in Tahlequah. A distance runner in college. He died in the line of duty a few months later."

"I see."

"Oh, by the way, Dr. Simmons. There's nothing scheduled for this room Thursday mornings."

"I'll be in the building by 7 A.M. Call me when he's hooked up. If he has any problems tonight, don't wait, just bring him in."

"Thank you, Sir." She smiled.

"No. Thank you. That little payback made my day." Simmons started to turn, then stopped. "Do you have your car?"

"No, Ronald had to go over to Fort Smith."

"Need a ride?"

Oh no, my cousin Larry is coming to get me."

"Who's your cousin Larry?" Simmons didn't even know why he asked. Marcy had cousins by the dozens.

"He's a police officer in Oregon. Got shot in the chest a few years ago in the line of duty, but he saved the governor's life. He's here to talk to the tribal police department about his experiences, get his picture taken, show off his medal."

That brought Simmons up short. He asked, "Larry Dyckman?"

Marcy stared at him. "How'd you know?"

"I was working in the E.R. that day. A bunch of people got shot in the same incident. Some came to me and Larry went to Epiphany Hospital."

"Wow!" She shook her head. "Small world." She started to walk away.

"I hope there won't be any fallout about this from Tacconelli."

Without turning, she said, "Mr. T. won the bet. As far as he's concerned, nothing else matters."

46. TREADMILL TEST

It is difficult to say which is better: a normal treadmill stress test on a patient who has no coronary artery disease, or an abnormal one on a patient with disease. Either way, the most important point is that, much like the house in Vegas, the treadmill almost always wins.

The primary purpose of any type of treadmill test is to diagnose cardiac ischemia. That is basically inadequate oxygen delivery to the heart muscle. As you may recall from the anatomy chapter, the coronary arteries surround and penetrate the heart muscle. They deliver oxygen, in the form of oxygenated blood, to the muscle cells. As long as there is adequate blood flow to all parts of the heart muscle, there is no ischemia, and, hence, no angina and no changes on your EKG.

You can have severely narrowed coronary arteries due to cholesterol plaques and have no symptoms, especially if you are not very active. When you are at rest, your heart beats slowly and still provides enough blood to the various muscles and organs throughout your body. As you become more active, your muscles and organs will require more blood and oxygen to perform their functions. In order to facilitate that increased delivery of blood, the heart muscle will have to beat faster and harder. Like any of the other muscles of the body, it too will require more blood flow. That means that more blood will have to flow through the coronary arteries each minute.

Much like a garden hose that is bent or squeezed at a certain point, cholesterol narrowing of a coronary artery will limit the amount of blood that can flow to that area of the heart muscle. If you increase the activity of your heart muscle in the presence of coronary artery narrowing, sooner or later there won't be enough blood flow to keep up with the increased demand for oxygenated blood. At this point, the heart muscle will cramp up and your EKG will show changes consistent with ischemia. That, in a nutshell, is the rationale for performing stress tests. You want to stress the heart by making it work harder and see if the coronary arteries are up to the task of supplying adequate blood to your heart muscle.

The basic treadmill stress test is fairly simple. You get hooked up to a harness which contains a bunch of EKG leads. These leads are attached to your arms, legs and chest. You get on the treadmill and start walking. Every three minutes the speed of the treadmill increases, as does the incline; you have to walk more quickly up a steeper slope. If you get to a certain predetermined maximum heart rate without developing angina or EKG changes, your stress test is declared "normal", which means it was an adequate study and it did not detect any evidence of ischemia. If you develop angina AND there are EKG changes suggestive of ischemia, your test will be reported as "abnormal". If you develop your usual chest pain and there are no EKG changes, your test report will state "chest pain without EKG changes." If you have no chest pain or EKG changes but you can't make it to your predicted maximum heart rate because you are on certain medications, your blood pressure goes too high or too low, you become too short of breath, you feel dizzy, or because you are in such bad physical condition--the twinkies defense--your test will be reported as "inconclusive".

When it comes to diagnosing coronary artery disease, no test is perfect, not even an autopsy. Standard exercise stress tests work better in males than in females. Patients with good exercise tolerance will be more likely to have an adequate study than those in poor physical condition. Certain medications can make it much more difficult to obtain an adequate study. The standard Bruce protocol exercise stress test has a sensitivity of 70-90%, which means that of all the patients with significant coronary disease who perform the test adequately, about 70-90% will have an abnormal result. The other 10-30% with significant coronary disease will have a normal or inconclusive result. These missed patients are known as "false negatives" because they have disease but it was not detected. In other words, the test result was negative but it shouldn't have been. Because of these "false negatives", imaging stress tests, which include nuclear stress tests and stress echocardiograms, were developed. Other reasons for doing an imaging stress test rather than a standard stress test include: an abnormal EKG at rest; exercise limitations such as arthritis, COPD, peripheral arterial disease or leg amputations; arrhythmias; previous stents or bypasses.

Nuclear stress tests, known in the business as "nuke treads", increase the odds of detecting cardiac ischemia. The procedure is more sensitive than a standard treadmill stress test; when you undergo a nuke tread, there are fewer false negatives. There are all sorts of permutations to the process, but the underlying theory is the same. First, you are injected with a nuclear tracer, which circulates in the bloodstream. Wherever blood goes, including the cardiac muscle, the nuclear tracer also goes. If there is inadequate blood flow to a certain part of the heart, the tracer will not light up that particular area. The tracer emits low-level radiation which is sensed by a scanner. The scanner hardware produces a film which shows the areas of the body where the tracer has circulated. Areas with good perfusion will light up with a bright orange, pink or purple glow. (Of note, the bright glow appears only on the film, not in your heart.) If there is no tracer, a dark spot is seen.

When you go in for a nuke tread, the tech or nurse will stick an IV catheter into a vein in your arm. Then they will inject thallium or another similar isotope into your vein. You will rest for fifteen to sixty minutes, then some resting images will be taken by the scanner. After that, you will perform the standard Bruce Protocol treadmill test for as long as you can or until you reach your predicted maximum heart rate. Or until you slide off the back of the treadmill like Wile E. Coyote. Or Larsen.

When you get to the point where you are working as hard as you can, they will inject more thallium. In a while they will scan your heart again to produce exercise images. The cardiologist and radiologist will then compare the two sets of images. If there is a matching defect in both the rest and exercise images, that most likely represents dead heart muscle, probably from a previous heart attack. If there are no defects on either rest or exercise images, the study will be read as normal. If there is a defect on the exercise images but not on the rest images, most likely there is an area of ischemia and associated coronary artery blockage. The results of these images, when combined with symptoms and EKG changes during exercise, increase the chance of finding coronary disease.

Sensitivity of the nuclear stress test runs about 80%, meaning 20% of patients with significant coronary disease will have a normal test, a false negative result. Specificity runs 85-95%, which means that of all the patients without significant coronary disease, 5-15% will have an abnormal nuclear stress test, a false positive result.

If you cannot exercise on a treadmill because of other medical conditions, you can be injected with dipyridamole or adenosine, both of which cause healthy coronary arteries to dilate more than diseased ones, thus resulting in better perfusion of healthy areas of the heart with thallium.

Stress echocardiograms are another tool in diagnosing ischemia. An echocardiogram is basically an ultrasound of the heart structures, just as a pelvic ultrasound is often performed to evaluate a pregnancy.

Wouldn't it be something if a baby is discovered in your chest during an echo? Sometimes you do find teeth. It's called a teratoma. The tech holds a transducer to your chest. The transducer sends sound waves through the skin and chest wall to the structures of the heart. As the sound waves bounce off those structures, the echoes return through the transducer to provide an image of the heart.

First a resting echo is performed, usually with you lying on your left side. In this position, the heart is closest to the chest wall, thus decreasing interference from adjoining structures. The echo tech will obtain images in multiple areas of the heart. He will evaluate your heart valves, to see whether they appear normal, whether they open normally without restriction, and whether they close normally without leaking. More importantly in this situation, he will also evaluate the motion of the wall of the heart muscle. If there are areas where the wall motion is impaired or absent at rest, most likely there has been permanent damage to that part of the heart muscle, i.e., a previous myocardial infarction. If all is well on the resting echo, you then undergo a standard treadmill stress test. When your heart is working maximally--when you are sucking gas and can't suck any more--or when you develop symptoms and EKG changes, you will again lie down and a repeat echo will be done. In theory, if there is significant ischemia, there will be localized or generalized wall motion abnormalities.

The sensitivity of a stress echo is about 85%, meaning 15% of patients with significant coronary disease will have a normal test, a false negative. Specificity is about 75%, meaning that 25% of patients without significant coronary disease will have an abnormal stress echo, a false positive.

For those who cannot exercise, often the protocol calls for the injection of dobutamine after the resting echo is performed. Dobutamine will stress the heart muscle by making it contract more forcefully, thus mimicking the effect of exercise. If you have an ischemic area in your heart, it will show up on your post-injection echocardiogram.

References:

1. Engel, Gregory, Froehlicher, Victor F. "ECG Exercise Testing." *Hurst's The Heart.* Ed. Valentin Fuster, Ed. Robert A. O'Rourke, Ed. Richard A. Walsh, Ed. Philip Poole-Wilson. New York: McGraw-Hill. 2008. 324-35.
2. Berman, Daniel S., Hachamovitch, Rory, Shaw, Leslee J., Hayes, Sean W., Germano, Guido. "Nuclear Cardiology." *Hurst's The Heart.* Ed.

Valentin Fuster, Ed. Robert A. O'Rourke, Ed. Richard A. Walsh, Ed. Philip Poole-Wilson. New York: McGraw-Hill. 2008. 545-52.

3. Chaitman, Bernard R. "Exercise Stress Testing." *Braunwald's Heart Disease*. Ed. Robert O. Bonow, Ed. Douglas L. Mann, Ed. Douglas P. Zipes, Ed. Peter Libby, Ed. Eugene Braunwald. Philadelphia: Elsevier Saunders. 2012. 168-82.

4. Udelson, James E., Dilsizian, Vasken, Bonow, Robert O. "Nuclear Cardiology." *Braunwald's Heart Disease*. Ed. Robert O. Bonow, Ed. Braunwald. Philadelphia: Elsevier Saunders. 2012. 293-300.310-12.

5. Connolly, Heidi M., Oh, Jae K. "Echocardiography." *Braunwald's Heart Disease*. Ed. Robert O. Bonow, Ed. Douglas L. Mann, Ed. Douglas P. Zipes, Ed. Peter Libby, Ed. Eugene Braunwald. Philadelphia: Elsevier Saunders. 2012. 227-9.

6. Morrow, David A., Boden, William E. "Stable Ischemic Heart Disease." *Braunwald's Heart Disease*. Ed. Robert O. Bonow, Ed. Douglas L. Mann, Ed. Douglas P. Zipes, Ed. Peter Libby, Ed. Eugene Braunwald. Philadelphia: Elsevier Saunders. 2012. 1214-6.

47. MINOR VICTORIES

Triage Nurse Winnie came into the hall, followed by a fiftyish man carrying a woman. Just finished talking to a guy with a broken toe, Simmons walked out of Room 11 and bumped into the man. Winnie turned to look at them before pulling the Bay 10 curtain halfway around the gurney.

"You can lay your wife here, Mr. McBride." She pulled the top sheet down and stepped aside.

"Sorry, Mr. McBride." Simmons stepped back to let him pass. The man nodded but never looked at David. He stepped forward and gently placed his package on the gurney. She moaned softly. Her legs flopped to the side. Simmons stepped up. "What do we have, Win?"

"Mr. McBride just walked in with his wife. She hasn't been able to walk or sit up for the past few days."

McBride turned and stuck out his hand to Simmons. "Ray McBride. This is my wife Carol."

Simmons shook hands with him, then reached over to shake hands with Ray's better half. "Hi, I'm David Simmons."

"You a doctor, David?"

"Yes, Sir, I am. David Simmons, M.D."

"Good. We could use a doctor."

Winnie said, "After I check her in, I'll get Roger to see her. He just came in and you're due to go home, aren't you?"

"In a while. I'll take care of these folks. I don't have anywhere to be tonight and I'm off the next few days. It'd be a shame to waste a perfectly good introduction and round of handshakes." He smiled at McBride, who looked down at his shoes. "How about a chair, Sir?" David grabbed a steel-rimmed chair and pulled it up beside the bed. McBride collapsed into it and then reached for his wife's hand. He looked exhausted.

Simmons thought to himself, *This should be a quick admission.* Aloud, he said, "I'll let Winnie get you checked in, then the nurse who has this room, I think it's Jenny, yeah, she'll be back to do her thing, then I'll be back to see you. How about a cup of coffee, Mr. McBride?"

"Thanks, that would be great. One for Carol too?"

"Afraid not, Sir. We may have to do some tests tonight, so it would be best if your wife has nothing to eat or drink until we know what we have to do." He turned to walk away, then stopped. "One other thing. Just so you know, your wife won't be going home tonight."

"We can't afford to stay here."

"Doesn't matter, Mr. McBride. We don't send home people who can't walk or sit up."

"Okay, then. Thanks."

"I'll be back in a bit."

****

"So tell me, Ray. What's been going on?" He looked tired, but Simmons got the impression that he'd been tired a lot lately and was used to it. Thanks to ten mg. of IV morphine, Mrs. McBride was sleeping.

"Carol can tell you better than I, David."

"Yes, I know. Let's start with you while she's sleeping, then I'll wake her up, we'll talk, and I'll examine her."

"Yeah. You're right. She needs her sleep. What with this pain and all, she hasn't slept more than a few minutes at a time."

Simmons nodded. "When did this start?"

"About a week ago, Carol got up one morning and said her back hurt. I tried to rub it for her, but she said that made it hurt more. She got dressed and headed off to Mrs. Rascon's."

"Who's Mrs. Rascon?"

"Oh. Carol cleans homes. Two days a week at Mrs. Rascon's and three at her next door neighbor's, Mrs. Treadwell. They live up on Jupiter Mountain, you know, the gated homes above Jupiter Valley. It's been a nice setup for her for the last two years or so. Carol catches the bus up to Jupiter Valley, then one of the ladies comes and picks her up."

"Hard work cleaning houses, eh?"

"We've both worked hard jobs all our lives, David."

"What do you do, Ray?"

"I've been a framer here since 1975, out of work only a couple of years in the late '80s. With this slowdown, though, I've been doing piecework downtown at a friend's lumber yard, building pallets."

"From what you said before, I take it you and your wife don't have insurance."

"Had it for about five years, but when Carol lost her job at a big real estate firm in town, that went away."

"How have you been getting your medical care?"

"Mostly out of pocket. My stuff has been on the job, so workman's comp covered it. Otherwise, I've been healthy, thank God. Until the last year or so, Carol's been going to Planned Parenthood for her female exams."

"What's been going on the last year?"

"The protests. She couldn't stand the things they shouted at her when she tried to go inside."

Simmons and Ray McBride talked for another ten minutes about this and that. Soon an ambulance crew came in and deposited a moaning thirtyish male with a splint around his lower leg in Bay 9, separated from Bay 10 by only a curtain. David half-listened to the report as the paramedics filled Jenny in on the history and his vital signs. A ten-foot fall. After the ambulance crew left, Roger Mallin came in and started examining him. His screams woke up Mrs. McBride. *Perfect timing.*

"Hi, Mrs. McBride. Remember me? I'm Dr. Simmons." She nodded slightly, then shifted her torso a little to see him better. That elicited another moan. Simmons knew from its brevity and breathlessness that it represented real pain, not melodrama, and that she'd had the pain long enough to know how to minimize it, even when groaning. A patient might start out with long-winded screams and agonized thrashing, but after a while, other than renal colic from a kidney stone, persistent pain teaches even a halfwit to keep everything as still as possible, vocal cords included. With real pain, every movement makes it worse. Even breathing.

"I've been talking with your husband for a while. If it's okay, I'm going to examine you. I'll probably ask you a few questions along the way." He pulled the curtain all the way around the bed so that the three of them were enclosed together. Ray McBride pulled his chair back to the foot of the bed, sat back down, and appeared to go to sleep.

Simmons started up at the top and worked his way south. He could see that Carol McBride had lost weight. She had some gum disease and a rotten molar. Maybe the weight loss was from her dental problems, maybe not. She couldn't sit up and he didn't want to raise the bed and cause her pain, so instead of listening to her lungs all over her upper back, he had her take a couple of deep breaths while he auscultated on the sides. Even the deep breaths caused involuntary groans.

When he slid the head of his stethoscope under her gown to listen to her heart, he overshot and bumped into something hard. Leaving the stethoscope head on her abdomen, he felt for the hard lump again. It was in the lower inner quadrant of her left breast. As soon as he felt it, Simmons knew he'd found the unifying diagnosis.

"How long have you had the lump in your breast, Ma'am?" Out of the corner of his eye he saw the curtain at the foot of the bed rustle, first one way, then the other. He knew the first was Roger leaving and the second Jenny coming in with some morphine for the tib-fib guy.

"There was a tiny bump there last February. I think I noticed it the first time right around Valentine's Day." She closed her eyes. Next door, a couple of x-ray techs wheeled the gurney out from Room 9 for some films. Simmons, still bent over, reached into her left armpit. Sure enough, a compact mound of hard lymph nodes.

He listened to her heart, determined that her liver and spleen were not grossly enlarged; a large mass in her lower abdomen turned out to be a distended bladder. He carefully palpated her spinal column to locate the source of her back pain. There it was, a deformed bulge, right in the midline at about T-10. That clinched it.

"When was the last time you were able to sit up or move your legs?"

"I've slept so badly my head is all confused. I think it was the day before yesterday. It's been about four days since I could get out of bed on my own. Ray's been carrying me to the bathroom and back. Doctor, I haven't been able to urinate since yesterday morning."

"Yes Ma'am. Jenny will be in with a catheter in a few minutes. That will empty your bladder. We'll leave it in so you don't have to get up to go." He pulled out his reflex hammer. No deep tendon reflexes in the knees or ankles. As he smoothed out her gown and pulled the cover sheet back up to her chin, Ray McBride woke up.

Simmons slid by his chair. "I'm going to go out and write a few orders, call a consultant and put in an order for a bed."

Ray looked up. "What did you find, David?"

"Give me a few minutes to get things going so you don't have to spend all night down here, then I'll be back and we can talk about what's going to happen."

As he walked out, McBride asked, "Is it okay if I stay with Carol tonight?"

"Absolutely. I'll see you both in a few minutes."

Simmons went out to his desk and dictated the H & P. He wrote a few orders, then put the chart in the unit secretary's rack. While he was on the phone with the on-call neurosurgeon, Jenny came over to his desk with a Foley catheter kit. She raised her eyebrows and Simmons nodded. After one more call, this time to a radiation oncologist, he headed back to Bay 10. The x-ray techs were just finishing up a few films on Carol McBride, a portable chest and an AP and cross-table lateral of her T-spine. Jenny had put in the Foley catheter. Mrs. McBride's bag held 800 cc. of dark yellow urine. Just as they left with the portable x-ray machine, before he could pull up a chair, a large red-faced man holding a Bible pushed his way around Ray's chair to Bay 9. As expected, he was a loud talker. Simmons, wanting to keep the McBrides' anxiety down to as manageable a level as possible, placed his chair up by Carol's head and motioned for Ray to do the same on the opposite side. There was no use trying to talk over the loud guy, so David kept his voice to a whisper. Their three heads were huddled together.

"Mrs. McBride, I want to ask you something. What kept you from seeing someone for that lump in your breast the past ten months?" Ray looked at her, hope in his eyes and despair in the set of his mouth.

"We tried a couple of times to go to Planned Parenthood, but the protesters, they were so loud and vulgar. They threw blood on a young girl. The TV people seemed to be out there every day, and, well, Mrs. Rascon and Mrs. Treadwell, they're both very religious. I didn't want them to see me on TV. I didn't want to embarrass them or the other ladies they have over for Bible study on Thursdays."

Ray spoke up softly. "The last time we went, there was this young guy with a bullhorn. He was on an elevated stage, kind of a scaffold, next door, up about ten feet, yelling at anyone who tried to go inside. People were pushing each other. It was crazy. A preacher fellow was screaming at the women who were trying to get through the crowd of protesters. The cops, they weren't doing much to help, just making sure nobody got too rough. Carol, like she said, she didn't want to end up on TV, get fired for trying to get a mammogram."

Simmons winced inside and hoped it didn't register on his face. "So what about AHCCCS?" That was Arizona's brand of Medicaid. Next door, the Bible guy was reading out loud. Simmons was tempted to tell him to lower the volume, but figured the best thing to do was to keep the McBrides occupied until they left the E.R.

Ray laughed bitterly. "Between the two of us, we make too much. My buddy offered to pay me under the table, but I thought that wasn't the way to go. Now I wish I'd let him."

The big florid man walked by into the hallway and started barking at one of the nurses. Carol grabbed Ray's hand. She whispered, "Honey, that's the preacher from the Planned Parenthood protest." Both Simmons and McBride sat up straight. Ray pulled the curtain aside and looked at the tib-fib guy. He shook his head and turned back.

"Yup, that's the one from the stage. He must have fallen off or it collapsed. Such sloppy construction, I knew that thing wasn't worth a damn."

"Mrs. McBride, they're going to take you over to get a cat scan of your spine, then you're going up to the ICU for the night. At some point you'll go down to get an MRI. A neurosurgeon, Dr. Toth, will be in later to see you upstairs. I'll be honest with you. I think the lump in your breast is a cancer, and it's spread to your spine. That's why you hurt so badly back there. He's going to look at your cat scan and decide whether you need surgery or radiation. I don't know if either will help with your legs, but it should help the pain. I'm off tomorrow, but I have a meeting here, so I'll stop by mid-morning, see how you're doing."

Just then the CT techs walked in. The large red-faced man pushed around them and ended up back in Bay 9, on the other side of the curtain, right behind Ray. He lowered the bedrail on that side, all the while talking loudly. After the techs left with Carol, Ray stood, then slumped back in his chair, discouraged and devoid of the smallest kernel of energy. Simmons extended his hand. "Good luck, Ray. Jenny will show you how to get up to the ICU. Your wife should be up there inside a half-hour. I gotta get home, I'm beat." They shook hands.

Ray summoned what little he had left. "Thanks, David. Thanks for everything." Suddenly he stood up, moved his chair to the side, and took two steps back, fast and hard. The bulge of the preacher disappeared from the curtain. He let out a yell, which was quickly followed by a loud scream from the tib-fib patient. Ray McBride smiled for the first time and walked out into the hallway.

48. HEALTH INSURANCE

Accident insurance was first offered in 1850 by the Franklin Health Assurance Company of Massachusetts. It provided insurance against injuries sustained in steamboat and railroad accidents. Insurance for illness dates from about 1890. The first employer-based disability policy was offered in 1911, to cover lost wages but not to cover medical expenses. In the 1920s, hospitals began offering coverage for medical expenses to individuals on a pre-paid basis, which led to the development of the Blue Cross systems in the 1930s. The first employer-sponsored plan for hospital services was developed for teachers in Dallas. Similar to modern HMOs, it covered them for all hospital expenses, but only at a single hospital.

At the same time that it was developing the Social Security system, the Roosevelt administration looked into the possibility of a national health insurance system, but opposition from the American Medical Association caused them to drop the idea.

During World War II, the government froze wages and prices. This, along with increased demand for goods and a decreased supply of workers, caused a shortage of labor. Although industry could not attract workers with higher wages, once the government declared that fringe benefits fell outside the wage freeze, employers offered sick leave and health insurance to increase their work forces.

In 1945, President Truman proposed a national health insurance system. Participants would pay a monthly premium to the government. During time of illness, the government would reimburse physicians and hospitals who participated in the plan and would provide cash payments to participants to cover lost wages. Although the public favored the plan, the American Hospital Association, the American Medical Association and the U.S. Chamber of Commerce all opposed the plan as socialistic. In the meantime, labor unions sought and gained employer-sponsored health care plans, which allowed industry to attract more and better workers. Because of the opposition from powerful special interest lobbying groups and the growth of employer-sponsored health plans, the national health insurance program never made it through Congress. Once the private sector offered health insurance, the public sector followed suit in order to attract the best employees. By 1960, three-quarters of all Americans had some form of health insurance.

Despite widespread coverage for employees, the poor and the elderly were not well-insured in the early 1960s. Before the passage of Medicare, only half of all seniors had any form of health insurance, and, despite lower incomes, paid two to three times as much as younger Americans. In 1965, President Johnson signed into law the Medicare and Medicaid programs. Soon Medicare was expanded to include dialysis for end-stage renal disease. Other chronic disabilities were also covered.

In the 1970s Sen. Kennedy proposed a universal single-payer system of health insurance but it was opposed by President Nixon, who wanted to encourage greater employer-sponsored coverage for employees through mandates and incentives. It came down to a debate between government-sponsored universal insurance vs. expansion of private sector coverage. Although there existed a great clamor for providing insurance for workers who could not afford coverage, the proposal died out without compromise or passage.

In his first term, President Clinton proposed a universal health insurance plan, which mandated that all Americans and all insurers participate; subsidies would be provided for those who could not afford the premiums. In order to spread the risk, the plan also included health-purchasing alliances, which would involve clusters of businesses and large groups of individuals. The insurance industry and employers' groups strongly opposed the plan. Because of this opposition, as well as that of the labor unions, who preferred a single-payer system, the proposal failed when the Republicans won control of Congress in the 1994 elections.

When President Obama took office in 2009, his administration made universal health insurance a top priority. His Patient Protection and Affordable Care Act, which followed in the footsteps of the Nixon and Clinton plans, mandated participation by all employers and all individuals and penalized those who failed to comply. In addition, it provided for individuals to buy insurance collectively to spread the risk. A public sector option, which would compete with the private sector insurers to cover those without employer-sponsored insurance, was strongly opposed by moderate Democrats and was therefore left out to assure passage. Given the majority that Democrats held in both houses of Congress, the bill passed easily, although not a single Republican voted for it. Since its passage in December, 2009, Congress has held a vote to repeal the PPACA six times and voted to defund or delay portions of it more than fifty times.

Health insurance is basically betting that you are going to get sick. Your health insurer is betting, with your money, that you won't fall victim to some chronic disease or an expensive acute illness or injury. Even though you are betting on illness, you don't want to get sick. So, in effect, you are betting hundreds of dollars per month and hoping you don't win the bet.

Right up until you are diagnosed with a serious illness, you can delude yourself into believing that your health insurer cares about you and your health. You pay your monthly premium; two weeks later you get a nice thin envelope in the mail. It contains another statement with the notation, "Payment Received--Thank you." You think, *They're so polite, this system is terrific. I couldn't be happier with my health insurer.* They bill, you pay. In some part of your brain, the wishful lobe to be exact, you have the notion that as long as you keep paying, you won't get sick. On that point you and your insurer have your fingers mutually crossed. It's almost like paying protection money to the mob.

Inside your head, a sweet female voice, Polly Purebred, tells you, "Keep paying your premiums on time, don't get sick, and everything will be just fine." In other words, give us your money, which we shall cheerfully accept, don't bother us, and we won't bother you.

Once you get sick, however, the delusion is shattered. Gone is the sweet young thing cooing inside your head. You start to get thicker, more menacing envelopes from your insurer. Now the voice inside your head is Boris Badenov. You can smell the stale vodka and caviar on his breath as he shouts out the only reasonably good news you will hear from this day forward, "THIS IS NOT A BILL!" His three-day-old beard rasps against the inside of your skull. The sound and the smell only worsen when you receive your first denial of payment, a decision quite possibly made by a high school dropout with an inseam IQ, that your lifesaving diagnostic or treatment procedures are not considered worthy of payment by your insurer.

Yes, everything is nice and friendly, right up to the time you go to your doctor with a new symptom. Right at that moment, before you undergo expensive surgery or medical treatment, before you undergo a single test, before you even have a diagnosis, your health insurer would be perfectly happy if you dropped dead in your tracks. You think, *But wait. What about all the ads in the media, all the "honored to serve" and "here for you"? Isn't any of that true? Of course it is. Health insurance companies are in business solely to help me, to save my life, to make my world a healthier, happier place. They have no interest in making a profit. Why would they?* That, my friend, is your brain's wishful lobe talking.

All the delays in authorization, all the requests for records, all the hoops you and your doctor have to jump through to get anything done, these are nothing more than their standard stall tactics, hoping you either get well on your own or die before they have to shell out. The former would be preferable, because then you can return to work and go on paying your monthly premiums. That sweet little Polly Purebred voice returns and it's back to business as usual. If that doesn't work out, well, the latter, sudden death, is much preferable to treating you for a chronic, expensive illness. If you die before you cost them too much, your survivors might even get a condolence card in the mail. So sorry your loved one passed away. We are here for you and honored to serve. Because we care.

I wish I had an answer for you when you ask, "How do I get my insurance company to pay my medical bills?" You would think that, having received your premiums on a monthly basis for years, your insurer would be glad to honor their side of the agreement. Not a chance. After discussing the ins and outs of the health insurance industry with people in the know, I can only repeat what I was told time and again. Never give up. Never stop harassing them when they deny payment. As soon as a denial arrives, fire off a letter of appeal. As soon as the denial of appeal arrives, fire off another. Each time you send a letter, call them as well and ask to speak to a supervisor. Keep going up the chain. That is your Obi-Wan Kenobi, your only hope. Sometimes it works, often it does not. Unfortunately, the bills start rolling in about thirty days after your surgery, when you are anything but ready to take on a business behemoth. The last thing you want to do is address conflict. However, if you don't, they will stab you wherever and whenever they can. That is who they are. Boris Badenov with a rusty ice pick.

Say what you want about Obamacare, it has eliminated that pre-existing illness crap. It is far from perfect, but we in the medical profession, hospitals and insurance companies have had this uninsured worker issue hanging over our collective heads for fifty years, and it was not getting any better. It is fascinating that, in over fifty votes to partially or completely overturn Obamacare, not one Republican congressman has come up with a workable, realistic alternative. Perhaps because there isn't one that all parties will accept.

If you remove Obamacare, you are back to where we were five years ago. If you are a member of the upper middle class with great health insurance, or you work for a branch of the government or a large corporation with great benefits, or you are on Medicaid or Medicare, you probably don't give a rat's ass about the upside of Obamacare and you would be perfectly happy to return to the good old days.

Unfortunately, that isn't going to happen. You have to start somewhere, and that's what this is. A start.

The ACOs, Accountable Care Organizations, are groups of doctors, hospitals and other health care providers who come together voluntarily to provide quality health care to their patients. Initially designed solely for Medicare and Medicaid patients, if the idea succeeds in providing improved quality of care while lowering costs, eventually it will be extended to those with private insurance as well. Physicians in private practice joined in droves, usually an ACO run by a local hospital, so that they wouldn't lose access to new and existing patients. Any time you are forced to either join an organization or go out of business, odds are you won't be happy down the road, especially when that organization's primary purpose is to save money, which really means paying you less money for your services. So, unless you are perched at or near the top of the pyramid, physicians should plan on working more for less money and not count on sympathy from the public.

There are those who feel that a universal single-payer system is inevitable. Perhaps they are correct, but when they cite England and Canada as examples that work, take a closer look. There are lots of Canadian physicians who work in the U.S. I doubt the reverse is true. Canadian expatriate doctors bemoan the multiple-payer system here and routinely sing the praises of the simplicity of the system back home. About fifteen years ago, I was discussing the topic with a colleague from Canada.

"So it's simpler in Canada?"

"Gosh, yes. No pre-authorization needed, you just show up, show them your card, and they take care of you. No bills in the mail afterwards, either, eh?"

"So if it's such a great system, how come so many Canadian docs come south to work."

"Because the system is going broke."

Another time he told me a story. He was doing a surgery residency, and was spending a couple months on the TCV surgery team. He heard that a friend's dad was in the hospital for chest pain. His diagnosis was unstable angina. Apparently the man had been sitting in a university hospital bed for two weeks waiting to have bypass surgery. There just wasn't any room on the O.R. schedule. My colleague asked the chief resident if they could go by and see how he was doing. When they arrived, the man was having chest pain, obviously in the throes of an MI. They took him to the O.R., bypassed him and saved his life. Had they not stopped by, he would most certainly have had an MI and possibly died.

Can anyone see that happening to an American in an American hospital, sitting around for two weeks with unstable angina? First of all, no insurance company or Medicare or Medicaid would allow a patient to languish in an expensive hospital. The hospital and physicians would soon be deleted from that insurer's list of providers. Secondly, it is just plain bad medicine to make a patient wait when lifesaving technology is available. This scenario is a lawsuit waiting to happen. Thirdly, O.R.s run when physicians want to operate, no matter what the time of day. An emergency is just that. Except in government hospitals, it doesn't come second after the preferences of the government employees working there. We Americans are used to having the best we can afford. With health insurance, everyone should be able to expect top-of-the-line care in a timely fashion. There is a significant portion of the American public crowing for single-payer health insurance. Be aware that it comes with consequences, not all of which are top-shelf.

As obstructive and silly as the Republicans have been about Obamacare, the Democrats and the Obama administration itself have been equally disappointing. It appears that once the website hurdle was "overcome"--if you've visited the Obamacare website recently and tried to enroll, that word will either make you howl with laughter or cry your eyes out-- that was pretty much the end of the White House tinkering with the system. There are numerous areas where the PPACA could be improved, be it through congressional bills or executive orders. For instance, why must all those insured have to carry obstetrical insurance? A fifty-eight-year-old woman is not going to have a baby, nor is a seventy-year-old man, the late Tony Randall notwithstanding. While some think the solution is to throw the whole thing out and start over, they have yet to convince the U.S. Supreme Court. It will be a difficult sell in Congress, even with the Republicans holding a majority in both chambers. One thing is for certain. If and when Obamacare is repealed, the insurance industry will throw every lobby buck they have at Congress to make sure that nothing comes down the pike to assist the poor and the uninsured worker. The fact that health insurance in the wealthiest nation on earth has become a political football speaks volumes about our priorities.

There are a few things I foresee. This is the only country on earth where health insurance is intimately tethered to employment. Eventually, that will change. Second, sooner or later there will be changes to the system that significantly slow the growth rate of the cost of medical care. As the establishment of ACOs for Medicare and Medicaid demonstrates, even the government realizes it has to do something to stem the ever-upward spiral of costs. In order for that to happen, however, the government will have to fund the National Institutes of Health and the Agency for Health Research and Quality. Without these two agencies directing research into improving care and lowering costs, expenditures will continue to move north, eventually bankrupting Medicare and Medicaid. That is my expert opinion. Anybody want to buy an icehouse?

49. NIGHT MOVES

"How long are we going to be at the hospital?"

"Not too long. I'm coming home after a while. You get to stay with some other kids tonight, then you come home tomorrow."

"I don't want to stay overnight. I want to come home with you."

"Don't worry. It'll be fun. All the kids there will be just like you."

"Oh." *Like me how?* he wondered.

"Why are we going to the hospital?"

"Because you have all these strep throats. The doctor is going to take out your tonsils, and that will make everything better."

"I had a lot of strip throats?" Murphy imagined red strips up and down his neck. He couldn't remember seeing that in the mirror. More importantly, he couldn't remember his sister making fun of him for having them.

"Strep throats. It's when you get a fever and your throat gets sore and you have swollen glands. You've had a few the last few years. This will keep you from getting any more."

"I promise I won't get any more strip, I mean strep throats if we just go home."

"It will be okay, Robbie."

They drove in silence for a bit, heading into downtown in the car. Murphy had no idea what a hospital was, but if they were going to keep him there all night, he knew it was a bad place. On TV, people were kept in places all alone overnight. In places called jails. And he knew it wasn't going to be okay.

"Is it going to hurt to take out my tonsils?"

"No. You'll be asleep. You won't feel a thing."

"Maybe I can take a nap when we get there and they can take out my tonsils while I'm asleep, then I can come home with you. I promise not to wake up."

"No, they have to do them in the morning. They give you something to make you sleep."

"A SHOT?" He had imagined that the procedure involved a screwdriver, a pair of pliers, and, of course, a hammer. Just like when Murphy Sr. "fixed" something. He didn't see how a shot could help.

"No. They give you a mask to wear, and you breathe in through the mask. Then you go to sleep."

"Does that hurt?"

"All these questions, Robbie. No, it doesn't hurt. It's a mask like Uncle Tim wears in his plane." Uncle Tim was a pilot for the Air Force, and whenever there was a pilot on TV talking into his mask, it was fun to pretend it was him.

"Did you or Daddy have your tonsils out?"

"No and neither did Margie." Mrs. Murphy was starting to anticipate, deluding herself into thinking that he might run out of questions.

"How come I'm the only one who has to have my tonsils out?" Robert was betting his sister had blamed him for something and thus it was determined that he get punished with a tonsillectomy.

"Here we are. Let's go, Robert."

The hospital was low-slung, grey and scary. Perfect for the blue-collar section of a growing industrial city in the '50s. Inside, they walked over to an area where an old lady sat. She pointed in the direction of the admitting office. After Mrs. Murphy signed a few papers, the cheerful young lady behind the desk picked up a phone and dialed. She chatted a bit, laughed, then said, "The last one is here." She put down the phone and smiled at Murphy. He was terrified. *The last one.*

"Hi, Robert. I'm Nurse Allen."

"Hi." There had been not one iota of support from Murphy's mother for any of his alternate plans, so, at least for the time being, he had decided to take the high road. A box of Kleenex on the desk reinforced him, as he thought of all those who had gone before him in a veil of tears, never to return home. Murphy gritted his teeth and, with dry eyeball sockets, followed Nurse Allen and his mother to his room.

"This is your room, Robert. You'll be staying here with three other boys tonight, and this is where your mom and dad can pick you up tomorrow afternoon." As Nurse Allen opened a drawer in the bureau, he looked around. Nowadays this setup is generally referred to as a "swamp", four beds and four bedside tables.

For some reason, he had brought a suitcase. Boxy, brown and constructed of the finest of cardboards, it contained a toothbrush. In the modern era, the first thing you do after recovering from strep throat is throw away your old toothbrush and buy a new one, but this was before you could go to Costco and buy a lifetime supply of toothbrushes for a dollar. In the '50s, people replaced toothbrushes less often than shoes. There was a tube of toothpaste, a pair of pajamas, and slippers.

Nurse Allen put his stuff into the drawer of a bedside stand and slid the suitcase under the bed nearest the door. Murphy was silently overjoyed with her choice of accommodations for him, as a plan was forming in his head. No inventory of your personal possessions like in the movies when you get out of jail or in modern-day hospitals. This was before surgeons started cutting off the good leg or removing the wrong kidney. It was a simpler time.

After a word of reassurance from Nurse Allen, Mrs. Murphy left to go home. Robert wasn't bothered by her departure, as he no longer saw her as an ally. He knew there was no way he could count on her to help spirit him away from the hospital in the trunk of the car. They had a station wagon.

In the movies, once the parents leave, the sweet nurse or teacher or headmistress turns into an unrepentant sadist bent on revenge for the death of her good twin. Nurse Allen continued with her kindly nurturing ways, thus arousing his suspicion even more. Murphy vowed not to sleep a wink.

Dinner was an early, mushy affair. The plops on the plate tasted vaguely familiar, but Murphy was unable to put a name to them. He imagined large vats in the hospital kitchen labeled "Meat", "Vegetables", and "Something Else". After dinner he and about a dozen other kids, all boys, sat on the floor in the dayroom and watched TV for a while. When a bell rang somewhere outside the dayroom, Nurse Allen came in and rounded everyone up. Murphy walked to his room and climbed into bed. Three other boys did likewise. After a bit, Nurse Allen came back in, arranged the sheets on each boy, and raised the side rails. To Murphy, the click of the rails sounded like the hammer being pulled back on a Colt .45.

"Nurse Allen, what time do we get up?"

"Your mother warned me about your questions, Robbie." She smiled. Murphy wondered if she had a knife concealed in her uniform. "Nurse Jenkins will be in to get you at 6:00 sharp, so you must get some sleep. You have a big day ahead of you." Again with the smile. Murphy wondered why he had to sleep if he was going to be asleep for the surgery. Then he realized the import of what she was saying. His eyebrows shot up into the Arch of Fear.

"You won't be here tomorrow morning?" Just when he was getting used to her. Another grownup deserting him. She rubbed his forehead and shook her head.

"No, Robbie, I have to go home to my family. Nurse Jenkins will be here at 11 P.M. I'll be back before you go home tomorrow." *As if*, he thought, *there is any chance I'll be here tomorrow.* The bed rail snicked shut.

"Okay. Thanks."

"Good night, Robbie. I'll see you tomorrow afternoon."

"Good night."

Murphy had always been a light sleeper, a trait that would torment him on a regular basis throughout his life but, on at least one occasion, keep him from prematurely entering the afterlife. He woke up when the 11:00 P.M. bell rang to signal the change of shift from swing to graveyard. It took a minute or two to orient. Apparently one of the vats in the hospital kitchen should have been labeled "Something Else + Chloral Hydrate". He was drowsy, slightly nauseated, and, when he crawled over the side rails, unable to land like a cat. The thump shot up from his butt to his neck, and he thought the smack on the tile would wake up everyone in the hospital. He could hear three separate sets of snores from the other victims. *You poor devils*, he thought. *I'll be praying for you at Holy Redeemer this Sunday.*

In later years, Murphy would never enter a building that contained potential dangers without first scoping out the various escape routes. Still a novice at age five, he was naive enough to believe that his only way out was through the front door. He considered donning his slippers, but knew that the noise might attract Nurse Jenkins, whom he believed to be the only adult in the hospital that night, she and Nurse Allen taking turns running the hospital every single day. He got down on hands and knees, stealthily crawled to the doorway, and peered around.

The hallway was bathed in dim light. Up the hallway to the right he could see a counter which was more brightly lit. He heard a woman's voice. From the cadence, he surmised she was talking on the phone. Probably with Nurse Allen, giving a report on him or planning the hospital meal vats for tomorrow. Women liked to talk about food.

Once engaged in phone conversation, he knew that women could talk for hours about anything and everything. It was a good time for a guy to do things he'd normally get in trouble for.

He turned and looked down the hallway to the left. Murphy remembered three or four doors on this hall between his room and the lobby. He started feeling sleepy again, but shook his head like a guy on TV who got cold-cocked with a rifle butt and started crawling down the hall to his left. His palms squeaked a few times, and he stopped and looked back. Nurse Jenkins was still discussing meal plans. Gritting his teeth, Robbie continued on down the hall until he reached the lobby.

From behind a potted plant, Murphy surveyed the huge expanse. There were clusters of chairs and a sofa set around a coffee table directly ahead, along the left side of the lobby. To the right he saw another hallway. *Probably goes to Nurse Allen's house*, he thought. Diagonally across to the right was the set of huge glass doors, and just to the right of them was a desk with an overhead light shining brightly. He crawled as fast as he could to the coffee table and hid behind it. The couch, a nubby brown example of late-'50s non-New York chic, beckoned to him. *Come, Robbie. Come take a nice little nap*, it said. *Wow!* he thought. *A talking couch.*

"I have to get out of here," he said aloud to the couch. "I have to get home." He double-gritted his teeth, pushing the loose one outward, shook his head again, and stood up. Before he knew it, he was running as fast as he could for the front doors. There was the scraping of a chair and movement to his right, from behind the desk. His conversation with the nubby couch had not gone unnoticed.

When he was less than ten feet from the glass doors, a big policeman in blue slid out from behind the desk and blocked his path. Murphy tried to slow down, then made a push to slide between his legs. The cop laughed and picked him up off the ground effortlessly. He held Murphy out at arm's length and examined him with a quizzical look.

"If you're going to escape, you have to be quiet." He laughed again, then looked over toward the coffee table. Still holding Murphy straight out, he walked over that way and checked behind the couch. "Who were you talking to over here? You don't by any chance have a fellow escapee, do you?"

Without hesitation, Robbie blurted out, "That sofa." He looked over at the brown nubby accusingly. Ratted out by a piece of furniture.

"So you found the little Houdini, eh, Tom?" Murphy heard shoes and a swishing noise coming up behind him. Flap, swish. Flap, swish.

"What's he in for?" Just like in jail.

"T & A at 7A.M." Murphy felt himself grabbed firmly around the waist from behind. He smelled lavender and Chesterfields as he was pulled backward and down toward a thick, warm, female body. The cop laughed again and let go. Murphy liked the cop, and he had a feeling he was in for a dose of reprimand from whoever had hold of him, presumably Nurse Jenkins. He wondered if nurses were allowed to administer spankings.

"Son, what's your name?" The cop reached over and squeezed his shoulder.

"Robertson Wetherill Murphy." Robbie gave the cop his cheesiest smile. A new plan was forming in his brain. Desperation was winning out over the chloral hydrate.

"Master Murphy, thank you. You made my evening. First escape attempt ever, thwarted by yours truly, Officer Daniel James Killeen. Should earn me a plaque over by the foyer." He reached out and shook Murphy's hand. "Don't worry, son. Hundreds of lads like yourself have their tonsils out every year, and every one of them does just fine and goes home the next day."

"We'll be heading back to our room now, Dan. Thank you." As she and Murphy turned, he gave it his best shot.

"Officer Killeen, I could stay out here with you tonight."

"Ha, Master Robert. Would that I could, son. I'm sure you could keep me fascinated all night with your tales of derring-do. Sadly, I'll be going home just as soon as my replacement shows up." He looked at his pocket watch, then at Nurse Jenkins."

"Oh, dear," she sighed. "Not again."

"He'll be along soon enough, Alice. Probably just overslept a bit."

"And we both know why, don't we, Dan?"

"Your brother is just having a bit of a rough stretch. He'll be fine. He's a good man."

Nurse Jenkins put Murphy down, but held onto his hand, and they walked back to the ward. He looked over his shoulder and waved to Killeen, wondering what constituted a rough stretch. Maybe something like a T & A at 7 A.M.

On the way down the hall to his room, Murphy became aware of the "Flap, swish" noise again. He stole a glance over at Nurse Jenkins legs and feet and realized the first sound was her shoe hitting the floor and the second was the sound of her white stockings rubbing against one another. He tried to look away but just couldn't.

When they reached the swamp, Nurse Jenkins hoisted him up effortlessly into his bed. While he was still getting used to being tossed around by big people, she pulled a white roll from her white uniform pocket and began wrapping tape back and forth across the top of the bed rails. It was pretty clear to Murphy that, whether he was truly the first captured escapee or not, Nurse Jenkins had aced the web weaving class at Black Widow school. Satisfied that he wouldn't receive a scolding or ear pull, he drifted off to sleep in his white cocoon.

A rattling in the hallway gradually brought Robbie awake. His three roommates walked past him. One of them, a boy of about six with glasses, eyed him curiously. He scrambled down to the bottom of his cage, from where he could see a double-decker steel cart just outside the door. Nurse Jenkins held the cart still while they climbed on to the top shelf. Then she came into the room and went to work on Murphy's web. In no time at all, the tape was wrapped up into a neat roll, which she stuck in her uniform pocket. Without a word, she walked back to the cart. At this point, there were four boys on top, all of them yawning and eyeing him slothfully. Murphy climbed up and over the side rail, and scooted over to the cart. He looked at the boys, then at Nurse Jenkins, who inclined her head and pointed at the bottom shelf. Burning with embarrassment, he climbed into the lower shelf space, and off they went to the operating room, Nurse Jenkins flapping and swishing her way ahead of the cart.

At the door to the OR, Nurse Jenkins stopped. Murphy peered out at her white stockings. He looked up. She was pointing toward the OR, staring straight ahead, silent. It gave him the willies. Obviously she was not a morning person.

To Murphy's surprise, there were about a dozen identical cots on wheels. All but five had kids lying on them. Some stared straight up at the ceiling while others raised their heads and looked over at the newcomers.

"Heads down." The voice came over a loudspeaker, sounding to Murphy like a robot from *The Twilight Zone*, which always gave him nightmares. A nurse walked over and helped the five climb up onto skinny tables. Murphy's had a placard at the foot with the number 7 printed on it. Sitting up on the table, he looked ahead into a large window with a dim light behind it. He could vaguely make out a head with a white nurse's cap sitting at a desk, holding what looked like a silver banana. Then he lay back.

"Boys," came the voice. It occurred to Murphy that, other than the three nurses, he hadn't seen any females since he arrived the day before. *Don't girls have tonsils?*, he wondered. "Nurse Berardi is going to put a mask over your face. It will smell a little funny, but I want you to breathe nice and slowly." A hand holding a mask hovered over his face. He took a few deep breaths and then he was gone.

He awoke with a start and tried to sit up. A voice droned, "Seven is up." *Seven-Up,* he thought. *Someone was going to get me chocolate ice cream and Seven-Up. A float.* His head hurt. Something else didn't feel right. A mask appeared, but this time it was jammed down over his face. He was gone again.

When Robbie awoke again, he was lying in his bed, his head propped up on pillows. There was no white tape to be seen. Mrs. Murphy and his sister were sitting in chairs next to the bed. Nurse Allen appeared over him, again with the smile. He thought, *The joke's on you, Nurse Allen. I'm getting out of here, but you have to stay.* Now his head and his throat hurt. It really hurt to swallow. *I bet a 7-Up float with chocolate ice cream would sure help my throat. Probably would make my head feel better too.*

"Robbie, you're finally awake! You've been sleeping so long I thought we might have to keep you overnight again. I'm sure Nurse Jenkins would love to have you." That made him sit up in a panic. He tried to speak, but his throat felt like it was glued shut, and no words came out. *Oh no, I'm ready to go home.*

Nurse Allen checked his pulse, felt his forehead, and then turned to Robbie's mother. "Robbie has been very busy since you left him here last night. He got to meet the night watchman, took a tour of the hospital, and slept in Nurse Jenkins' cocoon of tape. Then in the operating room he woke up early and got a double dose of anesthetic for his efforts." She turned back to Robbie. "All the other boys have gone home. I guess it's time for you to go too." With that she lowered the bed rail with a now-reassuring snick.

A little wobbly, he climbed down. He got into his clothes and the four of them walked out together to the front door. He shook hands with Officer Killeen and said good-bye to Nurse Allen. Moments later, he was fast asleep in the back seat of their station wagon, headed home.

50. GOING TO THE HOSPITAL

As an adult heading to the hospital for elective bypass surgery, most likely your mommy will not drive you in the family station wagon. However, since you'll be in for a number of days, it's probably a good idea to leave your car at home. Parking at hospitals tends to be scarce and pricey, and you will not be allowed to drive home anyway. If you know someone who drives well, it would be a good idea to ask them to drive you. Avoid bad drivers. Nothing is more embarrassing than showing up on a backboard in the E.R. after a car wreck, claiming that you're supposed to be admitted for bypass surgery. People will laugh at you, call you "Lucky".

Unlike young Murphy, usually you'll have an opportunity to ask all your questions before you arrive at the hospital. Some hospitals have a patient representative who will contact you a day or two before your admission. Some cardiac surgeons have a nurse or physician's assistant who routinely sits down with you and goes over the plan of attack. Often you will sign the consent forms at this time. If you are advised to bring ID and a credit card or checkbook with you, prepare to spend a little non-refundable earnest money. It's called a co-payment or a deductible or something. The mob should have it so good.

If you are having emergency surgery, most likely you are going straight from the cath lab to the O.R., so any decisions about your automobile are irrelevant. If by some strange turn of event your car is already parked there, just let the staff know; they'll have hospital security keep an eye peeled until someone can retrieve it. Postoperatively, you really don't want to have to worry about getting your car out of the impound lot. Arriving in a Winnebago, and that has happened more than once, will be more problematic.

There are a number of things you should not bring with you to the hospital. It may seem silly even to mention them, but guys have brought them before and guys will bring them in the future. Just make sure you aren't one of them.

No guns. Even if you are an internationally famous and wealthy celebrity, nobody is going to kidnap you or rob you. You will not have to shoot your way out, either. At least not here. In Russia or Venezuela, that's another matter entirely.

No booze, not even your trusty travel flask. If you need a drink that badly, let the staff know and they will give you meds to keep you from dancing the Dirty Frog with the little green men. If that fails, your doctor can write for beer or liquor once your surgery is done. Believe it or not, if you develop severe alcohol withdrawal, you can actually be served IV alcohol intravenously. Your highway to heaven.

No cigarettes. In case you just woke up from a long nap, Rip, smoking is no longer permitted in the hospital. Or anyplace else, for that matter. Somewhere down the line you might be permitted to smoke outside the hospital, but that won't happen until you are out of the CCU. Just ask and your physician will be glad to write for a nicotine patch.

No prescription meds unless you are in a research study. The hospital will provide you with whatever you are supposed to take on a regular basis.

No illegal drugs. Leave all bongs, crack pipes and works at home.

No vibrators, dildos or sex toys of any type. Only hospital-issue devices are permitted. If you really need one, someone can go down to the gift shop and get one for you. In some hospitals, the pink ladies come around with a cart full of goodies every morning.

No porn.

Don't bring your monogrammed gold lamé PJs and matching smoking jacket to the hospital. You can bring your lucky silver spaceman jammies, but don't expect to be able to sleep in them the first night or two, and you definitely can't wear them to the O.R. for the big event.

You can bring your cell phone, but leave the iPad, laptop and desktop at home. There won't be adequate space for your mini-Cray supercomputer.

No pets. You won't need Tippy, your "service dog". If your pet python Squeezer mysteriously shows up in your room, the hospital snake killer will make short work of him.

It is unlikely you will encounter the tape-on-the-bedrails maneuver, but every so often you may come across a guy handcuffed to the bed with a police officer nearby. Resist the urge to engage him in a philosophical discussion of the American legal system. The night before surgery can be as emotionally taxing for grownups as it is for kids. Guys will try to smoke in the bathroom, leave, hide in a closet ("Diane Sawyer! What the hell are you doing in here?"). These are not good alternative plans of action. In lieu of going AWOL, hit the call button and your nurse will gladly give you something to help you sleep. As a matter of fact, in terms of nervous anticipation, there is nothing wrong with taking a sleeping pill the moment you hit the bed and not waking up until after your surgery is completed.

Once you have gained access to the health care system, in particular, once you are hospitalized, and even more in particular, once you are hospitalized for heart disease, it really doesn't matter whether you are rich or poor, a celeb or a nobody, you should be receiving the same quality of care. Take comfort in the fact that you are just an average Joe, and thus are not an insider. When it comes to health care delivery, as a non-medical member of society, you are much less likely to have a bad outcome than is a health care provider or his family members. For the most part, you do not want to have special treatment. Blend in as much as possible. Your ass won't look any better than anybody else's hanging out the back of your gown. Unless, of course, you happen to be Cathy Lee Crosby, who apparently has "the best, absolutely the tightest, butt in New York City." Or did at one time.

These are a few suggestions that should seem obvious, but violations of each and every one of these have occurred and will continue to occur:

Do not play the "No Visitors" card. Odds are, if you think you need to go there, nobody wants to come see you anyway.

Do not use the phrase, "Well, I don't want to pull rank on you, but..."

Avoid answering phone calls when your nurse or doctor is in the room. For you, the only emergency phone call is the one your nurse makes to your doctor informing him that you are coding. If you think your phone call is truly an emergency, odds are you wouldn't know an emergency if it hit you in the face. Or shocked you in the chest.

From the cardiac surgeon to the nurses to your fellow patients, everybody in the hospital is on the same team. It's not the lions versus the Christians. If you are out and about in the wilds of the hallway, and someone needs help, help them out or get someone who can. You have a long recovery ahead of you, and you are going to need all the good karma you can muster.

51. DELUSIONS

Long cold grey tunnel. Big red boulder blocking the exit. Gotta move it, but I can't. Air's getting thin, it's harder to breathe. So tired, I have to lie down and sleep. And die. He stood there in the dark, looking down at his corpse, and felt nothing.

David Simmons awakened, oriented himself, and flicked on the bedside lamp. He reached for the marker, located the date on the calendar, and made an "X". That made three times in the past week. He lay in bed, savoring the luxurious comfort, until the alarm rang.

Sunday morning in August, Simmons's fourth weekend of day shifts in six weeks. He rose at 5:31, beating the sun by fifteen minutes. The temperature was already eighty-five degrees, headed for another monsoon seasonal one hundred five. He drank a couple cups of coffee, rinsed off in the pool and threw in a dozen laps. By 6:15 he was on his bike, backpack loaded with scrubs, his stethoscope and a delicious Fuji apple. The ride along the canal, mostly downhill, the rising sun at his back, was fast, warm and breezy. Dog walkers eyed him suspiciously as he sped by. A couple of Labs, one golden and one chocolate, dove off the path into the slow-moving green-grey water of the canal, of a single mind in their quest to retrieve a tennis ball slathered in drooly sand.

At the hospital, he took a quick shower in the on-call room, slid into his scrubs, chained the twelve-speed to the disability bar in the shower, and entered the E.R. right at 7 A.M. A fresh bike-and-coffee buzz hummed through every part of his body. David's partner for the day, Henry Alvarez, the early bird, had already picked up the cards on the players in the units and headed upstairs for rounds. The two night shift docs were awake and ready to go home. Karen Yamamoto was gathering up her stuff. Seth Emanuel handed off the three patients remaining from night shift.

"Bed 4's a guy with atypical chest pain, coming in for a rule out MI. He's been pain-free since he got here. EKG, chest x-ray and first set of enzymes are all normal. He should be going up in a few minutes. Bed 8 is a ninety-seven-year-old with uncontrolled A fib and belly pain. She's going to...", he looked past Simmons' shoulder, "nope, she's already in CT on her way up to the floor. Probably mesenteric ischemia. That new surgeon Hannebron will see her within the hour, decide whether to take her to the O.R. By the way, she is a full code. Bed 1 is a kid, fourteen, just came in with croup. Respiratory therapy's giving him back-to-back racemic epi SVN's and they're starting a line to give him some Decadron. Probably he'll turn around and go home."

"A fourteen month-old with croup is getting an IV?" Usually a shot of Decadron in the ass and a few breathing treatments was more than enough to fix a crouper.

"Nope. Fourteen year-old. No bark, but he has a little stridor. Fever of 105 too." An uneasy stirring in David's brain took him back to somewhere dark. *A little stridor.*

"Okay, I'll take care of him. Thanks."

"Thank you. See you tonight." Seth clapped David on the back and bolted. No doubt his wife was waiting out front. Seth was one of those hyperactive odd ducks who had to hike for an hour before he could fall asleep, even after a non-stop twelve-hour night shift. *Change-of-shift handoff,* Simmons thought, *as usual, the most perilous time of day for all parties concerned.* Simmons scribbled some orders on Bed 1's chart and handed it to the unit secretary.

"Good morning, Roberta."

"Hi, David. Whatcha got?"

"This is a sick one." Roberta sighed ever so slightly. Simmons was known for thinking everyone was going to die in the next ten seconds if his orders weren't processed immediately. Try as he might, it was impossible to modify his anal-retentive, control-every-aspect personality; he went over each order with her.

"I want two sets of blood cultures, the usual labs, and I have to speak with the ENT guy on call...", he looked up at the board, "is that today's call list?" Roberta nodded. "Okay, call Sherwood for me stat. That's priority number one." He walked over and looked at the kid in Bed 1. Skinny Asian teenager. Sitting straight up, breathing forty times a minute, shallow and retracting. For the most part, normal breathing requires an intact diaphragm and not much else. With respiratory difficulty, whether it be due to asthma, pneumonia, croup or any of a number of acute and chronic airway diseases, "accessory" chest and abdominal muscles help out, causing the intercostal (between the ribs) muscles to pull inward. David noticed he was holding a damp towel in his hand, so he pulled the SVN mask to the side. The kid was drooling. He put his stethoscope up to his neck and listened. Every time he inhaled, the scrawny teen's throat squeaked. Now there was a LOT of stridor. *Damn.*

Roberta paged him over the PA. "Dr. Simmons, I have Dr. Sherwood on 5501." Simmons picked up the nearest phone and punched the flashing light.

"Hi, Tom, this is Dave. Are you in-house? Oh, good. I've got a fourteen-year-old kid down here, just rolled in. Fever of 105, stridorous, drooling, breathing forty a minute." He listened for a minute. "Yeah, toxic looking. No, no bark. I'm thinking epiglottitis. We have a scope here. I'll get everything set up. Okay, see you in a few. Thanks." He ran in to talk with Bella, the day shift charge nurse.

"Bel, we have a bad one in Bed 1."

"The crouper?" She looked up from her computer, surprised.

"Fourteen-year-olds..." he caught himself. "I don't think he has croup, I think he's got acute epiglottitis. Dr. Sherwood's on his way down. Either the kid's going to get intubated nasally over a scope or we're going to be doing an emergency tracheostomy in Bed 1." He sounded more controlled than he felt. Or so he hoped. Croup, characterized by a barking cough and occasional stridor, resulted from a narrowing of the upper airway, the trachea, just below the epiglottis; it was a viral infection of infants and toddlers that rarely required anything more than exposure to cold air, some breathing treatments and oral or injected steroids. Epiglottitis, a bacterial infection in which the epiglottis, normally a thin flap, swells to five times its normal thickness and obstructs the patient's airway, was one of those rare emergencies where, no matter what you did and how well you did it, you could still lose a young, otherwise healthy patient in minutes.

"Would you rather I put him in the code room?"

"No, just leave him where he is. The less we move him around, the longer he'll be able to breathe on his own. And don't let anyone try to lower the head of the bed. This whole thing has to be done with him upright. Otherwise he'll either close off his airway completely or choke on his secretions. I'll grab the fiberoptic nasolaryngoscope; you bring the intubation cart over to Bed 1. Robbie, we'll need a consent form for the parents."

Bella was already on her way. She stopped and turned. "He came by ambulance. The parents aren't here, but an aunt is on her way."

"Okay, if the aunt doesn't get here in time, I'll sign the consent form. Nasolaryngoscopy with intubation and possible tracheostomy. Surgeon Sherwood. Oh yeah, page respiratory stat too." Simmons went into the back supply room, found the case with the nasolaryngoscope, and headed back to Bed 1. On his way, he noticed there were no new charts in the "To Be Seen" rack. *Thank God for small favors.*

Bella arrived with the steel intubation cart. On the lower shelf was the pump, one side for suction, the other to push air or oxygen, whatever was needed. On the top shelf was a plastic-covered sterile steel intubation tray, with a complete set of ET tubes, laryngoscopes, lube, topical lidocaine, and a plethora of weird forceps and clamps Simmons had never used. Sally, R.N.--that's how she answered the phone and referred to herself, "Sally, R.N."--arrived on the scene just as the patch phone rang.

Bella stepped back and said, "Sally, you assist Dave and Dr. Sherwood. I'll get the patch phone." She bolted for the communications area of the E.R. Simmons thought, *Right out of the blocks, like a sprinter.* Seeing her run, he realized everything was slowing down, the way it was supposed to. He turned to the kid in Bed 1 and shook his hand.

"Hi, I'm Dr. Simmons. Do you speak English?"

Before he replied, the kid lifted his mask and spit a small pond of saliva into his towel. A squeaky voice said, "Of course". *So something good did come out of the Vietnam war.*

 "What's your name?"

"Dung. Nguyen." *Dung*, he thought. *That means "brave" or "heroic" in Vietnamese.* Simmons had no idea how he knew that.

"Dung, you have a serious medical illness. This is your chance to be really brave." *What he and his family have been through back home, this is probably not the first test of his bravery.*

He nodded, and that made him choke a little.

"Try not to move your head or neck if you can help it. You have some swelling above your voice box that makes it hard to get air into your lungs. It also makes it hard to talk. A special doctor, Dr. Sherwood, will be here to help you very soon. He will place a tube in your nose and run it down your throat to look at the tight area. It will be uncomfortable, but if you are very brave, you will be okay. He will have to leave a tube in your throat so that you can breathe, maybe for a day or two, but maybe for as long as a week. Do you understand what I've told you?"

"Yes." Squeaky but firm, not afraid.

"Do you have any questions for me?"

"Can I go home soon?" Simmons was taken aback for a second, then he readjusted his perspective. This was the sort of question he expected from eight-year-olds and eighty-year-olds, as if they hadn't heard a word he said. This little guy had been so stoic and accepting that David had already begun to think of him as a clear-headed adult.

"As long as you have the tube in your throat, you have to stay here. Once the swelling in your throat goes away, that tube can come out and you can go home."

"Okay." Just then Tom Sherwood arrived. He held a scope case in his hand.

"I had to stop by my car. I remembered that the last time I used your pediatric scope here, the light source failed. Mine won't. Plus, mine is thinner. Just in case."

"Great, Tom. This is Dung." Sherwood gave David an odd look, but said nothing. "He is a very brave guy. I've explained what you are going to do, and he understands. There is an aunt around somewhere, but we haven't seen her yet. His parents aren't here."

"Okay. You and I can sign the consent and your nurse here, what's your name?"

"Sally, R.N."

"Okay, Sally, you can witness it."

Simmons looked up at the board. "I have to go see a patient. You need anything, just hit the light and we'll all come running."

"Good enough. Call one of the hospitalists to admit him when we're done. ICU, isolation room. Everyone get a blue mask on."

Simmons picked up a chart for a two-year-old with a chin laceration. Just about every little boy in the world, just as soon as he learns how to run, manages to plant his chin on a tile floor. The skin covering the vertex, the point of the chin, explodes into a nice, smooth oval that can be fixed with a five simple sutures. He wrote a few orders for the suture setup and handed it to Joe, the E.R. tech today.

While Joe was getting things ready, Simmons chatted with the mom and dad, who started out with the usual "We don't want any scars. We want a plastic surgeon for Little Roger." After calming them and assuring them that a scar was inevitable but would be small and virtually unnoticeable, and would not adversely affect Little Roger's future, he showed them the one on his own chin, closed by a G.P. in the late 50s. He stuck a wad of cotton soaked with cocaine solution into the hole in Little Roger's chin, taped over it, and promised to be back in thirty minutes.

He looked over at Bed 1. Sherwood was guiding the NL scope with what looked like a size 5 E.T. tube over it into Dung's nose. Everything seemed calm in that direction. David said a small prayer that the 5 wouldn't be too large. He sat down to dictate the charts left from yesterday. It was 7:30. *Man, what a fast fucking half-hour that was.* The patch phone rang again. Bella answered and took down the essentials of the patch. As she hung up the phone, she turned to Roberta.

"Robbie, code arrest by ground. Engine 107. ETA four minutes. We'll put them in the code room." She walked over to where David sat dictating.

"Dave, we've got a forty-eight year-old male in full cardiac arrest. He was..."

Simmons turned to look up at Bella and shook his head. "Let me guess. He was climbing Terrazzi Peak and collapsed. Henry's up in the units, right?"

Bella nodded, then shrugged her shoulders. "Of course. There were five traumas last night. You know him, he'll be up there for hours. Why?"

Henry Alvarez, thrice-divorced, once bald, was extremely proud of his weightlifter physique and his thick curly hair implants. He fancied himself the last of the great Latin lovers, and spent most of his time flirting with every XX chromosome specimen who came within wooing distance. On the other hand, Henry could knock out a row of TBS charts faster than any of the young guys. Until his partner finished his seduction dance in the ICU, Simmons was on his own.

"Nothing important. Is the family here yet?" The fire department would routinely call the next of kin as soon as they had a contact number from the patient or friends. When it came to rescues from the peak, by the time the meat wagon arrived, the family was usually here and waiting, anxious to see their loved one. Bella went over to her desk and placed a call out to the waiting room. After a few seconds, she put down the phone and nodded.

"The wife and daughter are out front. Do you want me to put them in the Consolation Room?"

Simmons thought this one over a bit. If they were on hand when the patient, obviously dead by now, was rolled into the code room, they would see he was flatlined and would burst into tears. While that would immediately and irreversibly change the tenor of the situation for the worse, they would know that he was DOA. The other option was to put them into the Consolation Room, a small soundproofed consultation closet down the hall from the waiting area. Once Simmons had pronounced the guy dead, accompanied by Bella or the social worker, he would go talk with them. This option had the benefit of maintaining calm in the code room, but families always assumed the patient was still alive on arrival, mainly because the paramedics TOLD them on the phone he was still alive, and if Simmons walked in and announced that their loved one had passed, they would assume he and the E.R. staff had screwed up a heroic and successful resuscitation effort by the men in the blue t-shirts. Simmons' instinct was to be Dr. Happy Face so everyone would get along, but over the past six weeks especially, he'd grown tired of playing the role of the bad doctor and covering for the fire guys' misleading the family.

"Would you get them some chairs in the observation corner of the code room? If it gets to be too much for them, we can always move them out to the family room."

"Well, we're going to be pretty busy when they get here."

"Bel, it takes the paramedics at least ten minutes to get from the station house to the parking area of the peak. Then it takes them at least twenty minutes to carry their gear up to the top of the peak, because that's where these guys always go down. Then they need five minutes to get him on a monitor and start an IV and begin resuscitation protocols. Then it's at least ten minutes hauling the guy down the peak on a stretcher. If he were still alive, they would have called for a chopper and brought him in that way. The fact that he's coming by ground tells me they just don't want the responsibility of pronouncing him. If they bring him here, they don't have to transport him to a funeral home or the county morgue. I don't blame them, but that's how it is. We won't have to do anything other than transfer him to the table, hook him up, do a little CPR, then pronounce him."

Bella stared at Simmons. "You're in a weird mood today." She was starting to dread working with him for the next twelve hours. Of all the E.R. docs, he was the most unpredictable, mainly because he changed from day to day and nobody ever got to know him. The more you tried, the harder he fought you.

"By the way, did they mention what rhythm he was in?"

She shook her head. "No, they just said they were continuing resuscitation efforts. He's intubated and has an IV running."

"Fifty bucks says he's been in asystole since they first got to him." Asystole, a.k.a. flatline, meant no electrical activity anywhere in the heart. You might survive a minute or two of that one, but after four minutes your heart and brain were heading inexorably downward toward a hole in the ground and tearful eulogies followed by lots of drinks and potluck funeral food.

"Whatever. Rough night?"

"Perfect night. Slept like a baby for eight hours. The dead hiker thing on a Sunday morning is a real buzzkill. Families understand it when the patient dies from a gunshot or an MVA, but when Dad heads out for a nice Sunday hike and drops dead, well, it's a little hard for them to get their heads around that one."

Bella summoned Megan the social worker and Sean the new nurse over the P.A. system. She told Megan to bring in the family; Sean drew code room duty. Two minutes later she called to David.

"They just pulled into the driveway." Simmons paused from his dictation and looked up. As he rose from his desk chair, he clicked on the microphone.

"End of dictation, David Simmons, M.D. on Ricky Richardson, number 445987." He grabbed his stethoscope and went to join the crowd. The wife and daughter were sitting on bar stools in the far corner of the room, positioned so they could see the cardiac monitor over the procedure table. Over a year ago, at her final review of the E.R., an efficiency expert had recommended this particular sitting area for family members. She also advised positioning the monitor at least six feet up off the ground, so that the loved ones would focus on it and not on the action on the table. She called it "The TV Effect". When she said it, she made quotation marks in the air.

"They're used to seeing monitors on hospital shows. They can relate to the appearance and the sound. It also allows them to think about something other than how bad the patient looks."

Wally Engels, who reportedly had wavered between an M.D. degree and an M.S.W., raised his hand.

"Yes, Dr. Engels?" He put his hand down and stood up. When he spoke, he looked down and around at his colleagues; his arms and hands made a swooping motion. *Help me out, guys.*

"I don't think the monitor is at all relevant. The families should be able to stand right next to the table and hold the patient's hand. Don't you think the family wants to see what's going on?"

"No, Dr. Engels. No I don't." The post-review vote by the docs was 13 - 1 in favor of raising the height of the monitor.

David went over and introduced himself to the patient's family. The ambulance team rolled in, looking like they'd just escaped from the steam room at the gym. Simmons thought, *A hot, sweaty hike up and down the peak to start their twenty-four-hour shift. I'd better keep my mouth shut.* As he walked over to the E.R. table in the center of the room, it crossed his mind that the wife and her daughter were the only ones present who didn't know she was already a widow. While the three EMT's slid the patient from the gurney to the table, Simmons backed up to where the paramedic, Guy Falcone, was giving his report, loud enough for the recording system and everyone in the room to hear clearly.

"This is Barry Sandberg, age forty-eight. He climbed Terrazzi Peak with two friends this morning. His companions said Mr. Sandberg seemed to have more trouble breathing than normal. They'd just reached the summit (*of course*) when Mr. Sandberg collapsed. One of his companions called 911. When we reached the scene, CPR was being performed by several hikers. We established an eighteen-gauge IV in the right antecubital fossa. Initial monitor showed asystole, so the patient was given a saline challenge of five-hundred cc. and sequential doses of epi and atropine. Fine V fib was noted, and the patient was shocked three times. From then on, his rhythm continued in asystole."

David looked up at the monitor. Still a flatline. He whispered in Guy's ear, "How long have you been working him?"

Without turning his head, Guy whispered back, "We're going on forty-five minutes now. He's had three rounds of everything and a liter of saline."

"Must have been a bitch of a hike down the hill with him. What's he weigh, two-twenty-five?"

"Two-forty at least, and he's 5'9" max. When you add in all the air in his gut from the initial mouth-to-mouth, it was like hauling a bowling ball. He almost rolled us off the trail a couple of times."

Sean and Bella flushed Sandberg's IV line and continued getting him hooked up. Simmons continued on softly, so the family wouldn't hear.

"You know, Guy, if you'd just pronounced him up on the peak, you could have saved yourselves a lot of supplies and spared the family the anguish. They think he's still alive."

"Doc", he took a breath, "Dave, we have strict orders not to pronounce in the field. It's not in our scope of practice. That comes from Deputy Chief Santiago himself."

"I know why you don't do it. We don't mind them coming in as DOA's, and we'll still do the disposition of the body, but it would be easier on everybody if you pronounced the dead guys dead. You're a Captain, run it by the DC. Maybe he can change your scope."

"That I can do, Doc. Probably not today, though. The DC and the Chief are playing in a golf tournament up in Flag." Simmons laughed into his hand. That would not be a pretty sight, the Chief and his D.C. and their godawful golf swings ruining the view of the majestic San Francisco peaks in the background.

"Yeah, maybe it can wait until tomorrow." He walked over to the patient, took his stethoscope from around his neck and listened to each side of his chest. One of the EMT's, Tony, was bagging the patient through the endotracheal tube, while a new guy was performing chest compressions. The monitor showed blips from each compression but nothing more. Simmons turned back to Guy Falcone. "ET tube is in perfect position. Good job." Intubating a patient with excellent lighting, lots of assistance and a raised table was relatively easy. A hot desert mountain trail was a different ballgame. Even experienced anesthesiologists who put tubes in tracheas every day had trouble intubating in the field.

"Thanks, Doc."

Simmons looked up at the monitor. Terry the respiratory therapist arrived and took over bagging duties. He asked, "Should we put him on the ventilator?"

Simmons shook his head and checked the clock for the official time of death. "Stop everything." In the observation corner, the wife and daughter were staring at the cardiac monitor. He walked over and reached for their hands.

"Mrs. Sandberg, I'm so sorry. He's gone." David had the briefest flash of hope that she would understand what he was saying and accept it.

"WHAT?" Her head shot up; bulging eyes stared him in the face. *So much for that idea.*

"I'm afraid your husband has passed away. I'm sure he had a massive heart attack and died instantly." He stopped, still holding their hands, waiting for it to sink in. If he could fit it in and not make it sound awful, he'd go on with, "I'm sure he felt no pain."

"How can that be? The firemen called and told us he was still alive." Simmons heard a rush of feet behind him. Normally the guys from fire would stick around to cool off in the E.R., rehydrate with some cold water, grab supplies to restock the ambulance, and flirt with the womenfolk. Not today, not with the widow getting all worked up. Mrs. Sandberg burst loudly into tears. Her daughter put an arm around her mother's shoulders while the woman rocked back and forth on her stool. Sometimes, before they left the code room, the family would want to stand next to the deceased, hold his hand, say good-bye. Simmons thought a little time-out in the Consolation Room would be better for these two. Then, later, if they wanted to, they could come back in for a last look. He suggested as much to the daughter. She nodded.

Bella came over. She and the daughter helped Mrs. S. up and out of the code room. Simmons made a few notes on the temporary chart and handed it back to Sean. He figured he'd give Bella five minutes, then head in to the Consolation Room to talk with the family. By then, most likely a few other relatives would be crowded in there as well. They could all have a fifteen-minute Q & A, then he could come back and sew up Little Roger's chin hole.

David walked out of the code room into the main E.R. area. Before sitting down to dictate, he looked over at Bed 1. Sally, R.N. was playing with the monitor, Snake Oil Joe the respiratory therapist was taping a tiny E.T. tube to Dung's nose, and Sherwood was packing up his scope.

Mission accomplished. Since this was purely an obstruction that was now relieved by the tube, most likely Dung wouldn't require a ventilator to help him breathe. That meant they could avoid sedating him if the tube didn't bug him too much. Because the tube was so small, he'd still have to breathe thirty or more times per minute; if he tired out, they could sedate him at night and put him on the blower so he could sleep. He picked up the top chart in his "To Be Dictated" pile and started talking into the microphone.

Sherwood put down his scope case and sat next to David with Dung's chart. When Simmons paused and looked over, the ENT specialist patted his arm and said, "That was a good pickup, Dave. A few more minutes and he would have needed a trach."

"Were you able to get the 5 E.T. tube in?"

"Almost had it, but he started spasming, so I switched to a 4.5 and that went right in. Tough kid. How'd you figure that out so quickly?"

"I almost lost one just like that ten years ago. I was working in this E.R. in a little rural hospital in Southeast Washington State. I ended up having to do a cricothyrotomy on him just as he passed out. Weird. Fourteen-year-old boy, same symptoms, Vietnamese just like this one. They could have been twins." The same odd look crossed Sherwood's face. He started to say something, but his pager went off. He looked at the number, then punched in four numbers on the phone and started talking. David went back to dictating.

After finishing two charts, Simmons decided it was time to face the music. He walked through the code room, across the waiting area, which was packed with the walking wounded, and opened the door to the Consolation Room. Every time he saw the words on the door, he expected to walk into the set of a TV game show. "Let's welcome our newest loser. He's David Simmons, an E.R. physician from Tucson, Arizona!"

The audience emits a loud "Ooooh".

"He's already having a bummer of a day!"

This time it's a chorus of "Awwwww."

"Then again, he's having a much better day than any of his patients!"

The "Hoorays!" explode.

"Danielle, what do we have for Dr. Simmons' consolation prize?"

Inside the room, about a half-dozen F & F's--family and friends--were sitting or standing. Once David walked in, all eyes riveted on him. He shook off the game show vision and walked over to where a twentyish guy wearing sunglasses was sprawled on the stuffed couch between Mrs. Sandberg and her daughter. Instinctively, Simmons knew this guy was going to play the role of the TIR--Truculent but Insignificant Relative.

"Hi, everyone, I'm Dr. Simmons. Hey, buddy, why don't you get up and let this nice lady here"--he nodded his head to an elderly woman standing to the right of the couch, probably the patient's mother, leaning on a black metal cane--"sit down."

The young man sat upright, ripped off his shades, and said in his most menacing voice, "He was my uncle, goddammit."

David shook his hand. "I'm very sorry for your loss, but why don't you get up anyway." Nephew looked around for support, found none, and stood up. Simmons helped the old lady, who looked to be at least eighty years old and couldn't have weighed more than eighty pounds, around the end of the couch and onto the sofa. Then he stepped back toward the door, opened it for Bella to leave, and closed it. Now it was just he and Megan. Simmons would give a short rendition of what he thought had happened to Mr. Sandberg, answer any questions, and let Megan take it from there. He leaned back against the wall right next to the door.

Rule Number One: Never let the angry mob get between you and your escape route. Had Caesar followed that dictum, there would be one less tragedy in Shakespeare's portfolio. Dying of old age was everyone's goal, but it didn't make for great dramatic material.

He began. "I spoke at length with Captain Falcone, the paramedic who was in charge of the rescue attempt of Mr. Sandberg. When he and his crew ascended Terrazzi Peak, they found him in what we call asystole, which means his heart was not beating and there was no electrical activity on the monitor. They did everything exactly right, including putting a tube down his throat to help him breathe, giving him fluids and the appropriate medications to get his heart started. For a brief period of time, he developed what we call ventricular fibrillation, which is usually a fatal rhythm. They then countershocked him and gave him other medications designed specifically for that rhythm. Mr. Sandberg's heart then reverted to asystole and remained that way, flatlined, for forty-five minutes. Despite the paramedic team's best efforts, he succumbed. Undoubtedly, he suffered a massive heart attack either on his way up the trail or just as he arrived at the top."

Mrs. Sandberg, by now much more composed--*Thank you, Bella and Megan*--spoke first.

"How could he have a heart attack? He hiked that trail with his pals every Sunday morning, right after breakfast! He was in excellent shape, he was down to a half a pack of cigarettes a day, and his blood pressure was doing really well on the new medications Dr. Elias prescribed." The rest of the family nodded in agreement. Simmons nodded too. He'd read an account of some famous shrink, maybe B.F. Skinner, sitting front row for a lecture. Every time the speaker made a chopping motion with his hand to emphasize a point, Skinner nodded and smiled. By the time the guy was done talking, he was chopping away like a rogue robot; his wristwatch flopped insanely back and forth. Nodding seemed like a good way to go. Simmons had seen it change the sentiment of a crowd from "He died and it's all your fault." to "He died despite your valiant battle with the Reaper."

Although he understood that rational thought under these circumstances was an impossibility for Mrs. Sandberg and probably for the rest of the crowd as well, his natural instinct to probe got the better of him.

"Well, I can't say for sure, but it seems his numerous risk factors for heart disease, the high blood pressure, the smoking history, combined with his obesity..." Mrs. S and her daughter both looked up.

"Obesity! How can you say he was obese? He was five-eleven and weighed less than two hundred pounds." Simmons' jaw dropped before he could stop it. He clamped his mouth shut and resolved to get out of there before he said anything else that could be construed as inciting a riot. "If you don't believe me, look at his driver's license." It occurred to David that you don't really get measured and weighed when you get your license. He could list himself as four feet tall and five hundred pounds and nobody would bat an eyelash.

"I'm so sorry. Of course you're right, Mrs. Sandberg. Nonetheless, I am sure he died of a heart attack. These things can come on without the slightest warning, even in your sleep. If you'll excuse me, I have a sick child to attend to. Megan, if anyone has any more questions, come get me and I'll do my best to answer them." All eyes were on poor David Simmons as he opened the door and eased himself through the doorway into the hall. Even the granny gave him the stink eye on his way out.

Simmons thought to himself, *I'm only an hour into it and it's already going to hell. Best I can hope for is a really busy shift that flies by.* He walked through the main E.R. and back to the suture area. What he found made him reassess the prospects for the day. Little Roger was snoozing away on the gurney. Big Roger and the missus were equally occupied in a big La-z-boy that Joe must have dragged from somewhere. Joe wandered in and smiled, giving David the thumbs-up.

Not even bothering to put down the gurney side rail, Simmons pulled off the tape with the cotton ball attached, gloved up, and in less than five minutes closed Little Roger's chin hole with five perfect 5-0 Prolene sutures. Just as he finished snipping the last one, Mrs. Roger woke up. When she saw Simmons bent over her little angel with a pair of scissors, she jumped up and tripped, bumping the side rail with her hand. Little Roger's eyes opened and he emitted a blood-curdling scream. He reached for Simmons, who stepped back, danced a merry little jig, and tossed the scissors on the suture tray. Big Roger, apparently accustomed to blood-curdling screams, just slept on.

"Joe, I'll go write up some discharge instructions. If you can throw some bacitracin ointment and a band aid on Little Roger's chin, I'd appreciate it. Be right back, Ma'am."

The rest of the shift went like clockwork. Simmons and Henry got into a smooth rhythm and plowed through sixty patients between them. Three trauma cases, all minor MVA's, barely took up any time. Simmons even got to spend a pleasant twenty minutes with a wiry seventy-year-old who'd worked on a table saw his entire life and was thoroughly embarrassed to show him a bag containing the severed distal phalanx of his right index finger.

"Been doing this since I was fifteen. First time I ever ripped stock without a push stick. Here's what I get. Like that J. Geils feller said, it serves me right to suffer." The old guy never flinched, just gritted his teeth and sat there calling himself a D-horn idiot.

"D-horn? You don't look like a drinker, you don't smell like a smoker, and you certainly aren't fat, so I'm not sure you qualify as a D-horn." Simmons raised his eyebrows as he sewed.

"Oh, so you versteh, eh?"

"Ein bisschen, ja."

"Okay, so I'm a run-of-the-mill idiot. Some days you're nothing special."

"Bestimmt!" and they both laughed.

Before he knew it, the clock read 6:30 and there were no new patients to be seen. David dove into the pile of charts in his TBD box. With ten minutes to go, he was down to the last one, his first patient of the day. He picked up the dictation microphone and began.

"This is David Simmons, M.D. dictating..." He stopped as he read the name at the top.

"Bella, the registration people out front must have stamped the wrong name on Dung's chart. This says, 'Doug Wynn'."

Bella turned to look at him. "That's his name."

Simmons shook his head. "No, it was Dung. Dung Nguyen. The Vietnamese kid."

"What Vietnamese kid?"

"The Vietnamese kid in Bed 1 this morning at change of shift. You know, the one who was on the verge of dying?"

"David," she laughed, "his name was Doug Wynn and if he's Vietnamese, he's the first blond-haired, blue-eyed one I've ever seen." She turned back to her computer and shook her head.

Right at seven, Karen and Seth walked through the front door. Simmons signed out his two remaining patients to Seth, two admissions all written up and waiting for beds upstairs. Henry checked out the unit players to Karen and turned to David.

"Great shift, Dave. Wish they were all that pleasant."

"Same here, Henry. Have fun in San Diego. See you next week." Simmons gathered up his belongings to let Seth get settled in. He started to walk away, but felt a hand on his upper arm. It was Seth.

"Dave, I was halfway up the summit trail at Terrazzi this morning when it hit me that the kid in Bed 1 probably didn't have croup. I almost called you, but I figured you were probably busy with him. I think I know what he had."

"Too bad you didn't call me. I could have used the help."

Seth looked concerned. "Why, how'd he do?"

"He died." Even as he said it, something stirred in the back of David's head. Seth went pale and put his hand up to his face.

Simmons said, "I'm just fucking with you. What do you think he had?"

"You asshole. That's not funny." *Probably not, but there's no way I'm passing up a setup like that.* "Epiglottitis?"

"Dinnnngggg! Sherwood intubated him nasally over a scope. He's up in the unit, and the last I heard, he was breathing on his own, without a vent. I'm heading up there right now to take a look at him. "As he turned to leave, Bella jabbed her finger into his ribs.

"The way the shift started out, I didn't think you'd keep it together enough to get through the day."

He smiled. "Rough start but a smooth ending. I'd rather have it that way than the other way around."

"If you have time, I'll buy you a beer."

"Oh yeah, I've got time. I've got my bike, so someplace close would work best for me. I can come back here and pick up my stuff afterward."

Bella smiled. "Let's go to Jake's." Jake's was a Mexican restaurant with a dusty old bar run by a second-generation Irishman from Kilkenny. It was all of a hundred yards from the E.R. front door. "I have to go upstairs and see my neighbor Moira. She's in with pneumonia. Meet you there at 7:30?"

A thought occurred to Simmons. "Perfect. I have to run upstairs to the unit, then maybe make a phone call. Meet you at the bar."

David ran up the stairs to the second floor, which housed what he called the ZOAs, the Zones of Action--the ICU, the CVICU, the O.R., the cath lab. Once inside the ICU, where shift change was in full swing, he scanned the board to locate the Nguyen boy. Nothing. There was, however, a Wynn in Room 4. He walked over to where the day shift nurse, Penny, was giving report to her night shift replacement, Amber. Two redheads in identical emerald scrubs. *Interesting.* The sign on the glass wall of Room 4 said, "Respiratory Isolation" and there were a few lines of instructions below. He stared through the glass at a fourteen-year-old blond boy with bright blue eyes breathing rapidly through a small ET tube taped to his nose. *Must be humidified oxygen, with all the fog in the tube.* Nothing else about the kid sank in. Simmons glanced down at the open blue chart on Penny's lap. At the top right corner of the nursing note page was the stamped ID. It read "Wynn, Douglas 446029". Below that was the date of admission and his age, fourteen years. Penny looked up at him.

"Hi, David. He's holding his own, his respiratory rate is down, and his sats are fine." She looked down. "I was wondering if we could get an order..."

"Sorry, but we're not following him officially, so I can't write any orders. You'll have to talk to Sherwood or the hospitalist group, or pulmonary, I guess. I just came up to see how he looked. Have a great night." He turned and walked out of the ICU.

Out in the hallway, Simmons navigated around the family of a trauma patient who had just come out of surgery, a t-boned MVA victim whose ruptured spleen was now resting comfortably down in the pathology lab. Simmons made a mental note to check in a couple days to make sure he received his pneumovax, which would protect the guy from dying of sepsis from a routine strep infection. Working his way through the dozen or so gathered outside the ICU door, all chattering away in Spanish, he temporarily forgot for a few seconds what he'd seen in Room 4. Then it hit him good and hard. *Jesus H. Christ, what is going on in my head?* At the top of the stairs he stood for a minute, then ran down to the first floor and out the side door to the parking lot.

He found shade behind a pillar, pulled out his cell phone and dialed 411, thinking, *I wonder if this is still how you get information.* To his surprise, the same universally nasal operator answered. After a few seconds, he punched the # key. He looked at his watch. *Twenty minutes before I meet Bel.*

"Hi, this is Dr. Simmons. Could you please connect me with the E.R.?" After a pause, he smiled.

"Hi, Gerry, this is Dr. Simmons. Yes, Dr. David, the Big City Know-It-All. Oh, it's been longer than that, more like ten. How are you? Good. Hey listen, is Trixie working tonight? She is? Great. May I speak with her? Oh, okay. She'll be there all night? No, I'll just call back in an hour or so. If you'd let her know I called, I'd appreciate it. Nice talking with you, too, Gerry. Have a good night. Bye." Simmons hung up and started walking across the parking lot to Jake's.

When he walked in, Bella was already sitting at the bar. Her hair was down from its workday bun; her scrubs were gone, replaced by a bright yellow sundress. As David sat down, he detected the fresh scent of "Angel".

"Sick neighbor, eh?"

"Oh, she's sick and up on 4A all right. When I went up to visit, she was down getting a CT. She kept dropping her oxygen saturations, so her docs were worried about a pulmonary embolus. I left her a note saying I'd bring her some posole before I go home. She can't get enough of it, eats it two or three times a week when she's well, every day when she has a cold. So I took a shower in the women's locker room next to the O.R., changed, and here I am."

"Angel?"

"I always carry an emergency supply." She smiled and held up a tiny atomizer. Before he could react, she sprayed a small dose into his face. "There. That's better. Now buy me a beer."

After squinting and sneezing a few times, David turned toward the bartender, Joe, a scrawny six-footer with a chronic cough, whose overall appearance fairly screamed "TB".

"Hi, Joe. We'll have a couple of Negras with limes, and some chips and guac."

Bella said, "Speaking of scrubs, I'm surprised to see you in here wearing yours. Usually you don't go anywhere in your work clothes, especially if it involves vices." Simmons looked down at his scrubs. Not bad for the end of a shift. A few drops of blood on his running shoes, but no sign of any other bodily fluids. Or solids.

"To be honest with you, I completely forgot. My riding stuff is pretty wet anyway. And I forgot my sundress." He looked around at the empty bar. "Hopefully nobody will notice."

"If somebody drops in and drops dead, you're screwed." Bella took a swig of her beer.

Simmons said, "Speaking of dropping dead, that Sandberg case was so sad. Maybe it was just me, but every one of those family members seemed to be suffering from the same delusion, that the guy was in great shape and had no risk factors for heart disease. It was a 'Folie a six'. They all seemed stunned that he could have a heart attack and die."

"People have to create and believe in delusions to make certain aspects of their life work." Bella glanced down at Simmons waistline, where his belly button formed a nice round hole in his gut donut.

David laughed. "What are you looking at? I ride my bike for at least an hour and swim in the pool for a half hour almost every day."

"Like I said, everyone has a delusion or two."

"I get that, but that stuff Mrs. S. said about her husband's height and weight. '5'11" and under two hundred?' That's just bending reality."

"What do you think the real numbers were?"

"I'd guess five-eight and Guy said he weighed two-forty. The fire guys are usually spot on when they hand-lift someone."

"Just before change of shift I took a look at the preliminary exam from downstairs by the diener on call. He was 5'9" and weighed two-thirty-eight."

"See? Out of touch with reality, and I don't think that was a temporary aberration brought on by the shock of the moment. She's even checked his driver's license, so she must have had some doubts. He's the one who fudged the numbers, so he was in on the charade too."

"Speaking of delusions, are you going to let me in on the Vietnamese gag?"

"Trust me, that was no gag. Until I upset Seth with an awful attempt at being funny, I couldn't have told you what that was all about. Now I think I have an idea. I have to make a phone call tonight that hopefully will shed a little light on that."

"Oooh, a clandestine phone call. How about a little hint?"

"The next time I see you, I promise I'll tell you the whole story, or at least my version of it."

"When are you making this mysterious call?"

"As soon as I finish this delicious guacamole, this frosty beer, this conversation with my lovely drinking buddy, and ride my bike home." Bella glanced at her watch.

"I'll make you a deal, David. I could use another beer or two. How about I buy a six-pack and come over in a bit. I have to drop some posole off with sick neighbor Moira, the dear, then I'll head over."

"Are you off tomorrow?"

"Yes, just like you. I checked. We have a 7 A.M. mandatory staff meeting, so, if I may, I'd rather stay on this side of town tonight." She looked at him quizzically.

"You want to stay with me?"

"More like stay at your place. Is the airplane bed available?"

"Always." *This day just keeps getting better and better.* "I was planning on floating in the pool for a while. Tonight's a new moon, and the Perseids are supposed to show around 3 A.M. I'm gonna pretend to stay up for them, right up until I fall asleep."

"I'd love that. You have a spare air mattress?"

He shot her his cheesiest leer. "Two singles and a queen."

"Make mine a single."

"BSO, Bel. Don't tell me you packed a suit too."

"I know the routine, remember?"

David walked across the street and retrieved his bike. His riding clothes were too soaked to reuse, so he wrapped a little red bungie cord around his right scrub pants leg and hopped onto the canal path. Even at this time of the day, the heat was atrocious. Within minutes his scrubs were soaked. At least the sun was setting at his back. As soon as he got home, he cleaned up the usual working weekend mess around the house, then jumped in for a quick rinse. He considered taking a shower, but the armpit sniff test came back negative. Sitting naked on the side of the pool in the lowering dusk, feeling anxious and excited at the same time, he placed a call.

"Trixie? Oh, great. Hi, Trix, this is David Simmons. Yup. It's been at least ten years. How are you? Oh, good. How's your buddy Stan? Oh, really? I'm sorry to hear that. He was a terrific guy. Yeah, I left Portland. I know, nobody ever leaves there. Oh, I moved around a bunch all over Arizona, been in Tucson for a couple of years. Working in an E.R. if you can believe it. Yeah, trauma center and all. I know, I feel bad for the patients too. No, I didn't call just to catch up, but I'm glad I got ahold of you. I wonder if we could talk about a case we worked together...."

Fifteen minutes later, as he clicked off his cell phone, he was surprised to see that darkness had fallen. He heard Bella let herself in. The light went on in the kitchen; he could see her reach up into a cabinet over the bar; after that she opened the freezer door. The light went out. A few minutes later, she emerged from the darkened house with one of David's beach towels wrapped around her. Cradled in her arm was a steel bowl full of ice and two Anchor Steam bottles. *Cold beer deliveredy on a hot summer night by a native girl in a sarong. More or less.*

She sat on a chaise longue next to him. He groped in the dark for his backpack, fumbled around inside and pulled out his Swiss Army. He opened the beers, handed one to her, and patted the cool deck next to him.

"Come on down, it's not too hot. I'll get the air mattresses out of the shed." Ten minutes later, they were floating naked side-by-side, looking up at a few stars peeking through the dissipating cloud cover. Bella dipped her hand in the water and steered closer to him. "This is what I miss most about being with you. The only way to spend a monsoon night outside."

"I seem to recall you liked me carrying you around in the pool in the dark too." He paddled over to the side of the pool and took a sip of his Anchor.

"That was also nice." By the glow from town, he could see her profile on the raft. There was a soft reflection of the Anchor bottle on her stomach. He had that months-old thought again. *Gorgeous, smart, funny, great bod, kids all grown up. What was I thinking?*

Bella changed the subject. "Are you seeing anyone?" *So much for the fantasy.*

"I went out with this one woman a couple times. She was okay. Second date, after dinner, she invites me in. I was beat, had to be back at work at seven the next morning, but I said sure. We walk into the house, there's a guy sitting in the living room with a drink, watching a baseball game on TV. Big smile, how's everyone doing? Not a care in the world. Turns out it's her ex. He has a key, drops in whenever, one big happy fucking family.

"Did they have kids? Is that why he was there?"

"Kids are grown and moved away. Turns out she's not even divorced, he just pays her money every month."

"What'd you do?"

"Are you kidding? An ex, no, not even an ex, with a key? I turned and ran. I was getting into my pickup by the time she reached the door to say good night. 'Thanks for dinner. I had a lovely time. Call me.' "

Bella laughed. "I'm surprised. That's sounds just weird enough for you."

"Even I have my limits. How about you?"

"You know me. No limits."

"No, I mean..."

She laughed again. "I know what you mean. I've been asked out a few times. Mostly cops and paramedics. Even my marathon trainer hit on me, which was kind of gross. I let them take me to concerts, cookouts, but that's pretty much it." They floated in silence for a while.

"I hope I wasn't interrupting anything by coming over tonight."

"Huh? No. I'm doing exactly what I would have been doing if you weren't here. The scenery wouldn't have been as nice, that's all. Why?"

"When I pulled into your driveway, there was a woman walking up to your house. As soon as she saw me get out of the car, she turned and walked away."

"What'd she look like?"

"Short brown hair, about forty, looked to be in good shape." Bella turned to look at him. "In the reflection from my headlights, I could see a wedding ring."

Simmons laughed. "That must have been Jan Taft. She's the town crier in the neighborhood. Walks around a few evenings a week, mooching beers and gathering gossip. She's sweet, harmless. Mostly just lonely. You never met her here when we were together?"

"Uh-uh, not even at the cookouts. So she stops by just to chat and drink beer? Maybe float naked in the pool too?"

"Oh, no. She's married. Her husband is the night supervisor at the city water works. Nice guy. Grew up in the neighborhood, knows all the history."

"Sounds lovely."

"Hey," David pointed to the eastern sky. "There's the new moon."

Bella spun her raft around and lifted her head. "Oh yeah. Nice that it's so dark out tonight." She turned her raft so they were facing head-to-toe. "Did you reach your secret contact on a secure line?" David laughed.

"Sure did. I had a nice long talk with Trixie."

"Trixie? Seriously?"

"Yes. Trixie from eastern Washington. She's an E.R. nurse in a small hospital. Actually, the place is so small that if you work the E.R. at night you're usually the house supervisor and probably the ICU nurse as well. I used to moonlight out there when I was a resident."

"Before you go any further, I need to form a visual of Trixie. Otherwise, I'll keep imagining an exotic dancer with a nursing cap on her head."

"Robust. She loved doing anything outdoors. Snowmobiling, bow-hunting, target shooting, swimming, hiking. She had a 'friend' named Stan, who worked as a lab tech, x-ray tech, surgical assistant, nursing assistant. They both had places about ten miles out of town. I couldn't tell if they were romantically involved, but they sure were attached at the hip. Did everything together. Trix just told me he died in a climbing accident a couple of years ago. He was one tough guy but a real sweetheart. It's too bad."

"Very interesting, Dr. Ruth. How did she look?"

Simmons laughed. "Oh, that. I found her attractive. Let's leave it at that."

"Fair enough. You have anything to eat?" Simmons got up, went inside, and made a couple of turkey sandwiches. He grabbed two more beers from the fridge. When he came back outside, Bella was sitting on a chaise, wrapped in her towel. They sat on the side of the pool and ate in silence. When they finished, David picked up the plates and took them inside the house. He came out and sat next to Bella.

"You still want to hear about the Vietnamese thing?"

"You want to talk about it?"

"I think I'm ready, but I'd be more comfortable floating."

"Okay, but it hasn't been an hour since we ate." They got back in and climbed on their air mattresses.

"My third and fourth year in Portland, I wasn't on call much, so about once a month I'd drive out to eastern Washington to moonlight. The money wasn't great, but it was a lot better than my resident's salary. More than anything else, I appreciated the change of scenery. There wasn't any hierarchy, the place was understaffed, and you never knew what you'd see. I think if I hadn't owed time to the public health service, I might have moved out there and worked for a few years in the E.R. full-time. Some of the best people I've ever worked with. It was such a comfortable place to be. Everyone, from the cafeteria cook to the urologist, showed up for any trauma and most codes. That's why you and I and everyone else work at Sabino; it's like a little country hospital in the middle of the city.

"So that's why you like working a full-time job and a part-time one? Change of scenery?"

"That, and I think if you stay in just one place too long, you tend to think about things and do things the same way every time. You get a little settled and less creative. At least I do."

"Okay, fine. Quit stalling and tell me. You promised."

David laughed. He drifted over to his beer and took a sip while still lying down. Some of it went into his mouth and caused him to choke. Most of it went down his nose. *That was brilliant.*

"See? God punished you for stalling." Bella took a sip of her beer lying down without incident. *How is it that she can drink lying down and I can't?*

"If you say so. Okay. It was August, I'm pretty sure it was exactly ten years ago this month. I'd drive up Friday evening, it took about five hours, work thirty-six hours straight, then come home Sunday morning. Around 7 P.M. one Saturday night this family of Vietnamese people comes rushing in. There were three of them, a mom, a dad, and a teenager, their son." Simmons felt like he was floating in midair on a psychiatrist's couch. He closed his eyes and rewound the phone conversation in his head. Although he knew he was talking aloud, he forgot that Bella was lying next to him.

"Trix, do you remember a case we worked together? A Vietnamese kid with difficulty breathing? I think his name was Dung Nguyen."

"Of course. That was so sad. Hard to believe it was ten years ago. Why?"

"I had a case today that reminded me of him. Did the kid walk in or did they carry him?"

"Neither. The father, Truong, ran in to get us. His wife, Ngoc, was outside in the truck with Dung. I took a gurney out to the entrance; Gerry paged you overhead. You and I and Ngoc pulled him out and wheeled him into the E.R."

Simmons interrupted. "I remember him sitting up gasping for air. Skinny little kid sucking in like a fish out of water."

"David, he'd stopped breathing entirely about five minutes before they got to the hospital."

"WHAT? He wasn't breathing?"

"He was dead."

"But I remember trying to intubate him after he stopped breathing. We lowered the head of the bed and I took a look with a laryngoscope."

"Yes you did, but you did that as soon as we got him into a bay. Gerry was doing chest compressions and I was hooking him up to the monitor."

"We didn't have any history, just that he couldn't breathe. That's right, he must have been dead. His mouth, his throat, everything was pale and dry, pale except..." Suddenly he remembered.

"Except, you said, he had a big round red foreign object just above his vocal cords."

"Yeah. At first I thought he'd choked on a raspberry or a marble. When I tried to pull it out with forceps I realized it was attached to his throat. I still didn't comprehend that it was his epiglottis." *That cold grey cave with the big red boulder blocking the exit.*

"Do you remember what you did next, David?"

"Now I do. I took a number eleven blade, without a scalpel handle, and cut into his cricothyroid membrane. Then I stuck a 4 or 5 E.T. tube through the hole. Then we started to bag him. Were his parents there for all that?"

"Truong was sitting in the corner the whole time. He never moved. Just as you started bagging Dung, Ngoc walked in. She was so excited. She thought we'd saved his life."

"Yes, we coded him for another half-hour. The whole time she thought her son was going to make it. She couldn't believe it when we stopped and he didn't wake up." The tiny father, Truong, just sat in the corner, the very essence of life sucked out of him, knowing the truth, unable to comfort his wife.

A thought occurred to David. "Trix, how do you remember their names so well after all these years?"

Trixie laughed, which startled him. "They lived near Eugene. The whole family were mushroom pickers. I don't know if you remember, but back then a lot of Vietnamese and Cambodians made a living harvesting wild mushrooms on the wet side of the state. They could get up to one hundred dollars a pound for them in the restaurants. It was very competitive. Every so often there'd be a battle between families and someone would get hacked to death. Anyway, that weekend they were visiting Ngoc's sister, Dung's aunt. She lives a few miles from my place."

"God, that must have been the last time they came out there."

"No. They moved out there with her sister a few months later. Both Truong and Ngoc were so grateful for our efforts. He works at a lumberyard in Chilton and does the landscaping here at the hospital. Ngoc cooks in the hospital cafeteria and at a little Chinese place here in town. They wanted to be near Dung. He's buried out at his aunt's place."

"Trixie, thank you so much. I can't believe I'd forgotten all that stuff."

"Pretty easy to block out something that traumatic, David. Hey, you said you had a case that reminded you of something. How'd he do?"

"Better than Dung. He's alive, intubated and doing well in the ICU. Same diagnosis. Epiglottitis."

"That's good, David. Listen, I have to go. It was real nice talking with you. Call anytime."

"Okay, bye. And thanks again, Trixie."

"You're welcome. Bye-bye."

When Bella spoke, he realized he must have told her the story while he was going over it in his head. "So that's why you thought our kid was Vietnamese?"

"Well, yeah. I mean Dung Nguyen and Doug Wynn? Can't get any closer than that." Suddenly he made another connection. "Bel, do you remember how'd I'd wake up all sweaty after a nightmare?"

"Oh yes. The first time it scared me to death."

"It was always the same dream."

"Seriously?"

"Absolutely. Always the same. I'm stuck in this grayish sandstone cave, long and narrow. I want to get out, but there's a boulder blocking the exit. A big red boulder."

"God. How long have you been having that dream?"

"Five or six years. At least twice a week. Had it this morning, as a matter of fact. The first year or two, I'd wake up screaming. It still scares me, but now I know enough to keep from screaming. Now I'm surprised if I go three days without it."

"You still wake up with the drenching sweats though."

"Yeah. I go through a lot of sheets. " *Probably best if I don't tell her about suffocating and dying every time.*

They floated in silence for a while. From the look of the clouds rolling in, there wouldn't be any Perseids sighting tonight. Simmons yawned. "I'm getting sleepy, Bel. You want to go inside?"

"Let's float for a while longer. It feels good out here; I have too much running around in me. You sleep. I'll wake you up in a little while." Simmons drifted off holding her hand. His last thought was, *What a weird fucking day.*

Bella smiled. While her eyes roved the skies, she went over David's delusion. As she fell asleep, she thought, *Finally, a layer of the Simmons onion peeled away. He's changing. There's a chance.*

52. THE EMERGENCY ROOM

The E.R. is about the least desirable port of entry into the cardiac surgery system, but for many of you, it is the place where you will be diagnosed with heart disease and begin your treatment. If you come to the E.R. with a previously healthy heart and are found to have coronary disease, you will be staying in the hospital for at least twenty-four hours, probably more. You may end up getting a treadmill stress test, a cath, an angioplasty, a bypass, or all four, but for sure a wallet biopsy is on the menu.

When it comes to the care of patients with chest pain or heart disease, one of the best things about a modern emergency room is the rapidity with which you will be admitted and treated. In some overcrowded urban E.R.s, it is not uncommon to wait hours to have your hand laceration sewn up or your miscarriage diagnosed. Every E.R. doc and nurse can recall a case where a guy checks in on a busy day with a weird, nonspecific symptom like weakness or nausea, sits down in the waiting room until an E.R. bed becomes available, and suffers a heart attack while watching the latest loser reality show on TV. Even if you survive, hospital risk management departments do not want to be on the hook for that one. It's a bad look. If it makes the news, and, let's face it, if you die, it's going to, someone, usually the triage nurse out front, is going to be looking for work elsewhere.

Whether you arrive via POV (Privately Owned Vehicle) or in an ambulance with a story suspicious for CAD, you will be placed in a room immediately. That's because every hospital who claims to be a "heart center" wants the bragging rights that go along with getting patients with acute coronary syndrome into the cath lab the fastest. According to the Department of Health and Human Services' Agency for Healthcare Research and Quality, once you enter an E.R. with ongoing chest pain, you should be started on thrombolytics within thirty minutes or undergo cardiac catheterization and PCI within ninety minutes.

As soon as you get to the E.R., unless the place is packed to overflowing, and even if it is, you'll be taken to a bed, undressed and placed on a cardiac monitor. The nurse or tech will check your blood pressure and pulse. A tech will do an EKG. Someone will start an IV and draw a few tubes of blood for lab tests. The techs from radiology will take an x-ray of your chest. You will receive oxygen through a set of nasal cannulas to unload some of the stress on your heart.

Sometimes just the administration of supplemental oxygen will relieve your chest pain. If you haven't already had a couple in the ambulance, a nurse will administer a nitroglycerine tablet sublingually (under your tongue). Likewise, if you haven't already chewed four baby aspirin in the ambulance, you will now. For persistent pain, you will receive IV morphine in successive small doses until either your pain is gone or a maximum dose is reached. According to some of the old-timers, there's only one appropriate dose of morphine--"Enough". You may also receive IV nitroglycerine continuously. By this time a physician should be listening to your story and examining you and your EKG.

If your story sounds good and your EKG indicates an MI or unstable angina, the E.R. physician will call a cardiologist, who will summon the on-call cath lab team. Sometimes you will receive a thrombolytic agent on your way to the cath lab, sometimes you won't. If for some reason a cath lab is not available and you are going to be transferred to another hospital, most likely you will receive an intravenous thrombolytic. In a weird sort of way, you are better off if your pain does not resolve in the E.R. If you continue to have chest pain, you are going to the cath lab or else you are going to be transferred somewhere that has the facilities to cath you right away.

If, however, your pain resolves with some nitroglycerine, oxygen and morphine, there is a fair chance you will be placed on anti-coagulants, admitted to the CCU and undergo a cardiac cath a little less emergently, as in later that day or the next morning. That means you get to sit in the E.R. until your bed is ready upstairs. That's more contact time with the rest of the E.R. patient population, which may include screaming hot yard apes, drunks, drug addicts wailing like assholes so they can score some prescription narcotics, meth addicts bouncing off the walls flicking MRSA pus in every direction, delirious trauma patients with head injuries, GI bleeders oozing red or black foul-smelling diarrhea into their beds, and Alzheimer's patients doing their best to escape from their restraints as well as their diapers. Not to mention that the change of shift is the most dangerous part of your E.R. visit, where sick patients tend to get lost in the shuffle. Sound like fun? Believe it or not, for E.R. staff that's part of the allure of the job. Not exactly an environment conducive to getting your heart right, but it will tend to keep you from worrying about that chest pain you had. Some E.R.s have special cardiac rooms, with lots of drawers and cabinets full of lifesaving stuff. Often they can be sealed off from the rest of the E.R. by soundproof glass doors. It can be pretty weird in there, watching all the aforementioned craziness going on outside but not being able to hear a thing. Weird but good. It's a lot like the Crying Room at the back of churches. You look back there and see all the kids making crying faces, but you can't hear a whimper. I'm not shot in the head with the rock bands or the guitar mass or all the Bible thumping, but I do love watching the Crying Room. It reminds me of silent films, without the subtitles. Anyway, the cardiac room is a good place to hang, because that glass door tends to keep most of the really bad bacteria and viruses on the outside. Your bedside visitors can also see everything going on out there, and they don't have to keep peeking out like perverts from the curtains around most E.R. beds. Triply important, their vantage point gives them stuff to talk about besides their collection of dead friends' CCU or O.R. horror stories, tales you really don't need to hear at this particular time.

"Helen said Sam woke up one morning and his big toe was gone. Someone snuck in during the night and cut it right off! Of course the hospital denied everything."

For good reason, your visitors may not bring along children, not even yours. Kids get bored very quickly with watching you lie in your bed. They would prefer that you do something exciting, like clutch your chest and writhe in pain. Watching you go into V tach and suffer a grand mal seizure is about the best entertainment a nine-year-old boy could hope for. Barring any excitement of that nature, they will begin to wander, opening drawers, climbing under your gurney, turning off the oxygen, playing with the light switches, and generally fucking with the system. It is a carved-in-stone rule that whoever is parenting them will give absolutely no thought to their pesky behavior, driving the E.R. staff up the wall with the urge to kill. In addition, children are dipped in a steaming vat of booger germs on their way out the schoolroom door every afternoon, sent off to infect as many adults as possible. So no kids in the E.R. unless they are patients.

Once the on-call cath lab team arrives, one or two of them will come down to the E.R. and take you away on your gurney. Your visitors will want to go with you, but, lucky for you, they can't. The E.R. nurses are left to explain why their presence in the cath lab is unnecessary and to tell them to go wait in the CCU waiting room or go home.

If you want to find the police in a hospital, head for the E.R. On any given night, one or more members of the local constabulary will be in attendance for any number of reasons:

1. After a motor vehicle accident, completing reports and possibly interviewing the survivors.

2. Visiting with the victim of an assault, taking pictures and getting a statement.

3. Evaluation and treatment of an arrested perp's alleged illness or injuries, a.k.a. stall tactics, prior to heading off to the hoosegow.

4. In response to a request from the E.R. staff to remove an unruly or felonious patient.

5. OFT (Ogling and fraternizing time) with the nurses.

With such a persistent presence of the men in blue in the E.R., if you are a master criminal with chest pain, wanted from coast to coast, you may want to don a disguise before you call for the ambulance. A big handlebar moustache with Groucho eyebrows will usually fool the most seasoned officer of the law. Most E.R. staff would prefer to have a police officer hanging around 24/7. In fact, it's not uncommon for a hospital to hire one off-duty.

At least ninety per cent of patients in an E.R. don't really have an emergency. Many if not all could just as easily follow up with their family physician or go to an urgent care facility or just stay at home and tough it out. You, with your unstable angina, might the only truly emergent patient in the whole place. So don't feel bad for taking up a bed. You deserve to be there and you are probably going to make lots of money for the hospital, its employees, and for the physicians who take care of you. You're a good guy.

It may not be the best place to start your cardiac journey, but it is better to start in the E.R. than to end there, whether it be to come in and die before you make it to the cath lab, or to bounce back after your bypass surgery because something has gone wrong.

53. TEN THINGS AN EMERGENCY ROOM PHYSICIAN CAN SAY INSTEAD OF "YOU'RE AN IDIOT"

1. Your toe isn't broken, and an x-ray won't make it heal any faster.

2. It appears you left two tampons in your vagina last month, not one.

3. Here's that prescription for antibiotics you demanded. They won't help your cold, but they may give you bloody diarrhea.

4. A 12-pack of Sudafed is not the antidote for drowsiness.

5. Rather than lifting up your lawnmower to trim your hedges, next time you might want to try a hedge trimmer. The hand surgeon should be here soon.

6. The next time your pit bulls start fighting each other, how about throwing cold water on them instead? The hand surgeon should be here soon.

7. There is no 20 on a 1-to-10 pain scale.
8. Superglue is not an appropriate substitute for an eye mask.
9. We don't have the correct prescription pad for crystal meth.
10. Your ass will stop buzzing when the batteries run down.

54. THE NIGHT SHIFT

When the lights go down in the unit or on the telemetry floor, who is there to take care of you? The night shift, that's who.

If you started this journey via the E.R., odds are you have already met some members of the night shift. Mother Nature has decided that when it comes to major medical events, they will usually take place on the night shift. That's when babies hatch, plaques rupture, coronary arteries clot, alcoholics seize and drug addicts overdose. That's what prematurely ages health care personnel.

For the most part, nurses and doctors and techs on nights look much like their day shift counterparts. Except, of course, for the forty-something nurse dressed all in black with the cat eye glasses framing those distant Martian eyes. Whereas on the day shift the tone of the department is set by the supervisor or director and the various administrative suits who lurk and annoy on a daily basis, the character of the night shift in a particular unit or ward is determined by the nurses who work there.

On the hospital floors and units, it is rare that you find a physician who actually works a night shift; any physician you see on nights is usually there by dint of being on call. In the E.R., docs tend to rotate shifts on a regular basis, so in terms of the night shift, they are more or less part-timers. Occasionally you will run into an E.R. physician who works night shifts only; either he has a unique home situation or he's a weirdo. I know. I was a little of both. E.R. physicians who work only nights start out pretty normal, whatever that is. Eventually the night takes over their personality and the dark side emerges. Powder on a day shift guy's upper lip is usually from a donut. Powder on a night guy's is something else.

If there are three eight-hour shifts available, the young party nurses tend to gravitate toward the swing shift, 3-11:30 P.M. That way they can sleep in and recover from the late-night trip to the bars. If there are only two shifts available, the socializing gig is more challenging. Young night-shifters with no kids will on occasion get together after work for breakfast and beers. Every hospital has a nearby dive which specializes in locally-tailored early-morning festivities. Here in

Phoenix it is margaritas and breakfast burritos. Occasionally you walk into the local dive and find a patient you discharged at 5 A.M. sipping on a draft at 8.

Assuming you don't fall asleep on the way home from that, barring a gall bladder attack, you are guaranteed blissful uninterrupted shuteye. Of course, there is always the casino. Nothing caps off a twelve-hour shift like a couple dozen tugs on the one-armed bandit.

Why would anyone want to work nights when they could work days and be in sync with the rest of the world? Some hate getting up early enough to be at the hospital and ready to work at 7 A.M. Some hate their family life so much they are willing to do anything to avoid it. Some have young children at home whom they care for during the day; their husbands handle the kids at night. Some work nights so they have time to play with their twelve cats during the day. Some do it merely for the night shift differential, which can be as much as twenty per cent.

Early on, it is pretty heady stuff to be on days and have the director of the department working with you, showing you the way it's done. You might think, *Someday I want to be a nursing director too, mentoring young nurses and guiding the department through happy challenges and positive growth, carrying out the mission and vision of this fine institution. Maybe I could even rise to the position of hospital vice-president in charge of nursing affairs.* After a few years of the grind, however, you realize, *Gee, being a supervisor of anything is nothing but dealing, day in and day out, with all the personnel issues from below while taking a raft of shit from above. I would never want her job. Her job sucks.* After a few more years, you realize that any contact whatsoever with the supervisor or the suits leaves you wanting to take a stat shower in the de-lousing station. That's when you move to nights. Fewer bosses, more independence, less butt-smooching. There's more equality on the night shift. The shit rolls downhill from a lesser height, so it has less momentum when it hits you in the face.

You won't find ass-kissers on the night shift. Occasionally a nurse or two will be doing nights while they attend grad school to get their Master's degree or doing their time as night shift supervisor before they move on to become day shift supervisor. In general, however, night shifters' ambitions lie outside the workplace. Those who aspire to greatness always find their way onto the day shift so their face is not forgotten by the director of nursing.

One thing for sure about night-shifters. They are all sleep-deprived. The moms with small kids at home will routinely go two or three days with no more than an hour or two of sleep per day, usually only while the tykes are napping. No matter how orderly your life, if you sleep during the day you will develop the night shift fog. Like living in the Pacific Northwest for a year or two, it creeps up on you. You never feel the fog settle in. You might notice its far-off edges while it gently envelops you. The massive urns of coffee that most night shifters consume on a daily basis don't cut through the fog, they merely intensify the edges of it; nothing penetrates fully, but actions or feelings that come closest to getting through just irritate you. When you bid adieu to the night shift, it takes a good six months before you feel the fog lift. Once it lifts, you can't believe how dulled you were. It's not just the sleep deprivation--it's your excommunication from society.

The esprit de corps on most night shifts is impressive. Anytime you have a supermajority of XX chromosomes in the workplace, it will never be dull, but on the night shift, when a true emergency arrives, everyone drops their egos and pulls together to get the job done. That in itself is easier than on day shift, where the powers that be prefer to slosh their personalized interference ladles into every bowl of soup. In terms of skill sets and experience, the night shift is always equal to and often superior to the day shift. They aren't second-stringers. You'll find nurses doing nights who have been down all the roads and have done time in a multitude of settings and specialties. They tend to be very independent as well. While the daytime charge nurse tends to hover, the night shift is often short-staffed, so the charge nurse is usually off helping one of the staff nurses with her heavy workload or assisting with the sickest patient. He or she will hear from a staff nurse only if something goes terribly awry. The team-building thing is noticeable on day shifts, when the nursing education coordinator is introducing the latest new protocol or form. Team-building on nights pretty much consists of surviving countless emergencies with your co-workers.

Much like a Vegas casino, in a busy urban or suburban E.R., there is no special nighttime mood lighting. You would have a better chance of getting a good night's sleep in an airport. On the floors, however, the room lights go down after your night shift nurse checks in on you and gets your vitals. It is a little eerie up there.

There aren't any ghouls working the night shift in the E.R. For the most part, that is. Every so often some patient disappears in the middle of the night. After a brief search, the charge nurse calls housekeeping, the chart disappears, and the bed is made ready for the next patient.

Undoubtedly you will encounter at least one witch or warlock. Have no fear. They tend to by kindly witches, interested in casting only happy spells.

Upstairs, however, in the units and on the wards, you will sometimes notice a nurse or tech on the night shift that just gives you the willies. When they crawl by your room, you pray that they don't stop at your door. Part of that is your evening meds. Part is the night shift lighting. Part is your gut being spot-on. Zombies, vampires, Son of Mengele. They all come out at night.

If you show up in the E.R. toward the end of the night shift, odds are that, unless you are dying or have to go to the cath lab, you will stay there until change of shift, usually 7 A.M, before being admitted to an inpatient bed.

55. THOROUGH

David Simmons was spending December in San Diego. He'd scheduled a Rheumatology clinic rotation, the easiest tour of duty available. Eight hours a day, five days a week. Like Dermatology, there were very few emergencies involving arthritis. Normally he preferred a higher acuity, but he wanted his weekends free to explore southern California. In addition, he'd heard from an intern that the attendings were very low-key and didn't bat an eye if you wanted to take a day off to ride up to L.A. and check out UCLA and USC. ICU attendings, surgeons and most medical subspecialists wanted you there day in and day out, rounding on the weekends, taking call, all the nonsense he'd get his fill of next year wherever he landed for an internship.

What he hadn't counted on was the quality of the women in San Diego, both at the university and out in the general population. The South was supposed to have its fair share of attractive co-eds, but in southern California, citrus wasn't the only species that grew on trees. Aside from the rare ball-buster, they also had a much better attitude here than on the East Coast.

For the first two weeks of the rotation, Simmons' attending in the clinic was an Irishman by the name of Ardan Butler. A strikingly handsome man of forty, he explained his name when they first met. "Ardan, from the word *ardanach*, which means 'high aspiration' in Gaelic. My father, who in fact worked his entire life serving a rich man, aspired for me to be something more than a butler. What if our last name were 'King'?" Simmons liked him immediately. When Butler invited him out to Hennessey's for a beer at the end of the day, he liked him even more. He had the gift of gab you expect from a son of Eire, but there was none of the usual reveling in the dreary morbidity of life. He gave David a few instructions.

"I want two days' notice if you are planning to be absent from the clinic. We reserve our new patients specifically for the medical student, so if you're not going to be there, we can reschedule them. I expect you to attend my annual Christmas luau on Saturday the fifteenth. My place is down the road in the Village, staggering distance from the dorm. So if you already have plans for that afternoon and evening, cancel them. Other than that, just be thorough."

"You mean in the clinic?"

"I mean in life. Clinic, work, play, love. Everything." They shook hands and parted.

The clinic scheduled ten patients per day, five before lunch and five after. The majority were classic or complicated cases involving some inflammatory arthritis or vasculitis. Between two and four new patients were booked per day. These were the ones Simmons was expected to see. After performing his history and physical, he would present to Butler and Artie Valenzuela, the second-year fellow. Then the three of them would go in to see the patient. Some days, especially Mondays and Fridays, Artie was gone most of the day doing consults on inpatients. If he found something interesting, he'd call down to the clinic and have David come up and take a look. Between the clinic and consults, he was seeing almost everything in the textbooks.

"There's so much more pathology here than in Virginia."

Artie nodded. "I know. I did my residency in San Antonio. We had nowhere near the number of good cases you find here. Partly it's the size of the catchment area. We're seeing cases from Tijuana all the way up to Orange County. People don't want to mess with L.A. if they don't have to, especially if they're going to need to come in regularly for gold shots or joint injections. But there's something else here too. Some epidemiologist will probably write a paper and win the Nobel Prize, and we'll be sitting there thinking, 'Of course! Why didn't I think of that?' Exposure to sea water or fish tacos or something like that."

Simmons was living in a dorm room on the medical school campus. Every day started with the short walk through a dull fog, which burned off by mid-morning. Coming back to the dorm at the end of the day before heading out to the beach, he was reinvigorated by the fragrance of the eucalyptus trees which dominated the campus landscape. On the warmer days, when he looked up, he could see the blue haze surrounding their crowns. He thought, *December in San Diego. I could get used to this.*

By the end of the first week, David had decided that if he stuck with internal medicine, rheumatology would be just the thing. Good hours, lots of interesting patients, challenging problems to solve. Of course, he swooned over every specialty while he was doing the rotation, then, fickle lover, moved on when the month was over. Psychiatry, neurology, general surgery, cardiac surgery, pulmonology--each had lured him with its siren song. He mentioned as much to Butler at Friday afternoon liver rounds. This week the three of them were celebrating the sunshine and surf at the outside bar in the Beach & Tennis club.

"Davey, let me tell you something about rheumatology. First of all, it's a specialty dedicated to chronic diseases and chronic pain. Your patients don't die, they just keep coming back to talk about their pain."

"But I've seen nothing but great cases."

"New cases. Right. This is a referral clinic. Private practice, you don't see all that many new patients. Just the same ones, over and over."

"Oh." So much for Simmons' visions of new patients with exciting new problems popping into his small but hip beachfront office on a daily basis.

"Here's how it works for a new patient, or let's say a patient that's new to your practice with active rheumatoid arthritis. That's our bread and butter. First, he's excited to see you because, unlike his previous doctor, you know how to cure his disease and pain. After about six months, he realizes that you are no better than the last bloke. Another six months and now you're the reason he's in pain all the time. Sound like fun?" He took a sip of his Black & Tan and smiled. "Of course, it beats sticking a hose up some guy's ass for a living."

"Amen to that." Artie Valenzuela lifted his glass. "Here's to never having to do another sig." The three clinked glasses and drank.

The second week passed. Between new clinic patients and Sam's inpatient consults, it was a cavalcade of stellar pathology. He saw Butler's point however. Every morning and afternoon, the waiting room chairs filled up with rheumatoids in various states of disability. Sitting down or getting up produced predictable groans. On Wednesday night, he had a nightmare where every patient who came in to the clinic--he couldn't be sure if it was for arthritis or leprosy--dropped a digit or an entire limb onto the floor. Simmons' job was to refasten the amputated body parts with glue and sutures. Just before he awakened in a sweat, there were dozens of patients standing in line, holding their limbs, waiting and moaning. *Okay, maybe a specialty with a little less of the chronic pain and disfigurement.*

The end of the second week, Friday the fourteenth, was Butler's last day in clinic. Simmons' first patient of the day was well-known to the clinic staff for his longstanding stable rheumatoid arthritis. He came in with horribly swollen joints throughout his body, especially his knees. Simmons had no clue as to why the guy had suddenly flared less than twenty-four hours ago. When he presented the case to Artie and Butler, his differential diagnosis included infection versus an acute flare of his RA. Artie added an obscure entity or two. Butler asked David what one test he would perform. Hoping to stick a needle into a joint, especially a nice fat one like the guy's left knee, he offered, "I'd perform an arthrocentesis of his left knee."

Butler, who was as puzzled as his two trainees by the patient's turn for the worse, shrugged his shoulders and said, "Why not?". He thought for another moment. "Davey, have you ever done one before?"

"No, sir, but I've watched a half-dozen, everything from knees to fingers to ankles."

Butler came back with, "Well, see one, do one, teach one. Sounds to me like you're overdue on the 'do one' step." The patient, lying on the exam table, lifted his head in horror. Butler patted him on the shoulder. "No worries, John. A blind chimp with one hand could hit that knee on the first stick," and walked to the door. "Artie, do you mind?"

"Not at all, Dr. Butler. Dave, ask Mrs. Teague to write up a consent form and get us a diagnostic arthrocentesis tray."

The knee tap was a piece of cake. When they were done, Butler came back in with a syringe, aspirated a few drops of fluid out of one of the tubes, and motioned for David to follow him. In the mini-lab next to the attending's office, he squeezed out a drop of the fluid from the patient's joint onto a microscope slide, and put it under a microscope.

"Ever used one of these, Davey?" Butler set up the scope while he spoke.

"A microscope?" *Is he kidding?*

"A polarizing microscope."

"Oh. No."

"What is it good for?"

Simmons brushed aside a brief flashback of Edwin Starr singing "War". "Analyzing crystals for gout and pseudogout."

"Tell me how you differentiate the two." Butler bent over the scope and began moving it around over the slide.

Thank God I reread this. Sweet Jesus, let me get this right. He went over it in his head for a good fifteen seconds before answering. "Start with a polarizing filter and a red compensator filter. Gout crystals are composed of monosodium urate and are shaped like needles. They are negatively birefringent."

"Explain."

"When aligned parallel with the slow axis of the red compensator filter they are yellow in color. When aligned perpendicular to the slow axis, they are blue."

"Good. Either someone's been doing his reading or he has an excellent memory from two or three years ago. You had me a little worried when it took you so long to answer. It would have broken my soft green heart to flunk you on my last day, but I would have. How about pseudogout?"

This time Simmons didn't have to pause. "The crystals in pseudogout are composed of calcium pyrophosphate. They are shorter than urate crystals, usually rhomboid in shape, and positively birefringent. When aligned parallel to the slow axis of the red compensator filter they appear blue, and turn yellow when perpendicular."

"Nicely done, Lad. Take a look." He stood up to let David position himself on the stool. After moving the slide around and rotating the compensator, Simmons jumped a little. He turned to his attending.

"Wow. He's got gout."

"Yes he does."

"I don't think I've seen it written anywhere, but I heard one of our attendings say that you never see gout in a rheumatoid. Am I right about that?"

Butler smiled. "Correct. That's what they say. Another example of a truism being anything but. What should we do with miserable John, who came in with RA, had a rookie stick a sixteen-gauge needle in his hot, swollen, sore-as-hell knee, and now has another pain-in-the-ass diagnosis to accompany him on his journey through life? "

Simmons thought for a few seconds. "First, before we do anything, we have to see what the Gram stain shows, make sure there's no obvious infection."

"Good God, I hope not. This poor bastard's already had a bad day."

"If that's negative, then we treat him for gout."

"Lots of choices."

"If it were only one or two joints, you could inject them with corticosteroids, I think Aristospan. But he's got involvement in at least a dozen, so I'd probably start giving him colchicine, 1.2 mg. p.o. to start, then 0.6 mg. p.o. every hour for six hours or until..."

"Until he shits his pants. It's brutal even for a normal active person. With his pain and misery and stiffness, he'd probably prefer the gout to the diarrhea. Let's do this. Have Mrs. Teague give him ten mg. of Decadron intramuscularly and start the colchicine regimen. He can stay here in the clinic until we close. If he's not dramatically better, I'll admit him overnight. He should be much better in the morning. Fair enough?"

"Yes sir."

"Okay, Boyo, you get that going. I'll see you back here at one."

When Simmons returned from lunch, John was already feeling a little better. It seems Artie Valenzuela ordered him a shot of Demerol to ease the pain. John's wife had called their son. When he showed up, he picked up his fragile dad as if he were a tube of styrofoam and carried him out to the car. Artie wrote up a couple of prescriptions and sent them on their way, to follow up in a week.

Artie handed the chart to David. "You did a nice write-up. For as bad as he looked coming in, that's a pretty good disposition of a weird case. I'll put John on the list for Rheumatology Grand Rounds. I think that's your last day here; if you present it, the mucky mucks in the department might take notice. That could be the difference between getting a residency spot here or ending up in Fresno. I'm going upstairs to see a consult. I'll call if it's anything interesting."

"Okay, Artie. Thanks for walking me through the knee tap."

"De nada."

Simmons walked over to the desk and picked up a chart flagged for him. There was only today's encounter sheet inside, meaning the patient had not been seen anywhere in the university health care system. The patient was a twenty-two-year-old female by the name of Shawna Appleton, with new-onset swelling of her fingertips. A nice break from the usual fifty-five-year-old tile setter with sore knees. While walking into the exam room, David reviewed the single page in the chart. When he flipped it over, he noticed a bright yellow circular sticker on the inside back of the manila chart, just beneath the patient's name on the tab. *I wonder what that means.* When he looked up at the young woman sitting on the exam table, he knew instantly. Blushing brightly, he stuck out his hand. Her hands remained on her thighs.

"Hi, Miss Appleton. I'm David Simmons, the medical student in the Rheumatology Clinic this month." The red-haired little knockout smiled at him the way she had done earlier in the week from behind her desk on the vascular surgery ward. Simmons realized his mouth was hanging open and shut it. *Say something, David.* "I, uh, I was wondering what this little yellow sticker on your chart means."

Shawna giggled. "I guess it means I'm an employee of the university. I'm a unit secretary on 2-B."

"Yes, I saw you up there the other day. Nice to meet you." Again he stuck out his hand. The patient did not return the gesture. "Oh, gosh. I forgot. You're here for swollen fingers." *You dope.* She lifted her hands off her lap and extended them toward him. Clearly she was not looking forward to having them touched.

"I type a lot, so it may be nothing more than that, but for the past month they've been really swollen and sore. Our head nurse, Angie Thompson, saw them last week and told me to come see Dr. Butler. Is he here today?"

"Yes, he and Dr. Valenzuela are here today. I see the new patients first, present the cases to them with my diagnosis, then they come in and figure out what's really going on." Simmons usually felt at his most comfortable when he went to the self-deprecating humor lines. This one didn't have much of an effect on her.

"I haven't met Dr. Butler yet, but Dr. Valenzuela, he's so nice."

"Yeah, they're both great to work with." He sat down at the desk and started taking notes. "So you say this started about a month ago?"

A half-hour later, David excused himself from the room. Artie and Butler were sitting in the attending office going over a consult. David looked over his notes and mentally organized his presentation. Soon Artie got up and left the office. Butler waved David in.

"So you're seeing Miss..." he looked down at a note on his desk, "Shawna Appleton?" He looked up at Simmons with a trace of amusement. David nodded. "My dear friend Nurse Thompson called and asked if we could squeeze her in before I rotated out of the clinic. I told her we had a particularly adept fourth-year medical student from that Jefferson fellow's university out East who would do a smashing job of evaluating her problem." Then Butler laughed, put his hands behind his head, and leaned back. "Please begin."

It took David fifteen minutes to go through the H & P. Given Butler's personal interest, he padded the presentation with more detail than usual. When he finished, Butler sat forward and made a few notes.

"Davey, what does the young lady have?"

"Well, she's kind of young, but she does type for eight hours a day, so Heberden's nodes secondary to osteoarthritis is a possibility. I think there's a form of psoriatic arthritis that affects primarily the DIP joints, but she doesn't have any psoriatic lesions."

"How do you know?"

Is this a trick question? "How do I know? I asked her and I examined her."

"You did, did you? Let's go take a look, shall we?" David opened the exam room door and let Butler precede him.

"Miss Appleton, this is Dr. Butler." Butler took one look at the patient, sitting on the table in her skirt and blouse, before turning to Simmons.

"So you examined her, did you?" He raised one eyebrow. He went to the supply stand, pulled out a sheet, and handed it to the patient.

"Please take off all your clothes, put this on, and open the door slightly when you are ready." Then he turned and walked out the door. David looked at Shawna, who wore a stunned look, and followed him out, closing the door behind him. Butler was waiting for him in the hallway. He was wearing a look of patient annoyance.

"Do you remember our conversation at Hennessey's your first day?"

"Yes, sir."

"Did I communicate my expectations to you?"

"Yes, sir."

"What were they?"

"Well, you expected me to show up at your luau, which I believe is tomorrow afternoon."

"Good. I brought in a Hawaiian shirt for you to wear. What else?"

"Be thorough."

"Yes. Were you thorough with Miss Appleton?" *Oh, so that's what this is all about.*

"Apparently not."

"Not apparently, Lad. Yes or no, were you thorough?"

"No sir."

"Listen, Davey. One thing you must always remember. Rheumatic diseases are not diseases of the joints. They are systemic diseases. Examine every part of the system. You let your exam slip because she's a cute little thing, you'd love to get into her pants, and you were embarrassed to check out her privates. I know, I've been there. That won't cut it. Sooner or later, letting your feelings get in the way of your job will cause somebody will suffer needlessly, perhaps die." He put his hand on Simmons' shoulder. "The door is open. I'll call you when I want you to come in." He winked and disappeared into the room, shutting the door behind him.

Simmons pondered that wink. *Is this whole thing a setup?* Hospitals are like small towns, where everyone knows what everyone else is doing. The word on Ardan Butler was that he was an inveterate playboy who rarely dated anyone twice. Even his one-nighters, sprinkled throughout the hospital, smiled at the mention of his name. *Some guys,* thought Simmons, *really know how to break it off.* That arrow had not made it to Simmons' quiver yet.

After about ten long minutes, the door opened. Butler stood in the doorway, sporting a tight little smirk. He motioned David in. Shawna was sitting on the exam table, holding the sheet over her chest. It extended down to her shins.

"Miss Appleton, please stand up and turn around." She did. Simmons found himself staring at her butt. He looked up at Butler, who could barely contain himself. Shaking his head, the Irishman asked her to bend over. When she complied, Simmons thought, *Thank God she can't see how embarrassing this is.* Then he realized, *Oh, yeah, this might be a little more embarrassing for her.*

Butler stepped forward. "I'm going to show young Dr. Simmons what I showed you in the mirror. Over here, David." With that, he parted her cheeks. On the right side, barely an inch above her anus, was a small red raised area covered with scale. Butler looked at David with both eyebrows raised. Then he removed his hands. The patient turned around and sat back up on the table. Her face was red, but she wore a tentative smile.

"We'll step out so that you can get dressed. When you are ready, please open the door." They left.

Out in the hallway, Simmons exhaled loudly. He realized he'd held his breath for the last minute or so.

Butler looked at him. "What was that for?" Then he smiled. "I know what you were thinking. You had this idea, based no doubt on my reputation around here, that I was going to put the moves on that sweet young thing, check out her attributes, shall we say. Nod your head if I'm correct." Simmons nodded.

"Oh, I might have, but my dear friend Nurse Thompson would have gotten wind of that, and sometime tomorrow evening I'd end up with a tiki torch stuck up my ass." David raised his eyebrows. "Yes, she'll be there. We are close. Very close." Butler gave him his lecher smile. "So what should we do with Miss Appleton?"

"Well, she has psoriasis..."

"How do you know she has psoriasis?"

"She has a psoriatic plaque in her gluteal cleft."

"Less than thirty minutes ago, you were telling me she didn't have psoriasis. I believe it went something like, 'How do I know? I asked her and I examined her.' "

"Fair enough. It looked like a plaque to me." *I can't believe I'm debating with an attending. At UVA, I'd be scrubbing bedpans at this point.*

"Look, this is an odd case. It's never business as usual when you are seeing physicians, nurses, unit secretaries, or their significant others. Don't assume anything when a colleague is involved. I think it's psoriasis too, but let's get an expert opinion. Send her to that room full of underworked doctors."

I'm almost afraid to ask. "Which room is that?"

Butler's eyes gleamed like an angler with an eight-pound summer steelhead on the hook. "Dermatology clinic, of course. What should we do today?"

"I'd get a simple AP view of both hands, see if there are any inflammatory or destructive changes, make sure it really isn't just osteoarthritis. She'll need some blood work, the usual stuff. CBC, chemistries, uric acid level, sed rate, ANA to rule out lupus, rheumatoid factor. Should we try to get an HLA-B27 on her?"

"Not at this point. It's only a coin flip even if she has spinal disease, which does not appear to be the case. Okay, time for me to go. You should plan on seeing her back in ten days, certainly before you finish up your month. Tom Gargan is coming on to attend here in the clinic; he loves stuff like this. Make sure you read every journal article he's ever written on psoriatic arthritis.

"By the bye, Davey. If you're going to spend your life in medicine, you might as well enjoy it. Act like an Irishman, or at least a Californian. You must move out here for your residency. You've already spent far too much time with those Puritan descendants out East. The only reason they moved to the States is that nobody wanted them to stay in Britain. Even the Brits tired of their dullness. Can you imagine?

"Here's the ugly truth. Some of your friends are going to have illnesses and chronic diseases. Some of those diseases will be the ones you treat every day. To be a physician and a human being, you must learn how to integrate your professional life and your personal life without confusing the two. It's not just about making a diagnosis and treating the disease process you've diagnosed. When it comes to rheumatoids, I get five times as many questions from patients about sex or golf as I do about the dosage of gold or prednisone. That's how it is. Diagnoses are unimportant to the poor souls who bear them. How they live their lives around those diagnoses, that's what's important."

"That's not how they teach it in medical school, Sir."

"I know. You're supposed to keep your feelings under lock and key when you are working, then magically unlock them and set them free when you're off the clock. Sounds perfectly perfect. Spend some time with any number of physicians and their families and you'll see how well that works."

"So I'm supposed to be a friend and a physician? Is that how it works? It was a nice speech, but I gotta know, do you have any relationships like that?" *I doubt it.*

"Why do you think Nurse Thompson and I are such close friends?"

Simmons said, "Oh." *You sly fucker, you got me again.*

"Anyway, I'm going to get you started. My dear friend Nurse Thompson is coming tomorrow evening, and she's bringing our Miss Appleton with her. Apparently the girl studies constantly and has no social life. One of her delusions is that going to medical school is a worthwhile goal. When you go back in, please let her know you'll be in attendance at my soiree tomorrow. Give her a chance to decide whether she wants the bloke who peeked down the crack in her ass on Friday to be wooing her with a mai-tai on Saturday. If she decides to come, I expect you to make her feel at home." He smiled and pointed at the door. "Good luck. According to my dear friend Nurse Thompson, Miss Appleton's other delusion is that you are nice. And cute."

56. THE TOUGHEST JOB

In medical school, we had a class with one of the senior surgeons. Good surgeon, excellent educator. In his opinion, the physician with the toughest job in terms of diagnosis was the general practitioner or family practitioner or general internist, i.e., the primary care provider

(PCP). Everybody took this in, but at that early stage in our training, bombarded on a daily basis with new hospital-based advancements in technology, I think most of us would have disagreed. After all, if a bunch of starry-eyed third year medical students could do one, how hard can it be to take a history and do a physical and figure out what was wrong with the patient? That was so old-fashioned.

After a few decades, it is obvious that he was absolutely correct. That is certainly the case when it comes to the diagnosis of coronary disease. Of all the guys who present to his office with chest pain, a PCP has to figure out which one probably has cardiac disease and should be admitted to the hospital or referred to a cardiologist. If the PCP overdiagnoses, i.e., diagnoses cardiac disease in a bunch of patients with esophageal reflux or chest wall pain due to a pulled pec muscle, he loses credibility and pretty soon the insurance companies are going to consider dropping him from their lists of providers. After all, even insurance companies that are very profitable can't afford to do stress tests and caths on every guy with any type of chest pain.

If he underdiagnoses, i.e., fails to diagnose cardiac disease in patients who present with chest pain, sooner or later one of them is going to die needlessly. That is considered poor form. If an overweight guy with a family history of coronary disease who smokes and has a total cholesterol level of two hundred fifty comes in complaining of typical exertional angina, even a PCP with a bag over his head will get it that this guy has heart disease and will refer him appropriately. If, however, the guy presents with an atypical story, he has to decide, without much objective data to help, whether the guy is likely to drop dead or needs to fart more often.

Conversely, cardiologists always get the diagnosis right, right after the cath. Neurosurgeons uniformly bat 1.000 when it comes to diagnosing a subarachnoid bleed within seconds of looking at the CT or the MRI. We Americans have a fondness and fascination for technology and experts. Subspecialists have to be proficient in their craft and know when to do what. Their judgment has to be razor-sharp when it comes to treatment. They get the publicity and a ton of praise from the patient and the family. The PCP, with the toughest job diagnostically, gets all the headaches, lower pay, and none of the glory. That may have something to do with the shortage of primary care physicians in this country.

57. WHO MAKES THE BEST DOCTOR?

"Good morning, Mrs. O'Leary. I'm Dr. Simmons. Dr. Taylor had to go home, so he asked me to review your chest x-ray and labs, then go over the results with you. Are you feeling any better after the breathing treatment?"

She nodded. "The treatment didn't help much, but the oxygen made a big difference. Now I don't feel like I'm breathing so fast."

"Right. Your respiratory rate was around thirty-five per minute when you arrived, and it's down to eighteen now. Your lungs don't have to work so hard to get enough oxygen. Your heart rate is down from one hundred twenty-four to ninety-three beats per minute, so that's a good thing too."

"How does my chest x-ray look?" She pulled the sheet up as far as it would go.

"Are you cold?"

"A little. You sure keep the air conditioning on high in here." Simmons reached into a bedside cabinet and pulled out a blanket.

"Rumor has it that the administration keeps it cold in here so we won't get sleepy. Wouldn't want our productivity falling." He smiled.

"Thanks. That's better. You were saying about my x-ray?"

"Yes. First let me ask you. Have you ever had a chest x-ray before?"

"A couple of years ago, in Chicago, Dr. Feldstein took one. I had a cold that wouldn't get better. I had a little trouble breathing, but nowhere near as bad as it was the past few days."

"And did Dr. Feldstein make any comments about that film?"

"He said it was normal. He gave me prednisone to take for a week, and I got better."

"I see. Well, this morning your x-ray shows an interstitial infiltrate throughout both lungs, which..."

"What does that mean?"

"Basically, your lungs look hazy. Interstitial infiltrates can be due to a number of processes, some of which are temporary and resolve on their own. Or they can result from more serious diseases. Were you ever a smoker?"

She laughed. "No way. My mother beat me good the first time she caught me smoking. And the second and third time too. After that I got the message."

"Good for her. That eliminates a number of serious diseases. I've seen chest x-rays with diffuse interstitial infiltrates from viral pneumonias, like influenza, from congestive heart failure, from tuberculosis or fungal infections, from asbestos, and from lung cancer."

"Well I doubt I have any of those."

"Right. There are also a number of illnesses lumped under the term idiopathic interstitial lung disease. That means they just happen, and an exact cause has not yet been discovered. There are theories that some are caused by inflammation, others by exposure to toxins."

"So what do we do now?"

"That painful blood test they took, out of your radial artery? That showed that your oxygen level was dangerously low. So, for at least the time being, you'll need to stay on supplemental oxygen. While in theory you could go home on oxygen..."

"No, we're just staying in a hotel room for now."

"...I would rather admit you to the hospital, have a pulmonary specialist see you, and decide how best to diagnose and treat this."

"Sounds good. Just one thing."

"What's that?"

"Get me a Jew."

"Excuse me?"

"A Jew. I want a Jewish doctor."

"Why is that?"

"Everybody knows, at least in Chicago they do. Jews make the best doctors."

Simmons thought for a moment. "Let me make a phone call. I think I've got just the guy for you."

Mrs. O'Leary smiled. "Guy, not goy, right?"

"Yes, Ma'am. I'll be back in a few minutes. Someone from Admitting will be over to have you sign a few papers."

A few minutes later, Simmons was on the phone.

"Shreiner here."

"Hi, Sol. This is David. I have a patient with an abnormal chest x-ray and marked hypoxia."

"Simmons, I'm not on call for consults today. It's Marcum."

"Sol, I really think this case is right up your alley. Plus, she wants a Jew."

"Well, then they can get Horowitz to see her. Besides, I'm not in the mood for a crabby old Jew lady. She'll be laying the guilt on thicker..."

"Her name's O'Leary. Her maiden name was Riley."

"And she wants a Jew, eh?"

"Says they make the best doctors."

"I'll be right over."

Two minutes later, Sol Shreiner walked in, dapper in his three-piece worsted wool suit.

"Now where is this fascinating woman?"

58. A GOOD LIFE

Savannah Keith watched her two girls get on the school bus, and waited until her little Tara, with the pigtails and the missing tooth, slid in next to the window and waved as the bus took off. She said good-bye to her neighbors and walked the half-block of brilliant autumn colors back to her brick neoclassical home.

It took about ten minutes to load the dishwasher with the breakfast stuff and turn it on. Right on schedule, eight o'clock sharp, there was the ringing of the house phone. Every Tuesday and Friday morning, she and her mother talked for about a half hour, Savannah listening while her mother recited the latest version of her hard life in Buckhead. This week her Dad was forgetful and snored; he must be getting Alzheimer's, or at least sleep apnea. *More likely,* thought Savannah, *he's getting a little too friendly with his Blanton's and branch.* Then came the breaking news of the day. Savannah's best friend from middle school, Ashley Riordan, was well down the road to changing her name back to Turner. Apparently Mike Riordan had found himself a younger version of Ashley and was now living the bachelor life, swanky penthouse apartment included, in Poncey-Highlands in the Fourth Ward. As soon as she heard the word "divorce", Savannah knew what was coming.

"You're so lucky, Savannah. Such a good husband, that Richard of yours. So unlike your father. What a catch." As her mother rambled on about the inconvenience of having to drive ten blocks whenever Kacey Whitworth hosted the bridge club at least once every three months, Savannah made a brief run-through of the plans for Saturday night. She had three good friends in the neighborhood. All four families would be converging here tomorrow night to celebrate Rich's fortieth birthday. Steaks and salmon on the grill, burgers and hot dogs for the kids, the neighbors bringing everything else but the cake. Margaritas to start, then a couple of the good bottles out of the cellar. She put the party planning on hold and willed her attention back to the phone conversation.

"Your father and I are going down to Pompano for some lawyers' convention Monday, but I'll be sure to call you Tuesday. He'll want to drive, of course. That should be an almighty adventure, me on alert every minute to make sure he doesn't fall asleep at the wheel and kill us both. Give the girls my love, and tell Richard I said 'Happy Birthday'".

They said their good-byes. No sooner had Savannah hung up than the phone rang. It was Jan Hayward from next door. This day was getting away from her.

"I'm on my way out to Harris Teeter. Does Rich like regular potato salad or German?"

"He likes German, but get the regular."

"Oh, I'll buy him a pint of German, then make a big bowl of the regular for everyone else."

"Jan, you don't need to go to the trouble. He'll be fine with whatever."

"No trouble at all. He's such a nice guy, he deserves a perfect fortieth."

"Okay, if that works for you. See you tomorrow night."

"Aren't you coming for tennis this afternoon?"

"I have to get my nails done for the party, and the only time Tracy can squeeze me in is at one, so I'll have to pass. Say hi to the girls."

She called and placed the usual order for Friday night pizza with Sammy and Tara, then checked to see what movies were available in the pay-per-view listings. It sure would be nice if Rich took off at least one Friday night a month so they could hang out as a family. As he explained it, doing Friday night call got him off the hook so they could spend every Saturday and Sunday together. It also kept him at the top of the pecking order for scheduling vacations. Sure made it hard to get together with the other anesthesiologists in the group and their wives though. Come to think of it, since Rich moved over to the Pain division and started taking call Friday nights, they hadn't been out at all with the others. Not that they had the time, what with all the neighborhood kid-friendly activities every weekend. On the upside, at least he wouldn't be out at the Copa on Friday nights with a girlfriend, like in *Goodfellas*.

Savannah looked through the pantry and the refrigerator, making a list of the things she could pick up on her way home from Nails With Tracy. They were low on pancake mix. She decided to go with a chipotle marinade for the steaks and a basic lemon and dill mayo mixture for the salmon. Oh, and of course, fresh buns for the burgers and dogs.

Next it was time to bake Rich's birthday cake. For the next hour and a half, she created a lemon layer cake with raspberry butter cream frosting, a recipe she found on the internet. It came out terrific, the frosting a bright cerise. Across the top in lime green script she wrote, "Happy Sunny Saturday", the same thing he always said when he served the girls their pancakes on Saturday morning, rain or shine. His favorite color combo, cerise and lime. She slid it into her cake caddy and placed it on top of the refrigerator, far from the sugar-seeking grasp of her girls.

Upstairs she sorted through her closet for a dress suited to the occasion. As an accent to the cake, she pulled out a Sarah Spaghetti Strap Bodycon dress in berry and tried it on. Her hips look fuller in it than she'd like, but she wouldn't have to wear a bra. For the Rich and Savannah festivities later, she went with a Dream Angels Lace Plunge Teddy in black, pink and white. In the mirror Savannah could see the background light filtering between her thighs. Not bad for almost forty. Thank God for all those crunches and twice-a-week tennis.

She wouldn't mind smoking some of that fat doob Betsy Moynihan gave her, loosen things up, might even slow Rich down a little. What initially intrigued her about him, his eternal optimism combined with his endless energy, now just wore her out. She wasn't in her late twenties now, she was almost forty. A slightly slower version of her husband would fit her needs just fine. A toke or two would do him some good, but Rich is such a stickler for a drug-free household, worried about the State board and sending the wrong message to the girls.

"It's a gateway drug, Savannah. Every drug addict starts out with marijuana."

"Sure, Rich. Using that logic, the ultimate gateway drug would have to be breast milk."

Rich with his anti-abortion arguments, not the least bit daunted about making decisions for millions of women, no matter what their situation, even if they've been raped or suffered sexual abuse at the hands of their drunken fathers. Even Rich's partners had a problem with his rightward opinions on social issues, never mind their wives. He had this unbending conviction about his beliefs. Deep down, he had his insecurities, but when it came to faith and morals, he was as certain as the pope. One thing for sure, she wouldn't have to worry about him going down the path some doctors take, cheating and drugging and drinking. Or would that be men in general?

His parents, bona fide southern Baptists, shunned every vice like a cancer, and instilled a frightening fear of frivolity in Rich and his sister at their estate in Lookout Mountain, Tennessee. Only one hundred twenty miles from Atlanta by auto, it might as well have been on another planet when it came to social issues. Rich still looked on Asians as not to be trusted, "after what they did to our boys in WWII". She admired his loyalty but wondered how someone born in the Vietnam era could be so immersed in the resentment felt by a generation earlier. Their first night together, she knew right away she was seducing a virgin. Absolutely inexperienced but his energy was intoxicating, as if he could fix any inadequacy with extra effort.

Now, their marriage. By all standards, good, stable and mostly fun. By reputation, Rich was an excellent anesthesiologist, who moved over to Pain Management six months ago without missing a beat. He doted on Savannah and the girls, always stepped up when it came to family activities, and was a good provider. He was more excited than the girls about their upcoming cruise to St. Maarten and Castaway Cay. Their home here in Raleigh, situated in the dead center of a safe, beautiful neighborhood, the house in Nags Head less than four hours away, perfect for a weekend trip, and the four-way share condo in Naples could host three couples for a golf getaway or a family vacation. No money worries. She had plenty of time to work out, keep herself in shape, not give Rich the slightest cause to look elsewhere.

It would be nice to go back to the O.R. though, floating or scrubbed in; in fact, that was where they met. There was that job at Regency Hospital, but Rich had nixed that, said you don't need to work, but if you want to, anywhere else but there, he couldn't put up with all the docs staring after her, joking around and trying to cop feels in the O.R. He knew it might happen, but he didn't want to hear about it and he sure didn't want to see it. Confident in everything he did, but just a little insecure when any man paid more than the usual attention, even that old Mr. Coughlin down the street with the fluffy eyebrows and hairy Hobbit ears.

No, she felt secure with Rich. Of course there was that one time, about six months ago. He came home, his prick all Bulldog red and raw, with some ridiculous story about spilling chemicals on it. Just in case, she'd talked with Betsy Moynihan, who knew a thing or two or three about divorce lawyers. However, once he'd finished his thirty-day sentence on ice, imposed without appeal by Judge Savannah, he'd been more attentive than ever; neither one of them ever mentioned it again. Some days, when Mother griped ceaselessly about Daddy, Savannah had the urge to spill the chemical penis story, just to see how she took it. So far she'd resisted, but one of these days...

At noon, right on schedule, the mailman deposited his daily offering out front. Savannah backed her Lexus RX out of the garage and stopped to empty the mailbox. There was the usual, circulars from the supermarkets, a pile of bills, and three envelopes addressed to Rich, birthday cards for sure. One other piece, a thick handwritten envelope for Savannah. She put the SUV in Park and opened it up.

CaryJane Williams had been her roommate and best buddy during their four years in nursing school at UGA. About eight months ago she'd taken a sabbatical from Gainesville and joined Doctors Without Borders. Wrapped within the two-page letter were a half-dozen photos of her with the locals in Antananarivo, Madagascar. *God, it looks awfully poor. She must be having so much fun.* CaryJane had tried to warn Savannah against settling down right away. When Rich proposed, she'd been even more explicit.

"Savannah, honey, you'll have plenty of time for that when you're thirty. Don't give up being young for a man. Come with me, we'll see the country, maybe the whole world in the next ten years." CaryJane had done exactly that, working as a commissioned officer assigned to the State Department in France, Japan, Australia and Argentina before signing on at Florida to teach in the Nurse Practitioner program there. She'd never married, but always sounded so happy and content when they talked. Savannah read the letter through twice, then sat looking at her home for a minute.

All this perfection in my life is rotting my brain. I have got to get back to nursing. If I keep on like this, I'll end up calling Sammy every week and bitching about my bridge club.

She returned the photos and letter to the envelope, then headed down the street, all the while pondering how she would tell Rich of her decision. The conflict raged in her head.

I have everything I've ever wanted, more than any woman could ask for. What's wrong with me?
Rich gets to practice his profession and have a family too. Why can't I?
Rich has given me so much. The least I can do is humor him and be a stay-at-home Mom.
Even though he cheated only once, he did break his vows. It was only once, right? He's not a serial philanderer like Daddy. Is he?
If Mother, Jan, Tara and Sammy all think Rich is so terrific, they can't all be wrong. What is it I see that they don't?
For God's sake, Savannah, you're married to him. They're not.

Back and forth she went. She'd almost talked herself out of the notion of working when she saw the billboard.

Nurses Wanted: Emergency Department, Surgery, Labor and Delivery, Intensive Care. Regency Hospital. 919-427-5555.

It is time, she thought, *for a change.*

59. DOCTORS' WIVES

Back in the days of Marcus Welby, the doctor's wife, whom he met in college or medical school, usually worked full-time in the office. Often she was a nurse, sometimes not. If she'd graduated from nursing school, you could count on her to wear her nursing school cap to work every day. Sometimes the cap was so omnipresent, so immutable in its permanence, a reasonable person could wonder whether she slept in it. Nurse or not, she took up residence in the doctor's office for two reasons. First, it helped to have family working in the business. Even sweet old secretaries weren't above ripping off the rich doctor. Equally important, it was good to keep an eye on the investment and the investment's lovely young employees and patients.

On the dark side of the Donna Reed story, the doctor's wife sweats and slaves and works full-time supporting her husband while he attends medical school. She figures they are building a life together and a career for the two of them, so the deal is that she works during medical school and perhaps residency, then, when he's actually making money, she can take some time off to start having children. It is no myth that every year there are more than a few wives (and a husband or two) who get served divorce papers on medical school graduation day. At this stage of the game, the doctor has virtually no net worth, probably has a fair bit of debt (for which, icing on the cake of pain, she co-signed), and will be working for the next three to ten years in a minimum wage job known as a residency. The doctor gets out of the marriage for a song, only to move on to his internship with the other medical student or nurse or unit secretary he's been banging for the past two years. Occasionally, Doctor He or Doctor She switches sides in the process. Often debated but never resolved is whether this is more or less humiliating for the doctor's ex-spouse.

Just as history tends to repeat itself, so the same scenario not infrequently recurs several years later, after the doctor has finished his residency and is starting to practice. Here, the alimony payout will be substantially higher, as he's been making some money, usually minimum wage, for the past few years, and his new job includes even better paychecks. Sealing the deal with a baby or two makes it more difficult and far more expensive to disentangle himself. Nonetheless, the lure of a new love conquers all. It happens every year.

Once our young doctor has begun to practice, especially if he starts his own practice and office, the smart doctor's wife takes a position in the office. Sometimes she's a nurse, sometimes she's the manager, but she is always the watchdog. Other women who work in doctors' offices see married doctors as eligible bachelors with a temporary encumbrance, his present wife, a.k.a. you. As a doctor's wife, there are two ways to go. There is plan A, living the good life, raising children, staying at home, and enjoying the ride as long as it lasts. Plan B entails more work, less glamour: maintain a daily presence in the office. In the old days, the doctor's wife often worked in the office because it kept overhead down. Nowadays, it is good to be there to provide the occasional sharp stick to the eye of any employee or patient who develops too much of a fondness for the doctor for their own good. The trick is to maintain order without resorting to a catfight. Unless the doctor's wife is getting a big cut of the royalties, it's best not to allow the office to become the setting for a reality show.

Three's a crowd, but three that always get along just peachy are power, money and sex. If one party has the first two, sure as shootin' someone's going to come along with the third. In most walks of life, in order for a married man to get into trouble with a femme fatale, he usually has a case of The Wandering Eye. Not so for CEOs, business owners and doctors. They've got the power, especially in the office. They've got the money, although "money" comes in various levels. They don't have to stick their heads out of their little turtle shells for more than a minute before someone comes hauling ass to help them out with the sex part of the triad.

If one day the doctor's wife walks into his office to find that it has been completely redecorated in a style that makes her gag and her hubby's cute little "Office Assistant and Decorator", stationed behind her prominent new desk, sports a new rack of comically oversized boobs, each one as large as a human head, it behooves the doctor's wife to be proactive in a stepwise fashion. Step 1: Pull out the smart phone and google "Attorneys, Divorce". Step 2: Schedule a house call with the locksmith. Then Step 3: Do I want to be a widow or a divorcee?

Visiting the home of a long-married doctor and his wife is like visiting the residence of any other kind of couple. Of course, there is a much better chance that when the wife answers the door with a saucy wink and hands you a martini, she is wearing her nursing school cap. Kinky.

Compared with office life or operating room life, where his every request will most likely generate a "Yes, Doctor", the doctor's home life is much more complicated. The stay-at-home wife, whose life revolves around yard apes, home and hobbies, is bursting with the latest news about school, the kids' extracurricular activities, plumbers, bills, landscapers, broken fingernails while playing tennis, lunch at a new cafe with the girls, electricians, PTA meetings, dance lessons, orthodontist appointments and wouldn't it be nice to put in a swimming pool so that I could have a pool boy? Worse yet, the doctor is expected not to simply listen and nod occasionally, but to actually participate in the conversation, admire the budding genius' finger paint masterpiece, examine the serious, serious black and blue from football, deny that the new dress makes her ass look fat. All the while he's thinking, *Boy would that dress look good on the hot new circulating nurse in the O.R., the one with the sugary drawl from down in Birmingham. It wouldn't make her ass look fat.*

Most doctors are more adept at dealing with injury and illness than they are with any other aspect of modern human life. When you do something all day every day and you get rewarded for it both financially and emotionally, it defines your comfort zone. You make a diagnosis, you write a prescription, you write an order, you perform a procedure, and everyone's happy with you. *I have saved another life. Next case, please.* So it's no wonder that doctor's wives, in an effort to get attention from the great diagnostician and healer, sometimes end up going to the malady card.

"I just don't know why I keep getting these headaches. What do you think, Dear?"

"I'm having the hardest time sleeping. Could you bring me home some Ambien samples?"

"I am so sick of this postpartum belly fat. I've been working at it for years but it just won't go away. Could you write me a prescription for some diet pills?"

"These weird palpitations. I get so dizzy. I'd better see a cardiologist, don't you think?"

At the very least, the doctor's wife will get his attention while he deals with her latest symptom, even if it's only for the time it takes to write a prescription.

Sooner or later, unless he wants to end up with four separate alimonies and countless child support checks going out monthly, the doctor will have to stick with one of his wives. Otherwise he'll be too broke to do anything but die.

60. DOCTORS' CLOTHES

Marcus Welby lived up on the summit of Physician Fashion Mountain. Back in the old days, doctors wore sport coats, slacks, brogues, button-down oxford shirts in white or blue, club ties and a stethoscope. Loafers for those carefree let-loose days. The sport coat was as essential as the stethoscope. A recent-issue Harris tweed was just the thing for hospital rounds. It said, "I am here to solve medical problems." Then, when he got home, Marcus changed into an older-model Harris tweed. It was identical to the hospital tweed, but with the added feature of patches on the elbows. It said, "I am here to solve domestic problems." Somewhere in the commute from hospital to home, he removed the stethoscope.

No, wait. That was Jim Anderson on "Father Knows Best." It's easy to confuse the two, especially at home, where there was no stethoscope to keep things straight. Jim had wife Margaret and kids Princess, Bud and Kitten at home. Marcus was a widower with considerably fewer domestic problems to solve.

Obviously, before you arrived in your office practice, you had to do an internship. If the TV show ran for more than one season, like *Dr. Kildare* or *Ben Casey*, which was essentially *Dr. Kildare* with chest hair, then you were doing a residency as well. During your internship, you were expected to wear white. Not just white, but a white double-breasted shirt-jacket affair custom-designed for style and comfort by Chairman Mao. After a particularly grueling episode, it was permissible to undo some of the top buttons so blood could flow to your head. Ben Casey endured many more grueling episodes than Dr. Kildare, so his special intern shirt was almost always open to his belly button. Once you finished your residency, apparently the white suit walked away by itself, to be reused by another starving intern or a patient in an insane asylum, or cut down and dyed baby blue and sent to Floyd in Mayberry.

Most of the time, Marcus Welby would wear a white coat in the office. Some were jacket length, known in the business as "short", some full-length, known as "long", as in "long white coat". Ingenious, eh? On occasion, just to keep things fresh and exciting, the kindly physician changed to a Floyd Jacket. Doc Welby was the fashion poster boy for "devil-may-care".

In the trenches of the O.R., everybody wears scrubs in one form or another. Surgeons, anesthesiologists, scrub nurses, circulating nurses, technicians. Usually the outfit consists of pants with a string tie at the waist, and a short-sleeved, v-neck shirt. In that milieu of unisex conformity, nothing gets the guys' attention like a scrub nurse who shatters the norm and shows up in a scrub dress. This practice came to a screeching halt when an epidemiologist (*epidemi* = the fucking problem; *ologist* = the guy who figures it out and, in some cases, publishes a paper, causing himself a shitload of trouble) traced infections in ICU patients to the exposed body parts of nurses wearing scrub dresses.

It's always been permissible (mandatory as well) to wear scrubs in the O.R. If you leave the O.R. without changing, you have to put on a long white coat. Whether that is to prevent O.R. goo from offending those timid souls in other parts of the hospital or to protect the O.R. from hospital goo remains unclear. Ask around. Nobody seems to know.

Your cardiologist may dress in a coat and tie most of the time and save the scrubs for the cath lab; outside his office, it is rare to see your cardiac surgeon in anything but scrubs. As a matter of fact, a cardiac surgeon spotted in civvies in the hospital is probably heading for a departmental meeting to explain what went wrong.

Who are the best-dressed physicians? First of all, let's be clear. Physicians will never be confused with fashion models, not even with lawyers. When it comes to doctors there is pretty much a direct correlation between dressing stylishly and managing money wisely. The smoothest dressers are usually the best businessmen. A guy who actually gets complimented on his clothing in the hospital is usually dressed by his wife. If she is smart, she is also managing the practice's and the family's finances. If you asked the average guy on the street which specialty of physician is the best-dressed, most would say plastic surgeons. They do dress well, as it is very important to exude an air of opulence and sophistication when charming women out of cold hard cash. However, in my experience, the best-dressed physicians are colorectal surgeons. They are also known as proctologists or proctological surgeons. I find it a tad ironic. You make your living hanging around colostomies and poop all day, but you look like you just popped out of a GQ photo shoot. I have never met a colorectal surgeon who didn't dress like a million bucks.

61. WHITE COATS

Med students always wear short white jackets, like a waiter in a restaurant with tablecloths and cloth napkins. Not as starchy, and always clean, as a med student rarely gets dirty. They are usually festooned with all sorts of unnecessary gadgets, like a Penrose drain through one of the button holes. The Penrose is a soft rubber tube designed to be placed in a wound to prevent the accumulation of fluid. It hangs at the ready, theoretically available as a tourniquet for an emergency blood draw or IV placement. In practice it is rarely used. They are there primarily to catch the eye of inquisitive women.

Women who want to know, "Can you tie me up with that thing?" or "How long before you're a rich doctor?" Stethoscope draped around the neck, also for quick access in life-threatening situations. Tuning fork in the pocket to test hearing and sensation in your feet. One or more paperback books stuffed with helpful information. These days, the books may be supplanted by an iPhone. You could probably supplant an entire medical library with an iPhone.

Intern white coats in academic institutions are almost always short, but in private hospitals with a few more perks, they can be long ones. Intern white coats start out clean, but, unless there is mandatory weekly laundry service or the intern is a tad fussy, by the end of the first month they should be camouflaged by all sorts of ink marks, food stains, and just plain body grime. Makes you wonder why they don't just issue interns dark grey coats and skip the preliminary white phase. Once they get over the thrill of being called "doctor", the smart interns lose the white coats and their name tags so that random hospital personages and visitors can't flag them down and pester them.

Residents function primarily as supervisors, so they get a long white coat, which they are supposed to keep clean. They see patients and assign them to interns and medical students, they read a lot, and they get medical journal articles for the interns, who are too busy and too tired to read them, and for the medical students, who read them and come away thinking they know what they are doing.

If you are a fellow or an attending, you can have your name, Dr. So-and-So, stitched onto your long white coat. It has to be above the left breast pocket. What if you reached into a breast pocket and there was actually a breast there? That'd be something. The embroidery is usually in black or blue, but the racier types prefer to go the red route, like those girls who wear bright red lipstick to let you know they put out. Having your name stitched on your long white coat used to save them the trouble of wearing a name tag, but nowadays, with all the security concerns, you might have to wear a clip-on photo ID. It's no longer a laughing matter if Jethro Bodine gets into the brain surgery O.R. and starts drilling someone's skull.

62. H & P

The H & P, also known as the history and physical, is the cornerstone of modern medical practice. No matter which physician, nurse practitioner or physician's assistant you see in the medical community, pretty much every interaction should start off with an H & P. In many cases redundant, in some cases lifesaving. The more difficult the problem, the more H & Ps you should expect to undergo. Any experienced physician will tell you that every member of the health care team is human, and details, sometimes crucial details, get overlooked. Whether it be asking you seemingly inane questions or performing intricate brain surgery, only through repetition does an individual practitioner decrease his miss rate, and only through repetition does the health care system avoid screw-ups that cost a life.

Step 1 in the H & P is the chief complaint. The question usually goes something like, "What brought you to the hospital (or office or emergency room) today?" Nobody should get pissed at you for coming back with, "An ambulance" or "My son's car." Even if he's heard that silly line a thousand times, it should still prompt a polite smile. If it doesn't, you may want to rethink your choice of a health care provider. Assuming, of course, that you have a choice.

After you deliver your snappy comeback, you should, in as few words as possible, state the reason for your visit or admission to the hospital. Something on the order of "Chest pain", or "I can't breathe," or "I fell out of a tree". Try not to blame your condition on others, as in "My wife gave me the worst headache of my life", or "My girlfriend gave me the crabs." The correct response from your physician to the latter statement will run something on the order of, "Oh, your girlfriend, eh? As if you've got a girlfriend. Next thing you'll tell me you've got a job too." Try not to waste everyone's time with some confabulated tale to explain the predicament into which you've landed yourself.

Once you have communicated your reason for being there, you and your provider will move on to the HPI, the history of present illness. Here is where your interviewer should get exceedingly obsessive about details. You start with a description of your chief complaint.

Let's say you have chest pain. You will be expected to tell him when this particular episode began, how severe it is, where it is located, places where the pain radiates (back, arms, jaw, shoulder, abdomen), what makes it worse (deep breath, cough, exertion, change in position, swallowing, smoking, sex), what makes it better (antacids, nitroglycerine, deep breath, swallowing, walking around in circles, sex). It is also helpful to know what other symptoms are associated with your chest pain (shortness of breath, sweats, nausea, vomiting, lightheadedness). Then you move on to whether this is a first-time event and if so, what you were doing when it came on. If there have been similar episodes in the past, the important details include how long you have been experiencing them, what you are usually doing when they come on, how long they usually last, what you did to get rid of them, and whether they are predictable. Beyond all the questions being thrown at you for the fourth or fifth time, feel free to share your thoughts. Everyone's description of a common disease is different, and so are the ways in which they deal with it. If you have a unique perspective on either of these, let your interviewer know. It shouldn't be dismissed or laughed at, and it might provide an insight heretofore undiscovered.

The third portion of the H & P is your past medical history, the PMH. Here you will be asked to recount every significant illness or interaction with the medical establishment since you were born. If your interviewer is thorough, you will be asked if you know how long your mom was pregnant with you, how you were delivered, whether you went home right away, whether you were circumcised, whether you got all your childhood immunizations, whether your tetanus shots are up to date, whether you've had the recommended adult immunizations. They should delve into every hospitalization, every bad reaction to a medication or food allergy, any complication from a procedure or surgery, pretty much every single thing that has happened to you from a medical perspective. The best thing about all this is that you have already gone over all this stuff with an intern, a resident, and at least one attending, probably three--your cardiologist, the cardiac surgeon, and your anesthesiologist. At this point, you should be able to spit everything out in your sleep. Seems a tad one-sided, everyone getting something from you, and you footing the bill. On the other hand, when you come to a teaching hospital, you usually agree to be interviewed, examined, and sometimes operated on by anyone working their way through the medical education and training system.

If you thought the HPI and the PMH were excruciating, the next part, the review of systems, also known as, you guessed it, the ROS, will make you want to jump out the window to escape. Basically, you start with your head and work your way through every symptom you could possibly experience in any organ system in any part of your body. This alone could take hours. I once took so long doing the ROS that they literally took my patient away to emergency dialysis. She thought she'd escaped, but I found her again hours later and finished.

After the ROS comes the family history. Here the med student will ask you about every relative you can remember and whether any of them had any illnesses. One good thing about this exhaustive climb up and down your family tree is that it doesn't have to involve a separate ROS for each branch. Theoretically. That and the possibility that it might save your life. Weird diseases run in families just like common ones, often for longer than anyone can remember. If you were orphaned at birth, this part of the H&P should be a snap.

Next on the menu is the social history. This is where you get to tell everything about your present life--your education, your job, your marital status, how many kids you have, whether any of them have an unusual disease. Your vices are fair game too. How many cigars or packs of cigarettes do you smoke on an average day, how long have you been smoking, ditto for alcohol use and drug use. For the most part, nobody should be making any judgments about your alcohol and drug use. Professionals don't take your habits personally. However, since most folks lie about their alcohol use, it is standard practice to take what you say and double it. That's usually closer to the truth than your answer.

Next comes a list of your medications and your allergies, whether to bee stings, rye grass, medications, or anything else.

Finally, what you've been dreading more than anything else, the laying on of hands, also known as the physical examination or PE. Especially for the youngsters, this can be the most challenging, embarrassing stage of the workup. Medical students of all ages, but especially the second- and third-year variety, have been known to poke patients in the eye, shove the tongue blade so far down their throat they gag, and caused major bleeding while examining their eardrums with an otoscope. At least the first few times through, most medical students assume a very grave, far-off look in their eyes while they try to palpate your thyroid gland. There's a lot of pretending they know what they're doing. It's easy to get flustered, so the goal in performing a PE is to memorize the progression, from eyes, ears and throat, all the way down to your toes. I was walking by a hospital room once when I heard one of my classmates declare, "My God, you have beautiful breasts!" I don't think he was talking to a guy.

Fiddling around with body parts is often an awkward time for both the student and the patient, mainly because the patient is picking up the "I'm terrified! Should I be doing this?" vibe from the student. Apparently my ineptitude was pretty entertaining, because early on, any number of my female patients giggled through most of the physical exam. The last step is the psychiatric evaluation; by that point it was obvious that they were not depressed, at least not while I was around.

God forbid the student should come upon what he interprets as "an abnormal physical finding". Occasionally he turns out to be correct, but most of the time he's interpreting normal heart sounds as a severe and rare murmur or a benign nevus (mole) as the first stages of serious, serious melanoma. That entails the raised eyebrows, the "Hmmn". Now the patient is really worried, even though he figured the kid in the short white coat hadn't a clue. That facial expression and the short interjection have him thinking something's up.

Patient: "What? What is it?"

Medical student, trying to mask his own alarm: "Oh, I'm sure it's nothing. I might have my preceptor come by and take a look later. Just a routine precaution."

The end of an H & P is usually anticlimactic for students. It's a thank you, good luck with your hospital stay, good-bye. It would be nice to have the credits roll or a curtain come down, but most of them want to head out and start their write-up of the H & P. I made it my practice to start an H & P about ninety minutes before the meal trays arrived, so that I could finish up and scoot out without much further ado.

"Thanks. See you later. Enjoy your yummy dinner."

For real doctors, the patient often has some unanswered questions, and this is a fair time to bring them up. If your examiner doesn't have the answer, they should be able to find someone with more gravitas to set you straight.

63. MEDICAL STUDENTS

If you are admitted to a teaching hospital or you are seen in a teaching clinic, odds are that you will run into a medical student at some point during your visit. Typically, after four years of college, medical students pursue a path through medical school that takes another four years. For the first year or two of medical school, they tend to be confined to the classroom, out of harm's way, memorizing basic science facts, listening to lectures, looking through microscopes, dissecting dead bodies (cadavers), pulling body parts out of a bucket of formaldehyde (pot cases), and looking forward to getting onto the wards at the hospital.

Sometime during their second year, they get their wish. About once per week or so, name tags affixed to their short white coats, which make them look like waiters out of an old movie set in the Stork Club, they get to invade the wards to interview and examine patients. Then they do an extensive write-up of what they have learned from you. This is a practice H & P. A long process, it can take hours, but, then again, you are in a hospital, and it's not like you are going to miss anything significant or fun while the medical student grills and gropes you. Unlike the interns, residents, and attendings, medical students are not paid to do what they are doing. They are paying for the privilege of learning how to be doctors. In most cases, they are paying a lot. This thing with the second-year medical student, though, is excruciatingly slow and detailed. Because it's practice. Not the real thing. Not for you. For the student.

Second year med students don't know the first thing about taking care of patients, but they're not expected to either; think of them as a blindfolded man evaluating a piece of art.

Try not to lose your patience. In the past, your kindly silver-haired all-knowing and confident private physician started out just as clumsy and clueless as the kid who is pestering you with all these questions. In the future, this kid or one of his confreres may be responsible for some very important lives: yours, your children's, or your grandchildren's. If you screw with it, karma can be a bitch.

Oddly enough, sometimes this second-year student workup can be beneficial to you. One time, while I was plodding through the H & P with an old gent from Roanoke, we got to talking about hiking at Peaks of Otter. He proudly mentioned his family's long tradition of moonshining in that area. Then he remembered one of his distant moonshining cousins who, while working on a construction crew, suffocated after minor blunt trauma to his neck. Turned out the cousin had a bleeding disorder that my patient shared. He was scheduled for some abdominal surgery, probably a gall bladder, which entails significant bleeding risks. I passed the info onto his intern, who, after informing me that I was an idiot, took credit for my detective work. So the guy went to surgery with replacement blood products on hand, and his outcome was uneventful. Sometimes, even a blind dog can find a steak in a dumpster.

Q: What's the difference between a third-year medical student and a bag of dog shit?
A: Nobody goes out of their way to step on a bag of dog shit.

Third-year medical students spend most or all of the year "on the wards" in the hospital. They do six-week clinical rotations in surgery, pediatrics, OB-GYN, internal medicine, neurology, and psychiatry. They do H & Ps, less comprehensive than those of second-year students, but more painstaking than those of the interns, residents and attendings.

Nurses catch a raft of shit from attendings, fellows, residents and interns on a daily basis, especially if the patient deteriorates. Downhill from them are the third-year medical students, and you can guess where at least a portion of that shit rolling downhill ends up. Second-year medical students tend to be left alone, unless they are dumb enough to interfere with patient care.

Fourth-year medical students are the smartest humans in any hospital. Just ask them. They are basically the medical equivalents of radio talk show hosts. They have learned a thing or two about patient care in their third year, but in almost all cases, they have absolutely no responsibilities. Fourth-year medical students do elective rotations, often in the specialties where they hope to get an internship or residency. Electives tend to be a walk in the park, so they have plenty of spare time on their hands. They run to codes and provide helpful suggestions to interns and residents, who would love to take a time out and squeeze their necks until their heads explode.

Nurse: "His heart rate is only 30 and his blood pressure is 50 over 30. Should we hang some dopamine?"
Fourth-year medical student, to whomever will listen, i.e., nobody: "Of course you should hang dopamine. 2.5 micrograms per kilo per minute."
Intern, who just last year was a fourth-year medical student and, now that he's actually responsible for the life of this patient, has just entered Game Show Contestant panic mode: "Dopamine? Dopamine. Ah, dopamine. So familiar, but I just can't put my finger on it. Refresh my memory. What does that do?"

In terms of your heart-related hospitalization, fourth-year medical students will sometimes interview you if they are doing an elective in cardiology, anesthesiology, or cardiac surgery. Occasionally, if you have a pre-existing problem that may impact your bypass surgery, something like COPD or a bleeding disorder, a subspecialty consult will be ordered and a fourth-year medical student may be sent to start the consult process. In the outpatient clinics you may be evaluated by one. Unless you want to be drowned in a vat of bullshit, avoid asking questions of fourth-year medical students. A little knowledge is a dangerous thing. Believe me, I was one once. A loaded gun waiting for someone to squeeze the trigger. Nothing more dangerous than a doctor with a license to kill who doesn't know how much he doesn't know.

Most medical students start out with perhaps a faint idea of how they want to specialize. Many just want to be doctors. Some are in it to save lives, some are in it because it runs in the family. Some like the idea of steady work with good pay for life. Through the four years of medical school, the vast majority of students want to help people. That's before they experience internship.

One of my classmates said, with a straight face, on the very first day of medical school, "I don't care what happens the next four years, as long as I end up with a plastic surgery residency." That made me sit up and take notice. Who thinks that far ahead on the first day of a new life? Not me. I was just happy to have my own microscope. I like to think he did not get what he wanted.

Like the nursing staff, medical students can be your advocate. While you may have the desire to step on them like a bug, they can make your trip through the inpatient or outpatient system safer and smoother. And, if they ask the right questions, they may save your life.

64. HAPPY JACK

Jack Henderson, M.D., the on-call intern for the cardiology service, walked into Room 416 at 4:55 P.M. Before the night was over, he would admit between five and ten new patients. Most were coming in for caths by the various attending cardiologists the next morning. His job was to take a history, perform a physical examination, and make sure everyone was ready to go to the cath lab. Most of those either went home in a day or two or transferred over to surgery for a bypass. The non-cath admissions would consist primarily of patients with congestive heart failure or arrhythmias; it could be anywhere from two days to two weeks before they went home from the hospital, if they made it out at all.

Occasionally there would be a longstanding patient of one of the older cardiologists admitted for any number of bizarre reasons, some social, some as vague as a tiny star in the Milky Way. These were the intern-killers. A daily litany of requests, fussiness beyond belief, and incessant complaints about having to be examined by the house staff and medical students. They expected personal service 24/7 from their private physicians only.

Mrs. Champagne in 416B had been a patient of Dr. Spotswood for twenty-five years. The admitting diagnosis was "weak and dizzy." Jack had the feeling this was going to be a dilly. As he walked over to her bed, all the curtains drawn, he could hear her on the phone, complaining about the room.

"I know the hospital is crowded, Miss Herbert, but Dr. Spotswood assured me that I would always have a private room. I was hoping for one of the suites." Jack surmised that Miss Herbert worked in Spotswood's office, doubling as a booking agent for his special patients. He hefted the Champagne hospital chart, a good five pounds of "weak and dizzy" admissions, and slid around the curtain. When Jack wanted to piss off a patient, he could don the pushy garb like nobody else, all the while flashing a dazzling, cheesy smile. Otherwise, day in and day out, his countenance could be most charitably described as "neutral". Hence his nickname, "Happy Jack". Irony at its best.

He'd learned that standing at attention until the patient was off the phone was an invitation to be pointedly ignored.

"Mrs. Champagne, I'm Dr. Henderson." He pulled up a chair and sat inches away from her. She pointed her index finger at him and then at the receiver in her hand. He dropped her chart on the floor as loudly as possible. "I'm here to do a history and physical on you."

"Can't you see I'm on the phone?"

"Yes, Ma'am, I can, but I don't care. I'm busy and I don't have time to wait." Jack held the record for patients checking out AMA (Against Medical Advice) the same day they checked in, nine in nine months. None of the other interns had more than two. He was going to do his best to make it an even ten. While this wouldn't endear him to Spotswood, a nice guy and an excellent clinician, Jack had no interest in specializing in Cardiology. In addition, the Chief of Medicine, a churlish bully named Hopper, despised social admissions and had no problem with Jack or any of the other house staff doing all they could to boot them out ASAP. He smiled and took out a notepad. "Now, in your own words, what brought you to the hospital today?"

"Miss Herbert, I am going to hang up now. There is a very rude young man in my room; I'll call you back shortly." Jack comforted himself with the knowledge that all the private offices turned off their phones promptly at 5 P.M. Miss Herbert had heard the last of this problem, at least for today. If only she knew how helpful he had been.

"What did you say your name was?" She glared at Jack.

"Henderson. Dr. Henderson." He smiled again, using yet another of his precious store of happy faces. Some AMA's were just plain hard work. Jack hadn't figured out what the last straw would be, but he was confident that it would arrive on the camel's back in the next ten minutes.

"Dr. Henderson, my name is Mrs. Lewis Champagne. My husband's family has been coming to this hospital since it was built. Their name is on the front wall of this hospital. I have been Dr. Spotswood's private patient for over two decades. Nobody examines me except for Dr. Spotswood. Therefore, I am discharging you from my care. I want you to call Dr. Spotswood and tell him to come see me immediately." She folded her arms and looked up at the ceiling.

"Mrs. Champagne, you've been assigned to me and my resident, Dr. Echols. We are responsible for your care while you are in the hospital this time." He paused and looked down at her chart on the floor for dramatic effect. "This is a teaching hospital. If you refuse our care, you will still be on our service. I won't force you to answer questions, I won't examine you against your will, but Dr. Spotswood still won't be able to write any orders on your chart. Those are the rules."

"I am going to deal with Dr. Spotswood and Dr. Spotswood only."

"Let me put it another way. I'm here all night. Dr. Echols is here all night. Dr. Spotswood will be at home, sleeping in his nice comfortable bed. If you die, and people make some serious efforts to die every day in this hospital, I'm the one who's going to save your life. Me and nobody else. So it behooves you to tell me everything, and I mean everything, about your medical history. Otherwise, I might not be able to keep you from dying."

The patient stared at Happy Jack with her mouth open for thirty seconds. Then she spoke through gritted old teeth. "Get out of my room. I am getting dressed and leaving."

Jack picked up the chart, pushed the chair back against the wall, and walked out. He thought to himself, *Number 10. Nobody will ever touch that.*

65. POST-CALL

"Jake. Jake. Wake up."

"Huh? Run in a liter of saline and give her an amp of D50. Call me back if she doesn't wake up." Jacques Willie Woods turned over on the couch.

"Jake. Come on. Wake up." Bernard Wormeley pulled on his arm until his fellow intern sat up and looked around.

"Oh, hi, Bernie." Jake ran his hand over his face and yawned.

"We're done in the O.R., Jake. You can go home now."

"Home? I can't go home. I'm on call." Jake looked around the TCV Surgery office, confused. "How'd I get in here?"

Bernie shook his head. "You were on call last night. Remember?"

"Remember? Are you kidding? I feel like I've been on call every night." He looked up. "I'm not on call? I can go home?"

"You'd better. You told me you were supposed to take Rita out to dinner at the Station House. You're meeting some old friend of yours from St. Joe. Get a move on, Jake. It's almost six, and you said your reservation is at seven."

"I still don't understand how I ended up in here." Jake stood up and pulled a wad of 3 x 5 cards from the pocket of his white coat and handed them to Wormeley.

Bernie looked at the cards, counted them, and said, "Jeez, you must have had a load of admissions last night. No wonder you're so beat." He looked at Jake. "I don't know how you ended up in here. All I know is you told me to page you when I was done in the O.R. with the post-op bleeder. You said you'd hold down the fort and field calls in the meantime. I paged you about ten minutes ago. You called me back and told me to meet you here. You don't remember any of that?"

"Uh-uh. Well, I better get going. I don't need to have Rita pissed at me."

Bernie laughed. "Right. You are dreaming. She's crazy about you. Hey, Jake. Thanks for staying. I owe you one." He slapped Woods on the back and headed out the door. "I have to go see a new admission. Try not to fall asleep on the ride home."

"Yup. Have a good night. I'll see you tomorrow morning, Bernie."

The walk to the house staff and student parking garage re-energized him. By the time he climbed into his car, he felt refreshed and ready for a nice meal and some music at the Station House. Wednesday nights were reserved for local jazz combos. That meant lively music. Open-mike folk night on Monday was about as stimulating as a fistful of phenobarb. And tonight's bonus is that nobody dances to jazz.

The ride from the hospital to Jake and Rita's townhouse, about five miles, took anywhere from ten minutes to a half-hour, depending on the time of day. Jake's ride home entailed a short drive on campus. The soothing scent of star magnolias in full bloom eased all his energy away. Once off the campus, the aroma of magnolia was replaced by fresh-mown grass. Here and there, held back by split-rail fences, horses stood and did what horses always do: nibble dandelions and stare at the road, daydreaming of galloping getaways leading to equine adventures.

He pinched his thigh a couple of times while searching the dial for something up-tempo. At last he found Ike and Tina doing "Proud Mary". To help stay awake, he started talking out loud to himself. "I can't imagine what it's like to spend every minute of every day with your spouse, especially on the road all the time like they are. Ike and Tina must have an incredible relationship to make that work."

As "Proud Mary" rolled down the river to its conclusion in the delta, Jake's thoughts slid from Ike and Tina to Tina, the new swing shift nurse up on the step-down unit. She liked to play up the connection to her namesake; while the flowing dark locks came naturally without the benefit of a wig or straightening process, she did favor the singer's leg wear. Woods had spotted her out with a couple of the other nurses at happy hour the week before--slinky black sleeveless dress and matching fishnets. He drifted off, thinking about how Tina would look when she shook it in that outfit. Nice dreamy visual, with Ike and Tina oozing out sultry background music, down that sleepy river, Jake expertly piloting the sternwheeler while he hummed along.

That soft float down the Mississippi suddenly turned into a wrestling match with the steering wheel. The old Mustang was angled into the roadside drainage ditch, still half-filled with rainwater. He managed to bring the car around and back up onto the road, but not before scraping the undersides but good. His brush with mortality released what little adrenaline remained. He held the wheel in a death grip the rest of the ride home. The rattling from underneath the Mustang reminded him to stay awake. The guilt helped too.

When Jake walked in to the bedroom, Rita looked up from putting on her lipstick. She stood up from her vanity and stared at him. He thought, *Man, she looks pissed. I must be really late. Either that or she's reading my mind again.*

She walked over to him and her face softened from shock to concern. "My God, Jake, you look awful." *Oh well, pity beats pissed.*

He fell back on the bed. "Yeah, really rough night. Ten admissions, lots of fever workups. The killer was a trauma this morning at ten. Guy who got impaled in the chest by a crowbar down at the railroad yard. Three hours of retracting for Naylor, then I had to hang around until

Bernie finished up in the O.R." He closed his eyes and fell instantly asleep.

"Jake. Jake." Rita straddled him and rubbed his sternum.

"Okay, give him a couple units of fresh frozen and two units of packed cells. Recheck his crit and coags and call me back." All this without opening his eyes. He started to snore.

Rita possessed what one of her tennis coaches had called "a sweet tenacity". While gradually increasing the pressure on his sternum, she gently pinched his earlobe between her long red fingernails. Jake twisted his head and opened his eyes.

"Oh, hi, Honey. Is it time to go to work?"

"Jake, how do I get ahold of Marsh? You can't go like this. You're out on your feet."

"Huh? Oh yeah, right. No, I'll be okay. Let me up and I'll take a quick shower."

"Are you sure?"

"I'm sure. Marsh drove seven hours from New York just to see us." He stood up and smiled. "You look terrific in that dress. We better go in your car though. The Mustang just started making a funny noise."

Rita had them to the Station House in less than ten minutes. The parking lot was only half-full. Jake walked around to open Rita's door.

"Looks good, Rita. We should be able to get a table without waiting too long."

"Oh, I called ahead. We have a booth in the back, away from the music."

"Perfect. Thanks, Rita." *God I love my wife.* She stood up out of the car and smoothed her dress, then ran both hands back through her blonde hair. Her tongue took a long ride over her teeth.

"You are welcome, Mr. Handsome. You can thank me properly at home tonight." *Good luck with that.* His legs felt like lead.

Inside, Rita spoke to the hostess while Jake scanned the bar. His face lit up when he saw Marsh, sitting on a stool. His back was turned, talking to a woman with black hair down to the barstool. Jake turned and waited for Rita to join him.

"I told Anna we'll be in here for about twenty minutes or so, then go to the booth. Is that okay with you?"

"Sure. Did you ask her if I could stand up during dinner?" He gave his wife his super charming smile.

"If you fall asleep, I'll nudge you awake."

He felt his left earlobe. It still hurt. "Nudge. That's what that was, a nudge?" He tapped Marshall on the shoulder. "Hey, is there a doctor in the house?"

Marshall turned. Since last Woods had seen him, almost a year ago, he'd grown a full beard. His skin was pale as snow. Marshall stood up, shook hands, and gave Jake a hug, then pecked Rita on the cheek.

"You look fantastic, Rita. Jake, you look like shit. Still great to see you, though." He turned to the woman on his left. "Jake, Rita, this is Sacajawea." She leaned her head around Marshall.

"Hi, nice to meet you both. Marshall has told me so much about you. So much." She turned back to the bar and sipped a glass of water. Jake gave Rita a look. *What is up with her face?* Rita shrugged and mouthed, "I'll find out." Marshall smirked; he hadn't missed the silent exchange. He motioned for them to sit. Rita slid around him and parked herself on the stool to Sacajawea's left and began talking with her. Jake leaned up against the bar but didn't sit down. He waited for Marsh to sit back down on his barstool.

"So how is Juneau?"

"Long dark winter. Good news is, we're about to begin our spring in two weeks. June 1. You want a drink?" He nodded toward his glass, what looked like a gin and tonic.

"Yeah. I'll have a draft." The bartender nodded and reached for a glass. "You look like you haven't been out of the dungeon for a few years. A little pale, Buddy."

"We actually have a tanning bed at the clinic, but I couldn't bring myself to use it. Going all pale and native at the same time."

"So you're enjoying the Indian Health Service."

"Yeah, it's fun. Best decision I ever made, working off the Public Health loan after my internship. I needed the break bad. The money is more than enough, and I get to fish for salmon pretty much every day. Chinook should be running up the rivers by the time I get back. Another year and I'll have enough saved to buy a boat with a cabin. Four weeks of vacation, I can go pretty much anywhere on the West Coast, from Nome to Cabo." He took a sip of his drink. "You ought to think about taking a year or two off. Plenty of surgeons would pay you good money in the private sector to assist. Once you get off the treadmill, life looks a lot sweeter."

"I think about it, Rita does too. But I'm pretty much set on going into TCV surgery. This rotation has beaten the crap out of me, but I love it."

"Jake, with the general surgery residency and then the TCV fellowship, you're looking at what, six more years after this one?"

"More like seven. You forgot the year of research in the middle."

"Jesus. You'll be an old man by the time you're done."

"Believe me, we've talked about it all month long. Rita thought I'd end up in urology or general surgery. She's with me on it, though. I'm lucky."

Marshall turned and looked at Rita talking with her new friend. "Get back to me on that part in about five years."

"So what are you and Sacajawea up to in New York?"

"Her folks spend about six months there and six in Anchorage and Seattle. They're yacht people, spend most of the summer sailing around Alaska, sometimes over to Hawaii."

"Are her parents Indians? Is that how she got her name?"

Marshall choked slightly on his drink. "Sacajawea Rosenberg?" he rasped. "No, they're big on Native American history. Her mom majored in anthropology at Columbia."

Jake ran that one around in his head. *Sacajawea Rosenberg.* He started to drift off to sleep, so he shook his head a little and took a sip of his beer.

"Are you going to take Sacajawea home to meet the folks? Lots of Native Americans in the Midwest. I'm sure it would be a mutually interesting time for all parties concerned." Marshall's father prided himself on being the exclusive car dealer for all of the Republican politicians in the St. Joseph area. His idea of ethnic diversity extended all the way to Nebraskans.

"We're heading to San Diego for a few days before we go back to Alaska. I'm going to add surfing to my impressive inventory of water skills. I believe our flight takes us right over K.C., so we'll pass within five or six miles of home. That's five or six miles straight up." He smiled. "Wondering at all about the scratches on her face?"

"Rita's on the job. By the time she's done with Sacajawea, she'll know at least one or two tasty info nuggets that you're not privy to. She is a trial lawyer, remember?"

"No doubt. Speaking of home, I can assume you still plan on doing your training here, then returning to practice in St. Joe or K.C.?"

"Oh yeah. We've met plenty of nice folks here, hang out with a few couples, but we both miss home. I honestly can't imagine raising our kids anywhere else. It was a great place to grow up, wasn't it?"

Marshall nodded. "Kids. Jesus. Well, in some ways I envy you. You're married to the girl you've always loved, you have the next seven years of your life planned out, and you know where you want to end up. Me, I'm barely capable of deciding what lures I'm going to use on those kings next week." With just a touch of smug, he added, "On the other hand, I am free as a bird. Once I've done my time with the IHS, I don't owe anyone a thing. I love it."

The hostess walked into the bar with menus. Rita nodded to her; Marshall settled up the tab and they went in to dinner. Jake gave it his best effort not to stare at Ms. Rosenberg's face.

Rita went first. She ordered the special, flounder stuffed with crabmeat. Sacajawea had a couple of questions about the ratatouille.

"It's not made with animal stock of any kind, is it?"

"No. All vegetarian, no meat products. It's pretty much what vegetarians order here. Very popular." The waitress, Marian, smiled. "It's the only thing on the menu that I eat."

"And no dairy products either?"

"There better not be any, or I've been lying to customers for over a year." She smiled again. Sacajawea frowned but went with it.
Jake ordered the pork tenderloin with roasted apples and mashed potatoes. Marshall went with the flounder special. As Marian walked away, Jake felt himself drifting off. He had the desire to put his head down and take a nap, just like after lunch in kindergarten.

Rita flicked his earlobe with her nail and announced, "We'd better get up and go listen to the band, or Jake will fall asleep on us." They all grabbed their drinks and started across the dining room toward the dance floor.

Jake needed to wake up. He sidled up next to Sacajawea. "This place was built by Hessian soldiers during the Revolutionary War. After they surrendered at the battle of Saratoga, Thomas Jefferson, who was the governor of Virginia, had the prisoners marched down here. They built a community, the Albemarle Barracks. This is the last of the barracks left standing."

Sacajawea, scratched face and all, turned to Jake with her first glimmer of interest in him. That spurred him on with his little history lesson.

"When the war ended, they were given the choice of returning to Germany or staying here. They all bolted into the Blue Ridge and married local women. It seems conditions in America were a tad more attractive than what they'd left back in Hesse-Kassel. At least if they stayed here, they wouldn't be forced to fight someone else's battles."

"So you know about the press gangs in Hesse at that time. Not bad, Jake."

"History major at KU. I focused on early American history, from the 1600's to the 1800's. On good days I still remember some of it." He noticed her hands for the first time. Scratches and divots up to the middle of her forearms, some old, some new. Fair bit of bruising as well. He couldn't wait to get home and hear the straight story from Rita. Hopefully he'd be able to stay awake long enough to get the gory details.

After standing for a few minutes listening to the jazz combo, Jake felt an irresistible urge to sit down. He whispered in Rita's ear and then walked back toward the table. The other three stood listening and chatting.

About ten minutes later, the band finished up their set and announced a thirty-minute break. Marshall, Sacajawea and Rita headed back across the dining room. Jake's head was not visible above the back of the booth. They found him lying face down in his mashed potatoes, his head turned slightly to the right.

Rita said, "Oh, dear," and slid in beside him. The others took their places across from the Woods'. Transfixed, they stared at Jake in his food.

Rita lifted his head up out of his food. Mashed potatoes slid down his face and onto his shirt. He coughed.

Rita said, "Jake." The young surgeon named after the great undersea explorer and the greatest center fielder of all time raised his head up just a little farther.

"Get an EKG and some lytes, then give him 0.25 mg. of Lanoxin IV. I'll be up there in ten minutes." Then he gently lay back down into his mashed potatoes.

At 5 the next morning, the alarm rang. Jake sat straight up in bed. Rita turned on her bedside light.

"Wow, what a wild dream. I was drowning in a vat of Cream of Wheat."

"Close. It was mashed potatoes."

"Did we go out last night to see Marshall?"

"You don't remember?"

It started to come back to him. He rubbed his hand through his hair. There was something crusted along the side of his face. He realized he couldn't hear out of his left ear.

"I remember something about an Indian princess. Pocahontas or something like that. Were we talking about American history?"

"Marshall's girlfriend's name is Sacajawea."

"Oh, yeah, that's right. Now I remember. She had scratches all over her face."

Rita stood up and put on her robe. "Good boy. Take a shower and I'll make us some coffee."

Fifteen minutes later, Jake walked into the kitchen. He was freshly shaved and had on a clean pair of scrubs. The hearing in his left ear had returned. He sat down across from Rita.

"Weren't you assigned to find out about the scratches?"

Rita laughed. "She's a go-getter, that one. I think she may be a little intense for your buddy Marshall."

"Yeah, seemed like high IQ, pretty serious."

"I'd say so. She graduated from Columbia when she was nineteen, then she got into the vegetarian thing and took an interest in raptors. That's how she ended up in Alaska, with a grant from some vegetarian foundation. She has this theory that if you feed infants a purely vegetarian diet, they'll grow up to be vegetarians and live longer. But they couldn't get permission to study humans until they do an animal phase first."

"Seriously, a grant to study vegetables?"

"No, worse than that. A grant to study vegetables and raptors. The grant is to teach raptors to eat vegetarian. Sacajawea climbs up into fir trees and tries to feed fruits, vegetables and nuts to bald eagle babies. That's how she got all the scratches on her face and hands."

Jake shook his head. Something shifted in his left ear canal.

"I did dig up something interesting. Something Marshall doesn't know."

Jake stopped short and smiled. *That's my girl.*

"She's not just a go-getter. She's the mother of all go-getters. You know how Marshall is looking forward to a week on the beach in San Diego?"

"Yes, he's going to take some surfing lessons."

"That's what he thinks. He's about to choke on that smug little smirk of his. Sacajawea's changed their airline tickets. They're going to St. Joe, by way of Kansas City. She wants to meet his parents. I'd love to see the look on his face when he figures that one out."

Jake walked out to the Mustang. He felt ready for another night on call. As he got in, Rita leaned out the door. "Looks to me like somebody went for an off-road adventure recently. Drop the Mustang off at

Ernie's in Fry Springs. I already called. He said he'd drive you up to the hospital and hopefully fix the damage by tomorrow night. Try not to fall asleep at the wheel again."

Jake laughed. Feeling like the village idiot, he backed out into the street and turned on the radio. Right on cue, there was Robert Palmer, living the good life, no doubt shirtless and shaved. Singing about how the women are smarter than the men. In every way.

66. HOUSE STAFF

House staff are the doctors-in-training who take care of you in teaching hospitals. They work in-house, in the other big house, the one without gray bars, hence the name house staff. To be eligible for an internship, you must attend four years of medical school and graduate with a Medical Doctor (M.D.) degree. In addition, you must pass the United States Medical Licensing Examination (USMLE), also known as the National Boards. There are three parts to the USMLE. Part 1, which focuses on the basic sciences--anatomy, biochemistry, histology, physiology, pathology, pharmacology--(a lot of ologies), is usually taken toward the end of the second year of medical school. Part 2, which medical students take in their last year of school, is comprised of the CK (clinical knowledge) portion and the CS (clinical skills) portion. The CK part consists of a day full of written questions about various diseases, their diagnosis and treatment. The CS portion involves taking a history and performing a physical examination on standardized patients. Inasmuch as each American or Canadian medical school has its own method of educating medical students, the USMLE is designed to guarantee a certain standard of knowledge across the board.

Once you pass Parts 1 & 2 of the USMLE and graduate from medical school, you head out for "training". At this point, you are authorized to practice medicine, but only with supervision. Everyone starts out as an intern or first-year resident. Some interns focus on a specific branch of medicine, like family medicine, pediatrics, surgery, or internal medicine. Others choose a rotating internship, where you do a month or two of everything in one year. At the end of that first year, you must take Part 3 of the USMLE. If you pass this final part, you are licensed to practice medicine without supervision, meaning you can "hang out a shingle" and treat patients in your own practice, you can work in a clinic setting, or you can "moonlight" to make extra money on nights and weekends in E.R.s and urgent care centers.

If you choose to stay in a residency, you continue to practice with supervision, but you also get to supervise underlings. At long last, after being bullied by interns, residents, fellows and attendings, not to mention nurses and x-ray techs, there are people you can boss around, namely medical students and interns. You can try bossing nurses and techs from various departments, but that won't go well. Upon completion of an internship, most residencies, including internal medicine, pediatrics, dermatology, neurology, obstetrics and gynecology, orthopedics, pathology, psychiatry, and urology last two to three years. General surgery usually goes four or five years after an internship.

After the residency, most physicians go out and start or join a practice. If you continue your training in one of the specialties, you end up as a fellow. For medicine and pediatrics, this would include subspecialties like endocrinology, cardiology, gastroenterology, nephrology, hematology/oncology, pulmonology and rheumatology. Surgery residents can become fellows in plastic surgery, TCV (heart and lung), or neurosurgery.

So the pyramid starts with medical students at the bottom. Next up are interns, followed by residents, fellows, and attendings. The attending physician is the one who heads the ward team. He can be an academic physician who teaches regularly, a physician with his own private practice who wants to teach house staff, or a combination of both. He is ultimately responsible for your care while in the hospital, even if you undergo procedures by physicians in other departments. If you already have a private physician, he may or may not see you while you are in the hospital. He can leave notes on the chart with suggestions for your care, but in a teaching institution, orders usually have to go through the house staff. This ensures that all orders are written by the same crew or their on-call colleagues. As in all walks of life, fewer cooks usually means fewer screw-ups. So don't ask your private physician to order this or that for your comfort. Ask your intern. You'll see him bright and early every morning.

In medicolegal terms, i.e., who you sue when you are pissed off, all medical students and house staff are considered "transparent". That means that when something goes wrong and the ambulance-chasers arrive on the scene, the attending is the guy who is ultimately responsible. He and/or his malpractice insurer are going to pay. While house staff may be named as co-defendants and may in fact be the real culprits, usually they are too broke for a malpractice lawyer to bother with them.

In the old days, interns and residents were paid almost nothing, but sometimes were able to live in housing in or around the hospital for free or next to nothing, and could take free meals in the hospital cafeteria. Judging by the starch content in their special white intern shirts, they got their laundry done in the hospital as well. Nowadays the money is better, but when you factor in the time they spend working in the hospital, their salary usually falls at or below minimum wage. Basically, while you are in the hospital, your life is in the hands of overworked, sleep-deprived, minimum wage workers. At times they may be crabby.

Like any other womb, the goal of residency training is to challenge you and protect you while you grow from who you were to who you are going to be. Education starts with the most protective of wombs, preschool and kindergarten, where the big challenge is learning to blow your nose and flush the toilet. In grade school and high school, there is still some protection afforded by your superiors, your teachers, while you learn to use your brain and learn to get along with your peers in ever-more challenging intellectual and social situations. College brings a whole new level of freedom, which sometimes can result in too much fun, with predictable consequences, but there is still a womb, the institution, and its environment, the campus, protecting you while expecting your best efforts.

Medical school, at least the first two years of mostly classroom learning, is more of the same, hopefully with far less fun thrown in. Once medical students start their clinical rotations on the hospital wards, they have to learn to get along on a completely different playground. In addition to dealing with peers and superiors, students have to interact with additional cast members in the play-- the patient and his family. The third-year medical student thinks he is learning to evaluate patients, but for the most part, he is subconsciously taking his cues from the intern who is there with him from the beginning. The fourth-year medical student, who, we have learned, is the smartest person in the hospital, functions as the quintessential Monday morning quarterback, tossing about pithy critiques of the decisions made by the guys in the trenches, with no responsibility whatsoever for the patient.

Once out of medical school, theoretically it is time to play in the big leagues, but interns still have the protection of residents and attendings while learning how to avoid making mistakes, or, better yet, how to avoid making the really big mistakes, the ones that kill patients.

One of the stated goals of medical education and postgraduate training is to weed out those who can't handle the stress. Even in medical school, some of the highest-ranked students in the basic sciences tend to fall apart during the clinical years. Others who were dim bulbs the first couple of years glow brightly on the wards in their third year.

Medical education is a boot camp, where one learns to function without sleep, or, better yet, to sleep on a pillow of mashed potatoes. It's about learning to make life and death decisions without agonizing, and then live with the consequences. Developing survival skills is essential, because, for the first few years, it is all about surviving. An intern knows he has arrived when he gets called about a patient, listens to the nurse's report, makes sound decisions and fires off a page full of sensible verbal orders, all while asleep. The next morning, he finds those verbal orders on the patient's chart with his name affixed to them, and he remembers none of it.

Most residents and residency program chiefs say the most important thing an intern learns is how to evaluate patients quickly and correctly and then go about saving their lives. Equally important, however, is learning how to work with nurses and ancillary medical services like radiology and laboratory and respiratory therapy. Interns learn how to work together as a team, but, for the first time, they are writing the orders; deservedly or not, they've risen a step above the rest in terms of authority and responsibility for the patient. An intern has to learn how to get what he wants done for the patient without pissing off the rest of the health care team. If he fancies himself as the King Bozo the Magnificent and acts accordingly, sooner or later one of the health care team members or, worse, her department supervisor, will go to his resident with a list of complaints about his behavior. At this point, the resident can assume one of three roles:

1) Mentor--he pulls the intern aside and tells him to wise up;
2) Sigmund Freud--he asks the intern how HE thinks he's doing;
3) Observer--he laughs, puts his feet up, and settles in for the show. "More butter on the popcorn, please".

As a patient, you can look at house staff in one of two ways: necessary evil or life saver. They are both. In order for them to become good or even excellent physicians, they have to care for as many patients with as many different disease processes as possible, during and after their residency training. The more patients they see, the better they become at diagnosis and treatment. If you are in a non-teaching hospital and something goes awry in the middle of the night, at least before your cardiologist or heart surgeon arrives, you will probably be seen by an E.R. physician or a night shift hospitalist, neither of which may know the first thing about your case. That may be better than an intern and resident who are caring for you on their service, or it may be worse.

You can console yourself with the truth that your kindly, caring, knowledgeable, in-control, silver-haired, suave and well-groomed private physician was hatched from the same basket of eggs that produced the nervous new intern or the couldn't-care-less resident, firing questions at you, waking you up for pre-rounds at 5 A.M., and doing his best to get you out of the hospital and your 3 x 5 card out of his pocket as quickly as possible. It may be uncomfortable, you might want to stick around and have nurses wipe your ass a few days more, and your attending might be going a little soft and agree with you, but the house staff guy is doing you a favor. The longer you stay in the hospital, for either medical or social reasons, the greater your chances of having bad things happen to you. The last thing you want is to become a statistic at the monthly Morbidity and Mortality conference. That's where physicians get together and discuss the patients who suffer an unexpected complication or die. In other words, the patients who end up at the bad end of the bell curve.

"Great case! Too bad for the patient."

When it comes to CABG surgery, if you are a patient in a teaching hospital with a TCV surgery program, odds are your bypass will be done by a TCV surgery fellow. He's a guy who's done five or six years of general surgery residency, and performed well enough to enter a fellowship. Your sternotomy--the part where they slice you open, then take a bone saw to your breastbone--may be performed by a senior surgery resident or the fellow. If you are at a teaching hospital like Cleveland Clinic or Mass General or Duke or any of the other well-known institutions, your surgery will most likely be supervised by a guy who's performed the procedure hundreds of times, publishes on a regular basis and is world-renowned. Otherwise he wouldn't be there. That's why you went to Mass General for your bypass in the first place. So, for the most part, you are going to be okay. Then again, you don't really want to be the on the receiving end of the first of anything a young doctor performs, especially a bypass.

Most cardiac surgery programs can handle a typical bypass with aplomb; if you have several confounding factors, like a bad pump from congestive heart failure, or terrible lung function due to COPD, or five previous bypass surgeries, you'll want to go to a big referral center, where they operate on patients with similar problems on a regular basis. Even if you don't want to go there, you'll probably end up there anyway, because nobody else will want to operate on you.

The powers that be in academic medicine have long maintained that house staff are absolutely essential to the running of a large teaching hospital. Economically, that is probably true. Paying a couple dozen interns and residents thirty-five to fifty-five grand a year is much cheaper than hiring hospitalists for three to four times as much to do the same job. House staff also are younger, hungrier, more malleable, and more tolerant of unfavorable working conditions than are older physicians. Unless strict protocols are in place and enforced, house staff will also order more tests than their more experienced colleagues. Again, that is why house staff are there: to learn what is necessary and what is frivolous.

When it comes to house staff, go with the flow. For the most part, they are going to get the job done quickly and efficiently. If you are having surgery in the month of July in a teaching hospital, the "quickly and efficiently" part may not be all that evident. That's when house staff graduate to the next level, from medical student to intern and from intern to supervising resident. Ask questions if something doesn't seem right.

Speaking of questions, if you are concerned about having house staff take care of you, and it's not an emergency situation, ask your heart surgeon to admit you to a non-teaching hospital. Most heart surgeons who are not full-time employees of a university hospital have privileges at several hospitals.

67. FOUR WORDS

Labor Day came on the first of September, and it was good-bye to summer in Seattle. John Paul Baker was the third-year resident in the ICU. His intern, Sanjay Chatterjee, west of the Mississippi for the first time in his life, was a walking medical textbook, knowledgeable and unfortunately proud of it. *It's only September,* John Paul thought. Constant rain and drear combined with an endless procession of death-proof octogenarians would wear Sanjay down just like everyone else. By December he would barely have the energy to crawl anonymously through the daily routine.

On day 1 of the rotation, while the rest of the world was busy pouring lighter fluid over charcoal briquettes, Baker and Sanjay had a sit-down. The intern had been in Seattle for exactly two months, but he'd already earned a reputation as a world-class know-it-all who held to a time-honored but incorrect notion that RNs were the personal assistants to MDs, ever at the ready to accede to their slightest whims.

John Paul wanted to nip this in the bud; an intern lynching in the ICU was a horrible thing to watch.

"Sanjay, not that any nurses in this hospital are willing to take your bossing them around, but the ICU is another animal completely. The nurses here consider themselves intensive care specialists. They have far more autonomy than the nursing staff on the floors. As long as they follow policy and protocols, they have the absolute support of the attendings who frequent this unit: pulmonologists, cardiologists, heart surgeons, anesthesiologists, the whole conglomeration of specialists who live and breathe critical care medicine and surgery." The Chatterjee lad looked at John Paul with mild all-knowing amusement, ready to retort as if this were a high school debate. *TIme to twist the knife,* thought Baker. "Not to mention that, even though they are not Harvard-educated physicians, not physicians at all, the nurses know more ICU medicine than you do."

Sanjay's eyes bugged out of his head. He gathered a full head of steam. "John, I know..."

Baker raised his hand commandingly. "If you are going to get through this month, and the rest of the year too, you will need to learn and heed these four words."

The steam dissipated in one exhalation.

"Yes?"

"Shut up and listen."

"I'm listening. What are the four words?"

The first week was chock-full of highs and lows. They saw a nice variety of pathology, from a twenty-five year-old biker with fulminant four-lobe pneumococcal pneumonia complete with bilateral empyemas requiring daily thoracenteses, to a fifty-something woman bleeding from every orifice and, thanks to a hefty dose of gin and tonics over the holiday weekend, possessed of not a single platelet.

Sanjay's admitting notes were flawless, to John Paul's eye the best he'd seen from an intern. As the supervising resident, normally he would throw in an erudite but irrelevant addendum. At the end of Sanjay's notes, he merely wrote, "Agree." and signed his name. The intern's eye exams were particularly thorough and enlightening, far beyond Baker's scope of knowledge; before work rounds each day, Sanjay would dilate the pupils of the new admissions and make sure the ICU nurses got a chance to see any interesting findings. Despite his personality, he was winning them over.

Things were not going so well when it came to young Dr. Chatterjee's interactions with various attendings and consultants. He had a penchant for opining more than a tad excessively in his daily notes, and, worse yet, disagreeing in writing with their recommendations. After checking with the other residents, it became obvious that this was the intern's modus operandi. On Friday afternoon Baker decided to wrap up the week with a little sweet and sour sauce.

"Sanjay, I am very impressed with how thorough you have been this week."

The intern smiled patiently with a look that said, "You seem surprised, Commoner."

"Especially your eye exams. A number of the nurses have told me how much they appreciate your teaching on rounds, showing them eye pathology," Baker raised his eyebrows, "particularly Melissa Bannister. Ophthalmologists don't hang out in the ICU any more than they have to. I know you plan on specializing in retinal diseases, but how did you acquire such a wealth of knowledge?"

"My grandfather was an ophthalmologist in New Delhi. He started taking me to the eye clinic on weekends when I was nine. I was proficient with the slit lamp within six months."

"You were seeing eye patients when you were nine?"

"He was mentoring me. He didn't want me to end up like my father."

"What did your dad do?" *Dishwasher, rendering plant lackey, ne'er-do-well?*

"Chief of internal medicine at the All India Institute of Medical Sciences in New Delhi. Then, when we moved to the United States, he rose to Chief at Beth Israel. As my grandfather put it, 'Jack of all trades, master of none.'" *Typical subspecialist's perspective,* Baker thought. *Denigrate the generalists until you need them to clean up your mess.*

Now for the sour.

"We do, however, need to talk about a problem that's been brought to my attention." Sanjay's head snapped back as if he'd been slapped.

"What is it, John Paul?"

"Sanjay, let me spell out a few things for you. The progress notes are not your personal diary. Try to stick to facts, and above all, refrain from criticizing the patient's attending and the consultants in the medical record. If you have a problem with their recommendations, do it face-to-face or on the phone. Stuff in writing never goes away. Even if you are right, winning a chart war is nothing more than a Pyrrhic victory."

"But John Paul, that's standard operating procedure at Harvard. Battle it out on the pages of the permanent record."

"Let me remind you that you are not, for this year at least, at the UVA of the North."

"The what?"

"The UVA of the North." He let that sink in a while. It felt good to watch the steam build and then dissipate. Sanjay sputtered but said nothing. Apparently, he'd finally figured out the four words.

"You are here to do two things. Learn and care. Learn as much as you can about real-life medicine so you can go back to Harvard with your internship certificate and your Part 3 National Board passing scores and begin your ophthalmology residency. Care for patients to the best of your ability. That's it. That's all you have to do. If you keep this up, the medical staff will grind your ass down to a toothpick. There are already plenty of reasons for them to dislike you. Don't give them one they can take to the Chief and get you tossed."

Sanjay looked at John Paul with disbelief. "Tossed? You mean terminated?"

"Tossed, terminated, shit-canned, fired, let-go. You'll get absolutely no credit for your time spent here. You'll have to start all over."

Sanjay pursed his lips and looked up at the ceiling. When he started to speak, he rolled his eyes back in his head. *That's a little creepy.* Baker followed his gaze upward.

"What do you mean, 'there are plenty of reasons for them to dislike you,'?"

Baker was ready. "There are three reasons why you are the perfect whipping boy for all these attendings." Sanjay sat back with his mouth clamped shut.

John Paul stuck his index finger into the air. "First of all, you are a foreigner. A foreigner with dark skin."

"John Paul, I'm an American citizen, as are my mother, father, two sisters and brother. I graduated first in my class both as an undergraduate and a medical student at Harvard University."

"The UVA of the North." Baker smiled. "I'm not saying any of this is fair or even right. I am telling you what I know. You stand out in this city full of Elmer's Glue-All white folks." Sanjay kept his mouth shut but shook his head incredulously.

Up went the middle finger to join its closest companion. "Second, you are smarter than any of us, particularly when it comes to textbook medicine. I have a sneaking suspicion that, if asked, you could quote me the entire chapter from Harrison's on Mrs. Sveringen's quinine-induced thrombocytopenia." At this, Sanjay thought a bit, then nodded. "The attendings know it and resent it when you come up with one of your morsels of minutiae, because you always turn out to be right."

John Paul stuck out his ring finger. "Third, you are here only for one year, after which you will go back to Boston and become a famous, well-published retinal specialist and make twice what any of these guys will. That pisses them off to no end. If you keep hassling them, they will ream you on a daily basis, knowing that you won't be around for two more years to screw them in return." He straightened his elbow so the three fingers were right in front of Sanjay's face.

"So that is how it is?"

"That is how it is."

With sad eyes he asked, "Can I go home now?"

"Of course. There's a party tonight right around the corner at Jill Aagaard's townhouse. She's a nurse in the CCU. All the house staff are invited. ICU and CCU nurses only."

"I'm sorry, but I don't think I'd enjoy myself. Besides, I have to study up on esophageal varices, then get here for rounds by seven tomorrow morning."

And finish the dish off with a touch of sweet.

"You can read all you want on GI bleeders tomorrow. If you show up at the party and stay for ninety minutes, you can have the day off. I'll round for you and then we'll meet up here to start call Sunday morning." Baker expected his intern to resist, but the kid's eyes lit up. He stuck out his hand.

"Deal."

That night, Sanjay showed up as promised. Surprisingly, he turned out to be a very entertaining storyteller, particularly when it came to anecdotes about the professors at Harvard Medical School. After about an hour, Melissa latched on to him. They spent the rest of the evening chatting and looking deeply into each other's eyes. Around midnight he came over and whispered excitedly in Baker's ear.

"Melissa wants me to walk her home!"

"Attaboy. See you Sunday, seven A.M. sharp." *Thank God. That should loosen him up a bit.*

Their second week in the ICU was a chaotic mess, but it still went more smoothly than the first. Sanjay the Smitten had a hard time keeping his eyes off of Melissa. Nonetheless, he did everything Baker asked of him and more. They were hustling patients in and out of the unit at a record pace, never leaving before 7 P.M.

By the time their turn to take call for the units came up on Saturday, things had begun to slow down. After admitting a couple of COPDers and a Saturday night special, a GI bleeder with the DTs, they both managed to grab a couple of hours of uninterrupted shuteye. Their last admission, a transfer, rolled in at 4 A.M. Sunday. Sandfrid Folstad, a sixty-eight-year-old apple farmer from Orondo, had been admitted to the Wenatchee hospital twelve hours prior and then rapidly deteriorated. He arrived via ambulance, paralyzed from head to toe and on a ventilator. Sanjay did his workup and wrote a page of orders. Around 5:30 A.M. he and Baker sat down with coffee to go over the case. Sanjay had all his ducks in a row, so they were done by 6:15. Then they rounded together on all twelve of their unit patients. At 7:30 Baker did a quick run-by to make sure everything was copacetic with the day shift nurses caring for the team's patients. He couldn't believe how smoothly the morning-after had gone.

David Simmons, a medical school classmate of Baker's, was up from Portland for a conference. He and Baker were going over to Bainbridge Island for the day. One of Baker's clinic patients ran an outfitting service less than a block from the island terminal and was providing all their gear gratis, including a nine-foot aluminum dinghy with a little electric kicker. The two were to meet at the ferry terminal at Colman Dock at 9 A.M. sharp. Baker sat down at his work desk and called to sign out to Kevin Spears. The CCU resident and his intern were on-call for the next twenty-four hours.

"Sanjay will check in with you before he takes off, probably around 11 or so."

"Sounds good, J.P. We're not going anywhere. By the way, how's he doing?"

"Better. I've been working with him on keeping his mouth shut. I'd like to take credit for his improvement, but it doesn't hurt that he's developed a romantic interest down here."

"Yup, nothing better than a little lovin' to adjust your attitude. Have fun over in Bainbridge. If you catch a lunker, keep it and cut me a slab. I'll kipper it on the beach and split it with you."

"Yah, sure, you betcha."

Just as he hung up, in popped Dr. Aaron Winkler, the noted immunoneurologist. As per his usual, he was rubbing his hands together like the town miser about to crack a waif's piggy bank. He leaned over Baker and whispered conspiratorially.

"Herman tells me we have a new Guillain-Barre patient in from Chelan County." Baker stifled a groan. Herman Feinbaum was Winkler's hired hand, an internist who had virtually no practice of his own and absolutely no personality. He made his living addressing the medical problems of Winkler's neurology patients and took ER call almost every night. It was rumored that no patient had ever kept a second appointment with Herman. Baker couldn't take the guy for five minutes.

John Paul closed his eyes for a second, then spoke. "First of all, Aaron, you might want to actually examine the patient. Then you'll want to talk with my intern, Dr. Chatterjee. He is not at all convinced that this patient has Guillain-Barre, nor am I." By the way Winkler was shaking his head and smiling, he could tell what was coming next.

"Nonsense. Herman told me the history is classic for Guillain-Barre. I've already called the pheresis team. They're on their way in. We should be running him by ten at the latest." Plasmapheresis was a process to rid a patient's blood of harmful immunoglobulins by filtering their blood through a dialysis-like machine, separating blood cells from plasma. Then the plasma is discarded; red blood cells are returned to the patient's bloodstream after being mixed with synthetic plasma products. It was all the rage for Guillain-Barre Syndrome and some blood disorders. Winkler had a three-year joint grant from the feds and a pheresis machine manufacturer to study one hundred patients. Alas, time was running out. In the past year, everybody who crossed the immunoneurologist's path had a puncher's chance of ending up on the pheresis protocol.

"Aaron, you might want to consider other diagnoses before relegating this guy to your study. Dr. Chatterjee has made an excellent case for tick paralysis or organophosphate poisoning being the culprit."

Winkler sighed knowingly, then ambled off. Figuring he had only one last arrow in the quiver, Baker caught Sanjay's eye and pointed over to Winkler, who was opening the door to Folstad's room. The intern nodded and bounded across the ICU. John Paul looked back as he left the unit. Sanjay had the neuron cornered, gesturing wildly like a coked-up orchestra conductor.

Monday morning, feeling refreshed after a day on the water and an excellent plate of razor clams with David at Ivar's Pier 54, Baker paged Kevin Spears.

Kevin asked, "Are you in the ICU yet, J.P.?"

"No, just got here. I'm in the lounge loading up on coffee. Anything to report?"

"Mr. Folstad didn't survive the pheresis."

"Aw, fuck. What happened?"

"I gotta go. We just admitted a big anterior MI and he's crashing and burning. Ask Sanjay. The kid stayed until 8 last night. Thank God, because we had a bitch of a day. Say what you want about him, he's a trooper."

"AOK." As he was about to hang up, he added, "I got one. A keeper."

Kevin mustered a weary cheer. "Finally, some good news. Bye."

Baker rushed up to the unit. For the first time, Sanjay hadn't beaten him to prep rounds. Through the glass door, he could see that Folstad's bed was empty. He dropped his backpack under the house staff work desk. For some reason, the apple farmer's chart hadn't accompanied him to the morgue down in the basement. He sat down and leafed through twenty pages of charts, handwritten notes and dictated summaries.

Oh, shit. It was clear that Sanjay had forgotten their discussion from a mere ten days prior. After Winkler's initial assessment note listing Guillain-Barre as the diagnosis and, surprise, emergency plasmapheresis as the treatment of choice, Sanjay had written a two-page dissertation on why he thought the patient had tick paralysis, which required nothing more than supportive care until the illness resolved with time, or organophosphate poisoning, which meant the patient should be receiving atropine and supportive care. The intern pointed out that plasmapheresis was not without its own side effects, even throwing in a couple of experiences from his time at Harvard, listing life-threatening complications some of his patients developed from the procedure. A classic chart war was developing, the kind Baker had foreseen when he first sat Sanjay down for the sweet and sour lecture.

He scanned the daily chart. The pheresis session, which should have taken a little over two and one-half hours, lasted only fifty minutes. At that point, Folstad's oxygen saturation dropped precipitously and he started producing copious volumes of lung secretions through his endotracheal tube. Predictably, soon thereafter his blood pressure dropped. A pulmonologist and a cardiologist were consulted to help with management. Given the old man's low blood pressure, pheresis was no longer possible, so the team unhooked him and left. Back to the progress notes. An 11 A.M. portable chest x-ray showed his lungs, which were clear on admission at 4:30 A.M., now resembled a field of snow, known in the business as a "whiteout".

Thereafter, at thirty-minute intervals, Sanjay had dutifully noted the patient's condition, what he had done to help, and why he thought the patient had deteriorated. Taken together, they provided an artful narration, carefully and rationally laid out for all the world to see. Occasionally, as the ship continued to sink, Winkler added a defensive line or two, justifying his decision to perform emergent plasmapheresis, just in case the patient actually did have Guillain-Barre. He signed off at 1 P.M.

"Please reconsult as necessary. We can continue plasmapheresis when the patient's hemodynamic and pulmonary status permits."

The way Baker saw it, either the patient had suffered some sort of immune response to the pheresis procedure, or there had been a toxic contamination of the machine, its tubing, or the replacement fluids. Nothing else could have produced such a rapid change.

Remarkably, Sanjay, Kevin Spears and the two consultants were able to keep Folstad going until almost 7 P.M. Herman, the attending of record, first showed up just as the patient expired. *Fifteen hours after the admission of a critically ill patient,* Baker thought. *Unfuckingbelievable.*

In a final turn of the screw of irony, Folstad's nephew arrived right after the cessation of life support for his uncle, whose heart was no longer beating despite a temporary pacemaker and a cornucopia of intravenous meds to support his blood pressure. Odolf Folstad served as the unofficial manager of Sandfrid's orchard. With harvest right around the corner, he'd decided to drive up to Spokane on Friday for some parts for one of the packing machines. He didn't get back to Wenatchee until early Sunday morning, probably around the time his uncle was transferred out. There was a verbatim report of Odolf's statement in the nursing notes.

"Uncle Sandy was restless the whole week. He always gets that way right before harvest, I guess because he worries about how it will go. There wasn't anything to do for the next day or two. He mentioned something about clearing out old pesticides from a shed we hadn't used in ten years or more. As I was driving away, I saw him riding his dirt bike over in that direction."

Son of a bitch, Sanjay was dead on. Folstad probably spilled a container of organophosphates on himself and didn't clean up right away. Had that history been available to the folks in Wenatchee, they never would have had to ship him here and the unlucky Scando would still be alive and kicking. Baker put the medical record back together and took it over to the unit secretary's desk. Just then Sanjay walked in. They sat down at their work desks. Baker handed him a cup of coffee.

"Long day-after, Sanjay."

"It wasn't bad. There was so much happening with Mr. Folstad, I didn't have time to get tired. I fell asleep as soon as I got home. So sorry to be late, John Paul."

Baker waved his hand dismissively. "Nothing happening. I'm glad you were able to sleep in a bit. I see from his chart that you were unable to follow my advice about a chart war."

Sanjay hung his head for a moment, then looked up at his resident. "Sorry about that too. I just thought Mr. Folstad deserved my best effort." He looked down again.

"Sure looks like he got it."

"You were right about winning a chart war. It is indeed a Pyrrhic victory." He looked up at the ceiling, then took a sip of his coffee. "That is, if I even won. Will there be trouble for what I wrote?"

Baker thought for a minute. "Doubt it. Winkler's an oddball, especially when it comes to his obsession with plasmapheresis. If anyone files a complaint, he'll probably get nothing more than a reprimand from the Board of Medical Examiners. Our chief shouldn't have any problem with your performance or your notes. Those farm folks out in the central valley aren't big on lawsuits, so not much of this should come back to haunt any of us, not even him."

"That is too bad. Mr. Folstad's death was entirely avoidable."

"Never hope for a lawsuit, Sanjay. I know it's hard for you to believe, but, sooner or later, one will be pointed at you, right between the eyes." He clapped his intern on the knee. "Despite the outcome, I am very proud of you." He looked over toward the nursing desk. "I believe a certain nurse is directing her baby blues your way. Go say hi, then we'll start work rounds."

Sanjay stood up with a big grin on his face. He started to walk away, then turned back toward Baker.

"John Paul, I really do try to adhere to your four words. I just thought of four more for Dr. Winkler."

"Oh, yeah?" The intern nodded and stuck out his palm with four fingers extended.

"I told you so."

68. CHART WARS

What exactly is a chart war? This form of paper conflict, unique to the hospital setting, is nothing more than two parties trading written blows over a patient or one of the patient's medical problems. There are three basic tenets of medicine that make chart wars inevitable:

1. Medicine is nowhere near an exact science. There is no single right answer, especially if there are confounding circumstances. For instance, a heart surgery patient with COPD will require a different treatment plan and will respond to a given treatment differently than will a heart surgery patient with AIDS.

2. Anything you do or prescribe to fix one problem has a fair chance of making another problem worse.

3. Every physician, especially every subspecialist, has a unique perspective on every medical problem. When treating a patient with lupus who has inflammation of the kidneys and the brain, a nephrologist (kidney subspecialist) has a different set of priorities than does a neurologist (brain guy).

If you are lucky enough to come into the hospital for bypass surgery, survive it, and go home in a timely fashion, good for you. That is exactly what happens to the majority of CABG patients in the U.S. If, however, a non-cardiac complication arises, often a subspecialist will be asked to consult on your case. He will make a recommendation or two, which most likely your heart surgeon or cardiologist or hospitalist will follow. If, for some reason, his recommendation causes a problem in another organ system, or if you develop a second separate complication, another subspecialist will consult. That's when conflict may arise.

At the center of all chart wars lies you, the patient, because without a patient, there is no patient chart and, hence, no chart war. Nor can there be a chart war if you are admitted, you get well, and you go home within the allotted time as determined by your DRG (Diagnostic Related Group). However, if you hang around the hospital too long and refuse to get well and go home, we then have the perfect scenario for a chart war. Endless days of rounding on you, ordering copious tests to figure out what's going on with you, then coming to a mutually-agreeable solution. Everyone gets frustrated, a.k.a., sick of the sight of you. Everyone wishes you would stop developing complications from their recommended treatments so that they can send you home or to the S.N.F. Most importantly, everyone wants to finish up with your case and get on with their happy lives chock-full of good little patients who have their surgery and go home on time.

By the time a chart war starts, well into your hospital stay, often the initial admitting physician is long gone and you are surrounded by dueling consultants. Just as the only lawyer in town will go broke but two lawyers will make a fortune, you must have two parties for a successful chart war. In a really juicy chart war, every time Consultant #1 leaves a brief note and an order on the chart, Consultant #2 will dash off a longer note explaining why Consultant #1's recommendation is a bunch of shit that will make the patient sicker and Consultant #2's job that much harder. According to Newton's Third Law of Motion, every action has an equal and opposite reaction. That's why Consultant #1 fires back that it was Consultant #2's recommendations that caused the problem in the first place. Everyone is covering his own ass. While wise men with nothing to hide will disagree face-to-face or on the phone, if you are going to cover your ass, you are going to have to document said ass-covering in the chart, specifically in the progress notes. A first class ass-covering can't take place without putting someone else's ass in the proverbial sling.

Early on in a chart war, it may be best for the primary physician to step back and not take sides while the two consulting asses duke it out in the progress notes. Interfering in their little pissing match offers as much chance of success as jumping between the snarling wet fangs of a pit bull and a Rottweiler. Meanwhile, once word of a chart war spreads through the hospital, you can count on a daily line-up of hospital staff waiting to read the latest entry. Nobody wants to miss out on a particularly juicy jab or a wily counterpunch. You, the subject of said chart war, will probably be completely unaware of the widespread interest in your chart. It is easy for gossipy onlookers to forget there is a human being at the center of this tempest.

If the chart war gets really testy, one or more consultants will pretend to take offense and seize the opportunity to sign off your case. The signoff note usually ends with, "Reconsult as necessary." or, even more fanciful, "I'd be happy to see this patient again if the need arises." Nothing could be further from the truth. Primary care physicians liken the slithering off of consultants on a case gone bad to a pack of rats abandoning a sinking ship. Sometimes they sum up the maneuver as, "Good riddance to bad rubbish." Other times it produces nothing more than a shrug of the shoulders, a sigh skyward, and then it's back to work.

Nurses can get involved in chart wars as well; sadly, for the most part they cannot write in the doctors' section or on the order sheet. Chart wars would be so much more fun to follow if nurses could just drop an occasional bomb or two in the progress notes. Given the constraints of tradition, if a nurse has a beef with a doctor about the care of the patient, she is limited to documenting the disagreement in the nursing notes, usually tying it up in a nice bow with the damning acronym, DANOG. "Doctor aware. No orders given." It means the nurse thought there was a significant problem with your care that one of your doctors didn't address. Like Ricky Ricardo's, "Five words, Lucy: Aye Yai Yai Yai Yai!", those five words say it all. They'll make any malpractice attorney drool with greed. Other parties may have quite dissimilar reactions. For instance, upon hearing those five words, hospital quality assurance staff, the ones who have to document and address any complication that prolongs your stay, have been known to fall on the floor and foam at the mouth. Somebody is about to take it in that ass they were so eager to cover.

Chart wars can be especially passionate in teaching hospitals. Interns and residents, who are charged with the responsibility for your overall well-being, resent consultants who drop condescending subspecialty trivia into the progress notes and resent even more the consultants' writing orders without conferring with them first. These young doctors-in-training often know all the facts about the disease in question but for some reason persist in the belief that this knowledge, applied judiciously, will rescue you from your present circumstances intact and grateful. In other words, they are clueless when it comes to Murphy's Law, karma, or human nature. Being relegated to the back seat of the decision-making jalopy after a long, frustrating night of prying you away from the Reaper's doorway wears at their sleep-deprived souls. That's when they forget two of the most important laws of medicine. "Primum non nocere", which means "Above all, do no harm". And "Si quid mali non tace." which translates roughly to "You can't do any harm if you keep your mouth shut." Into chart battle they march.

When it comes to treating sick patients, most old-timers long ago forsook their egos. They got to be old-timers by remembering three simple rules:

1. Get the job done with as little fuss as possible.
2. As long as nobody is doing anything really stupid, let it go.
3. Above all, don't engage in dick-measuring contests in the progress notes or on the order sheet.

If an old-timer gets involved in a chart war, look to his personal life for the reason. Perhaps the patient is an old friend. Perhaps the thirty-year-old son has moved back home because his latest entrepreneurial adventure, backed by Dad, has gone belly up. Best yet, perhaps the thirty-five-year-old daughter is getting a divorce and has brought her three ADHD pre-teens back home to live with Gramps and Granny "until we get settled in a place of our own". Family.

The optimal resolution to a prolonged chart war is a call by the primary physician for all combatants to sign off the case. If the primary physician doesn't sort things out, the consultants will continue to hiss and spit at each other and you will continue to circle the drain; one or more concerned parties (Nursing Department, Quality Assurance, Discharge Planning, Hospital Security) may ask a department head or the medical chief of staff to referee. That rarely goes well. He has to settle the fight without pissing off either side. Good luck with that. By this stage of the conflict, every consultant has invested his reputation, his pull, and his superior knowledge. In other words, he's knee-deep in ego. Usually, the guy who admits the most patients to the hospital or does the most teaching will get the better end of the chief's stick. Going forward, there will be gripes and grudges.

In the worst-case scenario, despite everyone's best efforts, you continue to decline, ending in permanent serious disabilities or death. That's when the chart war, which is part of the PERMANENT record, makes everyone look stupid. Morbidity and Mortality conferences and depositions before malpractice attorneys allow all parties involved an opportunity to see how their impassioned and authoritative opinions look in the rearview mirror of time, known in the business as the retrospectoscope.

"Doctor, I see here that your infectious disease consultant advised using an aminoglycoside antibiotic, yet you ordered a cephalosporin. Several days later, when the culture and sensitivities came back, the offending bacteria was found to be sensitive to aminoglycosides but resistant to cephalosporins. Twenty-four hours after that, your patient died of fulminant sepsis. May I infer from your course of action that you knew more than the double board-certified specialist?"

"There was a reason for that. Our renal consultant wanted to avoid the aminoglycosides because of pre-existing kidney disease."

"Ah, that would explain your terse comments in the progress notes. Interesting that, as a second-year resident, you felt the need to lecture your double-boarded subspecialty consultant in writing."

"That's not what I meant when I wrote that."

"Really? And here I thought I was pretty good when it comes to reading and comprehending. Then again, I tend to write what I mean and mean what I write. Thank you for enlightening me, Doctor. That will be all." Don't leave town.

It's even worse for the guy supervising the house staff, the attending physician on a case. When it comes to doling out the blame and the cash on a case gone bad, interns, residents and fellows are deemed "transparent". They are the glass doors in the hallway through which the wall safe at the end of the hall may be seen. Plaintiffs' attorneys depose them, perhaps even put them on the stand at trial, but they probably won't be part of the final judgment or settlement, mostly because they are broke, but also because they are trainees. Their supervisor, the head man on the case, the one who's supposed to keep them in line, he's opaque. He's the wall safe at the end of the hall. Often he gets dinged as much for doing a half-assed job of keeping the young whippersnappers on the straight and narrow as he does for the bad outcome.

69. CONSOLATION PRIZE

John Paul Baker was the second-year medicine resident on call for the units. The CCU was full of acute MI's; the only transfer out of there tonight would be on a gurney to the basement. The ICU had a couple of beds available, but the majority of patients in there were on the surgery service, so, unless one of them coded, he was going to have a fairly slow night. No room at the inn. His intern, Greg, barely out of medical school, already knew more textbook medicine than Baker and loved roaming the units at night, looking for missed diagnoses. By Halloween, all the residents had agreed to leave him on autopilot, and thus far, nobody had been burned. Greg hadn't paged a resident for help since the first week of August.

At midnight, Baker called each of the units, then the ER. All quiet. Barring a surprise of the worst kind, there would be nothing for him to do, at least for the next two hours. Two hours of sleep and, no matter what came in between 2 and 8, he'd be ready at 5 P.M. to drive up with Connie to Crystal Mountain for some night skiing. He stopped in to the Isolation Unit, where evil microbes ruled supreme, but Connie was off, so he spent five minutes chatting up the graveyard shift unit secretary, she of the mousy librarian look who diligently and precisely thumbtacked up a half-dozen naked guy pinups over her desk at the beginning of her shifts. She never failed to answer the phone with "Isolation, Meg Hart, Unit Secretary". He envisioned the scene in her apartment when it was just her, a man, and her allegedly impressive inventory of sex toys. Images of B&D sessions gone bad left him with a mild case of the willies.

He walked out into the street and stood still for a moment, letting the omnipresent winter mist dampen him a bit, then crossed over to the Lantana. Most house staff on-call rooms were barren, sweaty closets in the hospital with an overhead light, a bed, and a nightstand with a phone. The sheets were changed every day by Housekeeping, but most nights they went unused. The Lantana, though, that was something else. The art-deco masterpiece was built in the Roaring 20's by a lumber king for his loggers to use when they came into Seattle for a weekend. Booze and women were prohibited and the place was watched by off-duty cops, but it was cheap lodging with hot running water, so there was never an empty bed. An enterprising Turk built a giant dance hall less than a block away and supplied anything the boys couldn't get at the boardinghouse.

The old man died just after World War II, and his three sons, Puget Sound rubes turned New York bon vivants straight out of a Vanity Fair parody, sold every board foot of the empire, including the Lantana. The building served as an apartment house until the mid-1970's. There had been several deaths which didn't qualify as run-of-the-mill. A dance instructor left his wife and two-year-old daughter to go steaming around the world with a rich widow he met at the Fred Astaire studio. The wife plunged off the top of the building with the little girl in her arms. It wasn't the fall that killed either one--it was the garbage truck barreling down the street in the pre-dawn gloom. A car salesman from Tennessee drank too much of his homemade shine and then, in an Olympic-worthy feat of pretzelry, ate his .30-30. Then there was the curious case of the secretary found hanging by her pantyhose on New Year's Day in 1969. Per the international haunted house protocol, all four ghosts were routinely sighted working the night shift on the upper floors.

Under murky circumstances, the building ended up deeded to the Episcopalian Bishop, a frequent visitor to the hospital and the downtown nightclubs. After he turned the building over to the hospital in exchange for God-knows-what, it began yet another chapter as the house staff on-call quarters until such time as the planners would need the space for an office building or a parking garage. It was three stories tall, with a basement that served as the hospital library. The upper two stories were sealed off: Ghosts Only. On the ground floor, rooms for each of the on-call interns and residents were labeled as such on the doors.

Over the weekend, the hallway trim and doors had undergone a paint job. Baker could smell the oil-based enamel and thinner when he walked into the hall. Someone had put the brass labels back over the paint, but on the wrong doors.

He tried the door for the room he usually used, but it was locked. The brass plate now said "Surgery Resident". Relying on his deductive skills, he walked around the corner to the room usually used by the surgeons. Sure enough, it was now labeled "ICU/CCU Resident". The door was unlocked. Baker whispered a prayer of thanks, went in, took off his white coat, and sat on the bed. After calling both units and the E.R. and giving them his extension number, he fell back on the bedspread, asleep almost immediately. On-call sleep for him always involved swirling downward, into the coriolis of a flushing toilet.

John Paul was deep into a dream of rescuing a cute little Vietnamese telemetry nurse named Vicki from the clutches of one of the cardiology attendings, a notorious groper. He was ripping open the ragtop on the guy's 911 with a scalpel blade. It was hard work. In the dream, someone was trying to cover his head from behind with a pillowcase. In his bed, someone was working on pulling up his scrub top. That wasn't going well. A hand came around from behind and started working on the knot in his scrub pants drawstring. Somewhere deep in his subconscious, his conscious nose could detect a subtle scent with a hint of citrus, so he retreated back to the dream. His attacker was now working on his belt buckle. He considered flailing back with the #10 blade but was worried about popping the two warm soft balloons pressed up against his back. The scenario called for them to be full of napalm. Baker the hero.

A giggle stirred him. The scrub tie had lost the battle to the hand, and his scrub pants slipped down without a whimper. In his groggery, he eliminated the telemetry nurse, whose repertoire of laughter consisted solely of a titter. Next came "Isolation, Meg Hart, Unit Secretary." Unable to imagine her giggling without a fearsome snort at the end, his subconscious gave up guessing. Dream Baker woke up, and he and On-call Baker decided to join forces and go along for the ride.

"Do you like that, Marco?" Now he recognized the voice. He covered his laugh with a moan. It was Nancy from the day shift in the ICU, Chicago accent and all. While a tad shy at work, she had been linked romantically with more than one surgery resident, so, in the estimation of various medicine residents, she "went down like a ton of bricks", but not for them. Baker vaguely remembered a dream in which he rescued her from a surgical team. So chivalrous.

Things were heating up down below, what with the left hand providing a curious massage from the back forward, and the right hand directing a few frontal helicopter maneuvers. Nancy seemed surprisingly clumsy when performing procedures in the intensive care unit, but she had the subtle dexterity of a Vegas card dealer when it came to Baker's unit.

She began biting softly on his trapezius while tugging his stick shift around toward her. There was no obvious choice other than to follow. Now they were face-to-face in the dark.

"Hi, Nancy." She let go of him, pushed away, and almost fell off the single bed. He grabbed her wrist to steady her, then let go. She stood up and flipped the light switch.

"John Paul, what are you doing in here? This is Marco's bed." He considered the import of that, and had a vague image that he shooed away. She did the "Elke Sommer", covering her breasts with her hands. It'll drive any guy wild, and Baker was no exception.

"They changed the call rooms around, I guess. He's probably in the ICU resident's room." She pulled on her dress, a satiny wrap-around affair, and stood up. No undies. He was really warming to Nancy. "His door is locked."

"He never locks his door until..."

"Well, Nancy, let's review. He's practically engaged to that TV anchor lady up in Seattle. She probably drove down after the 11 o'clock news." She leaned back against the wall, looked up at the ceiling, and puffed out her cheeks as she exhaled. Then she looked back down at Baker.

Baker tried an icebreaker. "Is it okay if I pull up my pants now?" She giggled.

"Give it a minute or two. You don't want to hurt yourself." He looked down, then back up at her, and smiled.

"I think I'm going to need help."

"Dream on, Dr. Baker."

"Well, since we've gotten to know each other better, how about dinner sometime?"

"Oh, let's not start with a date. If you're not too tired, how about coming with me and Sarah and Laura. Laura's driving us up to Crystal to ski tonight. Or is it tomorrow night?"

As he slid his scrub pants up, Baker looked at his watch. "Tonight. I'd love to, but I promised Connie in Isolation that I'd ride up with her. Maybe I'll see you there."

"Not with her. Her partner tore her ACL in Vail last night. Connie flew to Denver this morning to help out the next few days. Probably won't be home before the weekend. She must have forgotten to page you."

"Well, then, I guess we are on for tonight." He smiled. "By the way, we'll be keeping this little interaction to ourselves, right? I'd prefer that the word didn't get out that I had you in bed with me in an on-call room and nothing happened."

"I wouldn't worry about that if I were you. I don't fancy myself as 'Nancy, that R.N. who went looking for one resident and ended up naked in bed with another.' I've already been romantically linked to half a dozen surgery residents in the past two years. Until I started working here, I didn't know that having a cup of coffee with someone meant you were having sex."

"Nancy, any hospital is pretty much like a small town. Not as much going on as everyone says."

"Then again, you did have a nurse show up uninvited in your bed." She laughed and opened the door. "Don't get up, I'll let myself out. Good night, Dr. Baker." As she left, she flipped off the light switch. Baker rolled over onto his back and smiled up at the dark ceiling. Out in the hallway, he heard three loud knocks on a door marked "Surgery Resident".

He thought to himself, *John Paul Baker, Consolation Prize.*

70. SEX IN THE HOSPITAL

Q: Will someone be having sex with me in the hospital?
A: A lot of someones will be having sex, but not with you.

At any given moment, more often at night than during the day, people are screwing each other's brains out all over your hospital. If you awaken at night and hear moaning in your room, most likely someone is getting it on with someone else right there. Do not look under the bed.

Actually, that isn't quite true. There is way more sex going on in your hospital than on those silly hospital TV shows, where everyone has to talk to everyone else about every possible melodramatic plot twist until you wish they would all shoot each other in the face. However, there is probably far less sex going on than you imagine.

Who's getting it in your hospital? Ideally, the guy footing the bill, i.e., you, would be the beneficiary of said hospital sex. After all, not only are you the one shelling out the monthly insurance premiums and the deductibles and the co-pays and all the other little charges that accumulate as if by magic on your daily bill, you are also the one suffering the most, what with your humiliating gown open in the back, your painful surgical wound, your Foley catheter, your silly cheap foam slippers that cost you and your insurance company $50.00 or more.

Wouldn't it be nice if your hospital experience were just like one of those steamy Playboy Channel (No, you don't even get Playboy Channel on the hospital TV. Not on your insurance plan anyway. Only Congress's health plan covers that.) fantasies where the smoking hot nurse comes in to give you a back rub, then can't contain herself any longer and peels off the 36D for some playtime between the sheets?

I think it would be nice. There are a few reasons why that probably won't happen to you. First, back rubs are no longer on the nursing menu. Second, by the time you can get it up after bypass surgery, your butt will be long gone from the hospital. Third, you aren't wearing a white coat.

If you want to see how the hospital sex system operates, rent a copy of *Coma*. In that movie, Tom Selleck plays Sean Murphy, a rugby player with all his teeth who is admitted to the hospital for a knee repair. Genevieve Bujold is a surgery intern who does his H & P and obviously develops a case of tepid hots for Sean. Unfortunately for our buddy Sean, Genevieve is doing Michael Douglas, the guy in the white coat. Not only does Sean not get the girl, he ends up in a coma (Coma. Get it?) because evil Chief of Surgery Richard Widmark is selling body parts, and, as we all know, Tom has some nice body parts, or at least he used to. Or maybe it's because he's flirting with Michael Douglas's girl. I don't mean to imply that if you flirt with a nurse or female physician or female anyone in the hospital you'll end up in a coma minus some essential body parts, but why push your luck? Besides, if a young Tom Selleck can't get any, what chance do you have?

Since there's no rush, let's pretend. Let's pretend you are tall, robust, handsome, rich, witty and possess about 5% body fat, rather than 40%. Better yet, let's go with the real you.

Time to check on Mr. Right. The day shift report says he's awake, alert, taking liquids, oriented X 4, has been up and in a chair, but hasn't walked yet. OK. Oh, God, look at that stupid grin. One hand under the sheets. "Pocketball", the hospital edition, from Season 4 of "Naughty Nurses". Hmmm. Only mildly balding, but a nice comb-over. "The Swoop". Bloodshot eyes, just like my ex. Patient breath with just the right touch of stale tobacco; remind me to wear a mask and bring in an extra supply of lemon swabs. Yum, nicotine stains on those strong, stubby fingers. No doubt the teeth have a nice tan as well. I like his third chin the best. Nice boobs. Poor baby, it has to hurt to suck in your gut like you're at Happy Hour at the Swizzle Inn. I'm working twelve-hour night shifts while my kids are home sleeping with my drama queen chronically depressed roommate. I get off here at 7 A.M., drive home while trying not to fall asleep at the wheel, just in time to see my kids off to school. I owe twenty grand on my nursing school loan and my ex hasn't paid child support in four months. My mom thinks I should boot out the roommate so she can move in and that almost sounds like a good idea. I've got a ten-page paper due next Monday for my master's class. I could sleep for a week at the drop of a hat, and this guy's coming on to me. What the hell. I'll lose my job, I'll be out on the streets, his Foley's crusting up, but hey, why not?

Put another way: No white coat, no sex.

I really have no idea how often people have sex in the hospital. Who surveys that? I do know that the ones caught doing it the most are usually house staff. Whether that's because they do it more often in the hospital--younger age, more stress, more hormones raging--or because they're not as wily as their older, seasoned counterparts, I have no way of knowing. I've walked in on only one on-duty tryst, and it was between a couple of forty-somethings, and not at all what I wanted to find in that supply closet, where I'd gone to politely expel some aromatic remnants of lunch at La Cucaracha. The young ones tend to pick places where they'll be caught, either in person or on videotape. Adds to the excitement, I suppose. Hang around a hospital long enough and gain the confidence of the nurses, and eventually they will show you a telemetry room recording of two people getting it on in an empty room. The first time I came across such a viewing, long before YouTube, my thought was, *God, I hope they strip the bed.*

Once you get out of the hospital, how do you know it's safe for you to have sex? First of all, if you don't have any desire, it's probably not time yet. It's not at all uncommon to be impotent for a while after bypass surgery. I mean real impotence, where you don't even get a piss hard-on early in the morning. Don't sweat that and don't reach for the Viagra just yet. The rule of thumb is that when you can climb two flights of stairs without stopping and you aren't sucking gas or having chest pain or about to pass out, you are ready to safely perform the Big Icky. These recommendations undoubtedly come from areas of the country where three-story houses are the norm. If you don't have access to two flights of stairs, I don't know long you wait.

Whatever you do, do not tell your partner or your doctor that you have chest pains during sex. If you do, I guarantee that every time you do have sex, from now until hell freezes over, your partner will spoil the afterglow with a worried look and, "Are you having chest pain?" Tell the concerned parties that you are having chest pain while climbing steps or while exerting yourself on a walk, but stay away from the sex part. Break this rule at your peril.

71. VACATIONER'S LODGE

"How much?" Robert Murphy looked at his watch.

David Simmons said, "Ten bucks an hour. Twenty-four hours, that's…"

"Three semesters of calculus, I know how to multiply. When will I see the fruits of my labor?"

"Next Friday. I'll throw in another ten to make it an even 250." Simmons the Magnanimous.

"Where are you gonna be?"

"I'm taking Mary Jo up to her roommate's wedding in Culpeper. We'll stay overnight at a motel there, get up early, and I'll be back to the room by 0900 Sunday morning."

Simmons had found work on a research study. Every weekend for six weeks, he bunked up free of charge in a room on the top floor of the Vacationer's Lodge, up on 29 North, just below Electricity Lane. 5 P.M. Friday through 5 P.M. Sunday. Ten bucks an hour, free room service, and all he had to do was supervise the participants in the study. He was explaining the research project to Murphy over beers at Nevermore.

He said, "A couple of Infectious Disease docs at the Medical School are working on the common cold."

Murphy wiped his mouth on the sleeve of his lumberjack-approved flannel shirt. "The common cold? What's there to work on?"

"They think someday they'll come up with a cure."

"Why bother?" Murphy hadn't caught a cold since the age of nine.

"A couple of reasons." David started counting on his fingers. "First, the common cold is responsible for more sick days in the United States, check that, in the world, than all other causes combined." Murphy raised one eyebrow. Simmons laughed. "Yeah, except for around here, even more than hangovers. Second, they figure that if they can come up with a cure for the common cold, some day they may come up with an immunization to prevent it. I know it sounds a tad farfetched, but that's where they started with measles, mumps, German measles, all of those. It's a big deal. Third, if they can figure out the mechanism for a cure for one virus, that opens the door for curing other viruses, some of the ones that don't just leave you feeling crappy for a week or two. Fourth, sometimes when you are studying one thing, you find the answer to a question that is much more important than the problem you are trying to solve." He took a sip. "Last but not least, research like this, funded by the NIH, keeps your lab going and your lab staff employed. Good for the economy in a small town like this."

"Okay. So where does a weekend at Vacationer's Lodge figure in?" The bartender, a guy named Willie who sported a ship tattoo from Subic Bay on his forearm, inquired about another round. David looked at his watch and shook his head. Murphy was headed for the bowels of Ackerman Library, so he declined as well.

"These two docs are trying to figure out how the common cold travels from one person to another."

"I've got that one. Just sneeze or cough on someone when you have a cold." Robert Murphy attributed his success at avoiding colds to his lightning reflexes and nimble feet around coughers and sneezers.

"Maybe, though some of the stuff they've looked at indicates that it might not be as easy as everybody thinks to transmit the virus that way. One of the most interesting things about clinical research is that if you take something that everybody knows is true and evaluate it objectively, sometimes you discover that what everybody knows is true is anything but." Murphy was deep into pondering this when Willie flipped an iced mug up in the air but missed it on the way down. David Simmons saw the whole thing and ducked his head just before the mug exploded on the brick floor. Everyone else at the bar jumped. Willie, who apparently had lost a screw or two from his brain pan during his time in the Philippines, looked around, grinned and took a bow. Simmons looked up over the bar before sitting up again. He sipped his beer, then turned to Robert Murphy.

"These two docs? I call them the Farfalle Freres." David was enrolled in an international cooking club that met once a month. "The Bow Tie Brothers."

Murphy guessed, "They both wear bow ties?"

"All the time."

"That's pretty good."

"That one came to me during my cooking class. We learned to make pasta."

All the scientific jabber was making Murphy feel a little intimidated, like he was the only one who didn't belong to the club. He countered with, "Just like J. Henry Matthews."

"Who?"

"J. Henry Matthews, law professor, judge, state representative and one-time gubernatorial candidate."

"He always wore a bow tie?"

Murphy said, "No, a necktie. There was an article in the Crier a few years ago. His daughter said she's never seen him without a necktie. Not even on Christmas morning when they're opening presents." He smiled.

"Seriously?"

"Serious as a heart attack."

"Oddly interesting."

"Okay, so back to the research. These two docs want to figure out how people catch a cold from someone else?"

David nodded. "Yes. This part of the study focuses on hand shaking."

"You're kidding." Murphy thought, *What the hell, rooting through the "counterculture fiction" in the basement of Ackerman was more fun with a beer buzz anyway.* He held up an index finger. Willie smirked, nodded, and fished out a fresh mug from the cooler. David shook his head. He had visions of swallowing broken glass in his beer and bleeding to death. By his third year, the typical medical student viewed every headache as an as-yet undiagnosed brain tumor. David was no exception. There was no symptom he experienced, no matter how transient or minor, that wouldn't inevitably lead to some form of horrible death scene, complete with a Hamlet-worthy soliloquy.

"This is what I do. My room is in the middle of the hallway, right across from the elevators. Every half hour, from 9 A.M. to 5 P.M., I call two rooms in the hotel. One is a donor, and one is a recipient. A donor comes out of a room to the right of me and a recipient from a room to the left. They meet in front of my door. The donor coughs into his palm, then shakes hands with the recipient. The recipient then puts his palm up to his nose and sniffs once, as deep as he can. Then they go back to their rooms."

"What the fuck is wrong with you people?" Everyone in the bar stopped talking and looked at Murphy, who was leaning back on his stool, staring at Simmons. When no fisticuffs broke out, they returned to their conversations. Willie waited, moving a toothpick from side to side with his tongue. The pensive puma, ready to leap into action.

"That's why they call it clinical research, Bub. This is relatively civilized. You wouldn't believe what they do to medical students in Texas. " Simmons knew the hand sniffing would get to his friend. Mission accomplished. Time to celebrate. He nodded at Willie. Another Amstel bubbled into a frosty mug. Simmons picked it up and eyeballed the bottom, searching for glass shards.

"Robert, believe it or not, researchers have won the Nobel prize starting with studies much less glamorous than this one. If their hypothesis turns out to be correct, theoretically you could prevent the transmission of the common cold by spraying some glop on your hands every few hours during the cold and flu season. Or just wearing gloves in public. Guys in research drool over getting in on the ground floor of something like this. Four donors and four recipients. Each pair meets four times each day. As cheap and simple a study as you could concoct, but brilliant nonetheless, and it could lead to a discovery that saves billions of dollars every year, not to mention thousands of lives if it pans out for influenza as well."

"I get the drool part." Murphy shook his head. "I'll do it, just this once, but you owe me."

"Of course." Simmons pulled out a twenty. "Beers on me."

Murphy was at Simmons' door at 8:45. He expected, no, hoped, that Mary Jo would be there. When David opened the door, he smiled and said, "She went home at midnight." He knew Murphy like a book.

"Dave, I'm not clear on one thing." Murphy rolled his bike into the room and parked it against the wall.

"What's that?" Simmons picked up a garment bag, put it over his shoulder, then grabbed his backpack off the bed.

"I'm not supposed to be here. You are."

"So?"

"So what if someone shows up to check things out?"

"The lab secretary was by last night at 5:00 to get everyone checked in. She'll be back tomorrow night at 5 P.M. for check out. I doubt she's gonna stop by tonight because she can't sleep. It's Saturday."

"What if one of the donors or recipients blabs?"

"Hah. They're all first year med students, getting paid to sit in a room and study. Nobody's going to screw up that kind of a deal. They won't even look at you." He handed Murphy the room key and walked out into the hall. "Besides, a first year med student is always stuck on page eight."

"Page eight?"

"As in, he doesn't know his ass from page eight."

Murphy laughed. "Okay. Have a good time. Say hi to Mary Jo for me."

"Thanks on the former. Probably not on the latter. She talks about you way too much as it is. You're on in ten minutes. The numbers and times are by the phone."

Everything went as slick as snot. After finishing up with Simmons at Nevermore on Thursday afternoon, Murphy had walked over to the library and checked out a half-dozen books. As soon as he was done with his first hall meeting at 9, he started with a collection of short stories by Updike, then moved on to a new Elmore Leonard novel. By 2 P.M. he was halfway through both and spent the next hour doing sit ups and pushups between trips out into the hall. Other than the pervasive smell of old cigarette smoke on everything, the room was fine. Murphy had opened all the windows and crisp April air flowed through. Around 4, realizing he had himself a batch pad for the night, he called his friend Diana. Her life consisted of school and volleyball, and any break from either one made her day. She said she'd pick up a six-pack and a pizza and come over by 9.

"Bring quarters. The bed features Magic Fingers."

David was right about the test subjects. As it turned out, they were not allowed to talk to anyone, face-to-face or on the room phone, for the entire forty-eight hours. Only one of them, D-3, a kid with overly-glossy curly hair and thick black-rimmed glasses, even looked his way during the cough-and-sniff sessions. The first time out, he gave Murphy a beady-eyed quizzical stare that lasted just a second too long, so Murphy shook his head and pointedly looked over at the recipient, R-3. He felt sorry for that guy, getting a spit slap every two hours from D-3.

Once the hallway sessions were done at 5 P.M., Murphy's job consisted solely of keeping an ear out for any noise in the hallway. Their end of the floor was partitioned off by a curtain from the rest of the rooms. The elevator across from Murphy's room was blocked from coming to their floor. Nobody was permitted to leave their room between 5 P.M. and 9 the next morning. Murphy couldn't imagine doing this for six weekends in a row, not even for fame, glory and good money. Diana showed up around 9:15. As instructed, she scratched three times on the door. Robert opened the door softly and she slipped in. "Hi. Hey, how'd you get up here? I forgot about this elevator being blocked."

She put down the pizza box, napkins, and a brown bag. "There was a sign in the elevator at this end, so I took the other one up. The curtain's a nice decorative touch. I felt so secretive slipping around it."

"Yeah, kind of silly. David says they'll actually mention that curtain in the report when they publish this study." He gave her a hug that Diana returned for most of a minute. They had tried dating a couple years ago, her freshman year, but her travel schedule with the team made anything other than random get-togethers every few weeks virtually impossible. After they finished embracing, Murphy stepped back. This was more awkward than he'd expected. "Anything going on out there?"

"You mean in the world?" She smiled.

"No. In the hallway."

"There's some weird smell coming from one of the rooms. The sign says D-3. It really reeked when I walked by."

"Smoke?"

"No, more like a chemical smell. I know I've smelled it before, but I can't place it. It'll come to me."

"Figures. There's one in every crowd." He filled her in on subject D-3.

"Well, hopefully we won't wake up to a fire alarm." That set Murphy back a step. He'd envisioned beers, pizza, a few laughs and then she'd head home. Diana was a regular at the sunrise Sunday guitar mass.

"I take it you brought quarters?"

"Oh, yeah. I won't be able to do laundry for a month." They both laughed. Robert pulled the six-pack from inside the brown bag.

"Lowenbrau! Nice. Where'd you get this?"

"Derrick works part-time for a distributor in Blacksburg." All five of the kids in Diana's family had names that started with "D". He couldn't remember all the names, but he knew that Derrick, the only one possessed of XY chromosomes, was studying pre-vet at Tech.

"They sell Lowenbrau there?" Murphy had gone down to Blacksburg once for the Commonwealth Cup game. From what he'd seen, he assumed that you couldn't buy anything but the big three: Bud, Schlitz and Miller.

"Don't wet your pants, Robert. Miller bought the rights to make Lowenbrau here in the U.S. Derrick says it's basically High Life with some spice thrown in, but it is free. He gave me two cases the last time I was home. Valentine's Day weekend. He said I should share it with somebody special, but not too special." She looked Murphy up and down, shook her head, shrugged and laughed. Now he was thoroughly confused. When it came to women, confused was Murphy's home address.

"So I'm special?"

"Not too special," they both laughed, "but you're the only special I know."

"What happened with the guy from the gymnastics team? Richard, was it?"

"'Great body, really handsome. Smart too, but so unworthy."

"More than most of us?"

"Shallow as a thimble of spit. I take very good care of my body, not because I want lots of guys looking at me, but because it feels good to be in shape. Here I am, trusting him enough to take my clothes off, especially with the lights on and everything, and the very first time we get naked he's staring at himself in the mirror instead of looking at me. I honestly thought he was going to lean forward and kiss his reflection. I'm tough, at least I think I am, but that night I cried like a baby."

"You cried in front of him?"

"No way. I got dressed, walked home, and cried in my bed."

"Sorry to hear that, Diana."

"Don't be. It only lasted a minute. I cry hard and fast."

They spent the next two hours chatting about mutual friends, her volleyball adventures, his upcoming graduation with an MBA and plans to do two years at Fort Drum. The beers and pizza went down smoothly.

Diana got up and went in to the bathroom with her backpack. When she came out, she was dressed in her orange and blue volleyball uniform.

"So we're going to burn off the food and beer with a little one-on-one?" He was lying up against the headboard.

"One-on-one. You'd need ten of your closest friends to keep up with me." She stood at the foot of the bed with her hands on her hips. "All the girls notice how you stare at me when you come to our games. I think the uniform gets you all hot and bothered. This is what I'm wearing. For now."

Murphy thought, *Who knew*? He tried a boyish grin, but ended up just screwing his face into a look of mild agony.

"I'm hoping you'll want me to stay for a while? Unless your graveyard shift girl is coming over at midnight."

"Nope, nobody else is on the schedule for this evening. Although if someone stops by with dessert, I have been known to be weak-willed."

"I got dessert covered, Mister." She crawled up the bed, all six feet of her, and straddled him.

"So, after all this time, we're really going to do this?"

"I don't know about you, but I sure am." She reached into her purse and pulled out a box of rubbers. "Let's get to it. There's a dozen of these things and I want to use them all up."

"Where'd you get those?"

"Coach Morrison insists we use them, in addition to whatever else a girl prefers. She says, 'An erect penis has no conscience.' I've had this box sitting in my bedroom for almost three years. I hope they're still good."

Murphy thought, *Ten bucks an hour, beer and pizza, and an Amazon volleyball delivery girl who wants to get naked with me. I have got to do more of these research studies*. They started making out on the bed. A question forced him to come up for air.

He asked, "Lights on?"

"No way. I'm not taking a chance on another guy screwing up my night." He reached over and flicked off the switch.

It was hard work. Diana was three years younger and in much better shape than Murphy. He thought, *I guess riding my bike around town isn't enough exercise*. When he first climbed on top of her, her abs were so solid he nearly slid off the other side.

"God, Diana, how many sit-ups do you do every day?"

Diana laughed. "We start practice every day with an hour of yoga. Core strength. Then there's the light weights with reps three days a week. Then swimming for an hour three days a week. Coach believes in us being in better shape than anyone else." She rolled over on top of him. Murphy felt like a doughboy being tossed around.

After a half-hour of bone-rattling, Murphy was ready to take a breather. It took another hour before Diana stopped to pause. Murphy said, "Thank God."

Diana laughed and kicked him in the thigh. "Wimp. Wait until I tell the girls."

The window drapes didn't quite close. He rolled over and looked at her in the slit of light from the parking lot. "You're not going to tell them, are you?"

She looked up at him and laughed. "Oh sure. 'He invited me up to the room that he didn't pay for, at the piss-elegant Vacationer's Lodge, and I was so flattered I rounded up a pizza, a six-pack, a box of rubbers and made a house call and fucked him.' Are you kidding me? I'd be 'Pizza Delivery Slut' for the rest of the season." Relieved, Robert flopped over on his back.

"Do you want me to get you up at any special time?"

"You're not getting off that easy. I'll come get you when I want you."

And she slid over to the far side of the big bed. Retired to neutral corners, he thought. Just like in a prizefight after a knockdown. He said a prayer for a two-hour mandatory eight-count.

****

They both woke up to the pounding on the door. It took Robert a minute to orient himself. He felt around for his pants. She was already up on one elbow with a smirk on her face.

"Sorry, Diana." He pulled on his pants and walked toward the door.

"Maybe it's the House Dick. Oh, wait, you're already here." She laughed and stood up. "Give me a minute. I'll get my stuff and hide in the bathroom."

Murphy waited until the bathroom door closed. There was a lighter knock as he opened the door. It was D-3.

The young medical student spoke up. "I'm sorry, I don't know your name." Murphy's nose twitched. The kid, now without his glasses but wearing a wet white washcloth on his head, gave off an aroma reminiscent of a pile of burning tires. Murphy thought, *God, I hope he's not cooking PCP in his room.* "I was wondering if you have any salve."

"Salve?" *Who the hell uses salve?* "What time is it?" He noticed D-3 was wearing some sort of bib over his pajamas.

"It's two-fifteen. Or maybe some cortisone cream? It's my scalp. I think it's melting!" *David was right*, Murphy thought. *This kid doesn't know his ass from page eight.*

"Okay, look. I'll see what I've got in my kit. Go back to your room, and I'll be over in a couple of minutes." He started to close the door.

"Thanks. I'm in D-3."

"I know."

He closed the door and turned. Diana was dressed. She picked up her shoulder bag and walked over to him.

"Looks like you're going to be busy for a while. I'll head home." She kissed him.

"Thanks. For everything. I had fun." He opened the door, looked out to make sure the coast was clear. As she walked past him into the hall, she bit him softly on the earlobe.

She whispered in his ear, "We'll finish this up. Tomorrow night, seven, your place."

"You mean tonight?"

She turned. "I may be coming to your place, but you're the one who's going to deliver." She winked and slid around the hallway curtain.

Still pondering the mysteries of womanhood, Murphy fished around in his backpack for his toiletry case. Inside he found a sand-crusted old tube of cortisone cream, probably from his last bad sunburn at the beach. He pulled on his shirt, surveyed the crime scene and left the room. Inside room D-3, his eyes watered. Between sneezes, he asked, "What've you been doing in here?" D-3 was patting his head with a wet hand towel. He still wore the plastic bib.

"I was straightening my hair. It takes three steps, with these chemicals." He led the way into the bathroom and pointed at the sink. "My chemistry lab partner in college developed them. He's an inventor." Rubbing his eyes and nose, Murphy examined the array of plastic bottles. He grabbed a Kleenex, ran some water over it, and dabbed at the corner of his eyes. D-3 put some more cold water on his hand towel and went back to swabbing his scalp. Tufts of wet black hair covered the towel.

"I think I must have fallen asleep during step 3. Or maybe I got my bottles mixed up. My contacts are burning my eyes and I can't find my glasses. My hair's falling out and my scalp burns."

Murphy walked back out into the room and proceeded to open all the windows. After a few minutes, he could open his eyes without the searing burn. He surveyed the room for the first time through clear eyes. His first guess was that a dozen badgers had gone ape shit trying to get out. Empty potato chip bags and textbooks covered the bed. The trash can was filled with empty Coke bottles. Trays of room service food were stacked next to the door. A small volcano of dirty clothes erupted from the floor of the closet. Apparently, research could get messy.

"How long have you been staying here?"

"Since last night. Why?"

"Never mind. Let's see the scalp." D-3 bent forward and removed his hairy towel, which by now was almost completely black. Murphy almost gagged on the kid's head.

"Jesus Christ!"

"What? What's wrong?"

"You have to go to the hospital." His head was almost completely bald. A few patches of scalp remained, and even those looked badly sunburned. Most of his head was a pink, glistening mass, oozing yellowish fluid. While Murphy watched, the patches of intact scalp sizzled and blistered, then evaporated. If this kept up, he'd be looking at brain in a few minutes. He walked over to the closet and turned on the light.

"Look, we have to do something to shut down the reaction or you're going to be headless pretty soon." He turned to D-3, fire extinguisher in hand, and pulled the pin. "Cover your eyes and your mouth and nose." He proceeded to cover D-3's head in carbon dioxide foam. After about thirty seconds, the smell dissipated. Foam dripped down his forehead onto the bib.

"Wow, that feels much better. Thanks!"

"I meant what I said. You have to go to the hospital."

"But then I'll be out of the study. Can't I stay? It's only fifteen hours or so."

"Are you serious, Kid? You've been scalped."

"But I'm here for a M.D./Ph.D. in microbiology and epidemiology. I want to be an infectious disease specialist. That's why I enrolled in the study. If I drop out, that's got to hurt my chances for a residency and fellowship."

"You seem kind of young to be in medical school. Mind my asking how old you are?"

"I'm nineteen, twenty next month."

"You're nineteen and you're in med school?"

 "I finished high school in three years and got my B.S. at Harvard in two." Murphy thought, *Jeez, this kid's a genius. It's a good thing you're going to be a doctor, you fucking weirdo. Otherwise, you'd starve.*

"Listen, trust me. You have plenty of time to repair your relationships with all those ologists. Right now, you've got to repair your head. I'm going to call you a cab, unless you want to go by ambulance."

"Oh, no. A cab's fine."

****

D-3, Murphy never did get the kid's name, was out the door and on his way to the E.R. by 3 A.M., Murphy thought about packing up the kid's stuff, but thought, *Fuck it, let the research people deal with the details.* He hit the sack and dreamed of rescuing Diana from a blood-spewing volcano.

By the time Simmons knocked on the door at 8:30, Robert had already showered and finished off a huge room-service breakfast. He'd been dreading the part where he had to explain why D-3 left the study in the middle of the night and was now undoubtedly warming a bed in the burn unit. Over his second cup of coffee, Murphy realized that R-3 was probably done as well. Would today be better or worse for him? One the one hand, R-3 wasn't going to make as much money as he'd planned, and any dreams of research glory were temporarily shelved.

On the other, he wouldn't have to look at D-3's scalp or sniff his snot any longer.

Murphy opened the door. "Hi, Dave."

"Hey. How'd everything go?"

"Sit down for a minute. I have to tell you something." He got Simmons a cup of coffee and some toast, then explained the D-3 episode from start to finish, omitting only his escapades with Diana. The PDS. It had a nice ring to it. When he'd finished, he waited for Simmons to bitch him out.

"God, Robert, I'm so sorry. If I'd known something like that was going to happen, I'd never have asked you to help me out. I should have warned you about D-3. I owe you big time." *Well*, thought Murphy, *that's certainly one way to look at it.*

"Listen, if you're free tonight, I'll buy dinner at the Virginian. The Sunday night steak and martini special."

"Thanks. Another time would be great. Tonight I have to make a delivery."

"Sure. Whenever you like. Well, I've got eight hours to figure out how to break the news to everyone. Wonder how this is going to affect the study."

"It'll be okay, Dave." Murphy smiled. "Bottom line, though?"

"What?"

"That aroma in D-3's room?"

"Yeah, Robert, what is that smell?"

"Whatever it is, it's not the scent of a Nobel Prize for the Bow Tie Brothers."

72. EVERYBODY'S EQUAL

"Hi, Marty!" He was older but not old, Jewish, and cynical. He played the goofball well, but Martin Lemon was by far the sharpest radiologist in the department. For Simmons, he was the go-to guy to read films before the dictations were available. Marty got a kick out of verbal sparring with David, as he was one of the few residents who wasn't offended by his warped sense of humor.

"David. How's my favorite goy boy named after the greatest Jew who ever lived?"

"Not bad. I had the weekend off."

"Good for you. Get laid?" Their usual Monday morning conversation.

"Nope. Spent the weekend moonlighting in Somerton. Friday night to Sunday morning." One of these days he was going to reply affirmatively to that question just to see how Marty took it.

Lemon didn't miss a beat. "I hear Playboy's doing a shoot next month. 'The Girls of Somerton and Their Sex Lives'."

"Yeah. More likely 'The Girls of Somerton and Their Six Kids'."

Marty laughed. "What can I do you for?"

Simmons handed him the films and the jacket. "Hot off the presses. Upper GI and small bowel follow-through. Guy with recurrent rectal bleeding, negative BE and flex sig. After all that, he's a tad flipped out about having his butt invaded once again, this time for a colonoscopy, so we're looking for alternative causes."

Lemon scanned the films for all of thirty seconds. "Meckels just above the ileocecal valve. Otherwise negative. Good study. Must have been done by Bart. Case closed." He handed the films back to Simmons. "Don't work too hard, David." As Simmons turned to go, he noticed a framed photo on the wall above Martin's desk, and stopped.

"What have we here?" Every member of Marty's wall of shame came with a good story.

Martin followed his gaze, laughed, and pulled the black-and-white off the wall. He read the brass plate at the bottom. "To Martin Lemon, M.D., Junior Gastroenterologist and a Tip-Top Ass Man." He handed the picture to Simmons.

"My wife found it in the attic this weekend."

There was a line of men in diapers, each one holding a letter-size white placard with a number on it. In the middle of the line, holding number 258, stood a portly gentleman. What distinguished him from the others was the turban, a good two feet tall and almost as wide. From the neck up, he could have passed for Mr. Softee's hirsute, unsmiling twin brother. Simmons examined the photo for a minute, then handed it back to Martin Lemon.

"That's how we lined 'em up for BE's. It was part of the Cleveland Institute's executive physical. Five thousand bucks for a week of testing. Some guys came back every year."

"Guys paid that kind of money for the privilege of wearing a diaper and getting their picture taken?"

"Oh yeah. Lots. I did that tour for three months. Every Tuesday morning, at least forty of them. From all over the world too. Needless to say, the photo was not part of the package."

"The guy with the turban, he's an Indians fan?" Lemon snorted. David thought, *Thank you for that.*

"That is the Sheik of Suloy, at the time the richest man in the world. Tiny island country ten feet deep in high-grade bat shit and sitting atop the world's largest platinum mine." He hung the picture back on the wall and looked at it for a bit. "That was a long time ago." Simmons patted his shoulder. Then Lemon turned and looked up at him with sad eyes, shaking his head. "Every year, as soon as he was done, he'd waddle as fast as he could to the bathroom. Never made it in time. Not once."

"A barium enema every year. Did you ever come up with an even remotely significant diagnosis?"

Marty grinned. "Absolutely! 'Very poor sphincter control.' The richest guy in the world, crapping in his diaper. In Cleveland."

73. DIFFERENT RULES

The old man stirred. He tried to sit up. A woman in scrubs gently restrained him until he stopped struggling. She leaned over him until her mouth was no more than two inches from his right ear.

"Relax, Senator. You're in recovery now. I'll page the Doctor. He wants to talk with you." He nodded, then opened and closed his mouth several times. The Nurse placed the end of a straw between his lips. He sucked on the ice water until she withdrew the cup and straw and placed them on the side table. He fell back to sleep.

"Senator?" The Doctor shook the old man gently. He snorted once, then licked his lips. The doctor thought, *You know, from this angle, he really does look like a duck. I never noticed it before. The cath lab ladies are right.* He shook him again. This time the old man turned over on his back and opened his eyes. The doctor held the Up button on the console until the head of the bed was upright at almost ninety degrees.

"Oh, hi, Bob." The Senator yawned, then smacked his lips together. He looked around. The Nurse appeared on his right, holding the cup of ice water. He smiled groggily, then opened his mouth. She put the tip of the straw to his lips and he sucked again. After a few seconds, the Nurse took the ice water away. The Senator gave her a glare, tried to say something, then closed his eyes again and started to snore. The Doctor pinched the old man's big toe as hard as he could. *Enough of this.* The old man's eyes fluttered open.

"Senator, I have to leave for an important appointment very soon, but I wanted to let you know how things are. If you'd like to go over our options, we can do that now or you can come in to the office tomorrow." The old man nodded. *Let's make this short and sweet. Maria will be waiting in the classroom, watching the clock while she plays with her little friends.*

"You've developed significant atherosclerotic narrowing in the coronary arteries of your transplanted heart." He stopped to let that sink in. The Senator blinked a few times, worked his lips together, and nodded again. The Doctor took that to mean he understood. He started to say something when the old man spoke up.

"Balloon or bypash?" He wrinkled his eyebrows, and made as if to sneeze, but nothing happened. Then he rubbed his nose. *That's the morphine,* the Doctor thought. It had taken twenty of MS plus ten of Versed to put him to sleep. The cath lab nurses gave the Doctor repeated looks when he'd told them to push more. The old man had a chronically high fidget factor and whined incessantly about pain during his procedures. After the last bump of Versed, he snored contentedly and his oxygen sats stayed up around 90%. Nonetheless, the charge nurse insisted on increasing the oxygen flow through his nasal prongs. *Whatever.*

"Well, Senator, the narrowing is almost perfectly concentric." Again he paused.

"Conshentric, like a shircle?" *Make that morphine and a set of dentures missing in action.*

"In a way. You have calcium deposits throughout your arteries. I suspect that, despite all the anti-rejection medications you've been given, you're experiencing some inflammation in your heart. That inflammation tends to attract calcium, resulting in very tiny arteries." He pinched his thumb and forefinger together to form a pin-sized opening. *Teensy-weensy. That young trophy wife of yours with the double-D's should know all about teensy-weensy.*

The Senator moved his lips around, trying to free them up. "Sho the balloon then."

"I'm afraid not. First of all, I could barely get a guide wire down into your coronary arteries. There's no way even our thinnest angioplasty catheters or stents would fit."

"Another bypash, then?"

"There again we have a problem. Dr. Hemlich just reviewed your films. He says there's no place where he can graft into your coronary arteries." The Doctor made an effort to push his right index finger between his pinched-together left thumb and index finger. "Too narrow."

"Jeshush Chrisht Almighty." He shook his head, then looked upward. "Shorry, Jeshush." He returned his sluggish stare to the Doctor.

"Senator, we tried both VEGF and FGF on you when you still had your native heart, to grow those collateral arteries. As you may remember, there was no response to either. Nor to the synthetic integrin injections. There's no reason to believe that any of those would work on your cadaver heart either."

The Senator was wide awake now, all business. He grabbed the turquoise cup off the bedside stand and inserted his dentures. "Well, Bob, what else have you got to offer then?"

The Doctor pulled a chair over and sat down. "While you were sleeping, I talked with the chairman of our Cardiology department. We considered all the options short of another transplant. Neither of us felt the odds of finding a perfect cadaver donor match were very high. Even if that were to happen, your chances of survival would be pretty slim."

"And?" He raised his right eyebrow and smiled with the left half of his mouth, his favorite look. It was the one he flashed while conjuring up one of his legendary deals across the aisle, the look the magazines usually featured when he landed on the cover.

"There are some promising trials ongoing in Canada and in Europe."

"Something experimental, eh? You like the idea of that, don't you, Bob, making me into a guinea pig." *More like a guinea duck.*

"Senator, from our perspective, it is the only option we believe has a reasonable chance of saving your heart and keeping you alive."

"Okay, shoot."

The Doctor took a deep breath. "Dedicated stem cells."

"Stem cells, eh? You mean I'd have to have a sample of my bone marrow taken? My brother-in-law Tommie Lawlor had one of those for his chronic leukemia. Said it felt like they were twisting a corkscrew into his back. He swore he'd never go for that again." He gave the Doctor the look again, as if daring him to suggest he do just that.

"Actually, Senator, after all the anti-rejection medications your bone marrow has been exposed to, I'm pretty certain your stem cells wouldn't work anyway. No, we'd need undifferentiated stem cells from a fresh source."

"Where are you going to get that?" Gone was the deal-maker face. The old man from the thirty-first parallel was genuinely curious. In the Senate, he usually knew well in advance what sort of offer would end up on the table. This was something else.

"Let me give you a little background, Senator. In conjunction with a couple of biotech firms out in California, the French have developed a way to direct undifferentiated stem cells straight to the coronary arteries. Once there, they cause new collateral arteries to grow and the existing ones to open up and allow more blood flow around blockages. In some cases, they've been able to increase blood flow by as much as forty-five percent. That should buy you a few years, at which point there will probably be newer, more effective technologies available."

"Sounds good. Let's get to it."

"Well, there is one major hurdle. We're a branch of the federal government, and, as such, we have to follow each and every federal law."

"Which law specifically are we talking about, Bob?"

"The law regarding the use of embryonic stem cells in federal facilities." *The one you campaigned for back in Bush 43's second term, saying that only God had the right to create life. The one that got you on all the Sunday morning news shows for six weeks running, quoting the Bible and frothing at the mouth.*

"Embryonic?" The old man scratched his ear and frowned slightly. Then his head shot up and he glared at the Doctor. "You mean those human embryos? You want me to take the stem cells stolen from unborn babies by some science fiction Satan? Mad scientist offspring? In my body? Are you out of your mind?"

"Senator, they've been shown to work exceptionally well in most cases. In addition, there's no chance of rejection or other inflammatory reaction. Preliminary results from the study in Canada are very encouraging." He spread his hands helplessly. "Perhaps you should think on it, talk with your wife and your minister. If you decide to go ahead, I'm sure our Director would be glad to call the White House..." He pictured Maria, smiling when she climbed into her seat in the minivan.

"The White House? What the hell have they got to do with this?" His face glowed, hot as the center of the earth. There was no apology to Jesus this time.

"Well, as I said, Senator, your law against the use of embryonic stem cells requires a specific bill or order for each exceptional case. President Price has expressed support for embryonic stem cell research. I'm sure he'd be glad to issue an Executive Order allowing you to receive..."

"Allow me? He's an ASSHOLE! Why does he get to decide whether I live or die?"

"It's either that or you can run a bill through both houses of Congress. That might take a bit longer." *The publicity would be interesting too.*

"Listen, there's time. Not much, but some. We can't get started today anyway. Your limo is waiting outside. Go home and think about it, let me know in a day or two. I have to go pick up my daughter at her school." The Doctor stood up to leave. He could already hear her singing the latest song she learned in pre-school, stumbling a little over the words but never slowing down, never stopping to correct herself.

"Oh, yeah, your daughter. Maria, isn't it?"

"Yes, Maria." He felt himself tighten up.

"How's she doing?"

"Still having lots of seizures. They got all of the tumor, thank God, but there's so much scar tissue left behind in her brain."

"Bob, you'd think all those overpaid research doctors and pharmaceutical companies hauling in all those obscene profits could get together to come up with a drug to control a little girl's seizures." He shook his head.

"Well, there's a lot of promise in purified marijuana preparations for children with seizures..."

"Hell, Bob, you don't want your little girl getting hooked on that stuff. Next thing you know, she'll be out on the streets turning tricks for heroin."

Did he just say that? The Doctor took a deep breath, then went on.

"...but Congress won't allow the pharmaceutical companies to research its benefits. There's also a couple of pediatric neurologists up in Toronto who are doing great things with stem cells. They've been able to regenerate healthy brain tissue that replaces the scar tissue. Anna Marie and I might take her up there this summer."

"Be careful, Bob. Those Canadians, they don't play by the same rules we do down here. They're a little out of control. If you want my opinion, they could do with a little reining in from Parliament. Well, you get along now. I'm thinking this stem cell thing might be just the ticket to keep me going. I'll call you tomorrow." The Nurse reappeared and began removing the EKG leads from the old man's body. A thought occurred to the Senator.

"Say, Bob, are they doing any of this stem cell research up at McGill?"

"Yes, Senator. I have a classmate from medical school up there who is involved in the study I mentioned. You might have to pay for it, since you aren't a Canadian citizen and therefore ineligible for free care. And usually American health insurance companies won't pay for experimental treatments, especially on foreign soil. Why do you ask?"

The Senator emitted that short chuckle of his, usually reserved for face-to-face interviews on television, the one that implied, *I've got something up my sleeve, little lady. Wouldn't you just love to know what it is?*

"Bob, Congress's insurance plan doesn't have any of those limitations. We make the rules, so our rules are different. I was just thinking. If I go up there and receive the injection, I won't have to deal with that fool at 1600. My Missy would dearly love Montreal in May." He gave the Doctor his deal-maker look once more. "Just something to think about, I guess. Well, good night, Bob."

"Good night, Senator." The Doctor turned to leave.

"Oh, Bob. One more thing."

"Yes?"

"Jesus loves you. You and your little girl." The Doctor turned and walked away.

74. GOOSE, HONEY, PASS ME SOME OF THAT SAUCE

"So you're wrapping things up here pretty soon?" Scott Echols arranged the crease on his pants, crossed his leg, shot his cuffs, and smoothed his hair, which was perfectly coiffed, never moved, and was never in need of smoothing. This was his sit-down-in-a-chair pattern. Now close to forty, his omnipresent smile consisted of perfect teeth and crinkles at the corners of his eyes.

"Sooner or later." David Simmons sipped his Coke and put the can down on a side table. The old scratched but incredibly comfortable leather chair beckoned to Simmons to yawn, lie back and close his eyes. To combat the urge he clasped his hands behind his head and twisted a couple times to the left and right. "This month here on Pulmonary, then a couple of months out in Portland and Seattle doing Dermatology and Cardiology, then San Diego for Rheumatology, then back here for Critical Care, Anesthesia and Cardiology, then graduation in May." Scott smiled and nodded.

This was Simmons' second rotation with Scott Echols. A year ago they had spent three weeks together on the same rotation, Scott the second-year resident leading the team and David doing his Internal Medicine clerkship as a third-year student. Scott started rounds every day with a new joke, a necessary skill he had honed to perfection in his previous life as a used-car salesman and a sales trainee with IBM before finding his way to medical school. David liked working with him; for Scott, there was no time for blame, but there was always time to work together to find a solution to the latest screw-up. His attitude wasn't shared by the other house staff, many of whom saw their residency training as nothing more than a three-year chance to suck up to the faculty in hopes of obtaining the golden ticket, a subspecialty fellowship. Neither friends nor lovers nor hapless medical students would stand in the way. Life was cheap in the pyramid system.

"I just got back from Salem, but rumor has it that your compadre on this rotation is doing time on a ventilator in the ICU?"

"Yeah. Josh Bartram. He caught Guillain-Barre from one of his Neurology patients. He's starting to turn the corner, but they're saying he probably won't be back to work before the first of the year, if then. He's supposed to start a surgery internship in July. If he graduates, that is. Already has a spot in the ENT program at Yale." Another nod and smile from Echols.

David continued, "The dean of students wanted one my classmates to bump up their Pulmonary rotation from the winter to this month, but Dr. Haskins said no."

"The chief always wants three students each month from October through March. Flu season. The consult load skyrockets." Scott uncrossed and re-crossed his legs, once again going through his routine. "So, Dave, it's just you and me."

"And the fellow, right? Dr. Scoma?"

Scott laughed. "This must be your first month on a subspecialty consult service."

"Well, I did Psych consults, but it was just five students and the shrink. No house staff or fellows."

Scott patted his hair. "You and I, David, we're the engine on this service. The fellow will be around to do some teaching when we, I mean you, present the cases to Dr. Babacan, the consult service attending this month. Mostly, though, Scoma's doing procedures during the day. The good news for us is that he has to handle any emergent consults that come in at night. So as far as our daily routine is concerned, Tony Scoma is there primarily to interpret for Dr. Babacan, who, despite an education at Hopkins and Columbia, is becoming less and less fluent in the English language. Another few years and I suspect he'll be back to speaking entirely in Turkish."

"Is he the one with the moustache and the white hair?"

"That's him. Must be close to seventy now, but he looks closer to ninety. He was the Pulmonary division chief for about ten years, but now all he wants to do is teach and do research on atypical pneumonias in his lab. His big thing now is TTA's for diagnosing pneumonia. One of his lab assistants told me he's working on a new kind of catheter.

"What's a TTA?" David had worked up his share of pneumonia cases last year during his Internal Medicine clerkship and had amassed a trunk full of abbreviations since day one of medical school. This one didn't sound familiar.

Now it was Echols's turn to clasp his hands behind his head. He stretched his legs out. "TTA. Trans-tracheal aspirate. You stick a catheter through the trachea," he raised his head further back for a second to show off his windpipe, "pull out the needle inside, and suck tracheal secretions through the catheter into a syringe." Simmons shivered.

"Wouldn't it be easier to just have the patient cough into a plastic cup?" That was the time-honored method for obtaining a sputum sample.

"Easier, of course. If you're lucky enough to get a pure sample of infected sputum from the lower respiratory tract, and if it isn't contaminated by mouth flora on the way out, no problem. If the sputum culture grows out a variety of bacteria, you don't know if they're all in there because you've got all sorts of bacteria in your lungs or because the sputum picked up saliva contaminants along the way, for example, in your mouth. These days, with all the drug resistance, bacteria like Acinetobacter and Serratia, things that you would normally ignore in a culture report, are dangerous pathogens that can kill you if you don't treat them with exactly the right antibiotic. So there's the medical reason for TTA's. And of course, there's the financial one."

"Financial?"

"You can bill for procedures like a TTA or a bronchoscopy. A researcher who comes up with just the right catheter for TTA's can make a ton of money, not to mention future research grants for his lab." Scott raised his eyebrows and smiled. David always found it odd when medical people mentioned money as a driving force. He expected that in business and law, especially when you considered the types that went into those professions, but not when it came to caring for the sick. He said as much to Echols.

Scott patted his hair. "Your naiveté is touching. Let's go."

They stood up and walked down the hall to the Pulmonary division office, where Scott introduced him to the secretary and showed him where to pick up the new consults. He took Simmons aside.

"Try to check in here at least twice in the morning and once after lunch. The secretary will page you if she gets a stat consult, but generally she's too busy to page you for the routine ones. Let me know if you get overloaded and I'll go see a couple, just to get them started. I'll make some preliminary recommendations, but you still have to do a formal consult on each one and see each one in follow-up before we round every day, okay?"

"Sure. I'm here to work and learn." David turned to go. "I'll get started on these two and page you when I'm done."

"One last thing, Dave. This month you are a consultant. You don't have any direct responsibility for any of these patients. We make recommendations, and the medical or surgical team decides what they want to do. Despite the workload, it's supposed to be a fun month." He smiled, shook Simmons' hand, and went to answer a page. David walked out of the office.

****

It took a day for David Simmons to get the hang of the consult service. On the one hand, the workups were incredibly detailed, especially regarding Pulmonary history, and took him much longer than he'd expected. On the other, once he'd presented the patient to Drs. Echols, Scoma and Babacan, and they'd discussed the case and made their recommendations, his job was incredibly simple, just like Scott had said.

After David saw the day's consults, he'd run them by Scott, who usually went with him to the patient's bedside to point out pertinent historical and physical findings. He was such a laid back guy, especially on this consult service, it was easy to forget how sharp he was. Thanks to Scott's insights, by the time they met with Drs. Scoma and Babacan, Simmons' presentations were much more informative, flowing, and, most importantly, concise. That left more time for the fellow and attending to add their knowledge to the case. Scoma turned out to be an excellent teacher, especially when the case involved TB or fungal lung infections. He had just finished up a three-month stint out at the sanatorium. Babacan was a little difficult to understand, but it was not as much of an issue as David had been led to believe.

Although the workload was much heavier than he'd initially expected, Simmons felt he was having by far his best experience on a medical rotation. As the only student on the service, he got all their attention. While he preferred to have another student or two on a rotation with him, the four of them were cruising along so well that he didn't miss Josh's company at all. Since they had consults to follow on every service in the hospital, he was also able to get to know the nurses on a number of the wards he'd never visited. As a consultant, he'd review charts and examine the patient. Because there wasn't any order-writing involved, he was considered much less of a pain in the ass for the nurses to deal with. Whenever a third-year student, chart in hand, approached the ward desk, a collective groan would circulate among the nurses. They knew from experience that the medical team had found something new and useless for them to do. Simmons thought, *When I grow up, I'm going to be a consultant.*

The other nice benefit to being on a consult service was that Liver Rounds were held every Friday afternoon, rather than only on the Fridays when the team was not on call. On their first Friday, Scoma regaled them with the latest stories from out at the sanatorium. The hospital had recently picked up a federal contract to detain and treat noncompliant TB patients from all over the East Coast. So Blue Sky, once the hospital devoted solely to Central Virginia consumptives, now housed on the locked wards, as Scoma put it, "the worst of the worst, the hardest, bloodiest coughers, the skinniest federal inmates in the U.S.." Babacan's English improved dramatically over beers, especially when he poured forth on the final model of his TTA catheter. Just before the end of their session at the Rattrap, he announced that five hundred of them would be arriving the following Monday. This particular catheter's special feature was a ninety-degree angle on the flexible catheter about halfway down its length.

"Normally, you insert the catheter and needle into the trachea at a right angle--here he demonstrated with a pen against their table--then angle both downward at forty-five degrees, then withdraw the needle to aspirate secretions. With the Babacath, you still insert at a right angle, but, instead of angling the needle and catheter downward, risking a tear in the trachea, you merely remove the needle and the soft, flexible catheter flips downward on its own. You get a guaranteed optimal positioning every time, and virtually no risk of a tracheal tear." He looked around proudly at the other three and hoisted his mason jar.

"To the Babacath."

****

Monday arrived. Simmons had three new consults to present that afternoon, and he noticed a change in the attending's demeanor. Suddenly Babacan was proposing a TTA for every consult involving a pulmonary infection. It didn't matter how straightforward the case, how obvious the diagnosis and treatment should have been, Simmons found himself writing, "Strongly suggest TTA to be performed by Pulmonary consult team."

On one particularly simple case of pneumonia, when Simmons questioned the need for a TTA, Babacan was ready for him.

"According to a study published in 1967 in the New England Journal, transtracheal aspiration is a safe procedure." *Safe for the guy doing it*, thought Simmons, *maybe not so safe for the guy in the bed.*

On another occasion, when Scoma argued that a bronchoscopy would be more effective than a TTA, Babacan cut him off with, "A study of TTAs reported in the Archives in 1974 demonstrated correct diagnosis of the pathogen in ninety percent of cases of pneumonia."

This caused Scoma, who wanted to do as many procedures as possible, to advocate for a bronchoscopy on just about every patient. By Wednesday, the air of collegiality that had wafted through the first two weeks was replaced by a toxic cloud of heated disagreement. When Simmons mentioned to his resident the sharp uptick in recommendations for invasive procedures, Echols told him not to get involved.

"Like I said the first day, just present the case and listen and learn. Let them duke it out. In this fight, you want to be a spectator with a front row seat, not the referee. You get into the ring, and you'll get sucker punched from both sides."

By the end of the week, Babacan had clearly won the battle. Five of their consults had received TTA's, with the Babacath of course, and only one underwent bronchoscopy. Scott Echols kept a tally of all invasive procedures. On Friday morning he showed the results to David.

After Simmons looked over the figures, Scott smiled and said, "I think I'm pretty impartial. From my perspective, the bronch was indicated and only one of the TTA's was justified. Since Tony's doing all the TTA's, he's probably okay with the volume."

"You really think he's okay with this?"

"Unlike academia, in private practice you try to get the most bang for your buck. Time is more critical for a busy solo practitioner who doesn't have a ton of house staff to coordinate the workup. So some of the extensive, step-by-step workups we do here would never be done in a private hospital. That's especially true for a consultant. When a generalist consults you, you'd better come up with a quick route to the answer. Otherwise, he won't consult you anymore and you are out of business. Tony gets to practice a procedure he'll probably employ on a regular basis when he is out in the cold cruel world."

The atmosphere was a little lighter the following week, but Simmons could still feel a subtle animosity between Scoma and Babacan. Again, Scoma advocated for only one bronchoscopy during the week, while Babacan urged the medical teams to let him perform ten TTAs. Around mid-morning on Friday, Scoma started in with a laughably bogus cough. By noon, claiming illness, he had gone home for the weekend. When Babacan cancelled Liver Rounds for that afternoon, David was thrilled. A couple days away from the feuding would make his remaining time on the service much more tolerable. He and Scott walked out of the hospital together at 5 P.M.

"Dave, I'm sorry it's so tense on the service. Normally the whole month goes pretty much like your first week. The important thing is, you're getting to see a lot of pathology. Don't even think about this situation this weekend. Sooner or later, it'll resolve itself. Things always work out in the end."

After a perfect September weekend, Monday afternoon was busy, with David presenting four new consults. Everyone seemed resigned to getting through the last week, and the tone was subdued. Babacan, who looked like he'd lost five pounds since Friday, spent most of rounds trying to clear his throat and hardly spoke. Scoma did all the teaching. Shockingly, neither the attending nor his fellow recommended an invasive procedure on any of the four. In his little black book, Scott was also keeping track of how many Babacaths were used. After two weeks, of the original five hundred, four hundred eighty-seven remained.

Tuesday morning, Scott paged Simmons at 7 A.M. "Dr. Babacan was admitted by the chief of Pulmonary last night. Fever, shaking rigors, and an infiltrate on his chest x-ray. I'm here in x-ray with Tony. Come on down and we'll take a look at his films from last night and this morning." David hurried down to the main inpatient x-ray reading room. The Welshman, Evans, was reading this morning. He threw two sets of chest films up on his board and picked up his dictation microphone.

"The next patient is Babacan, first name Alper." He turned to Scoma with a questioning look.

"Yes, he came in last night. Fever, chills, hypoxic, abnormal film." Evans turned back and recited Babacan's patient ID number into the mike. Simmons was surprised that the number was a new one. He hadn't thought about it previously, but he'd expected that an attending in his seventies would have been admitted to the hospital a time or two over the previous thirty-five years, and thus would own an old patient ID number. Evans swiveled in his chair to look at David.

"How'd he look yesterday?" David was in awe of the guy's accent, and this was one of those rare radiologists with any interest in disease processes, rather than just their appearance on an x-ray. Simmons the purist found this reassuring.

"He looked like he'd lost five pounds or more over the weekend. He wasn't coughing, just trying to clear his throat." Evans looked at him for a few seconds, then swiveled back to the films.

"On his admission film from twenty-two hundred hours last night there is a tiny right middle lobe interstitial infiltrate partially obscuring the right heart border. His images from 6 A.M. this morning show a diffuse interstitial pattern in both the right middle lobe and the lingula. Given his symptoms, I interpret this as an atypical pneumonia. You all know the differential, but, given the rapidity of onset of his symptoms, tuberculosis and viral etiologies are less likely. More likely to be a bacterial pathogen. If he was having trouble with secretions but couldn't cough, either he has some form of upper airway obstruction or he's too weak to cough."

As the three left the reading room, Scoma turned and said, "What are the odds?"

After stopping off at Babacan's office, they walked together to the telemetry ward. David asked, "How come he's up here?"

Scott said, "Two reasons. First, an old guy with a pneumonia almost always has PVC's, and it's not unusual for an elderly person with pneumonia to develop atrial fibrillation. Second, and probably more important, this ward has one of the four VIP suites in the hospital." He turned to look at Scoma. "Are you really going to use that?"

Scoma looked down at the box in his hand. It was white cardboard, with the word "Babacath" printed in bold blue letters on the face. Then he looked at Echols and Simmons.

"A patient who is constantly exposed to resistant bacteria but can't produce sputum? It would be hard to come up with a more suitable patient. I really don't have a choice. I have to do it." He smiled. "Unless one of you wants to." As if on cue, the other two stepped back. David had seen a half-dozen TTA's and, about a week prior, had performed one. His patient had looked terrified as he injected a little lidocaine under the skin. Simmons wondered why he had volunteered to perform the procedure, then remembered that he didn't volunteer, Babacan told him to do it. Other than the poor guy's bulging eyes, the procedure had gone far more smoothly than he'd expected. The patient coughed weakly as the catheter went in and coughed again as he withdrew the needle and the catheter presumably snapped downward. Simmons aspirated thin hazy secretions into the syringe.

As he was withdrawing the catheter, the patient finally coughed forcefully. A gelatinous dollop of brown sputum the size of a quarter flew out of the patient's mouth and stuck to Simmons' forehead. He was about to wipe it away, when Babacan produced a sterile culture swab and a glass microscope slide and rubbed each over the snotball. Then he handed David a Kleenex and told him it was okay to wipe it off. A couple days later, the TTA report came back as "Mixed Flora", meaning it was worthless, but the forehead sample grew 4+ Strep pneumoniae.

They entered Babacan's room as a team. Standard hospital bed with a fancy wooden headboard, lots of chairs, a nice view of the East Range across the street, no visitors yet. The place smelled like old sweat and Pine-Sol. Covered by a thin sheet and a light blue hospital gown, Babacan had shrunk to the size of a table-top Halloween scarecrow. His thick white hair stuck out in all directions. Beneath the oxygen mask, the black moustache framed parched lips. He gurgled slightly with each breath. When he saw the team enter, he smiled weakly.

Scott bent over the old man and pulled the oxygen mask down below his chin. From the breast pocket of his white coat he produced a couple of lemon swabs and ran them around the inside of Babacan's mouth, then held a cup of water with a straw in it so he could sip. Babacan nodded and closed his eyes. Echols replaced the mask over his mouth and nose. In the meantime, Scoma had set up the TTA kit and began donning a pair of sterile gloves. He spoke softly.

"Dr. Babacan." There was no response, no indication he's been heard. In a louder voice, he said, "Dr. Babacan." This time the old man's eyes opened. He looked up at Scoma on his left side. David had positioned himself on the other side of the bed. "Dr. Babacan, the respiratory therapists haven't been able to obtain a sputum sample from you. Given your exposure to resistant bacteria here in the medical center, I think this would be an appropriate time for a transtracheal aspiration to obtain an uncontaminated sample." David wondered if Scoma was getting in a dig for all the inappropriate procedures Babacan had recommended, but one look at the fellow's eyes told him he was trying to be as respectful as possible. *Good for you,* he thought. In Scoma's place, David wasn't sure he could have exhibited that much restraint.

For the first time, Babacan moved his right arm. He pulled his oxygen mask down and rasped, "Get the hell out of here with that thing." He stared at Scoma as he replaced the mask.

Scoma said, "Sir, you have an atypical-appearing hospital-acquired pneumonia." Babacan shook his head and closed his eyes. Now Scoma was pissed. "But what about the Babacath?"

Without opening his eyes, Babacan pulled the mask to the side and wheezed, "No more TTA's. Throw them all away."

As the three walked out of the VIP suite, David asked, "Is he serious? Throw away his invention?"

Scoma said, "You heard him. All five hundred."

Scott looked down at his little black book, thumbed through the pages and smiled. As he smoothed his hair, he said, "Four eighty-six."

75. RESEARCH

If the odds of your contracting a disease or experiencing a side effect from a treatment are one in a million but you're the unlucky one, the odds really don't matter to you. That is, unless you like the idea of wandering about with a sign around your neck that says, "Look at me, I'm one in a million!"

Modern medical research is often directed toward answering the question, "Is the treatment in question more likely to lead to a certain desired result than pure chance, other existing treatments, or placebo?" If the answer is "yes", then that treatment will most likely become widespread in use and extremely profitable. If the answer is, "No, you twit", the treatment will most likely be thrown on the scrap heap of discarded research. Or, better yet, shelved for a few decades, then trotted out as a cure for something else. When taken by pregnant women to prevent morning sickness, thalidomide, the scourge of the '60s, caused flipper limbs in newborns. Over the past few decades it has enjoyed a resurgence in popularity as a possible treatment for various inflammatory diseases such as rheumatoid arthritis and Crohn's disease. It may turn out to be a valuable tool in the treatment of cancer as well. If you look long enough, sooner or later you can find a niche for just about any drug.

In the early chapters of the story of American medicine, research was often performed almost as a hobby, squeezed in after office hours in tiny labs and garages. Outside of a few major research centers, funding was scarce or nonexistent. Now it pays the bills, with funding coming from deep pockets like pharmaceutical companies, medical foundations, the federal government and venture capitalists. Modern medical schools couldn't run without research money. You can be the worst teacher in the world, but if you have a knack for obtaining large chunks of cash for research, medical schools will line up to offer you lab space, cushy clinical hours and a fast track to tenure. It's not uncommon for medical schools to be included in patents for medications or devices invented in their facilities.

When people hear the word "research", one of two things often comes to mind. For the financially-oriented, it means "money", as in lucrative patents, startup companies, and hospital expansion. Total nominal spending on pharmaceuticals in the U.S. was about $375 billion in 2014.

To the pet lovers of the world, research means toxic chemicals injected into the conjunctiva of monkeys and dogs for the purpose of discovering a new anti-aging formula or a better wrinkle cream or longer lasting mascara and lipstick. Animal rights organizations are proud of their impact on animal research in the industrialized nations, particularly the U.S. However, given the financial incentives, you can bet that the guy who doesn't blink an eye at killing an elephant for its ivory would jump at the chance to run a profitable research lab in some third world country far from the inquiring eyes of investigators.

Pharmaceutical companies probably prefer that scenario anyway. Less attention from the world media and far easier deniability.

At the basis of all research is a problem that requires a solution. A researcher encounters a common problem and asks himself, "How can I fix this more quickly, more easily, less expensively?"

Some questions are answered by a simple clinical trial, pitting two treatment options against one another. Often one of the options is a placebo. Surprisingly, some of the best studies of a treatment option, whether it be a medication or a procedure, come years or decades after the initial discovery of said treatment. In this scenario, cost, hospital length of stay, or complications spur the later research study. It is always a good idea to review "time-honored" treatments on a regular basis. The biggest risk to the patient is the placebo arm of the trial, where the patient volunteers to possibly forego the standard of care.

Particularly when the search is on for a new medication, some questions require significant time in the lab, mixing chemicals to find just the right compound for a common condition. For someone to spend most of their time in a lab rather than seeing patients, you have to have deep pockets available. That's why so many drugs are discovered by pharmaceutical companies--full-time lab guys. Once they discover the drug, then it's on to the medical schools and major medical centers for drug trials involving animals and eventually humans.

Research studies, surgical and non-surgical alike, often require animal testing first. The use of living animals for research goes back as far as Aristotle in the fourth century B.C. The Moors in twelfth century Spain tested surgical procedures on animals before applying them to human patients. In the 1880s Louis Pasteur proved the germ theory of infection by giving anthrax to sheep. A decade later Ivan Pavlov used dogs to demonstrate conditioning. The history of modern medicine is rife with examples of how animal studies have benefitted mankind. Even now, it is virtually impossible to introduce a new medication or procedure without a round of animal studies to demonstrate effectiveness, safety and superiority over other treatment options.

Man's relationship to animals seems to become stranger and more schizophrenic with each passing generation. Now more than ever we dote on our pets. As Seinfeld put it, people walk around cleaning up dog poop; a visitor from another planet would rightly assume that the dogs are in charge. We dress dogs and cats in silly costumes and put them on YouTube., where millions will watch in fascination. In a life-threatening situation, you wouldn't want a dog owner to decide who lives, you or his pet. We allow dogs to breed, even pay high prices for specially bred dogs, yet we euthanize more than a million dogs every year. The same holds true for cats. We jack off bulls and racehorses for their sperm, then sell it for millions of dollars, while slaughtering upwards of forty million cows for food every year. It is estimated that tens of thousands of racehorses are shipped off each year to slaughterhouses in Canada and Mexico. Millions of us gleefully chow down on veal saltimbocca yet decry the conditions under which calves are reared. Chickens can be raised in tiny chicken jails or allowed to run freely across the range, but they're all going to have their heads chopped off. Backed by strong research from prominent veterinary schools, the vegetarian movement swears that methane from livestock is a major contributor to U.S. greenhouse gas emissions. Yet, if you hang around the frozen food section of a vegetarian market, you will find vegans, the purest of the pure, buying frozen soy shaped to look like chicken legs.

You would assume that surgeons who practice surgical procedures on dogs are not big dog lovers. You would be wrong. There are countless general and vascular surgeons who say they love the family dog but have no problem using canines to improve their surgical technique or to develop a new procedure. As with any new technique, there will be casualties. Some certifying courses like ATLS offer an optional dog lab. While the thought of experimenting on and possibly killing a living animal makes me sick to my stomach, I've participated and it made me a better physician when it comes to resuscitating dying humans. Many surgical programs require a resident to spend an entire year in the lab. Is it ethical to practice on a "stray" animal in order to save countless human lives? Modern medicine has answered that one with a resounding "Yes".

Luckily for us, so far, nobody has reported back that God is a dog.

Besides answering a question, there are plenty of incentives for pursuing research. It pays the bills while paving the way to a tenured position at a medical school or research foundation. You may end up the beneficiary of a lucrative patent. No matter how many times you've been through it, it is still a kick to see your name in print, especially if you are the lead author on a lead article in a prestigious peer-reviewed journal like the New England Journal of Medicine. Everyone is different, and so are their motivations.

Whatever reason a medical researcher has for venturing into research, somewhere deep down, in the farthest corner of even the blackest heart, there is the desire to save....

76. LIVES

The alarm went off at 6:00, still dark. He'd been sleeping on his right side, and when he turned to hold Sally for a moment, cupping her breast in his hand, she stretched and wiggled back into him with her butt. David smiled, then realized he was heading for a tardy slip if he allowed this nonsense to progress one wiggle further. He passed on a smooch to her neck that would have sent them both to Wackyland and rolled over and up to the sound of the old bed creaking.

A groan from down below Sally's feet reassured him that Bertha was sleeping up top, not underneath the bed. The mutt had made the move up onto the bed a couple weeks ago, presaging yet another bed collapse; the slats would slip from their precarious perch on the bowed frame sides, and the box spring, mattress and occupants would crash to the floor, creating a thunderous boom that would rattle windows throughout the old house. The dog had used up more than her share of lives and was finally learning to stay away from potentially lethal situations.

"Where are you going, Simmmmonnns?" From the change in her voice, he could tell she'd turned toward him. Dave the Doppler Effect Expert.

"You know where." The ancient pine floor, stripped for decades of any sheen or splinters, offered all the warmth of an ice rink. He sat down on the side of the bed and reached over to the chair for a fresh pair of socks.

"Come back to bed. It's too dark and cold to go anywhere." *Correct.*

"I gotta go. I have to pick up Kenny by 6:30."

"Kenny." She paused, the actress timing always perfect. "Right. Come back to bed. I want you to shove my face down in the pillows and fuck me like an animal. Then you can go pick up Kenny."

That seemed sensible. He thought about Kenny standing on Allen St., waiting. Kenny had found them this weekend job. Four hours Friday afternoon, eight hours each on Saturday and Sunday. Easy farm work, no nights, no hassling with the public or a boss.

"We have to be out there by 7. Busy day."

"Busy day caring for lab dogs." Simmons winced. He thought of them as dogs, not lab animals.

"I thought about Mia and her pups all night."

"Not all night, Buddy Boy." She giggled. Around midnight there had been a prolonged session involving a glass of godawful homemade wine, a bong hit and Sally's soft palate. Like a spoonful of sugar, the other two had helped the wine go down.

"I'll be home by four. If the offer still stands, I can come by and mess up your bed."

"Sofa. In the front window." A pause. "With the curtains open." She was conceding, but then again, for her it was always about winning the war, opening skirmishes be damned. Future JD/MBA dealmaker. Or was it just some homework for a human chess game assignment from her Transactional Analysis class? Either way, playing the pawn suited Simmons perfectly.

"Then you can take me out to the Barn for a steak. My sister sent me a new outfit from New York and it is sexxxxyyyyy. It's date night."

"OK, Baby." After he got his jeans and work boots on, he stood up and grabbed his sweatshirt and jacket.

"You know, they're going to die."

"Who's going to die?"

"The dogs. All of them."

"Maybe not." He felt a little chill. Leave it to Sally to mess with his illusions.

"David, you're working at an experimental animal farm! Sooner or later, you know one of those surgeons will fuck up and each and every dog and cat out there will bleed to death or die some other horrible death." From the index card over the entrance to each doghouse and the plethora of scars, he could tell that a few of the dogs had been out there for years, surviving countless surgical procedures. It grabbed at his chest, the way it always did when he thought about it. Were they luckier or unluckier than the ones who died? He cheered up a little when he remembered Mia licking her newborns yesterday afternoon.

"I like being out there. Everything but the eventual outcome. What's wrong with being nice to them? What did they do? They're entitled to have some fun while they can." *Christ, I sound like a Little Golden Book for three year-olds. David and the Experimental Puppies.*

"You are doing something good. I just hate to see you putting your heart and soul into such a tragic job. Why don't you and Kenny do something truly kind and set them all free?"

"Not part of the deal, Sal." David was making steak money out there, and he had already violated the terms by telling her about the job. Top secret facility, like a Nike missile base. "They probably wouldn't even leave, and anyway, if they did, one of those hillbilly dogcatcher shitheads would just round them up, kick'em a few times and bring them back. They'd get paid again, we'd lose our jobs, and whoever replaced me would probably treat them way worse." Every Friday, Kenny bought a box of dog biscuits.

"Only following orders, eh, Herr Leutnant? Suit yourself." She rolled over in bed and pulled the covers over her head. Bertha gave him the stinkeye, then put her head back down with a don't-bother-me groan. He walked out.

He got to the corner of Harding and Allen right at 6:30. By the time Kenny got settled in with his lunch and the box of biscuits, the heater was blowing reasonably warm air and most of the frost was sliding down the windshield the windows. Kenny looked over at David, David waited, then Kenny sighed and reached for his seat belt. In another minute they were on their way through town.

Eventually Kenny asked, "Anything new?" Simmons went out on Friday afternoons to service the tractor, store the sacks of Chow, and get the report from the full-time staff. After Lukas and Buford headed home for the weekend, he drove the tractor around the rows of doghouses to say "Hi" and see the new dogs.

"Mia had four pups yesterday morning. Looks like each one was from a different dad."

"Mia? Who's Mia?"

"Mia Farrow. You know, Frank Sinatra, *Rosemary's Baby?*"

"Dave, come on. No fraternizing with the inmates."

"Sure thing, Doggy Cookie Man." Before they closed up shop on Saturday and Sunday afternoons, David would drive the tractor up and down the rows. Kenny stood on the back and tossed each dog a biscuit, all the while crooning a medley of Broadway show tunes from his childhood.

"It's not the same. You've got a name for every one of them. I bet you named the puppies already." He looked over at Simmons, who stared straight ahead at Brown's Mountain in the distance. *Willie Boy, Stinger, Betsy Ross and Martha Jefferson.* "Why do you have to personalize everything? Please keep it simple. If Lukas finds out, he'll kick our asses out of there. I need this job to pay my bills." On one occasion, Simmons slipped up and called a dog by name. Lukas had given him the eye but said nothing.

Simmons thought for a moment, then said, "How about we bring them home with us in a few weeks? Lukas said they can't hang on to pups to wait for them to grow." It dawned on him for the first time that if they couldn't keep them there, something must happen to them.

"Jesus, David, you're crazy. If you get me fired, I swear I'll kill you." Simmons smiled. "And that'll mean no more weed, either." Caught off guard by this last threat, David took a curve on 20 South too fast and they skidded across the road on a patch of ice before he regained control. Sally loved her weekend weed.

David drove in silence until they turned off the highway. Kenny got out, unlocked the gate, and waited for the big Lincoln to slide through on the mud and ice, then closed the gate and fastened the padlock. After Kenny got back in, Simmons came to a decision.

"Fuck it, I'm taking them home tonight. Marybeth Patterson raised dogs when she was a kid. She'll know how to handle them. If we leave them here, they'll die or get killed. Lukas won't care. Buford said he's been out of town for the past three days. He doesn't even know they're alive." Kenny looked up at the ceiling and said nothing.

Up at the main building, Kenny took their lunches inside while David fired up the tractor. He offered to let him drive, but to no avail. Kenny was afraid of the tractor but had no trouble hauling ass on that big Norton with his frat brothers. Simmons, on the other hand, had a dread of motorcycles occasioned by a laydown and acres of road rash from an ill-timed encounter with a Suzuki crotch rocket at the age of fifteen. Tractors were slow, possessed of four fat wheels and seldom turned over.

From his seat up on the tractor, he could see into the burn barrel. Three leather collars sat on top of cut-up cardboard boxes. The tags had been snipped off, probably were sitting in the trashcan at Buford's house. The deal was that the farm accepted only animals from other counties, never from Albemarle. In theory, they were all strays.

Kenny was dicking around inside the building, probably taking a crap or playing charades with the monkeys. David left the tractor idling, got down and started jogging in a steam cloud down row 4. *Willie Boy, Stinger, Betsy Ross, Martha Jefferson.* Two boys, two girls. In his head he rolled through a list of friends, placing each one of the pups in a loving home full of students. *So this is what it feels like to be a social worker.* Midway down the row he bent over and gave Sam Snead, one of the old-timers, a running pat on the head. At the last house on the left David Simmons stopped and looked down.

Mia was outside, shivering, wet and whimpering. Her chain was wound up around the stake and the doghouse. She was unable to move, just lay on the ground staring up at David with the most pathetic look he would ever see. Helplessness. Humiliation. Failure. Just out of reach, frozen in a puddle of ice, mud and water, lay the four puppies. Willie Boy, Stinger, Betsy Ross and Martha Jefferson, curled up together for warmth that could not be had.

Numb and automatic, he knelt down next to Mia, thinking that another two feet of chain and those puppies would be alive and sucking on her teats inside the doghouse. Drained of energy, Simmons stood up, holding Mia, and walked around the house until the chain was unraveled. He let her down gently in the doorway and gathered up the dead little dogs. As he put them in the pockets of his jacket, he could feel their wetness soak through his sweatshirt. Mia slunk into the house and curled up on the floor, her back to him, shivering. Simmons walked back toward the shed that held the pickaxe and shovels.

77. CARDIAC CATHETERIZATION

Cardiology Joke:

Q: What are the indications (reasons) for a 7 A.M. cardiac cath?
A: An insurance card, a femoral pulse, and an 8 A.M. tee time.

The term "catheterization" means sticking a synthetic tube into one of your tubes. It can refer to placing a Foley catheter into your urethra and thence into your bladder. It could refer to the insertion of a plastic tube through your mouth or nose into your esophagus and then into your stomach. Technically speaking, anytime you have an IV catheter inserted into a vein, you are undergoing a form of vascular catheterization. In this chapter, "catheterization", also known as a coronary arteriogram or angiogram, and commonly referred to in the business as a "cath", means the placement of a catheter into one of your peripheral arteries and advanced through your aorta for the purpose of squirting dye into your coronary arteries and heart chambers.

While the treadmill test and all its variations are designed to demonstrate your heart's functional status and exercise tolerance, the primary purpose of the cardiac cath is to provide a map of your coronary arterial system, with special attention to areas of narrowing or blockage. It delineates both the function and the anatomy of your heart. It is the final necessary step before undergoing a CABG, because no reputable cardiac surgeon will operate on your coronary arteries unless he knows which ones need to be bypassed. In the future, CT scans or MRI's may suffice to locate your coronary lesions, but for now, the cath is the gold standard.

Cardiac caths in search of coronary disease are usually performed for one of the following reasons:

1) You have a positive stress test;
2) You have a normal stress test, but, based on your history of symptoms or some other finding, your cardiologist strongly suspects you have coronary disease;
3) Your stress test is indeterminate, meaning that you are unable to reach your predicted maximum heart rate;
4) You present with unstable angina or an MI. Although there are still some hard-headed old-school cardiologists out there, it is generally considered bad form to stress a patient who very well might drop dead on the treadmill.

A cardiac cath is designed to demonstrate the location and severity of your coronary narrowings or blockages. Armed with this anatomic information, your cardiologist can decide what form of treatment is most suitable for your lesions. Options include medications, PCI or bypass surgery. In other words, not everybody who undergoes a cath, even if he has coronary disease, will end up on the operating table.

Many of the greatest discoveries in medicine were complete accidents. While not exactly accidental, the history of the cardiac catheterization had a particularly juicy start. In 1929, a German physician named Werner Forssmann decided that it would be possible to thread a catheter from a peripheral vein in his antecubital fossa (crook of his elbow) into his heart. He enlisted the help of an operating room nurse who had charge of the necessary sterile supplies. She agreed to help, but insisted he perform the procedure on her, rather than on himself. The wily Forssmann agreed. First, he restrained her on the O.R. table. The conversation probably went nothing like this:

"Oooh, Dr. Forssmann, what are you doing?"

"Relax, mein Fraulein. This is just to remind you not to move while I am inserting. Do not worry."

"Worry, Herr Doktor? I am not worried. Ich liebe die Kinky!"

Then, while pretending to operate on her, he anesthetized his forearm, cut into his own antecubital vein and inserted the catheter. He then untied his assistant, who by this time was putty in his hands.

"So brave, Dr. Forssmann! So brave and so masterful. Ich bin putty in your hands."

Together they walked to the radiology department, where, under fluoroscopic x-ray, he guided the catheter into his right ventricle. An x-ray was then taken with the tip of the catheter in his right atrium. Over the next twenty years, Dr. Forssmann allegedly worked as a cardiologist, a urologist, a Nazi, a prisoner of war, a lumberjack, and a little country doctor. Apparently he had a hard time holding down a job.

Dickinson Richards, an American, and Andre Cournand, a Frenchman who became an American citizen, worked together in New York. They recognized the importance of Forssmann's discovery; in the early 1940's, they were the first to use cardiac catheterization as a diagnostic tool. They studied the effects of trauma on the heart, the changes associated with congestive heart failure, and the effects of various drugs on the function of the heart. Their work was particularly important in developing techniques for diagnosing congenital heart disease in children. They shared the 1956 Nobel Prize in Physiology or Medicine with Werner Forssmann. Wouldn't that have been an embarrassing Oslo moment, Wernie showing up in his Third Reich uni, my nocturnal door-knocking amigo Narvid all red-faced and tongue-tied?

The insertion of a catheter into a peripheral artery for the purpose of diagnosing diseases of the aorta, an aortogram, was developed by a physician named Egas Moniz in Lisbon, Portugal in the late 1920's. He is credited with the discovery of radioarteriography, for which he was thrice nominated for the Nobel Prize. Always a bridesmaid, he never won. Don't feel sorry for him, however. He did win for the discovery of leucotomy, a brain procedure used to treat several forms of severe mental disease. He is thus also known as the father of the lobotomy.

By the early 1950s, the introduction of the Seldinger catheter technique made the procedure much safer and almost routine. In 1958, Frank Mason Sones, a pediatric cardiologist at the Cleveland Clinic, was performing an aortogram on a young man with rheumatic heart disease. As the catheter was advanced up toward the root of the aorta, the tip accidentally flipped into the opening of the patient's right coronary artery. Before the tip could be withdrawn back into the aorta, a large dose of dye was injected. The patient's heart immediately stopped. Dr. Sones yelled at the man to cough. He did, and his heart restarted immediately. This was the first documented selective coronary arteriogram. After this, Dr. Sones figured out that a smaller dose of dye could be safely injected into a coronary artery.

Because of this discovery, again a complete and almost fatal accident, the world's first CABG was performed nine years later at the Cleveland Clinic by Dr. Rene Favaloro. By the way, it is standard operating procedure to have you cough if your heart stops and the monitor shows asystole or ventricular tachycardia. So, if your heart makes a bad rhythmic choice and your cardiologist tells you to cough, you'd better do it. It could save your life. If you don't, at the very least you'll get punched in the chest or zapped with the defibrillator. Keep It Simple.

In contrast, almost fifty years later, there should not be anything accidental about your coronary cath. Your day will start with a ride to the hospital. You can drive your own vehicle to the cath, but you won't be allowed to drive it home. Nor are you allowed to go home in a bus, a train, a taxi, or an Uber without a responsible party along for the ride. While a limousine is a possibility, the celebratory sunroof and a bottle of Dom will be appropriate only if your cath is completely normal. Barring that, get a friend or loved one to drive you there and wait for you. Start to finish, the whole thing should be done in five hours max. You always want to be first on the schedule so that lunch at home is a distinct possibility.

Your cath adventure in the hospital will most likely begin with a wallet biopsy in the finance department. Bring along your driver's license or similar form of photo I.D., a credit card (not a debit card, unless you want your bank account emptied), and your health insurance card. The clerk will run down all the pertinent info regarding your upcoming bill. Given your situation, about to undergo a potentially life-threatening procedure, none of this will sink in or make any sense to you, but they have to cover their asses.

Unless you had blood tests performed the previous day, you'll go to the pre-op lab to have some blood withdrawn from a vein. The usual labs include a CBC, to make sure you have enough red blood cells and platelets. They will perform what is called a "type and screen" or a "type and hold". This will be important only if you bleed excessively and require a blood transfusion. Some coagulation studies will be done to make sure you don't have a congenital bleeding disorder. You might say, "Well, I've never had any bleeding problems." That's what all the bleeders say right before they exsanguinate (bleed to death) during a procedure. In terms of blood chemistries, they will check your potassium level. If it is too high or too low, your heart will have a much greater chance of developing an abnormal rhythm during your cath. They will also check your BUN (blood urea nitrogen) and creatinine levels, both of which are indicators of your kidney function. If these are elevated, there is a risk that the dye injected during the cath will cause further kidney damage, which in the worst-case scenario would leave you traveling to a dialysis center three times a week for the rest of your life.

Next you will go to the EKG lab. You might think another EKG is unnecessary, but your cardiologist wants to make sure you haven't had a significant cardiac event since your last EKG. If you haven't had one recently, they will probably also take a chest x-ray, to be sure you don't have some weird congenital abnormality that will complicate the cath. Additionally, it would be nice to know if you have active TB or a ravenous cancer devouring your lung.

After the pre-op testing is completed, you will head to the cath lab waiting area. Here a nurse or tech will have you sign some consent forms. You'll be on a cardiac monitor during your cath, and anytime you are monitored, you must have a port for access to your venous system, so she'll put a saline lock into a vein on the back of your hand. Should you suffer any untoward events, drugs can be given quickly through the saline lock. Here is where you also change into the ubiquitous open-backed hospital gown. If you have never experienced this fashion statement, welcome to the world of potential humiliation.

There are two sets of string ties. Of absolute importance, do not forget the lower set. Should you happen to be the owner of crummy health insurance, you may be issued moth-eaten duds. Not a big deal. However, if the lower set of ties are missing or shortened to the point that tying them and securing your butt from public view is impossible, speak up. In cheap hospitals they will secure the nether porthole with tape. Nothing good can come from air on your derriere; your day is only going to get worse. Once gowned and supine (lying on your back) on the gurney, it is time to hurry up and wait.

If you are fortunate enough to be the first case, congratulations. You will have a definite starting time. If you are not first, the starting time is listed as "TF", as in "to follow". That means if the case before you runs longer than expected, you sit and wait. We'll assume it's your lucky day and you are Numero Uno. Pretty soon you will be wheeled in a chair or on a gurney into the cath lab. The staff prefers the gurney. If you are feeling healthy, either option is humiliating, but the third option, the one that makes the most sense, walking in under your own steam, is frowned upon by the risk management department. We'll assume you ride the gurney, a cold steel table on wheels. Interestingly, it's the same device used to move stiffs around the morgue.

Once in the cath lab, you get to meet the staff. The nice thing about the cath lab is that it's a closed system, behind formidable doors. All the nurses, x-ray techs and lab techs have a job to do, which is to get you in, get your cath done without any complications, and get you out. No random rubbernecks allowed. You are helped with the slide across from the gurney to a different cold slab, the cath table.

To keep things nice and sterile at the catheter insertion site, you will have to be shaved and prepped. Occasionally this task is performed in the waiting area, hopefully behind a drawn curtain or closed door. Usually, however, you can expect to be shaved in the cath lab. Up goes your gown, a towel or two is placed over your groin area and then partially retracted. This is where a half-dozen women, give or take a guy or two, get a peek at your dick if they so choose. If you are shy about that sort of thing, you can comfort yourself with the knowledge that, unless you are a urologist or spend considerable time in a bath house, in which case you have other things to worry about, each and every one of the cath lab staff have seen many more dicks than you have, and yours holds as much fascination for them as an uncooked Hebrew National. Or a peanut shell, depending on circumstances.

The prep razors are usually the old-fashioned double-edge variety. Some institutions use betadine scrub, an iodine-based foaming solution, as the shave cream. Others use plain foam shave cream. Many use nothing. Don't worry. The shave prep rarely causes nicks or cuts. Accidental penectomy is almost unheard of. Some hospitals prepare for the worst and shave both sides, in case entry on the right is difficult. That leaves you with a Hitler moustache, except that it's above, rather than below, your proboscis. Other places simply shave the right side, hoping for the best. I don't know what you call that result, but it is definitely a lopsided look. After the shave job, the nurse will cover you back up. While this is going on, especially if you are the first case of the day, various staff members will be getting the injection setup ready and making sure the x-ray equipment is up and running. You will be wearing EKG leads so that your heart can be monitored during the procedure.

This is a good place to make a suggestion. There are plenty of busy, noisy hospital departments where it is perfectly acceptable to fart loudly in public. Nobody in the E.R. will so much as raise an eyebrow when you let one rip. If you are unconscious or semi-conscious on the table in the operating room, even with all the volatile anesthetic gases present in potentially dangerous quantities, no one will begrudge your lighting one up. If you are a post-op patient on a surgery floor, a deafening butt bazooka is considered a prerequisite for your discharge home. In contrast, the cath lab is a quiet sanctuary of sanity. The lighting is dim, almost intimate. There may be some soft, soothing music playing in the background, but ambient noise is at a minimum. Unless hot flashes are pervasive among the staff, airflow will be adequate but not excessive. While there may be an acoustic ceiling above you, you are lying on a hard table, which can make any proximally generated noise echo like a gunshot in Carlsbad Caverns. In addition, you don't want anything, solid, liquid or gas, spoiling the sterile field down there. Consider pinching your cheeks for the duration. If you don't, you'll be remembered as "The Farter". That should be enough of a deterrent; think how much worse it will be if you are scheduled for a return engagement.

When the lab setup is complete, the torero, your cardiologist, will enter. He should be masked, gowned and gloved. His hands should not be shaking. Nor should he be wearing a bullfighter's hat. He is, however, "wearing the lead". The lead, which prevents excessive exposure to x-radiation, is a smock of shiny material weighing approximately a thousand pounds. It is one of the main reasons cardiologists stop doing caths and stick to noninvasive cardiology. After a few pleasantries and a question or two as to whether you are currently having any chest pain, one of the staff will pull off your groin towel. Your cardiologist will then scrub your groin with betadine and a foam brush for a while. Then he'll lay out a series of sterile towels to cover your dick and keep it out of the action zone.

Most cardiologists will ask you if you are allergic to lidocaine, a local anesthetic known incorrectly to the general public as novocaine. Often you'll be offered a combination of medications, something like morphine or demerol for pain relief, and some type of benzodiazepine from the Valium family for relaxation and sedation. If you are the nervous type, accept the offer. If you are the curious type and want to see what's going on, stick with the lidocaine. The monitor showing the injection of dye into your various arteries will be located above you and to your left. If you ask nicely, your cardiologist may be able to angle the screen so that you can watch. After the sterile prep is completed and the towels are laid in place, your cardiologist will palpate your femoral pulse. He'll inject lidocaine into the skin. The first shot of lidocaine will burn. Subsequent injections will cause pressure, perhaps a temporary dull ache.

Once the area is numb, he'll perform the "femoral stick", inserting a catheter with a needle inside it into the skin and artery. At this point, you should feel a mild pressure or nothing at all. Depending on the insertion set, he will then remove the needle and advance the catheter. He may insert a dilator through the catheter to open up the insertion site a little wider. After the dilator is removed, a wire may be threaded through the catheter and the original catheter removed. An introducer, known as the "femoral sheath", will be threaded over the wire; the wire is then removed, leaving only the sheath in place. Some cardiologists prefer to suture the sheath in place, but most do not. In the majority of cases, that femoral artery stick is all that will be required. You may receive blood thinners like Integrilin or Plavix before the cath, to prevent clots from forming.

In some cases, where the cardiologist is worried about disease in your heart valves or high blood pressure in the pulmonary arteries, he will also want to perform a right heart cath. In order to access the right side of the heart, he will place a similar catheter in your femoral vein, which is right next to the artery. An important point is that "right heart cath" and "left heart cath" refer to the chambers of the heart, not which side of your body the cardiologist sticks to gain access. Shockingly, there are physicians who think a right heart cath requires a stick on the right side of your body and a left heart cath requires a stick on the left side. I even crossed paths once with a cardiologist who thought the same way.

Once the femoral artery introducer is in place, the cardiologist will thread various catheters up your aorta and begin squirting dye into various arteries. There will be shots in your right coronary artery, then several in your left main and its offshoots, the left anterior descending and the circumflex. Some of these will be done with the camera recording from various angles so as to best visualize the entire artery; there is a good chance each artery will be injected more than once. There will be a shot of your left ventricle and sometimes the proximal aorta, the portion closest to your heart. Most cardiologists will also inject your LIMA, the left internal mammary artery, because the LIMA is preferred over a saphenous vein graft if you require a bypass of your left main, left anterior descending or circumflex arteries. Less commonly, if there is significant disease in your right coronary artery or one of its branches, he may also inject your RIMA, the right internal mammary artery.

While most patients will experience little or no discomfort during the injection of dye into the various coronary arteries, some will feel burning during one or more of them. Surprisingly few patients complain during the injection of the left ventricle or the aorta, both of which involve significantly larger boluses of dye. Many patients will feel a burning discomfort during the LIMA and the RIMA studies; it is so common that your cardiologist or one of the cath lab nurses will usually give you a heads-up just before the injection of these arteries. It shouldn't last more than a few seconds. In addition, some patients may feel chest, abdominal or back pain during the injection of dye into an artery with a particularly tight blockage.

As in every other aspect of heart disease, no two patients have an identical cardiac cath experience. Some procedures go as smooth as silk. Easy femoral artery stick, easy threading, easy entry into each of the coronary artery ostia (openings), no arrhythmias, no adverse reactions from the dye injections, no problems with post-procedure bleeding. Others are what is known in the business as a "thrash"; every step of the procedure is complicated, from difficult sticks into femoral arteries that are narrow or full of calcium, to difficulty getting the catheter tip into one or more of the coronary arteries, a tear in the wall of a coronary artery, life-threatening arrhythmias or bleeding that requires transfusions. Most caths fall somewhere in the middle and require little or no post-cath care beyond some observation time on a monitor.

Once all the dye studies have been completed, your cardiologist will remove the catheter from the sheath, then the sheath itself. There is now a hole in your femoral artery. Like a garden hose with a hole in it, the liquid contents of your artery, blood, will tend to leak out. If there is nothing restraining it, that blood can shoot pretty high in the air.

Fortunately, the muscle layer in the wall of the artery will contract, shrinking the size of the hole. In addition, your cardiologist will place firm pressure on the insertion site for ten to fifteen minutes. In some cases, one of a variety of substances will be injected into the puncture site to plug the hole in your artery. Studies have shown the efficacy of several of these preparations in terms of arterial bleeding and recovery time. They are almost always used after an angioplasty.

The actual cath procedure may take anywhere from thirty to sixty minutes. Obviously, the pre-op waiting time, the prep time, and the post-op observation time will be much longer. If you are in and out of the hospital within four hours, that is a good day. You should prepare for the worst-case scenario, in which you are there all day or have to be admitted to the hospital for a complication or for angioplasty or bypass surgery that same day or the next.

Complications of cardiac catheterization include:

1. Pseudoaneurysm of the femoral artery. Blood leaks out of the lumen of your femoral artery and causes swelling between the layers of the artery wall;
2. Bleeding at the insertion site causing a hematoma (black and blue) to form;
3. Arrhythmias during placement of the catheter or injections of the coronary arteries and left ventricle;
4. Chest pain and possible heart attack during injection of the coronary arteries;
5. Infection of the puncture site or of your heart valves;
6. A dissection (tear) in the wall of one of your coronary arteries;
7. Air embolism: introduction of air into an artery or vein;
8. Allergic reaction to dye;
9. Blood clots in any of the arteries or the left ventricle;
10. Stroke.

Even in the hands of an experienced cardiologist, any of these are a possibility. However, most likely you will experience either no side effects or a mild hematoma at the puncture site in your groin. Arrhythmias are common and usually self-limited, meaning they resolve on their own. However, if you frequent locker rooms in the buff, you might get a comment or two on your new hairdo. I shall address that particular situation in another book.

References:

1. Kern, Morton J., King, Spencer B. III. "Cardiac Catheterization, Cardiac Angiography, and Coronary Blood Flow and Pressure Measurements." *Hurst's The Heart.* Ed. Valentin Fuster, Ed. Robert A. O'Rourke, Ed. Richard A. Walsh, Ed. Philip Poole-Wilson. New York: McGraw-Hill. 2008. 467-90.
2. Davidson, Charles J., Bonow, Robert O. "Cardiac Catheterization." *Braunwald's Heart Disease.* Ed. Robert O. Bonow, Ed. Douglas L. Mann, Ed. Douglas P. Zipes, Ed. Peter Libby, Ed. Eugene Braunwald. Philadelphia: Elsevier Saunders. 2012. 383-429.

3. Sette P, Dorizzi RM, Azzomo AM "Vascular access: an historical perspective from Sir William Harvey to the 1956 Nobel prize to Andre F. Cournand, Werner Forssmann, and Dickinson W. Richards." J Vasc Access 2012. 13(2):137-44

4. Bourassa MG "The history of cardiac catheterization" Can J Cardiol 2005. 21(12):1011-14

5. Sassard R, O'Leary JP "Egas Moniz: pioneer of cerebral angiography" Am Surg 1998. 64(11):1116-17

6. Fusar-Poli P, Allen P, McGuire P "Egas Moniz (1875-1955), the father of psychosurgery" Br J Psychiatry 2008. 193(1):50

7. Cheng TO "The cough that resuscitated Dr. F. Mason Sones's first patient undergoing selective cine coronary arteriography" Catheter Cardiovasc Interv 2004. 63(3):398

8. Sheldon WC "F. Mason Sones, Jr. --stormy petrel of cardiology" Clin Cardiol 1994. 17(7):405-7.

9. Captur G "Memento for Rene Favaloro" Tex Heart Inst J 2004. 31(1):47-60.

78. AFTER THE CATH--DECISIONS, DECISIONS

Now that you have undergone cardiac catheterization, your cardiologist has all the information he requires to decide the next step in your treatment.

In over ninety percent of cases, your cath most likely shows one of three categories of findings:

1. There are either no significant stenoses or very mild ones which would best be treated with medication and will require no further intervention;
2. You have one or more significant lesions that will require angioplasty with a stent or bypass surgery, but they can be done on an elective basis, i.e. later in the week or beyond;
3. You have one or more significant stenoses that will require angioplasty or bypass surgery urgently or emergently.

In situation #1, hooray for you. Tell Habib the limo driver to crank open the sunroof and chill that magnum of Dom posthaste, because you, sir, are going HOME! In situation #2, most likely you will be discharged home, perhaps on some additional medication. In situation #3, you will be admitted to the CVICU. Depending on scheduled procedures and the urgency of your stenoses, you will either go back to the cath lab or the O.R. that same day or the next.

Excluding bizarre rarities, it takes most experienced cardiologists and cardiac surgeons all of five minutes to review cath images and decide what needs to be done. No matter which category you fall into, your cardiologist will be able to outline what he thinks should come next, often before you even leave the cath lab. Any cardiologist who performs angioplasties will usually favor that option over surgery. They are less invasive and thus less likely to cause complications, and there is no need for general anesthesia. In cases where angioplasty is too risky or unlikely to succeed, he'll recommend bypass surgery. At this point, you might be thinking, *Finally, we get to the part of the bypass book that deals with the actual bypass.* No, Sport, not yet we don't. Apparently I'm under the impression that I'm getting paid by the word.

While some cardiologists may ask you if you have a preference in terms of cardiac surgeons, most will just tell you which group he uses and then call them. Like most physicians, he has reasons for his referral preferences. Hopefully it's because of a good track record, not because of kickbacks or because he has a crush on a particular surgeon. If it appears that your surgical needs are more elective than emergent, it will probably be a few days before you have to return for surgery. Sometime before surgery, you will meet the guy who's going to operate on your heart. Depending on the time frame, it may be in the cath lab waiting room right after your cath, it may be in his office, or it may be just before you are rolled into the O.R. Whenever and wherever that occurs, you can be sure your cardiac surgeon has already looked at your cath films before making the commitment to perform bypass surgery on you.

79. ANGIOPLASTY AND PCI

Angioplasty is a procedure designed to open up narrowed areas (stenoses) in arteries and veins. Like a cardiac cath, it is usually performed in the setting of a percutaneous puncture, i.e., a needle stick in your femoral artery.

The first human to undergo percutaneous angioplasty was an elderly woman with a severe blockage of a major artery in her thigh, which was causing pain and gangrene. Fortunately, she refused the usual treatment, amputation of her leg. In early 1964, an interventional radiologist by the name of Charles Dotter at the Oregon Health Sciences University passed several catheters over a guide wire and successfully dilated the stenosis. Her circulation improved dramatically; the gangrene resolved and she lived without symptoms for over two years. Known as the "Father of Interventional Radiology",

Dr. Dotter was nominated for the Nobel Prize in Medicine in 1978. Incredibly, he did not win. Had he been nominated ten years later, when angioplasty had become the standard of care, it probably would have been a slam dunk.

Angioplasty of a coronary artery was first performed by Dr. Andreas Greuntzig in Switzerland in 1977. By the mid-1980s, PTCA (percutaneous transluminal coronary angioplasty) was being performed on patients with angina at hundreds of hospital centers around the world. In the mid- to late-1980s its use became more popular in patients with unstable angina as well. Usually referred to nowadays as balloon angioplasty, this procedure falls under the general heading of PCI (percutaneous coronary intervention), which also includes rotational atherotomy (roto-rooter), laser atherotomy, stent implantation, and brachytherapy (use of radiation to re-open stents or vein grafts that have developed stenoses). Of all these interventional options, balloon angioplasty with stent placement is by far the most common.

When angioplasty became all the rage for treating stable angina in the 1980s, you were obligated to have a cardiac surgeon stand by in case the balloon caused a rupture of the coronary artery. Experts predicted that angioplasty would replace bypass surgery within ten years. In other words, ninety percent of the work that most cardiac surgeons lived on would disappear. Obviously, the limitations of angioplasty soon became clear and that never happened, but in the meantime, cardiac surgery groups started branching out to smaller hospitals and smaller towns, to get while the gettin' was good. Similar to septic system installers, trying to make the most of a fading market. Good studies showed that while angioplasty is at least as good as medications at relieving stable angina, bypass is superior to angioplasty when it came to preventing MI or cardiac death down the road. You might think that relieving angina would prevent heart attacks and death. Oddly enough, that's not the case.

The angioplasty procedure starts out the same way and in the same place as a cardiac cath. In fact, if you have signed a consent form for angioplasty before your initial cath, it is permissible to perform it right then and there, especially if a critical stenosis is demonstrated during your cath. Before the fun starts, your cardiologist will administer intravenous blood thinners. Once the femoral sheath is in place, he will advance a catheter and inject dye to locate the stenotic lesion. He will then advance a thin guide wire through the stenosis. Over this guide wire he will thread a deflated balloon catheter. The balloon will light up on x-ray so that he can position the balloon right in the middle of the stenosis. He will then inject a mixture of dye and sterile water into the balloon to a pressure over five times normal blood pressure. If all goes well, and it usually does, the pressure of the inflated balloon will compress the plaque and open up the narrowed area of the artery. A post-procedure injection of dye will demonstrate that the artery is now open.

If your physician believes in their effectiveness, and most cardiologists do, he will insert a catheter with a stent positioned over the balloon. Stents are metal mesh tubes that are placed over the angioplasty balloon and then expanded. In theory they stabilize the area of the angioplasty and hopefully prevent re-stenosis of the artery.

Unlike after a diagnostic cardiac cath, often your femoral sheath will be left in place after an angioplasty and you will be admitted to the CVICU. The sheath is not removed immediately because of the possibility of re-stenosis or clot formation, which would necessitate an emergent return to the cath lab to reopen the blockage. Later that day the sheath can be removed in the CVICU and a pressure clamp or plug inserted into the puncture site to prevent bleeding.

So you've had a wire and a couple of catheters shoved up into your heart and then a balloon was inflated under incredibly high pressure to squeeze open your coronary artery. What could possibly go wrong?

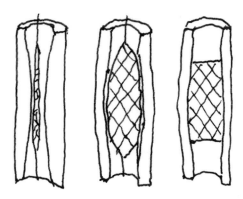

BAC/FMP

Angioplasty balloon and stent positioned in coronary artery narrowed by plaque (left)
Balloon inflated, expanding stent and dilating occlusion (middle)
Balloon deflated, then removed, leaving stent in place (right)

1. All the same things that could go wrong during a diagnostic cardiac cath;
2. Coronary artery perforation caused by the guide wire. Surprisingly, even though this leaves a tiny hole in the wall of your coronary artery, usually you don't need any urgent intervention;

3. Rupture of all or part of the wall of your coronary artery. Your usual systolic blood pressure is about 120 mm Hg. The pressure inside the angioplasty balloon is anywhere from 75 to 500 mm Hg. That's a shit load of pressure, Kemo Sabe. An actual rupture of the wall can be seen when dye is injected after the balloon is deflated. The dye leaks out! Uh-oh. This requires emergent surgical repair, so you will earn a bypass after all. Of note, your cardiologist will still get paid, so you don't need to lose any sleep over his financial situation and how your adverse outcome will impact his lifestyle. A bunch of perforations, however, could land him afoul of various insurance plans. Though they may proclaim their deep concern for your well-being, health insurance companies do not giggle with glee when they have to pay for emergency bypass surgery just because your cardiologist has a habit of rupturing coronary arteries.

If your angioplasty is elective (usually for uncontrolled angina), successful and free of any complications, most likely you will not require any further surgical interventions. If, however, you came to be on the cath table because you were having a cardiac emergency, such as unstable angina or an MI, you may not get off so easy. In some cases, the PCI reopens the acutely blocked artery, but you may have other critical narrowings in the same or other coronary arteries. In that case, you will be heading to bypass surgery pretty soon.

You might hear some chatter about bare metal stents (BMS) versus drug-eluting stents (DES). BMS is just what you imagine, stainless steel originally, now more often cobalt, and nothing more. A DES has the same underlying structure as the BMS, an expandable metal frame, but it is covered with a polymer which contains one or more drugs. The idea is for the drugs to elute (release) into the wall of the artery over time. One of the drugs is an immunosuppressive, which is designed to prevent inflammation caused by the accumulation of various types of white cells around the stent, which your body treats as a foreign body. The other drug is usually an antiproliferative, which prevents the growth of smooth muscle cells around the stent. Either of these processes, inflammation or proliferation, will tend to thicken the wall of the artery and lead to restenosis. Obviously, you don't want that. What you want is endothelialization, whereby the stent becomes part of the endothelium (inner lining) of the artery wall. Various studies have shown the superiority of DES over BMS when it comes to restenosis, so odds are that your stent will be a DES. To summarize, after the stent is placed and the artery reopened, you want endothelium, not muscle cells, to grow around the stent.

When you are discharged from the hospital after your angioplasty, most likely you will be taking clopidogrel (Plavix), and enteric-coated aspirin (ECASA), two platelet poisons. These medications will help prevent clot formation around the new foreign body, the stent, until endothelialization is completed. Studies have shown that the optimal duration of therapy with both agents is twelve months from the time of stent insertion. If you tolerate the treatment without side effects (most commonly bleeding) for the initial twelve months, some experts recommend another eighteen months of therapy.

References:

1. Weitz, Jeffrey I. "Blood Coagulation and Anticoagulant, Fibrinolytic, and Antiplatelet Drugs." *Goodman & Gilman's The Pharmacological Basis of Therapeutics.* Ed. Laurence L. Brunton, Assoc. Ed. Bruce A. Chabner, Assoc. Ed. Bjorn C Knollman. New York: McGraw-Hill. 2011. 849-71.
2. Douglas, John S. Jr., King, Spencer B. III. "Percutaneous Coronary Intervention." *Hurst's The Heart.* Ed. Valentin Fuster, Ed. Richard A. Walsh, Ed. Robert A. Harrington. New York: McGraw-Hill. 2011. 1430-8. 1442-4.
3. Popma, Jeffrey J., Bhatt, Deepak L. "Percutaneous Coronary Intervention." *Braunwald's Heart Disease.* Ed. Robert O. Bonow, Ed. Douglas L. Mann, Ed. Douglas P. Zipes, Ed. Peter Libby, Ed. Eugene Braunwald. Philadelphia: Elsevier Saunders. 2012. 1270-82.
4. Payne MM. "Charles Theodore Dotter: The father of intervention." *Tex Heart Inst J.* 2001. 28(1):28-38.
5. Freidman SG. "Charles Dotter and the fiftieth anniversary of endovascular surgery." *J Vasc Surg.* 2015. 61(2):556-8.

80. PROTOCOLS

People in the medical profession, or, rather, the medical industry, have been talking about medical protocols since the 1970s. They got a sharp boost in interest when DRGs and HMOs came along. DRGs are diagnostic related groups. When you are admitted to the hospital, say, for pneumonia, the hospital and physicians who care for you are paid a set fee for the entire hospital stay rather than for each day you are there or for each procedure performed on you. This DRG may be increased depending on your age, other medical conditions you have, or certain complications that may occur during your stay. HMOs are health maintenance organizations, those providers of care to whom you pay your monthly premiums. Protocols tend to focus on safety, good outcomes, shorter hospital stays and lower costs; in other words, the best bang for the buck. If you are going in for heart surgery, you want to undergo as few tests as possible. Your insurance company also wants that. If that's what you want, the simplest, quickest, safest, most effective surgery and hospital stay, you want to go to an institution that has a protocol in place that is pretty much inviolate. That leaves as little room as possible for human error, either by omission or addition.

There are certain scenarios where protocols are most effective:

1. Training programs where there is a tendency for house staff to fill pages of charts with orders that aren't necessary;
2. Big egos who think they know best and persist in doing things the way they always have, even in the face of scientific research that proves otherwise;
3. Physicians who may practice at multiple hospitals and are subject to different routines;
4. Cowboys, a.k.a. doctors who know the science, but ignore it in favor of trying something new and unproven;
5. Hospitals with a focus on research, where adherence to protocols can make or break a research project;
6. HMOs where protocols ensure that patients do not get lost in the system during their workups;
7. Sleepy physicians who might forget to write an important order, necessitating a call in the middle of the night for clarification. "Did you really mean to omit that?"

81. TWO-FER

Simmons was on his west coast swing, to see the cities, experience the lifestyle, and hopefully score an internship. Portland in October, Seattle in November, and finish up with some warm weather for the first three weeks of December in San Diego before heading home for the holidays. He'd lucked into the Dermatology rotation on the hill in Portland, not knowing a thing about the department. To his way of thinking, a city where precipitation reigns supreme for nine months of the year hardly qualifies as a hotbed of skin pathology. Once there, he found he'd stumbled into a gold mine: pasty Scandos with an insatiable appetite for solar exposure. Every Memorial Day they burst forth, semi-naked and loaded to the gills on two-carbon fragments, mushrooms and Pakololo, in a three-month frenzy to get as sunburned as possible, supplemented the rest of the year by weekly visits to the tanning beds. Much like "teetotaling" Utah Mormons and their success at making more money off of booze than anyone else, Portlanders squeezed the maximum amount of dermatologic sun damage out of the minimum amount of exposure to toxic UVA and UVB rays.

Portland was the first city he'd visited west of the Mississippi. Life ran at half-speed compared to out East. You couldn't swing a spring chinook by its tail without hitting a state park. People hiked and camped in the rain and even the girls didn't bitch about it. There was more than enough nightlife to go around, for humans and vampires alike. At least during the winter, the bloodsuckers could roam freely during the day as well, knowing they wouldn't have much trouble avoiding lux solis. Between the Derm clinic and touring the wet side of the state on the weekends, October flew by. The next thing David knew, he was on the bus to Seattle.

When he'd called the student affairs office at UW, he had about four or five rotations in mind. Anesthesia wasn't one of them, but, again, it was available. So he cancelled the anesthesia rotation he had scheduled for March in Charlottesville and looked forward to passing gas on Puget Sound. Clayton Lightfoot, one of his interns at UVA, advised him on evaluating places to land after graduation.

"If the students and the residents are nice but the interns are assholes, cross it off your list. When the majority of interns act like they could tear your head off and suck out your brains, the system is designed to stress them to the point of homicide. I bet when you look in the mirror, you see a cheetah staring back at you. I look at you and see a toucan. Your best chance at survival in that particular type of jungle is to fly high and safe over the big cats and their bloody ground skirmishes." It took a while to recover from that piercing deflation of his ego balloon, but after jettisoning his admittedly hilarious self-delusion as an alpha male, David accepted the advice and started eating Fruit Loops for breakfast.

At OHSU, the students were terrific, easy to get to know. The attendings were as well, professionally laid back, into sailing, hiking and acting hip. The residents were nowhere to be seen, presumably lounging in the library. The interns were busy, helpful, and very much into the Pacific Northwest lifestyle. Salmon, coffee, beer, music. UW was another story. The students were great. The attendings tended to be polite but remote. The residents wore an affable numb weariness he associated with slogging through a year of hell and coming out the other side in one piece. The interns, however, were wound as tight as piano strings; Simmons didn't see toucans or any other prey surviving in that milieu, let alone thriving. UW was considered a hot shit place for internal medicine, surgery, and a bunch of subspecialties.

Had Simmons known how stiff it would be, he probably would have opted for a month elsewhere. Fortunately, anesthesia was one department where, as long as you saw the pre-ops and showed up for the cases, nobody was going to ride your ass for not knowing the minutiae of every anesthetic medication. He didn't cross Seattle off his list, but he knew he wouldn't end up there.

Another plus about the anesthesia rotation was that the two fourth-year students virtually never got in each other's way. While one guy was doing pre-operative evaluations and consults, the other worked cases in the O.R. Each week they switched assignments. You also worked with a multitude of attendings in the O.R. rather than the same guy day in and day out. The O.R. supervisor simply wrote your name in on whatever cases she chose. Simmons was there to see as much as he could and do whatever they told him. Trying to decide where to go in a strange environment was one headache he was glad to avoid. In the meantime, he got to experience Seattle during the rainy season, see if it was something he could take for a month, let alone three years.

Fate smiled upon him and he scored a single room in the medical school dorm. The guy who was supposed to bunk with him came down with mono the last week of August and headed home to Billings for the semester. On his second day in town, while ambling down Alaskan Way at sunset, puffing on a juicy Dannemann, he noticed a dozen fishing poles sticking out the waterfront windows at the Edgewater. *When in Rome...* He bought a cheap pole and equally cheap tackle at GI Joe's.

On the weekends he took the bus downtown and fished early either right by the Edgewater or down the way at Pier 62. Most afternoons after work he'd trot down to the Montlake Cut and fish in the blurry sunset for whatever came his way. One afternoon he spotted an old fellow with glasses paddling a red canoe across the cut toward a row of houseboats near the Seattle yacht club. He mentioned him later that night at a reception for the new students on the rotation.

One of the attendings asked him, "Have you ever heard of the Scribner shunt?" It was the standard vascular access for dialyzing patients with kidney failure.

"Sure. I got to assist on a couple on my surgery rotation."

"Well, that's him. That's Scribner." *Wow.*

From there on out, it seemed a day didn't go by when he didn't come across some attending with a book, disease or device named after him. He started compiling a list of famous physicians he encountered or simply eyeballed. Simmons felt grateful to be able to hide in the anesthesia department, which owned its own share of big names but was significantly less intimidating than on the wards. Even in the O.R., the big name surgeons left him alone and were content to suck the souls out of the students and interns working at the south side of the table, below the neck.

It was Thursday of his first week. He'd drawn pre-ops and consults. After about the fourth consult on Monday, he had the routine down. Review the patient's chart, see the patient, ask all the usual questions, do the physical exam, which was limited to upper airway, heart and lungs, and write it up. Then he'd run it by the senior anesthesia resident, Tom Wofford, put a note on the chart, and it was on to the next one. The anesthesia pre-op workup made much more sense to Simmons than any of the other models he'd experienced. Very practical, much simpler than on internal medicine or pediatrics, but overlooking a detail could mean the difference between a routine case and a death on the operating table. The acuity of the setting grabbed him. Once again, Superficial Simmons was falling briefly in love with a new branch of medicine.

David ate lunch with Nadide Karadag and Mike McCreary. Mike was on his third year surgery clerkship at UW and was planning to do his internal medicine residency in Spokane, where his wife's family lived. They'd struck up a conversation on the general surgery ward on Simmons' first day. Nadide, a former Turkish junior girls weightlifting champion, now a fourth year student at the Ankara University School of Medicine, was in Seattle for a urology elective, hoping to land a spot in the residency program next year. There had never been an XX chromosome in the UW urology program, but she was not one to stand on tradition.

"The intern was having great trouble retracting the fat man's adipose so that the famous Dr. Tillamook could remove the kidney. He was without sleep and had a bad angle, so I reached over and gave it a moderate tug. The exposure was now much better. The intern was very angry. He told me to get out of the way. I told him if I wanted, I could extract his windpipe and crush his balls." Nadide put down her fork and squeezed both hands into fists. Then she emitted her best dead-lift grunt and went back to eating.

Mike laughed. "I'll bet Tillamook loved that."

Very pleased with herself, Nadide smiled. "He said it was nice to work with a real man in the O.R. for once."

That caught David off guard. "He said that? He called you a man?"

"He can call me anything he wants, if in the end I have a residency position in this urology program."

While they finished eating, he mulled the import of having to crush someone's balls and rip out a windpipe or two to get a residency slot. Though reputed to have powerful beaks, this was not the stuff of toucans.

After lunch, David walked into the anesthesia department office. There were six pre-ops listed on the board behind Myrna Dominguez's shipshape desk. As the department's coordinator for surgery, she made sure every inpatient pre-op consult was on the board by noon. Students, interns and residents divvied up the pre-ops and consults. All work was to be done and logged in to Myrna by quitting time, 5 P.M. Monday's cases were handled Sunday afternoon by the anesthesia resident on call. Ditto for emergencies at night.

"Hi, Myrna. Wow, what did you do with your hair? It looks terrific!"

The dowager cracked a rare smile as she patted her black bob. Display of her teeth was not high on Myrna's list. "Why, thank you for noticing, David. My niece is training to be a stylist at the beauty school. I drove up after work last night and she used me as a model." She touched every item on her desk, then looked back up at Simmons, satisfied that nothing had moved while she spoke.

"The boys at the disco will be all over you this weekend."

"Oh, the discos are too young for me, David. However, I am considering attending Salsa Sunday at the American Legion." She patted her coif once more, but this time without the smile. Back to business.

"That'll be fun. Say, does your niece do men's hair? I'm in serious need of a haircut this weekend."

"Oh, yes, they're open for business all day Saturday. The 48 bus will take you up there." She jotted on a notepad. "Here's her name and number. I'm sure she'd be delighted to take you on." Myrna replaced the notepad to its assigned spot on her desk.

"Thanks. What have we got today?"

"Well, it's Thursday, so...Oh, I forgot, this is your first week. It feels like you've been here longer." Myrna touched her eyebrow, correcting his start date in her mental log book. "On Thursday afternoon most of our consults are for GYN surgery and pediatrics. Lots of those cases are in for only twenty-four hours, so the O.R. schedule on Friday is basically BTLs, PE tubes, and emergencies." BTLs, bilateral tubal ligations, better known as "tying your tubes", took an hour at most. Induction of anesthesia usually took longer than the placement of PE tubes for infants and toddlers with chronic middle ear infections. Both were considered "clean" cases, with little or no pus and rarely any bowel involvement.

"Here, take these two. Foxman and Howell. BTLs first thing tomorrow. Oh, look at that. They're in the same room, 312-A and B." She handed the sheets to Simmons, then stood up and wrote his last name next to the two patient names on her board. The anesthesia residents referred to her office as the "War Room"; there was no doubt in anyone's mind that, should circumstances require it, Myrna could plan an invasion of a belligerent nation on that board.

"Thanks, Myrna. See you in a bit."

"Take your time. There won't be much of a workload this afternoon. I'll page you overhead if anything interesting shows up. Dr. Wofford will handle the rest." The way she said it left no doubt as to who made the decisions in the department. David exited the office and walked over to the GYN floor. It was good to have some work to do right after lunch. Otherwise he might have to head to the library and pretend to read with his eyes closed.

It was David's first visit to the third floor. In anticipation of a big surgery day Friday, the GYN ward was abustle. Women were being wheeled off to have one procedure or another performed in the x-ray department. An elderly patient walked the hallway, her Foley bag hooked to the back of the wheelchair she leaned on for balance. Simmons didn't hear any primal screaming or "Push!", so he assumed either it was a slow day for hatching babies or Labor & Delivery was located somewhere else. Room 312, a semi-private, was halfway down the long corridor on the left.

David walked in to find two attractive women in their late thirties lounging in bed watching "General Hospital" on the TV. A box of See's candies lay open on the table between the two beds. When he walked in, they turned their heads, then sat up in bed and smiled. *Synchronized, like a rally squad.* He addressed the woman in the bed nearest the door.

"Mrs. Foxman?" He held out his hand. " I'm David Simmons. I'm here to do your anesthesia preoperative evaluation." They shook.

"Nice to meet you, Dr. Simmons." She smiled, reached over, and pulled shut the curtain that separated the two beds. From behind the curtain, David heard a stifled giggle. *Well, this should be fun. Everybody's in a good mood.* Most of his pre-ops had been cranky old guys with prostates the size of softballs or anxious middle-aged fatties moaning in tempo with the pulsations of their chock-full o'stones gallbladders. This held the promise of a far friendlier encounter. He pulled the rest of the curtains around her bed for privacy and sat down.

"As I understand it, you're here for a tubal ligation?" Another giggle could be heard from Mrs. Howell in bed B.

"Oh, yes."

"Good. How many times have you been pregnant and how many times have you delivered a baby?"

"Four for four. I was the good girl." She winked at Simmons. After a brief rustling from behind the curtain, a nougat square flew up and over, landing on the sheet covering Mrs. Foxman. She picked it up, took a bite, then dropped it in the trashcan. "Yuck."

"So, no miscarriages, no abortions, no twins or triplets."

"No, none of those. Like I said, I was the good girl." She nodded her head toward bed B.

From bed B came, "Oh go fuck yourself." Then a giggle followed by choking.

"Are you okay over there, Mrs. Howell?"

After a few coughs, she said, "I'm fine. Which is a lot better than Miss Prissy's going to be just as soon as you leave." *Oh, a catfight? Better stick around, just in case someone gets hurt.* "Why don't you ask her why all the girls in high school called her Latexia Pretzelina?"

David looked at bed A. "Why?" Nothing like a puzzle to bring Simmons brain back to life. Mrs. Foxman pursed her lips and squinted, as if expecting a blow to the head. The answer to the riddle came from bed B, that voice behind the curtain.

"It's because she always had a dozen rubbers in her glove box and could bend her legs around any guy in her VW." At this, both women started laughing.

"Let me guess. You two know each other." Now the two of them were howling. *Screw it.* He stood up and opened the curtain between the two beds, then moved his chair to the space between the foot of each bed. "It might save us all a little time if I interview both of you at the same time. Feel free to correct any inaccuracies your friend might blurt out."

Mrs. Foxman spoke up. "Oh, Dr. Simmons, we're in no rush. Nothing to do but wait for surgery tomorrow morning. But, if you prefer, we can do this together."

"How did you decide to get your tubes tied on the same day?" That caused the loudest outburst of laughter yet. He waited for them to settle down.

Mrs. Howell in Bed B straightened up first. "Dr. Simmons, we didn't decide it." *A court-ordered double spaying?*

Bed A (David gave up on trying to keep their names straight in his head and decided on the take-out Chinese route. One from Bed A, one from Bed B.) added, "Who in their right mind would choose to have their belly cut open?"

"So if you didn't make the decision, who did?"

Bed B giggled. "Our husbands."

David was confused. "Can a husband force his wife to have her tubes tied in the state of Washington? I don't think men could get away with that in Mississippi, let alone up here." *Seattle is more sophisticated than that, right?*

Bed A spoke up. "No, silly, they can't force us. But they did make us an offer we couldn't refuse." *Now we've got crime bosses with Anglo-Saxon last names.*

Bed B took over. "Neither of them wanted any more kids, so it was condoms or the pill, which frankly scares the tar out of both of us at our age, or the you-know-what." She raised her right hand and made a scissors gesture with her index and middle finger. "Snip snip." At that, they both laughed. "Ooooh, it might hurt to get their little nutty buddies cut on."

Bed A reached over into the See's box, selected a piece of chocolate, and held it up to the light. "We said we'd both get our tubes tied if we could come in together and if they...," She reached over and shook hands with her friend, "sent us on an all-expenses-paid vacation to Vegas!"

"Woo-woo!" shouted Bed B.

"David injected a downer into the otherwise highly energized conversation. "Ladies, you won't want to travel for a week or two, in case you develop fluid in your abdomen after the procedure. That can be very painful. Besides, it's not a good idea to fly too soon after any kind of abdominal or pelvic surgery. There's a higher risk of blood clots in your legs and lungs."

Bed B looked over at her BTL buddy, then at Simmons. "Oh, we're not going for about ten days. Besides, we're not flying."

"Oh, driving?"

"No, silly. We're taking the bus."

Bed A chimed in. "Go Greyhound, go Greyhound, and leave the driving to us."

"Vegas, eh? You like to gamble?"

Bed B puffed up her hair. "Well, maybe a little slot action. Mostly we're going to see the sights and look for...." She giggled and looked over at Bed A.

In unison they crooned, "Ellllvisssss".

David pondered this for a moment before asking, "You realize he's dead, right?"

"Of course, silly. We're going the weekend of the Elvis competition finals. All those men dressed up like the King, with their deep voices and their dreamy hair." Bed A shivered at the thought.

"I hope it's fun. Maybe you can talk your hubbies into sending you on a bus ride to Graceland sometime. I hear it's fascinating, and his ghost sometimes makes a cameo appearance." Their eyes lit up. "Of course, you'll probably have to trade another surgical procedure for an offer you can't refuse." He looked from one to the other.

Of but one mind, they sang out, "Boob job!"

82. COMPARTMENTS

Richard Keith climbed into the Escalade and opened his leather dopp kit on the passenger seat. From the console between the seats he pulled out a black velcro wrist ammo holder with six empty elastic cartridge loops, and strapped it onto his left forearm as tight as he could. The veins in his hand and wrist bulged like Schwarzenegger's. Next he fished around in the dopp kit until he found a glass bullet snorter. After a long pull on the contents, he dropped the bullet into the breast pocket of his scrub top for easy access.

"Whew! Righteous nose candy. Thank you, Jesus!" He screamed as the pharmaceutical grade coke made its way into his frontal cortex. Dr. Keith started up his SUV and punched a couple numbers on the iPod docked on the dashboard to his right. In a few seconds he was singing along to "Can't You Hear Me Knocking" while he filled the cartridge loops with six 5cc. syringes. The milky white liquid contrasted nicely with the black holder. He tapped the iPod Pause button.

He ran his index finger around inside his nostrils until the tip felt a little numb, then rubbed the finger up and down on the skin between the ammo holder and his left thumb. He felt the tingle of the cocaine penetrating the dermis. The "painful vein", already swollen from the pressure of the constricting ammo holder, was ready to go. He reached into the dopp kit, pulled out a fresh 21-gauge butterfly, and, after rubbing the area with an alcohol wipe to remove the booger germs, smoothly inserted the needle into his vein. He loosened the ammo holder to allow his veins to flow again. Within seconds he had peeled off the backing from an Opsite and placed the clear plastic dressing over the hub of the butterfly, securing his IV access in place.

"Goodbye, Richard Keith. Hello, Keith Fucking Richards." With that, he hit the play button and backed out of the hospital parking lot. The cocaine made him chatty; he began talking to himself in between belting out the lyrics.

"Forty years old in less than twenty-four hours. Imagine that." He eyed himself in the rearview mirror. "Not bad, you holy devil!" While steering the Escalade through the surgicenter parking lot, he pulled out one of the syringes, attached it to the butterfly's purple port of entry, and slowly pushed the milky liquid into his vein. After 1 cc., he stopped. Even though he was the Birthday Boy, he didn't want the celebration to begin until he was safely on the I-540 headed to

Durham and his first party of the weekend. He punched the telephone button on the steering wheel. "Call home."

"Keith residence, Tara speaking." His seven year-old was working on her answering skills. A few weeks ago she'd seen some old movie from the '40s and made switchboard operator her latest career choice, displacing dolphin trainer. Neither Richard nor Savannah had the heart to tell her the job no longer entailed pulling out and pushing in the wires capped with multicolored switches.

"Hi, Honey, it's Daddy." He popped another 1 cc. It calmed the cocaine edge so he could talk slowly and rationally. In the Friday rush hour traffic, he had a good forty minutes before he got to Sunny's apartment.

"Hi, Daddy! Happy Birthday!"

"Thank you, Sweetie. It's not until tomorrow, but you're the first to wish me a happy birthday."

"Yayyyyyy!"

"I wonder whose birthday is next?"

"Tarrrrrrra's!"

"It is?"

"Yesssss!"

"And how old is Tara going to be?"

"Eight!"

"Oh, and are we going to have a bunch of boys over for Tara's birthday party and just sit around eating bugs and playing video games?"

"No! We're going to Castaway Cayyyyy! On the Disney boat!"

"That sounds like fun. Can I come too?"

"Daddy always has to work. Especially Friday nights."

"Oh, well maybe I can ask my big boss if I can take Friday night off."

"Okay! Then you can come too." There was a pause. "Are you coming home now?"

"No, Tara, it's Friday night and Daddy's on call. But I'll be home tomorrow morning before you wake up. Matter of fact, I'll wake you up with a kiss and pancakes in bed."

"Strawberry, please, with a chocolate smiley face."

"Well, as long as you said 'please'. Can I speak to Mommy, Honey?"

"Here she is. I love you, Daddy."

"I love you too, Tara. Tell Sammy I said hi." For the next five minutes, Richard Keith spun his wife a web about his day at the surgicenter and his upcoming shift at Regency Hospital that night. All the while, he mulled the upcoming week-long cruise to the Caribbean. Seven days of cruising, relaxing, playing with the kids in the pool, seeing a few sights, a couple of rum drinks. Leave from Cape Canaveral, down to St. Maarten. Savannah gets to shop her heart out in Phillipsburg, maybe they can fit in a rhino boat trip from Sapphire Bay and a day trip to Anguilla to see Mr. Benny. Then head back up to San Juan; there must be something to see on the Puerto Rico stop other than San Juan itself. Then comes the pièce de résistance, Castaway Cay for a Tara birthday special.

In Castaway Cay, nothing but fun for him and the two precious gems his beautiful wife has given him. Savannah can do a spa day while he and Tara and Sammy bake themselves to a perfect crisp at the Pelican Plunge and Spring-a-Leak. Then, while the girls wiggle their little tushies at the dance party with Lilo and Stitch, he and Savannah can grab a couples massage in one of those cabanas on the beach. *Speaking of baked, it's cooking time.* He reached over, found his one-hitter, and took a small toke of pakalolo. He was careful not to overdo it and end up coughing in his wife's ear. *Greedy greedy makes a hungry puppy.*

"Sounds like I'll be in the O.R. most of the night with a couple of leftover cases from today. With any luck, I should be able to catch some sleep around two or so. No, I'm not on trauma, but I am pulling all the non-trauma emergency cases. I should be home by 7:30, just in time to make pancakes for Tara and Samantha so you can sleep in. Yes, I sure will. Anything else? Okay, traffic's getting tricky, I'd better go. Love you too. Bye." He tapped the phone icon and turned his iPod back on. With the extra-dark window tint, nobody could see him, especially as the sun dropped below the pines in front of him. He raised his sun visor and thought out loud as he drove.

"Best thing I ever did, getting into Pain Management at the center. Better pay, easier work, and no O.R. time. Better yet, call is nothing but checking messages on my phone in the morning. 'If you need a refill of your meds, please call back Monday morning after 8:00 A.M. If you have a pain emergency, please go to your nearest emergency room.' And make sure they call your fucking primary care doctor for your 'pain emergency', not your pain anesthesiologist. Pain emergency. Are you kidding me? What is this world coming to?" He tapped 2 cc. in, saw that only one remained, said "What the hell," and finished with a quick plunge. The nod feeling came on; he sat back, relaxed, making sure he kept his eyes open and tapped the brakes from time to time. The feeling of deadness in his hands and face made him laugh.

"Friday night vacations. God I love 'em. Vitamin D, vitamin C, and vitamin Sunny. One from column C, one from column D, one from column S." With a quick twist, he removed the empty syringe and replaced it with a fresh one. *Number two.* His brain was still sharp, he was keeping track of the syringe count, so Richard rewarded himself with a 1 cc. bump. With the Disney trip all set in his mind and Savannah taking care of the barbecue plans for his birthday party tomorrow night--eight adults, twelve kids, and everyone within walking distance in case there was too much booze *(Duh, really?)* or the kids got too tired--he could focus on the upcoming festivities in Durham.

Start off with a quick, violent make-out session, reaching under her shorty kimono, the cerise one with the lime trim, to caress, then pinch, her tight little body. Then Sunny sticking out her hand, palm up. Very task-oriented, that girl. He drops the bullet into her hand, whereupon she goes into her bedroom, shuts and locks the door--as if he cares where she hides her stash--and refills his Friday night bullet from her "Party-Favor Pilfer Program for Poor Residents", her name for it, not his.

Then it's time for a special birthday dinner. Cold pearl sake with a frosty Sapporo and a perfect teppanyaki of shrimp and scallops, his favorite. Only after all her work is done in the kitchen will Sunny Sumiko Anderson allow herself to indulge in the vitamin C. She prefers hers in tidy thin lines on a mirror. A couple of those and it's off to the races; hungry angry vicious non-stop fucking for hours on end. Early on in their romance, if you could call it that, he'd tried to nod off. After all, he's almost forty. She shoved a fifty mg. Viagra into his mouth and pinched his lips together until he swallowed. Thereafter, he popped half a fifty just as he walked up the path to her apartment. She fucks his brains out until 2, then kicks him out. Thoroughly satisfied and ready for sleep, he drives the five miles to Regency and finds a call room to catch a few hours--with a 4 cc. bump to ensure deep sleep--before heading home.

He checked his dopp kit. Two strips of three Ultra-Thinz rubbers. After their first Friday night vacation, exactly six months ago, come to think of it, where all the coke-fueled fucking left him raw and bloody, he'd showed up the next week with rubbers. Sunny laughed at him.

"You stupid ass. Do you think I'd trust a horn dog like you not to knock me up? I've been on the pill since I was fifteen."

"I'm not worried about that. It's all the friction. My penis bled for three days. I told my wife I spilled some chemicals from work on my scrubs and they soaked through." Savannah had laughed and told him too bad he wasn't wearing a condom when the toxic spill occurred, and, oh, by the way, did he contact the EPA and request his willie be designated a superfund cleanup site? Anyway, she said, a few quiet nights would be nice. Richard had breathed a sigh of relief and slept like an unknowing baby. That is, until the few quiet nights turned into a few quiet weeks. After exactly thirty quiet nights, his very proper Georgia wife jumped his bones like a twenty-year-old fresh out of county jail. He'd already decided to include a six-pack of rubbers on the contents list of his Friday night vacations kit. The month-long dry spell from Savannah's sweet body hammered that idea in stone. "Thou shalt not fuck around unprotected, Dumbass."

After his explanation, Sunny said, "Poor little Richie's wiener, all scabby and sore." With that, she'd grabbed a pencil from the bedside table and snapped it across his Viagra-emboldened erection. Then she laughed again and climbed on top of him.

He took the exit onto I-40 west. Traffic was still crawling, and as the night lowered, he began to feel sleepy, so he snorted a little one from the bullet. He resolved, as so many Friday nights before, that from now on he'd wait an extra half-hour before leaving the surgicenter, to let the traffic die down, but he knew his impatience would betray him again and again. This was Sunny's last year of residency. Come July, she'd be heading back to Seattle and out of his life. When he'd find another resident with her cooking skills, her enthusiasm for marathon once-a-week sex and her access to pure vitamin C, well, by that time he'd need a hundred of Viagra just to get himself up out of bed in the morning.

That got kindly Dr. Keith musing on retirement. Probably around sixty, assuming the girls could find their way through college and grad school or else get married by then. He and Savannah could do some real traveling then. Keep the place in Raleigh or downsize and move to a condo closer in, near the university. Their place in Nag's Head would be paid off long before then, and they'd be well on their way to paying off the four-way share down in Naples.

The traffic continued to drag through the fall colors along I-40. He tapped his way through syringe number two & most of three. At the exit to the 147 he saw the reason for the sluggish pace. A Navigator, black or maybe just a dark color, in the late dusk it was hard to tell, lay on its side in the rain ditch. Richard's headlights lit up the reflection of a silver parking sticker on the back bumper. In the glare it was tough, but he thought he picked up the bright blue ID sequence: DW-957. The design looked eerily like the one on his bumper, the official doctor's parking lot permit that read DW-714. He grabbed his handy notebook and wrote down the sticker number. *I'll check it out with surgicenter security on Monday morning.* An MVA in a vehicle with a doctor's parking sticker was sure to get back to Medical Staff at the center, not to mention the state Board. Richard hoped it wasn't anyone from his group. That could really screw up his workload, especially the call schedule.

The ride up Durham Freeway took only ten minutes. He was parked outside Sunny's apartment complex in another five. After tapping in the final cc. from number three, he pumped in a few cc.'s of heparin to keep the butterfly from clotting. Then he curled the tubing setup around the needle site and covered the whole thing with a few wraps of royal blue Coban. It wasn't to hide his works from Sunny--she thought he was an idiot to go anywhere with an IV hanging out of his vein, but she didn't care, it wasn't her problem--but it kept it from getting caught on things during their bone-rattling gymnastic sessions. After removing his ammo holder, he shoved the dopp kit under the passenger seat, got out and started up the walkway.

God, tomorrow night's going to be so much fun. I can't wait to see what kind of birthday outfit Savannah's come up with. As he climbed the stairs two at a time, his heart quickened in anticipation of Sunny's embrace.

Everything went exactly as he imagined it, from the pink kimono to the outrageous sex, punctuated by hoovers from Sunny's mirror. Just as Richard began settling into an exhausted drowse, her bedside alarm went off.

"Time to go, Cowboy." She hopped out of bed and yanked the sheets off his naked body.

"Aw, come on, Sunny. It's my birthday. Just a couple of hours?"

"Not a chance. You know the rules." He got up and dressed in his scrubs. On the way to the front door, Sunny dropped the repacked bullet into his pocket. "Drive safely." In the open doorway, she kissed him, then pushed him away. "It's none of my business, but you might want to re-think your Friday night vitamin D playtime. That stuff can be dangerous, even in your experienced hands. Plus, the Board's always poking around anesthesia departments. Now go home to your family."

"That's why I only indulge on Friday nights. By the time the Board gets to me on a Monday morning, all the vitamins are out of my system. I appreciate your concern, but believe me, I'm very careful. It's all good." Sunny shook her head and closed the door.

Once out in the cool night air, Richard Keith woke right up. He realized the benefit of getting out of Sunny's apartment. A couple of hours of sleep at Regency and he'd be ready to drive home, twenty minutes tops on a Saturday morning. He loved the smell of Savannah on Saturdays when he bent over to wake her up with that first cup of coffee.

Fully awake, excited even, Keith hopped into his vehicle. He felt his heart pounding. There had been a few more lines tonight than usual; it would be tough to fall asleep like this. *It was sweet of Sunny to worry about me. She must think I'm taking a big risk.* He reached under the seat for his dopp kit. By the time he left the parking lot, the Coban was off his wrist and number four was attached to the hub of the butterfly tubing.

Richard got back on the 147. He figured he had about ten minutes before he got to Regency. Just as he was popping in the first cc., a deer appeared out of the woods on his right and bolted across the highway. He slammed on his brakes. Instinctively gripping, he pumped the entire syringe into his vein. He thought about pulling over for a few minutes, but decided that would be risky, he'd probably fall asleep; there was a good chance the Highway Patrol would stop and inquire.

To help keep awake, he turned on his iPod full blast. The guitar solo on "Sister Morphine" came through loud and jangly but, given Richard's circumstances, just a tad slow. He backed it up a few until "Start Me Up" came on. *That's it. Start me up, Baby.* Feeling friskier, he set the cruise control at fifty-five and started jiggling to the music to stay awake.

Sunny. Imagine her thinking I don't know my way around a syringe or two of Diprivan. If Michael Jackson had hired me instead of that cardiologist, he'd be on tour today. He stopped fighting the drug swirling through his bloodstream to his brain, and let his eyes close. *Just a few seconds won't hurt.*

"Single occupant, male, thirty to forty. He's breathing, but not moving otherwise; it looks like he's unconscious. Seat belt and shoulder harness are on, airbags deployed from steering wheel and passenger dash and door. Vehicle has minor damage to front end, is lying on its right side. Engine is not running, no odor of gasoline noted. That's right, northbound on 147, just south of exit 12A."

Keith heard the trooper's report as if from behind a cloud. He opened his eyes and turned his head toward the flashlight beam. His left hand was jammed at an odd angle into the lower spokes of the steering wheel; the butterfly tubing, still attached to syringe number four, dangled downward toward the passenger airbag. Dusty smoke floated in the air. *Must be the airbag propellant.* His clarity of thought felt reassuring.

"*Ah, shit, he sees the butterfly. Better go with the chemo story. Then again, after all that coke we did, probably doesn't matter what I say. Gotta keep Sunny's name out of this or she'll be screwed too.* He nodded his head toward the trooper and cleared his throat. "I'm okay, officer." *Looks like I'll be heading down to Atlanta for a six-month rehab stretch. Better call Steve Samuels today. I think he said his brother's family transferred to London for a year. If his place is for rent, Savannah and the girls can move in there so they can visit on the weekend. Or they can stay with her parents. Her mother's always liked me. I better take a look at the schools in that part of town.*

The state trooper climbed up onto the driver's side and reached down. As he yanked the door up and open, a new thought came to Richard Keith. *I wonder if that rehab clinic has any female residents.*

83. ANESTHESIA

Anesthesiologists are usually at or near the top of the list when it comes to physicians committing suicide, particularly by injection, right behind those crazy shrinks. Given their familiarity with the agents on which they usually overdose, you have to wonder whether they intend to kill themselves or simply get overconfident and accidentally O.D. Either way, the good news for you is that they virtually never kill themselves while on the job.

The word *anesthesia* is of Greek origin, *an* meaning "without", and *aisthesis* meaning "sensation". The goal of anesthesia is analgesia (pain relief), amnesia (no memory of the procedure), muscle relaxation, and unconsciousness. To achieve these goals, physicians will employ a single or multiple agents, including anesthetics (local or general), sedatives and hypnotics, muscle relaxants, paralytics, and narcotics.

If you can come up with a safe, effective way to relieve pain, the world will come running to your door. It's been that way for centuries. Except for the occasional oddball, no human prefers a painful procedure to a painless one. Likewise, if you can invent or discover an agent that gets people high, it will always be popular. Ironically, usually the discovery of the high precedes the use of the agent for nobler purposes.

Long before the Three Stooges were administering general anesthesia with a ball peen hammer, healers and physicians employed numerous herbal preparations. Alcohol, most likely in the form of beer, was used as an anesthetic at least as far back as 3000 B.C. in ancient Mesopotamia. While they may not have enjoyed perky barmaids in kilts, they did worship a goddess of beer by the name of Nin-kasi. Around the same time, the Sumerians, the dominant society in that region, began harvesting poppies for their opium content. In ancient Egypt, various plants, including the mandrake, were grown for the purpose of obtaining anesthetic compounds. In the Old Testament, mandrake root was referred to as the "love plant" because it allegedly enabled barren women to become pregnant. Mandrake is also the source of various hallucinogenic compounds, known as tropane alkaloids, including atropine, which is used in eye drop form for pupil dilation, and scopalamine, which is used in patch form to prevent motion sickness.

By around 300 B.C., the Chinese were probably using various herbal compounds to induce general anesthesia during procedures. During the Renaissance, European surgeons combined tropane alkaloids with opiates to induce general anesthesia. Inca medicine men reportedly chewed coca leaves and then spit into wounds to provide local anesthesia. Cocaine, the active ingredient in coca leaves, was isolated in the 1850's. It was used extensively for local anesthesia. At the suggestion of Sigmund Freud, cocaine was first employed in eye surgery by an Austrian ophthalmologist named Karl Koller in Vienna in 1884. Prior to that, eye surgery was extremely difficult to perform because of the involuntary blinking activity of the eye. Around the turn of the century, cocaine and opiate narcotics were first used via the intrathecal (inside the spinal canal) route to prevent surgical pain in a specific region of the body.

Early Arab writings mention anesthesia via inhalation. In the 13th century in Italy, a father-and-son team of surgeons perfected the "soporific sponge". A soporific is anything that causes sleep. They combined various herbal fluids, derived from mandrake root, hemlock and poppies. A sponge was placed in the mixture and allowed to absorb as much as possible. The sponge was then allowed to dry. Just before surgery, the sponge was moistened and held under the patient's nose, producing unconsciousness and analgesia.

The most famous general anesthetic, ether, was first synthesized in the Middle Ages. It was noted by Paracelsus in the 16th century that chickens who inhaled ether were rendered unconscious and felt no pain. Something that makes a lot of people a lot of money or something that makes a lot of people giddy will always be popular. It became a very popular recreational drug in the early nineteenth century. During Prohibition, ether, specifically diethyl ether, which could be inhaled or drunk, was extremely popular as an intoxicant. Its effect as an intoxicant is similar to that of alcohol, but more potent.

In 1772 Joseph Priestley discovered nitrous oxide. In 1799, Humphrey Davy, an inventor, inhaled some and began to laugh, so he nicknamed the compound "laughing gas". It was an immediate hit at "laughing gas parties" for the British upper class. Around the same time Davy discovered the analgesic (pain-relieving) properties of nitrous oxide, but more than four decades passed before it was first employed as an anesthetic in a surgical procedure, a dental extraction. To this day, nitrous oxide is still used as an inhaled general anesthetic, in both the operating room and the dentist's office.

Two major steps forward in the development of general anesthesia occurred in 1846 at Massachusetts General Hospital, a major teaching center for Harvard Medical School. William Morton, a Boston dentist, employed ether to induce general anesthesia in a patient who then underwent surgery to remove a tumor from his neck. The operating theater was later named the "Ether Dome". Shortly thereafter, Dr. Oliver Wendell Holmes, Sr. coined two terms, "anesthesia" for the state of unconsciousness, and "anesthetic" for the agents that cause it.

Chloroform, which most of us know as the stuff bad guys put on handkerchiefs to knock out hapless good guys and dizzy blondes in movies, was discovered in the 1830s. Almost immediately it gained worldwide popularity and played a starring role when Queen Victoria gave birth to Prince Leopold. Because ether explodes, makes you puke and leaves you with a terrible headache, and because chloroform kills people, both were gradually replaced by newer, safer inhalants. By the late 1960s, both agents were abandoned for surgical procedures. Of the older inhalants, only nitrous oxide is still widely used today.

When it comes to cardiac surgery, the optimal combination of anesthetics provides unconsciousness, muscle relaxation, analgesia and amnesia. In addition, you want to avoid anesthetics that cause arrhythmias and hypotension or hypertension. Because the situation is ever-changing during bypass surgery, especially when the bypass pump is used, anesthetics with a short half-life (stay in the bloodstream and have an effect for a shorter period of time) are preferred. That way, if something changes dramatically, the anesthetic can be replaced with another agent that will not worsen the situation. Every anesthesiologist has his preferred drugs to use in different situations. Some will use inhalants, some will use narcotics, some will use sedative/hypnotics.

The most important job of an anesthesiologist occurs before you enter the O.R. He'll review your chart, ask you a slew of questions, and examine you as part of his pre-anesthesia assessment. This is designed to identify risk factors for complications during and after surgery. He will focus on:

1. Your AIRWAY. He wants to be sure that if you have abnormalities of your upper airway (congenital abnormalities, dentures, previous surgery on your mouth or throat, radiation therapy), he can plan for them so that intubation is safely accomplished. Likewise, if you have pre-existing lower airway disorders (asthma, COPD, recent lung infections, any chronic lung diseases) he can employ anesthetic agents that won't make your lung problems worse; he'll be ready to use bronchodilators if necessary.

2. BLOOD status. He'll want to know whether your blood hemoglobin is normal, too high (polycythemia) or too low (anemia). He has to estimate the amount of blood that will be lost during the surgery. Toward that end, he'll ask whether you or anyone in your family has ever experienced excessive bleeding during surgery or in the course of normal activities like shaving. He'll need to know your blood type (O negative, A positive, etc.) and determine whether enough blood will be on hand for replacement should the need arise.

3. He'll want to know about CO-MORBIDITIES, pre-existing illnesses you may have, such as diabetes, heart disease, lung disease, anything that will require special treatment during surgery. He'll also perform a CLINICAL exam. This will involve recording your height and weight, listening to your heart and lungs, and reviewing your EKG and chest x-

ray. These will all play a role in his decision as to the types and dosages of anesthetic agents he uses.

4. He'll ask about DRUGS you are taking. This includes prescription and over-the-counter medications, alcohol, tobacco and recreational drugs. It is very important that you be open and honest about your use of the latter three. It could mean the difference between life and death. He'll ask about the DETAILS of previous surgeries and anesthetics you may have been given in the past. It is most important that you tell him about any allergies to medications, especially when it comes to those drugs he may administer during and after surgery.

5. He will EVALUATE the overall picture.

6. He will ask whether you are FASTING, and, if so, how long it has been since you last ate or drank anything. Again, it is vital that you provide honest answers to these questions. A full stomach provides far different risks than an empty stomach, and anesthesia must be tailored to your specific situation. If you don't believe me, just watch *The Verdict*. You don't want some personal injury lawyer making millions while you lie in a coma in a nursing home simply because you lied about the dozen donut holes you inhaled on the way over. He'll also make a determination of your FLUID status, whether you are well-hydrated, dehydrated from diuretics or starvation, or fluid overloaded because of kidney or heart failure.

7. He will GIVE an overall assessment of your physical status and GET written consent from you that allows him to give you anesthesia.

See what happened there? ABC's all the way through G. How fun is that? Ideally, this assessment should be done before you enter the O.R, but not more than a day or two in advance. If you are admitted to the hospital the night before, your anesthesiologist should see you that evening. Should you be admitted the day of surgery, he will probably perform his assessment in the pre-op waiting area. In the rare case of a life-threatening emergency bypass, he will interview you in the O.R. If you are already unconscious, he will attempt to interview any family members who are on hand.

Once in the O.R., the anesthesiologist will administer medications, either via inhalants through a mask or intravenously, to knock you out. This is called "induction of anesthesia". Once you are unconscious, he will use paralytics and/or other anesthetics for the purpose of putting an E.T. (endotracheal) tube down your throat. This is known as "intubation". Almost certainly he will place a large catheter into your internal jugular vein on the side of your neck. This is necessary for the administration of large volumes of fluids or blood products as needed, and can also be used to monitor the pressures in your heart. If you require any further intravenous anesthetic agents, and you will, he can give them to you through this catheter without reaching into the sterile operating field to get to the IV in your hand or arm.

Once things are underway, some surgical procedures require constant adjustment of fluids and meds to keep you stable, while others are relatively simple and require nothing more than the occasional re-dosing of the same meds to keep you out cold.

If your CABG is performed without the use of the bypass pump, i.e., "off pump", your anesthesiologist will be much busier than if your surgery is done "on the pump". If you are on the pump, the perfusionist--the pump runner--does a lot of the work to keep things stable, so your anesthesiologist may spend much of the time reading the stock tables, boning up on continuing medical education, searching for that special someone on Match.com or Ashley Madison, or playing Scrabble on his iPad. If your anesthesiologist is part of a recognized group practice at one or more hospitals, he's not wearing a multicolored headdress when he performs his pre-anesthesia assessment, and he's not taking the occasional hit off your nitrous oxide mask in the O.R., odds are he is in good standing and won't have any trouble getting you through surgery and into recovery.

References:

1. Patel, Piyush M., Patel, Hemal H., Roth, David M. "General Anesthetics and Therapeutic Gases." *Goodman & Gilman's The Pharmacological Basis of Therapeutics.* Ed. Laurence L. Brunton, Assoc. Ed. Bruce A. Chabner, Assoc. Ed. Bjorn C Knollman. New York: McGraw-Hill. 2011. 527-50.

84. CARDIAC SURGEONS

Heart surgeons, also known as TCV or thoracocardiovascular surgeons, tend to be the sharpest tools in the surgical shed. You might think that plastic surgeons would be the smartest, as they make women look more beautiful and are surrounded by large-breasted babes all day long, or eye surgeons, who make a fortune removing something smaller than a dime, but you'd be wrong. If you have to rely on a surgeon to treat a non-surgical condition, a TCV surgeon is your best bet.

No more do you see guys like Johnny Bench's TCV surgeon. He saw a spot on his lung and removed it. When it turned out to be coccidioidomycosis, a.k.a. valley fever, allegedly his comment was, "He was lucky. It could have been cancer." If the Hall of Famer were truly lucky, he would have ended up with a surgeon who knew how to work up a solitary pulmonary nodule in a non-smoker before he dove in and hacked out a perfectly good lung lobe. Then again, surgeons operate. That is what they are trained to do, and that is what they are paid to do.

Then again, had his routine physical exam by the team doctor not included a chest x-ray, which we know now is virtually worthless in asymptomatic patients, especially non-smokers, the spot on his lung would never have been detected and he would never have undergone surgery.

Then again, had he seen a physician in Phoenix or Tucson, they would probably have written off the spot as cocci, which is as common as dirt in those cities, and sent him home. Location, location, location.

Ironically, at the time, there were tests for tuberculosis and histoplasmosis, both of which were negative in his case, but apparently none for cocci. Now there is. Timing, timing, timing.

85. CAN YOU TRUST YOUR HEART SURGEON ?

In 1939, an Italian physician by the name of Fieschi sought a procedure to decrease the frequency and severity of anginal attacks in patients with coronary artery disease. He figured that if he ligated (sewed shut) the left the internal mammary artery (LIMA), which supplies blood to the chest wall, he would send more blood to the heart muscle via the coronary arteries and the collaterals. His results were much better than even he expected. Three-quarters of the patients had significant improvement in their anginal symptoms. One third were cured of all chest pain. LIMA ligations were adopted by numerous medical centers as a cornerstone in the treatment of angina.

Twenty years later, a group of heart doctors at the University of Washington in Seattle decided to critically investigate the value of the LIMA ligation procedure. They performed the LIMA ligation in eight patients. In the other nine, they performed a sham surgery; they made an incision in the patient's chest but did not ligate the LIMA. The patients who had the sham procedure had just as much relief of their symptoms as did the ones who underwent the real surgery. For more than thirty years, surgeons have overwhelmingly chosen to use the LIMA to bypass lesions in the left main and left anterior descending arteries.

Do you really need coronary artery bypass surgery? The question has been batted around by cardiologists and statisticians for decades. While there haven't been many big studies involving sham surgery vs. bypass surgery, there have been numerous studies pitting surgery against medical treatment for coronary artery disease. While every study tends to produce slightly different results, it is clear that bypass surgery is better than medical treatment for patients with significant disease in their left main coronary artery and for patients with significant three-vessel disease with angina. Likewise, if you are having a heart attack and an occluded vessel can be demonstrated, either bypass surgery or PCI works better than medical therapy alone.

Again, you will not fall into the hands of a cardiac surgeon unless your cardiologist thinks a bypass would be better than PCI or medical therapy. Additionally, your cardiac surgeon will have to agree with that assessment before he is willing to take you to the O.R.

References:

1. Cobb LA, Thomas GI, Dillard DH, Merendino KA, Bruce RA. "An evaluation of internal-mammary-artery ligation by a double-blind technic." *NEJM.* 1959. 260(22):1115-8.

86. THE SURGICAL SCRUB

The threads you wear into the O.R. are called "scrubs". This term does not refer to third-stringers on the high school football team. It probably has something to do with the fact that once you get into these clothes, you go and do the scrub. At this point you put on a surgical mask as well. The scrub consists of opening a sterile plastic pack which contains a sharp plastic arrow and a brush. Designed by Chairman Mao, the arrow was initially used to obtain information via the fingernails. The surgical powers-that-be adapted this to uncomfortably remove dirt from under the fingernails. Should a medical student or new intern employ the arrow in a manner deemed unacceptably wimpy, it is the prerogative of a senior surgical resident, or, more likely, a hoary old surgeon, to instruct said novice in the appropriate use of the arrow. While no longer intended for obtaining spy secrets, it can on occasion cause the removal of a fingernail. The so-called brush, in reality an array of short ice picks, has a foam rubber backing loaded with betadine, an iodine mixture that kills everything with which it comes into contact. If you are allergic to iodine, there are substitutes, but you will never escape the wussy label.

After making a show of picking every microbe from under every fingernail, you then proceed to the actual scrub. This particular form of betadine, known as betadine scrub solution, when mixed with a little water and scrubbed on your hands and forearms, produces copious mountains of foam. The foam is a bright mustard yellow, a shade or two more colorful than the bubbles you see after a wave recedes from a beach. Fish pee. You stand at a sink that can easily accommodate a human body and scrub away at your skin, every inch from your fingertips to your elbows, for a full ten minutes. If you go less than ten minutes, the invisible scrub watcher will know; giant superstrong mechanical Dr. No hands will descend from the ceiling and deposit you into the sink and hold you there. A river of betadine will flow from the wall and cover you for ten minutes. Scrubbing with betadine is bad, but drowning in it is worse.

The entire time you are scrubbing you must keep your hands up in the air above your elbows, so pit bugs won't roll down your upper arms and drip onto the sterility of your forearms. What if pit bugs crawl down from their cozy spots in your pits and then crawl UP your forearms? Again, if the craggy old chief surgeon sees you scrubbing with less than ferocious efforts and your epidermis isn't tumbling into the sink like shards from a punctured pink inner tube, he or the operating room head nurse--in the old days, Viking guys would turn over their most hated prisoners to the Viking gals--will proceed with a demonstration of how you get rust off a battleship. Then you rinse your hands, wrists and forearms with water from a faucet. Sterile water? Sterile faucet? Scrub with a sterile brush, using sterile soap, in a sterile manner, and then rinse with tap water?

Once you have rinsed, still with your hands held up *come il papa* before your masked face, you back your way through the swinging door into the operating room, where the motto has always been, *A chance to cut is a chance to cure.*

87. SCARECROW

"I can't believe we get to watch Dr. Naylor do a bypass! Did you know that Halsted wrote in his memoirs that Naylor was his favorite resident ever?" Ricky Gooch pulled off his tortoise-shell glasses and wiped them on the hem of his scrub shirt. When he put them back on, they slipped down on his nose. He reminded himself to get some of those ear things to hold them in place.

David Simmons sighed. "First of all, Naylor doesn't do bypasses. They're all done by Cartwright and Kaplan. This is a resection of a pulmonary artery aneurysm with a possible lobectomy. And no, I didn't know that Naylor was anyone's favorite anything. I can't imagine that. Have you ever been in the same room with him?"

"Not yet. But my granddaddy Venable came here for a thymectomy back about twenty years ago. He said Dr. Naylor was the best chest surgeon in Virginia."

"Your grandfather had a thymectomy?" Removing a thymus from an old man wasn't exactly your commonplace surgery. "What was that for?"

"He caught, I mean, he was diagnosed with myasthenia gravis at the age of 65. Dr. Naylor took out his thymus and everything got better. At least for three more years. Old Doc Randolph in Kenbridge said he could either come here to Dr. Naylor or else go see this one surgeon up at Johns Hopkins. If he went anywhere else, he might as well grab his Army .45 and spin the Russian roulette wheel." Ricky pushed his glasses back up. A couple of days ago, when the two fourth-year students were just starting their TCV Surgery elective, Simmons counted the number of times Gooch adjusted his glasses. Between 8 A.M. and noon, it came to one hundred eighteen.

"You might want to get some adhesive to put on your glasses so they stick to the bridge of your nose. How'd you keep them from falling down all the time when you assisted during surgery clerkship last year?"

"Aw, Dave, they were new last year. The hinge here on the left," he took them off and shoved them to within an inch of Simmons eyeballs, then wiggled both hinges repeatedly, "has gradually relaxed. I just need to get some of those ear things."

"You know, if you go over to that eyeglass shop next to Roy's Buddy Buddy on West Main and tell them you're a med student, they'll probably repair it for free."

Ricky eyes widened. "That's a great idea! Thanks, Dave." Simmons knew he'd never get there. At the end of the year, Ricky Gooch would certainly be voted "Most Likely to Forget to Graduate." Despite all his nervous energy and his high school reputation as the fastest sprinter in Lunenburg County, when it came to getting stuff done, he was always a lap or two behind everyone else. Some of his classmates just left Ricky to dangle in the wind and take his lumps. A small minority propped him up whenever they could. Simmons, ever the enabler, fell into the latter group.

David nodded. "Don't mention it. By the way, Robert Slaughter...".

Ricky gave David a look that said, *You know I don't understand Chinese.*

"...he's the TCV Fellow on Naylor's service this month. the guy in the long white coat who rounds with us every day?" The Gooch lad's mouth formed a perfect O. "He recommended we read the chapters in Sabiston on pulmonary artery aneurysms and lobectomies tonight. Naylor never talks to medical students, but Robert said he would pimp us a little, give Naylor the impression we know what we're talking about. As he put it, 'A chance to shine.' "

Through a frowny face, Ricky asked, "Does it have to be Sabiston? I have such a hard time reading it. The glare from those shiny pages makes my eyes tired."

"Read'em with sunglasses, then. Naylor wrote one of those chapters, I'm not sure which. He may not pimp us, but if you don't quote his chapter, he'll notice." Getting noticed by the chief of TCV surgery for the wrong reasons was never a good thing.

"Sure. Got it. Great idea, Dave. I'll do that tonight before I go to bed." Simmons had a vision of Ricky bursting into the Surgery Department Library at 5:00 tomorrow morning to skim the chapters before the procedure.

"And remember, Ricky. We have to be at the TCV O.R. scrub sink at 6 A.M. sharp. You don't want to be late."

"We get to scrub in?" Ricky pulled off his glasses and excitedly rubbed them again. For the first time, Simmons realized that he pulled them off by the left earpiece. *That might have something to do with Ricky's rickety hinge.*

"Scrub, but not in. According to Robert, Naylor insists on everyone scrubbing before coming into his OR. But don't count on getting to glove up. We're there just to watch."

"Okay, but I got dibs on Dr. Naylor's side of the table." *Not a problem,* thought Simmons. *I want to be as far away from that crabby old bastard as possible.*

That night, Simmons read each chapter twice, then went through a third time and wrote down everything he couldn't remember on 3 x 5 cards. He fell asleep reading them.

David arrived at the scrub sink ten minutes early. The only person more fearsome than Naylor was Mrs. Watkins, the O.R. supervisor. On their first day in the O.R., she personally instructed each and every third year medical student in the proper ten-minute scrub. It was basically lift your fingernails with a plastic pick, wash your hands with a betadine sponge for five minutes, scrub them with the abrasive side until they bled, then rinse away all evidence of the crime. Once you passed, she entered your name on a card in her file box, which resided permanently on a shelf above the scrub sink. Mrs. Watkins reached for the box and thumbed through the cards.

"Simmons, eh? Simmons, David, or Simmons, Thomas?"

"Thomas Simmons is in practice in Piney River. He graduated seventeen years ago, Ma'am." Like Naylor, Mrs. Watkins was getting on in years, and her memory was slipping, but it firmly retained the drill on how to squash a lowly medical student like a bug.

"I know that! Now get to work and show me you haven't forgotten how to wash your hands."

"Yes, Ma'am." Simmons dove into the task; the senescent supervisor barked commands when his technique wasn't up to snuff.

At 6:10, Ricky rushed in, red-faced and out of breath.

"I'm so sorry I'm late, Mrs. Watkins. I got lost coming from the Surgery library."

Old lady Watkins peered at him over her glasses. "I remember you. You're that Gooch boy from Victoria, aren't you?"

"Yes, Miz Watkins. My sister's married to Roland Payne, your cousin Henry's grandson."

"Oh, yes, that's right." David looked up to see the supervisor contorting her face into what passed for a smile. "How are they doing?"

"They moved over to Newport News this summer. Roland's a welder at the shipyard and Amelia's working as a secretary. They're going to have their first baby in a couple of months."

"How nice for them! Be sure to give them my best. Is your Daddy still a representative in the state assembly?" Ricky pulled off his glasses to clean them and nodded. "You tell him we surely appreciate all his committee's done for our hospital."

"Yes, Ma'am, I will." Ricky put his glasses on and reached for a scrub packet.

Son of a bitch, thought Simmons. *That's how he's managed to stay in school.* To put it mildly, there wouldn't be any Dr. Gooch delivering the valedictorian speech in May.

By six-thirty, both students were standing with their backs against the wall of TCV O.R. Number 2. The room supervisor, a fortyish woman named Michaels, gave them their instructions.

"Stand over there by the supply cabinet. You'll be able to see all the prep work by the team. When it's time to move in toward the operating table, I'll come over and let you know. I'll put a stepstool on each side of the table. If you use them," she smiled, "Dr. Naylor insists you keep your hands behind your back. Inside your scrub pants."

"In my pants?" Simmons made it a point not to question routines, but, even for an institution drowning in tradition, this one was way out there.

"In the past, some students on step stools have accidentally touched a sterile gown. He doesn't want any ungloved hands anywhere near the operative field. If you don't want to do that, you can try to see what's going on without a stool. I have to say, though, that unless you're 6' 5" or more, the step stool is the way to go." She raised her eyebrows.

Both students nodded. This was humiliating, but there was no point in trying to change a rule etched in stone. Except for Ricky pulling off his glasses a half-dozen times, they watched but didn't move much over the next fifteen minutes. The patient was rolled in on a gurney, the team slid him over to the operating table, and the anesthesiologist went to work with his syringes and catheters. Within two minutes, the patient was unconscious and intubated. The scrub nurse shaved the patient's chest and abdomen, then scrubbed everything with betadine. When Naylor walked in with his hands up in the Pope position, Miss Michaels supplied him with a sterile gown and gloves. After he moved into position, everyone else took their places. Robert Slaughter stood across the table from Naylor; he and the TCV Surgery chief pulled open the sterile drapes and laid them across the patient's body, leaving only the middle of his chest exposed.

Miss Michaels, who would serve as the O.R. float nurse, supplying instruments from the storage cabinets as needed, picked up two step stools and positioned them for David and Ricky. Then she waved the students over.

Simmons strode across the room to stand on the stool behind and slightly to the left of Slaughter, up toward the patient's head. After fiddling more than usual with his glasses, Ricky Gooch took up his position behind and to the right of Naylor. As if on cue, both students put their hands behind their backs. And into their pants.

As Robert Slaughter and Naylor worked, the TCV fellow threw a few questions Simmons' way. David had hoped to be able to refer to the 3 x 5's in his breast pocket, but he had only two hands, and they were doing time in the environs of his butt. Nonetheless, he did a fair job of knocking Slaughter's softballs for singles and doubles. Then Slaughter asked a question of Ricky. That's a hanging curve. Simmons thought, grand slammable. Ricky got it right, but then he kept on talking, right in Naylor's ear. The surgeon stopped exploring and looked up at Robert Slaughter for a good five seconds. Slaughter nodded. The pimp session was over.

To compensate for his handless situation, every minute or so the future Dr. Gooch tilted his head back violently, shaking his glasses back into the A position. Obviously he hadn't availed himself of glue, tape, the "ear things", whatever they were, or Simmons' advice. Once, on her trip around the table, Miss Michaels adjusted the glasses for him, then whispered in Ricky's ear. He nodded, but a couple minutes later, he resumed his spastic head jerk.

By this time, Naylor and Slaughter were deep inside the patient's thoracic cavity. A third-year surgery resident standing next to Naylor gently retracted the lung up and to the side, while an intern across the table yanked with all his might on the poor guy's mediastinum in the opposite direction. Some thoracic surgeons had progressed with the times and used a specialized spreader, a thoracic model of the "iron intern"; Naylor stuck with the tried-and-true methods, in this case the brute strength of underpaid minions. David craned his neck over Slaughter's shoulder as much as he dared, but still couldn't see any of the action. He looked at Miss Michaels as she walked by, but she just shrugged and shook her head. *Sorry, Bub. You're out of luck.* He realized Ricky's vantage point on Naylor's side of the table was far superior.

Ricky Gooch craned his neck as well. He began to wobble, and David thought, *Uh-oh, he's up on his tip-toes.* Suddenly he pitched forward.

His chest was stopped by Naylor's right shoulder, but his glasses continued on, flying straight for the action. They bounced off the mediastinal retractor and disappeared into the patient's thoracic cavity. Except for the anesthesiologist and the patient he was bagging, nobody moved or breathed. Simmons looked up to see Ricky staring down into the abyss whence his glasses disappeared, his chin resting firmly on the shoulder of Naylor's no-longer-sterile gown.

After about ten seconds of immobility, Ricky's head still perched like Blackbeard's stuffed parrot, Naylor reached in and retrieved something solid with his curved Kelly clamp. In a perfect 8 A.M. to 1 P.M. fly fishing backcast, he flung the tortoise-shells up and back, over his head. Accompanied by the Kelly, they slammed against the wall halfway up. Off came the offending left hinge and earpiece. Everything clattered to the ground and lay still.

Naylor looked straight ahead at Robert Slaughter. "Miss Michaels, I'll need a new gown and gloves." The supervisor grabbed a pack of each and came over to Naylor's side of the table. She gently pulled Ricky down off his step stool and steered him over to stand against the wall. Seemingly in shock, Ricky stared down at the two pieces of his glasses. Miss Michaels moved the stepstool off to the side and went about getting Naylor all steriled-up again.

Once re-gowned and re-gloved, Naylor turned back to the patient. Still nobody had moved. He requested and received a new curved Kelly. As he was about to dive back into the dissection, he said, "Miss Michaels, replace the scarecrow into a more stable position."

"Yes, Dr. Naylor." Michaels put the step stool back to where it had been. She then put a gown on Ricky, told him it wasn't to be considered sterile, and led him back to stand on the step stool. After positioning an IV pole on either side of him, she proceeded to wrap the excess gown shoulder material over the arms of the poles and clamped them in place with a couple of towel clamps. She bent over and locked the wheels on each of the poles. *Ricky hanging there*, Simmons had to admit, *does look like a scarecrow doing duty in the cornfield.*

The next three hours went along in silence. Every so often, one of the team would steal a glance at Ricky. For his part, though blind as a bat when it came to reading or distance vision, he kept his eyes locked on the operative field. After the skin incision was sutured, the patient was wheeled out to the ICU and everyone left the O.R. Simmons thought about leaving him there, but figured the cleaning crew wouldn't know what to do with him, so he came back and undid the towel clamps.

Ricky stepped down, peeled off his gown, and retrieved his glasses. They walked out together.

"So, how was it, watching Dr. Naylor ply his trade?"

Rickland Byrd Gooch wiped his glasses off, held them up to his eyes, and looked at David. "That was amazing. He really is the best chest surgeon in Virginia!"

Simmons patted Ricky's shoulder. "And the meanest."

Ricky nodded. "That too."

Simmons looked at his watch. "Hey, Ricky, it's only 11:30, and we don't have to be back until 1. Let's walk over to West Main and get your glasses fixed. Then we can get a hot dog and some cheese fries at Roy's. I'll buy."

"Boy, that would be great, Dave. Thanks."

"My pleasure. By the time we get back, you'll be a legend around here. I've never bought lunch for a legend before."

88. THE OPERATING ROOM

The O.R. (operating room) is like no other department in the hospital. In most places, you start out with a problem or a wound or a baby inside you and you are there to get help in healing it. In the O.R., you enter with an intact body and before you get to leave, a masked man is going to cut into you, sometimes remove body parts, and do a lot of sewing. Ironically, when you are admitted to the hospital for a CABG, or any surgery for that matter, most of the action and a large portion of your billing activity occurs while you are asleep. That may seem unfair. After all, you are on the hook for the bill, but everyone else gets to watch.

Once your cardiologist and your cardiac surgeon decide you need a CABG, sooner or later you will end up in the operating room. If you are a typical guy in your 40s or 50s, maybe even your 60s, there's a pretty good chance this is the first time you've undergone surgery.
Given the frequency that C-sections are being performed these days, if you are a woman, it's probably not your first time in this particular rodeo arena.

No matter how scary it is to contemplate being put to sleep and then having your chest cavity opened, it would be a lot scarier to have all that plumbing work done wide awake. Very few bypass patients scream like the turbaned saps in *Indiana Jones: The Temple of Doom* when the bad guy with the weird eyes and the goofy horned hat pulls their hearts out of their chests. At no point during the surgery will your heart be removed from your body. So don't worry about the surgeon donning some bizarre headgear, lifting your heart, still beating of course, over his head, and spouting a monologue of gibberish. It's not often a surgeon removes an organ, works on it, and then puts it back where he found it. Despite what Crazy Aunt Millie says, her cataract surgeon did not remove her eyeballs from their sockets, not even for a few seconds. That's why nobody refers to her as "Reliably Sane Aunt Millie". (Cut to Aunt Millie in the background, nodding her head and whispering, "Oh yes he did.")

In the business, your CABG surgery is referred to as a "cabbage". I could explain why, but my goal is not to belabor the obvious, so I'll let you figure that one out. When they first started doing these procedures in the 1960s, the common term for bypass surgery was "aortocoronary bypass" or ACB. Your friends or family members who have undergone a CABG will usually refer to it as a "triple bypass" or "quadruple bypass". This usually refers to the number of vessels that were bypassed. That seems a tad dramatic. Be a tough guy and just call it a "bypass". There is a certain nobility in acting like you've been there before. Besides, you might have the most life-threatening situation, severe left main disease, and require only two bypasses, one to the LAD and one to the CIRC, whereas a guy who requires five bypass grafts may have more lesions but each one is less than life-threatening.

How does your cardiac surgeon know how many bypasses you will require? When he goes over your cath films with your cardiologist, they'll look to see how many blockages there are. Then they'll look at each vessel just beyond the blockage, to see if each one is large enough to graft an artery or vein around the blockage. Tiny vessels with blockages usually can't be bypassed.

The strongest indications for a CABG are as follows:

1. Significant left main disease;
2. Significant 3-vessel disease involving the LAD, CIRC, and RCA;
3. Significant diffuse disease not amenable to any form of PCI;
4. Patients with CAD who have poor left ventricular function or diabetes mellitus.

What exactly constitutes significant disease? Historically, any vessel with a stenosis of fifty percent or greater is considered to be significantly narrowed. Patients in categories 1, 2, and 3 above will do better with CABG than with medical treatment. Some studies have looked at the subset of patients with stenoses of seventy-five percent or greater. If you employ this latter definition of significant disease, CABG surgery is much more effective at eliminating angina and preventing MI and cardiac death. When you talk about fifty percent stenosis, you are saying that the cross-sectional area of the coronary artery is reduced by one-half. That may show up on the cath images as the width of the dye being cut in half by a single plaque or it may appear as concentric narrowing by as little as twenty-five percent all the way around.

Say you have a normal coronary artery whose lumen is 1 cm. in diameter. The radius, R, is one-half the diameter. The cross-sectional area of the lumen of that artery is Pi R squared. One-half of 1 cm. is 1/2 cm. 1/2 cm squared is 1/4 square cm. Multiply that by Pi, which is 3.14, and you get a cross-sectional area of 0.785 square cm. If you have a plaque that takes up fifty percent of the lumen in one view, you have removed one-half of the lumen, and your cross-sectional area is now down to 0.392 square cm. However, if you have cholesterol or calcium buildup all the way around the arterial lumen, a thirty percent circumferential narrowing will reduce the cross-sectional area to 0.392 square cm. So a thirty percent narrowing, if concentric, can cause a fifty percent decrease in the cross-sectional area and the blood flow in a coronary artery. Thoroughly confused? Good. Now you know how it feels to be a physician reading a medical journal article and trying to figure out what all the numbers really mean.

The first CABG was performed in 1960 at Albert Einstein Medical Center in the Bronx. Dr. Robert Goetz and Dr. Michael Rohman inserted something called a Rosenbach ring from the cut end of the LIMA into the side of the RCA, and then tied sutures circumferentially around the ring. The actual bypass took less than a minute and did not require a bypass machine. When the patient died nine months later, at autopsy the anastomosis (the connection between the arteries) was still open, but a cholesterol plaque had occluded the LIMA above the anastomosis. It is reported that Dr. Goetz never performed another coronary bypass surgery.

In 1964, Dr. Vasilii Kolesov in Russia performed the first LIMA to coronary artery bypass using routine suture techniques. Over the next five years, he performed more than thirty coronary bypass procedures. While most of the anastomoses were sutured, he also pioneered the use of coronary artery stapling. His work was dismissed by both American surgeons and his Russian peers, who felt that surgery was not a viable option for the treatment of coronary artery disease. Fifty years later, now that robotic surgery is becoming more widespread, there is once again interest in stapling rather than suturing.

In 1967, Dr. Rene Favolaro of the Cleveland Clinic used a saphenous vein graft to replace a stenotic area in a patient's RCA. Basically, he cut out the narrowed area and inserted a piece of vein. Later he used the saphenous vein to bypass stenoses, in the manner widely used today. Since then, the CABG has been the mainstay in the treatment of coronary artery disease. According to the CDC, in 2010 almost 400,000 CABG procedures were performed in the U.S. So, even though you are the only one on the operating table, you are not alone.

For a routine, scheduled cardiac bypass procedure, you can usually check in the morning of the surgery. In the old days, you would come in the night before and have all sorts of blood tests, an EKG, and a chest x-ray. In most cases, everything would be fine, and you'd just lie in bed waiting to go to the O.R. Once in a while, some hospital would come up with a bright idea like, "Hey, why don't we put in a bunch of lines and catheters before you go to the OR? That way, you'll be all ready to go once you hit the O.R., and we can save time and money." As in most of medicine, but even more so when it comes to the O.R., time IS money. What they found was that the rate of infection in those lines and catheters went up, because the most sterile place in a hospital is the O.R., not the patient's room. Even worse, they found that it took much more time to perform these procedures on a patient who was awake. Thus, the OR staff would be standing around with their collective gloved thumbs up their collective butts while some poor schmuck was trying to stick something into a very anxious patient.

About the only time you should expect anything to be stuck into you while you are awake might be a Foley catheter if you've had a history of prostate problems or surgery or radiation. Then you might get a preop visit from a urologist. Even then, however, it is much easier to stick a Foley in a sleeping, relaxed patient than one who is awake and fidgety.

Like the visit to the cath lab, on your way to the O.R., expect to stop first at the billing office to sign a bunch of papers and fork over some do-re-mi. Then you usually go up to preop, where you are assigned to a numbered waiting alcove. Behind a curtain you will get undressed and don a hospital gown. The preop nurse may draw blood if it hasn't been done before, and she'll start an IV in your hand, forearm or antecubital fossa, the crease on the inside of your elbow joint. A tech will do an EKG to make sure there haven't been any changes since the last one. Much like before an execution, your visitors will be allowed to stop by and shed a few tears. Middle Eastern funeral wailing is discouraged. Your surgeon may stop by, unless he is already in the O.R. When it's your turn to bat, your nurse will wheel you in to the O.R., where a throng of gloved and masked people are waiting. It's not a good idea to watch the *Twilight Zone* episode "The Eye of the Beholder" or the movie *Johnny Got His Gun* before coming to the hospital for any type of surgery.

Once in the O.R., you'll be assisted in sliding from the preop gurney to the O.R. table. If it's cold in there, and often it is, you'll be covered with warm blankets ("Ahhh"). The anesthesiologist usually serves as the Master of Ceremonies, and your surgeon might be there to say "Hi, Patient!" before he heads out to scrub. Since he and everyone else in the OR is wearing a mask (they better be), you'll have to take the masked man's word as to his identity, because unless he operates with an eye patch or has Groucho eyebrows. nobody is truly recognizable behind a mask. That's why cartoon bandits wear those silly hankies with the eye-holes in them.

At this point, the anesthesiologist tells you to count backwards from one hundred. There are a multitude of anesthetic agents available for use during cardiac surgery. When you think of anesthesia, probably you picture yourself inhaling some sort of gas from a mask held over your face by another guy with a mask, presumably--hopefully--an anesthesiologist. While there is a wealth of anesthetic agents available for IV use, some anesthesiologists still use the gas type. Some guys use narcotics, like morphine or fentanyl, some use benzodiazepines from the Valium family. Another popular anesthetic for bypass surgery is propafol, which is the medication that killed Michael Jackson. Fortunately for you, The King of Pop's physician won't be administering it, and, better still, the guy who's using it on you knows what he's doing.

Once you are unconscious, the anesthesiologist puts a mask on your face, bags you a couple of times with an ambu bag, and injects some muscle relaxant/paralytic. This is to keep you from puking all over him when he goes to intubate you. He'll take an endotracheal (ET) tube, lube it up, and put in a stylet to allow him to direct it. He'll gently tilt your head back, insert the laryngoscope into your mouth and down your throat; way down. It's a good thing you're not awake for this part.

The laryngoscope has a long smooth blade to open up your upper airway and a light that allows the anesthesiologist to see where he's shoving that smooth blade. Once he sees your vocal cords, he will slide the ET tube down through your vocal cords into your trachea. When it is in the correct position, out comes the laryngoscope. He'll inject some air into the cuff, a balloon at the end of the ET tube that helps to hold the tube in place and prevent aspiration of vomit into your lungs, and remove the stylet. Then he'll bag you a few more times through the ET tube. Now your airway is secure and the rest of the O.R. staff can get to work.

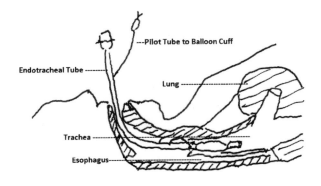

BAC/FMP

You will require a Foley catheter so that your bladder can empty. You might require a fair bit of IV fluids for various reasons, the usual being to boost your blood pressure. Some of the anesthetic agents may cause urinary retention; to prevent your bladder from exploding, the catheter will allow free drainage of urine as it accumulates. It also keeps your urine from dripping down the side of the operating table, where quick-moving O.R. staff would slip in it. In addition, it is much easier to keep track of how much urine you are producing. If your kidneys are not processing fluids properly, diuretics can be administered to prevent fluid overload to your heart and lungs. During the surgery you want fluids going in and fluids coming out, and you want to keep track of both.

Often the Foley catheter is inserted by an OR tech or nurse. He will swab the head of your penis with betadine solution. If you are uncircumcised, he will have to retract the foreskin. Then he will shove the catheter into your penis, through your urethra, past your prostate gland and into your bladder. Once the tip of the Foley is in your bladder, he will fill the balloon at the tip with saline via an injection port. The balloon is there to prevent the catheter from falling out. Then the catheter is connected to a plastic bag with volume calibration. This bag is hung below the level of your bladder to enhance gravity drainage.

Occasionally the catheter is placed by an OR nurse who volunteers for Foley duty, especially the difficult insertions. Call her Brunhilde. She may have issues. On your way into the OR, if you notice a stout woman with a shoe horn and hammer, be concerned.

The anesthesiologist will place a central line in your internal jugular (IJ) vein. In experienced hands, this takes about ten seconds. Sometimes rookies will miss the IJ and accidentally stick the carotid artery, the main artery supplying oxygenated blood to your brain. That is undesirable at best. Depending on the size of the catheter, it can cause a small temporary leak in the carotid, a big longer-lasting leak resulting in a big hematoma, or complete obstruction of the carotid. Most experienced anesthesiologists have placed hundreds, if not thousands, of IJ catheters. Through this single catheter, fluids, blood products and medications can be administered. He can also insert a Swan-Ganz catheter, which measures pressures in your heart and allows him and the surgeon to make decisions on administration of fluids and meds.

A respiratory therapist or a cardiovascular tech will place a small catheter in your radial artery, which is located on the volar (palm) side of your wrist near the base of your thumb. This is one of those procedures that is much easier for the therapist to accomplish, much less painful for you, and much less stressful for both when you are anesthetized rather than awake. This catheter will allow your blood pressure to be continuously monitored in real time, making the traditional blood pressure cuff unnecessary. If things get dicey, it is also an excellent source of arterial blood, which can be used to measure your oxygen level, your carbon dioxide level, and your acid-base status.

A nasogastric (NG) tube may be inserted through your nose, down your esophagus and into your stomach. This, when placed to suction, will remove gastric secretions and help to prevent aspiration, whereby stomach contents come up through the esophagus and down your trachea into your lungs. It will also keep your stomach and part of your small intestine from getting too bloated. Some of the older anesthetic agents can cause abdominal swelling.

If required, the assisting surgeon, usually a general surgeon or a physician's assistant, will harvest one or both of your greater saphenous veins. Often one is enough. The longest vein in your body, it runs from your ankle up the medial (inner) aspect of your calf and thigh to your groin. In the old days, it was harvested by opening your entire leg from ankle to thigh, tying off both ends, and removing the vein intact. Nowadays it is removed much more quickly and safely by inserting a scope at one end, running the scope up inside the leg, tying off the vein top and bottom, and removing it intact with the scope. Instead of a long scar, you end up with two or three tiny scars.

The assisting surgeon may also perform the sternotomy, whereby he opens your chest with a scalpel and saws through your sternum (breast bone) with an electric bone saw. *Say what?* Then he'll insert the Iron Intern, a sternum spreader that allows better visualization of the heart. Prior to the invention of said spreader, medical students and interns were required to pull on metal retractors for the entire duration of the surgery. God help you if you let it slip at a crucial point in the procedure. As a surgeon, you knew you'd made the big time when you came up with a retractor (which, of course, you named after yourself) that was used by other surgeons on a regular basis.

"Hand me the Montgomery Deaver, Marge."

By this time your surgeon should have finished his scrub, re-entered the OR and been gowned and gloved. Then he gets to work. Usually it has already been decided whether your procedure will be "On Pump" or "Off Pump". In the past, virtually all cardiac surgery was performed "On Pump". Your heart was chilled and paralyzed so it didn't beat. Your blood was taken from the right side of your heart and run through an oxygenator, in lieu of your lungs, and a pump, in lieu of your heart. Together these were referred to as the cardiopulmonary bypass machine, or heart-lung machine. Then the oxygenated blood was returned to your body through a tube inserted into your aorta.

The heart-lung machine is run by a fellow known as a perfusionist, because he is responsible for perfusing your body with oxygenated blood. Generally, this makes the anesthesiologist's job easier: he can peruse the stock tables while the perfusionist perfuses your body. The benefit of this "On Pump" procedure is that the heart is easier to work on, i.e., a target standing still rather than a moving target. The biggest drawback is "pump head", whereby the patient suffers foggy thinking and memory loss, either transiently or permanently. "Off Pump" or beating heart surgery, which was developed in part to combat pump head, involves sewing the bypass grafts onto the heart while the heart is still beating. No bypass machine (thus, no perfusionist), no chilling or paralyzing the heart, less severe brain damage. Since the heart is still beating, surgeons will often use a pair of devices, one to position the heart for the best possible exposure, the other to temporarily stabilize the part of the heart being operated on. About two-thirds to three quarters of all CABG procedures are still done on pump.

There is a great deal of debate among heart surgeons as to which method to use. Some surgeons perform almost all of their procedures off pump. Others use the off pump method only as a last resort. How do the rest decide? Maybe it's a matter of best-of-three rock-paper-scissors.

Or maybe:

Referee: "Doctor Peterson, call it in the air."
Surgeon: "Heads."
Anesthesiologist: "Come on, tails!"
Perfusionist: "Come on, tails!"
Referee: "Heads it is."
Surgeon: "Off pump."
Anesthesiologist: "Rats."
Perfusionist: "Ditto"

If you are undergoing on-pump bypass, the surgeon will stick one needle-catheter into the superior vena cava, which drains the brain and upper body, and one into the inferior vena cava, which drains the lower portion of the body. This will allow blood to be drained from the venous system. Alternatively, a single venous catheter is inserted into the right atrium. A third catheter will be inserted into the aorta just above where it exits the heart, to allow blood to return to the body in an oxygenated state. Basically the blood is removed via the venous system, pumped through an oxygenator, and then returned via the arterial system. Fluids and blood products are used to prime the pump so that air is not returned to your body.

Once the bypass machine has begun operating, no more blood will pass through your heart. The body's temperature is brought down to prevent damage to other organs. The aorta is cross-clamped and cold fluids with high levels of potassium are infused into your heart. The potassium causes your heart to stop beating. That's right, your heart does not beat during the procedure. Since no blood is running through the coronary arteries, if the heart were to beat, the heart muscle would become ischemic and eventually die. That would tend to thwart the efforts of everyone involved. Often, cold fluids are applied directly to the heart to ensure that all parts of the heart are cooled. In some cases, the body is not cooled, but, except for the simplest forms of bypass surgery, this tends to lead to increased complication rates. Blood is thinned with heparin to prevent it from clotting while it is outside the body.

The surgeon can now begin sewing in the bypass grafts. The basic idea is to place a graft from the aorta to the coronary artery distal to (beyond) the blockage. Thus, blood can run through the bypass graft freely rather than stalling at the blockage. For blockages in the left anterior descending artery, most surgeons will free up your LIMA, which has been studied for patency during the cardiac cath, and attach the free end to the target artery just distal to its blockage. Occasionally your RIMA will be used for right coronary artery bypasses. For other blockages, the saphenous vein is used.

Once the grafts are all sutured and shown to be watertight, your body can be warmed, the aorta cross-clamp can be removed, and all blood returned to your body. After your heart starts pumping again, the venous and arterial cannulas are removed. The grafts are checked for flow and stability. If your blood is too thin, it may be treated with protamine, which is designed to reverse the effects of heparin. The pericardium is sutured, large drainage tubes are placed in your mediastinum and sutured in place so that they exit your body just below your solar plexus. Your sternum is wired back together and the surgeon or his assistant will place either staples or subcutaneous sutures, which lie underneath the surface of your skin and will dissolve. All anesthetics are discontinued and you are slid onto a gurney with all your tubes, lines and catheters. Most likely you will be bagged by the anesthesiologist as you are whisked away on your steel and wheeled magic carpet to the CVICU.

References:

1. Ressler, Ladislaus, Rubens, Fraser D. "Cannulation Techniques for Cardiopulmonary Bypass." *Atlas of Cardiac Surgical Techniques.* Ed. Frank W. Sellke, Ed. Marc Ruel. Philadelphia: Saunders. 2010. 12-24.
2. Konstantakos, Anastasios, Sellke, Frank W. "On-Pump Coronary Artery Bypass Grafting." *Atlas of Cardiac Surgical Techniques.* Ed. Frank W. Sellke, Ed. Marc Ruel. Philadelphia: Saunders. 2010. 29-44.
3. Pusca, Sorin V., Puskas, John D. "Off-Pump Coronary Artery Bypass Grafting." *Atlas of Cardiac Surgical Techniques.* Ed. Frank W. Sellke, Ed. Marc Ruel. Philadelphia: Saunders. 2010. 47-60.
4. Vassiliades, Thomas A. "Endoscopic and Traditional Minimally Invasive Direct Coronary Artery Bypass." *Atlas of Cardiac Surgical Techniques.* Ed. Frank W. Sellke, Ed. Marc Ruel. Philadelphia: Saunders. 2010. 61-80.
5. Morrow, David A., Boden, William E. "Stable Ischemic Heart Disease." *Braunwald's Heart Disease.* Ed. Robert O. Bonow, Ed. Douglas L. Mann, Ed. Douglas P. Zipes, Ed. Peter Libby, Ed. Eugene Braunwald. Philadelphia: Elsevier Saunders. 2012. 1239.
6. Sabik, Joseph F. III, Lytle, Bruce W., "Coronary Bypass Surgery." *Hurst's The Heart.* Ed. Valentin Fuster, Ed. Robert A. O'Rourke, Ed. Richard A. Walsh, Ed. Philip Poole-Wilson. New York: McGraw-Hill. 2008. 1504-5.

7. Konstantinov IE "Robert H. Goetz: the surgeon who performed the first successful clinical coronary artery bypass operation" *AnnThorac Surg.* 2000. 69(6):1966-72

8. Haller JD, Olearchyk AS "Cardiology's 10 greatest discoveries" *Tex Heart Inst J.* 2002. 29(4):342-4

9. Berry D "History of Cardiology: Vasilii Ivanovich Kolesov, MD. The story of a pioneer in coronary artery bypass surgery" *Circulation.* 2007. 116(23):1136-8

10. Olsen DB "Dr. Rene Favaloro" Artif Organs 2012. 36(6): 501-4.

11. Captur G "Memento for Rene Favaloro" *Texas Heart Inst J.* 2004. 31(1):47-60.

89. THE VINEBERG PROCEDURE

The Vineberg procedure has been performed on as many as fifteen thousand patients worldwide. Developed by Arthur Vineberg, a cardiac surgeon at McGill University in Montreal, and first employed in the late 1940s before coronary arteriography was widely available, it involved freeing up the LIMA and implanting it directly into the muscle of the heart's left ventricle. Although not universally accepted by the cardiologic and cardiac surgery communities, it did relieve angina in many patients. Once coronary arteriography was available, it was possible to demonstrate that the procedure increased blood flow in the distal portion of the left anterior descending coronary artery.

You would think that cutting an artery and shoving the business end of it into a muscle would cause a lot of blood to leak out around the insertion area or cause a big blood clot. In fact, it is not uncommon to cut an artery and have no bleeding at all, at least for a while. That's because the wall of the artery has a layer of smooth muscle, the tunica media, sandwiched between the outer tunica adventitia and the inner tunica intima. When the artery is transected, or cut at a ninety-degree angle, the muscular layer constricts, narrowing the lumen of the vessel. If the artery is cut at an angle, the muscular layer is disrupted unevenly and thus can't constrict adequately. Surgeons have long noted that a freshly cut artery will not bleed for anywhere from a few minutes to over an hour.

In addition, it turns out that the coronary arteries send out perforator branches that penetrate the heart muscle and bring blood (and, of course, oxygen and glucose) to the muscle cells that lie beneath the surface of the heart.

So basically, Vineberg freed up the LIMA from the chest wall, cut the end, tied off the end of the LIMA, dug a tunnel in the heart muscle next to the LAD, and made a small hole in the side of the LIMA closest to the LAD. Then he shoved the LIMA into the tunnel and sutured it in place. His theory, which he tested on animals from 1946 to 1950, was that blood would flow from the hole in the LIMA into small vessels known as sinusoids, and thence into the LAD. There was no actual surgical connection between the LIMA and the LAD. This was all done before he could even visualize the LAD through angiography. He just knew that people with bad angina tended to have disease in their LAD at autopsy.

After undergoing the Vineberg procedure, patients tended to have good relief of their angina. Somewhere between ten and twenty thousand Vineberg procedures were performed between 1950 and 1975. One study from the 1970s showed that, seven to ten years after surgery, three-quarters of the LIMA's were still open and forty percent were filling a major coronary artery. Once cardiac surgeons had cardiac caths available to better define the coronary vessels, the results improved; about ninety-five percent of Vineberg LIMA's were open at seven years after surgery. One patient who underwent the Vineberg procedure using both the RIMA and LIMA was found to have both grafts open and functioning exactly as normal coronary arteries. Twenty-seven years later.

References:

1. Shrager JB. "The Vineberg procedure: the immediate forerunner of coronary artery bypass grafting." *Ann Thorac Surg.* 1994. 57(5):1354-64.
2. Michaels AD, Chou TM. "Images in cardiology. The Vineberg procedure." *Heart.* 1999. 82(5):569.
3. Marx R, Jax TW, et al. "Vineberg graft: flow reserve of bilateral implantation after 27 years." *Ann Thorac Surg.* 2001. 71(1):341-3.
4. Raftery EB, Oram S. "Evaluation of the Vineberg Procedure." *Brit Heart J.* 1969. 31(3):389.

90. RECOVERY

O.R. time is very expensive. For most surgical procedures performed in a hospital, once your surgical wounds are closed and dressed, you are moved to a gurney, then wheeled to the recovery room. After cardiac surgery, you bypass the recovery room and go directly to the CCU (Coronary Care Unit) or the CVICU (Cardiovascular Intensive Care Unit), known collectively as "the unit". Usually these units also hold nonsurgical patients admitted for ACS or MI. Some places have a separate ICU solely for heart surgery patients. Henceforth we'll lump them all together and call it the CVICU. Most cardiac surgeons do not want their nice clean bypass patients in the medical-surgical ICU with general surgery patients, featuring open or infected wounds, or medicine patients, with pneumonia, gangrenous limbs and MRSA.

Usually you will arrive in the CVICU still anesthetized, as the anesthesiologist would prefer you not awaken and start gagging on your ET tube in the hallway or the elevator; that makes for an awkward, aesthetically unpleasant situation. Anesthetized means asleep and still intubated. Usually the anesthesiologist and/or respiratory therapist will be bagging you, i.e., using an ambu bag to push oxygen through your ET tube into your lungs. If you are already breathing spontaneously when you reach the unit, there is a most excellent chance that you will be extubated (have the ET tube removed) just before or just as you awaken.

If you are not breathing on your own, you will continue to have your ventilation assisted until you awaken. Sometimes you will require assistance with your breathing for a longer period of time on a ventilator. A wealth of information is available in textbooks and journals on the variety of ventilators available and all the clever ways they can be utilized, but the important thing is that a ventilator is nothing more than a machine to push oxygen into your lungs at a predetermined rate, volume and pressure. Although major changes for the better have been made over the past few decades, breathing with a ventilator when you are awake is not like normal breathing. Some patients can relax and go with it, while others just never get the hang of it and have to be sedated so they don't fight the vent. Sedation tends to prolong the time you are on the vent, which is a bad thing. The longer you are on the vent, the greater the risk of infection, pneumothorax (collapsed lung), and blood clots. If they don't kill you, all of these complications will prolong your hospital stay.

Especially if your surgery involves the bypass machine, there is a good chance you will experience transient myocardial depression (TMD). This phenomenon, characterized by dysfunction of your ventricles, usually occurs within the first four hours after bypass is completed. Most of the time it is something detectable only through echocardiogram or nuclear imaging. Occasionally your blood pressure will fall, requiring medications to give it a boost. There are lots of theories about the cause of TMD: capillary leakage, warming from your hypothermic state during bypass, bleeding into your mediastinum, and inflammation. The fact that it seems to occur more after on-pump procedures than after off-pumps suggests that inflammation caused by exposure to the bypass machine and recovery from your cool-down may be the key players.

Although massive post-op mediastinal bleeding requiring transfusions of more than ten units of blood occurs in only three to five percent of cases, like all "rare" complications, if it happens to you, it's a big deal. Because exposure to the bypass machine has a tendency to lower your platelet count and inactivate the ones remaining, patients done off-pump have a lesser chance of requiring transfusions.

Your lungs are the commonest cause of morbidity (illness) in the first forty-eight hours after surgery. When you are on the bypass machine, your pulmonary arteries and veins are not perfused by blood, and your lungs are allowed to collapse. When you come off the bypass machine and your lungs are reperfused, they are reinflated with oxygen and you start to breathe on your own. In most patients a certain degree of collapse, called atelectasis, remains. While this usually doesn't cause a problem, in some patients vigorous suctioning of their lungs is necessary to get their blood oxygen saturation levels up to normal ranges. In chest and abdominal surgery, atelectasis is the commonest cause of fever in the first twenty-four hours postop. Other common causes after bypass surgery include pericarditis (inflammation of the outer lining of your heart), pleuritis (inflammation of the outer lining of your lung), and blood clots in your veins, particularly in your legs and pelvis.

Once you awaken, you will meet one of the most important people in terms of your survival and your length of stay. That would be your nurse. More accurately, you will meet the nurse assigned to care for you. Her job is to give you the best possible care so that, once again, you can get out of the hospital as quickly as you can. Her job does not consist of catering to you or your family. That is a subtle but important difference, and it is truly baffling how many patients and families do not grasp it. There is a significant portion of the American public that thinks of a hospital as a hotel with nurses.

Except when you are sleeping, the goal is increasing activity first, preventing complications second, and providing comfort third. While numerous experts will tell you that a comfortable patient is more likely to recover well, when it comes to recovery from surgery, you would much prefer a bare-bones hospital with a shorter average length of stay (LOS) over a plushy one with a longer LOS. The longer your length of stay, the more the complications. The first thought you want to have when you wake up after the surgery is to get your ass out of the hospital as soon as possible. Your nurse is the single best person to help you achieve that.

When it comes to patient behavior around nurses, the rules are simple:

1. Do what your nurse tells you to do.
2. Keep your hands to yourself.
3. Don't poop in the bed.

Whether you are awake or still anesthetized, as soon as you arrive in the CVICU, your nurse will begin an assessment of your body and your lines. The lines consist of a central venous catheter, usually located on the side of your neck and running through the internal jugular vein. The IV catheters that are inserted into a vein in your hand or forearm are known as peripheral lines. There are probably several IV bags running into the various ports on this central line. There is usually some type of chest tube or mediastinal tube hooked up to suction, to drain blood from your wound and prevent your lungs from collapsing. You may still have an ET tube running into your mouth to breathe for you. There may be an NG (nasogastric) tube entering your nose and ending up in your stomach, designed to suck out excess gastric secretions and air until your guts start working again. There is probably an arterial line in one of your wrists. There is almost certainly a Foley catheter draining urine from your bladder. There may be compression hose on each leg to prevent blood clots, and in some cases these have tubes connected to air pumps. The nurse has to check each one of these lines and make sure everything is connected correctly and working as designed.

Visitors usually are not allowed in until the nursing assessment is completed. The pushier your visitors are to get into the room, the longer they will end up waiting. Advise your visitors that the nurses pretty much run the show 24/7 until you leave the hospital. It's set up that way because they know what they are doing.

Once you are fully awake and breathing on your own, if your ET tube has not been removed, the respiratory therapist will deflate the cuff around it. The cuff is designed to keep the tube in place in your windpipe (trachea) and prevent stomach contents from regurgitating into your lungs (aspiration), which can cause pneumonia and/or death. Then he'll pull the tube out. As the tube comes out, prepare to cough and gag a bit. This is an uncomfortable process, but you'll live. Depending on how thin your blood is and how long the ET tube has been in, a trail of clots, crust and disgusting slime may follow it out. If you ask nicely, you may be permitted to keep your ET tube as a souvenir. Afterwards, the RT will set you up with supplemental oxygen, usually via nasal prongs.

If you have pre-existing lung disease, or if your surgery required a thoracotomy (causing a lot of pain that restricts your breathing), or for some other reason you are not breathing well on your own, you may have to stay on the ventilator for a few hours or overnight. If you have severe lung disease or experience any of a number of complications during surgery, you may be on the vent for a week or more. Before the tube is pulled, you will be given a chance to breathe on your own through the ET tube. If that works, then your ET tube can be pulled. It is much better to leave the ET tube in for a while than to pull it prematurely; if the tube is out and you start having significant difficulty breathing, someone will have to sedate and paralyze you and reinsert it. That move counts as a major screw-up when it comes to the insurance companies and regulating agencies like JCAHO, not to mention that any time you have to be reintubated, there is a slim but definite chance of serious complications. If you have to remain on the ventilator overnight or longer before you get extubated, there is a good chance you will have to undergo testing of weaning parameters.

THE WEANERS

Weaning parameters are a series of torture maneuvers disguised as measurements to determine how well you can breathe on your own. Over the past few decades, they have been shown to predict who will breathe well spontaneously and who will not. First, the respiratory therapist turns off the ventilator. Then he or she measures your respiratory rate, which is the number of times you breathe per minute. The more effective you are in bringing oxygen into your lungs, the more slowly and deeply you can breathe. He then looks at the oxygen saturation of your blood. This is measured by that hinged plastic clip on the tip of your finger, or, if you still have one, the catheter in your radial artery. Normal healthy patients have an oxygen saturation above ninety-five percent. Yours should be at least ninety percent on a standard amount of supplemental oxygen. Then they look at your tidal volume, which is the volume of oxygen you take in with each breath. If you are in pain you will tend to take in less with each breath, and your breathing will be shallow and rapid. Then, if all this stuff is in line with guidelines, you may undergo a measurement of your negative inspiratory force, or NIF.

Literally and figuratively, the NIF sucks. It looks awful and it feels worse than it looks. The respiratory therapist disconnects your ET tube from the ventilator tubing, then he connects a gauge to the end of your ET tube. The gauge measures how hard you try to suck air into your lungs. Your job is to inhale when there is literally nothing to inhale. Patients have likened it to trying to breathe with a very thick, very stiff plastic bag shoved down their throat. Many of them thought they were going to suffocate during the test, which lasts only a few seconds but feels like an eternity. It is much easier to make less of an effort to inhale, but if you go that route, you will most likely fail the NIF. It may be six or twelve or twenty-four hours before you get another try, and then you'll have to do the NIF again. The longer you are on the ventilator, the more likely complications will occur. In addition, your in-hospital recovery and rehabilitation can't begin until you are off the ventilator and breathing on your own. Suck it up.

If you have any degree of COPD and continued to smoke up to the day of surgery, right about now you are wishing you'd quit years ago. When you are awake, every minute on the ventilator seems like an eternity, doesn't it? Four words, Bub. I told you so.

Once you are off the ventilator, you may be placed on supplemental oxygen via nasal prongs for a day or so. These are much more comfortable than a mask, but can still be annoying. If they dry out your nostrils too much, the nurse can place some antibiotic ointment in your nose. With these on and a mobile oxygen tank, you can move around.

LET'S GET THE SHOW ON THE ROAD

The life of a newborn is basically eat, sleep, poop. Your life on the first postoperative day is pretty much the same thing, without the eating or pooping. There are a number of reasons why you will feel weak and tired. First, depending on how fast you metabolize and excrete the anesthetics used during surgery, you may have a bit of a drug hangover. When you come out of heart surgery, or any surgery for that matter, you might be volume-depleted (dehydrated). If you've ever experienced significant dehydration, you know that your energy level is pretty low. In addition, the surgical procedure and the anesthetics may temporarily screw up your autonomic nervous system (ANS).

Normally when you sit up or stand up, gravity causes blood to pool in your legs and feet. This tends to make your blood pressure drop a bit. Lower blood pressure means less blood flows to your brain. A significant decrease in blood flow to the brain causes lightheadedness. If your ANS doesn't do its job, your blood pressure stays down and you experience "orthostatic hypotension". If your ANS is up to snuff, it will cause your leg arteries and veins to compress, thus returning more blood to your heart. In addition, it will increase your heart rate, so that more blood can be pumped per minute by your heart. These two adjustments allow more blood to flow to your brain. Your lightheadedness is prevented or alleviated, and you don't end up in a heap on the floor, with strangers exchanging significant looks and speculating as to how much you have had to drink.

To get your recovery started, the nurse will raise the head of the bed. In the modern hospital, there is an electric button she pushes to accomplish this. It is a gradual rise, not the toaster effect with the "Boing" you see in Roadrunner cartoons. If you wanted to raise the head of the bed in a movie, say, *Dr. No*, the robot-voiced head tech would command over the PA system, "Elevate HOB." There would be some spooky mechanical sound, then the schmuck tech, the one with the buck teeth and thick glasses, the one who invariably gets blown into the air later on, would reply, "HOB elevated". Back to the hospital bed. Odds are you will feel a little lightheaded, at least for a short period of time. Depending on how much your heart rate increases and your blood pressure decreases, she may give you some IV fluids. That will expand (increase) the volume of blood flowing in your blood vessels, allowing your heart to work less intensely to keep your blood pressure up.

If you survive "Elevate HOB", you can move on to the dangle. The dangle refers to your left and right legs, not the other one. This involves swiveling in the bed until your legs are hanging over the side. Some hospitals have a protocol for measuring your heart rate and blood pressure at one and three minutes. Whether there is a protocol or not, a smart nurse always measures these "orthostatics" and records them. This is just one further step in the process of getting your ANS to work normally.

When I was eighteen, my grandfather, who had severe rheumatoid arthritis, developed an infection in his elbow joint. He was hospitalized, sick as a dog, basically bedridden for over a month. Somehow he survived the infection and the antibiotics. On the day of discharge, he stood up to get dressed and dropped dead. He had developed blood clots in his legs and pelvis from inactivity. Upon standing, they broke off, floated up his vena cava to his heart, passed through his right atrium and ventricle, and lodged in his pulmonary artery. The fear of one of these migrating blood clots, a pulmonary embolism, is why you will get up and walk from POD (post-operative day) #2 onward. If you're smart, you'll push to get up on POD #1.

On your first walk, you may or may not be in pain, you may or may not feel dizzy, but you will feel weak as a kitten. Your walks in the CVICU, with your butt hanging out the back of your hospital gown, will usually involve a wheelchair, an oxygen tank, and almost certainly an IV pole. Don't worry about anything but that wheelchair you are pushing in front of you. Someone, either a nurse or an aide, will handle the other stuff. You might give a little thought to the bag connected to your Foley catheter as well. For this exercise, that "closed gravity drainage" bag should be hanging somewhere on your wheelchair, below the level of your bladder. Never let it out of your sight. If you do, the resulting tug on the Foley will remind you that your wiener is in constant peril.

The first walk is usually down a hallway or in a loop around the unit. Normally it would take about a minute, but that first time around, it'll seem the length of three football fields and will take anywhere from five to twenty minutes. Take your time, as nobody cares how long you take. It's probably better for you to walk more slowly for a longer period of time. Don't be surprised if you have to stop, take a breather, perhaps even sit down in the wheelchair for a bit. Older folks often can't make the whole walk and have to be wheeled back to their beds.

Normally this would be humiliating, but this is one of those times when you are too weak to give a rat's ass about humiliation. In some hospitals, when you finish that first post-op walk, the nurses gather round and give you a group golf clap. It might seem silly to onlookers, especially when the staff throws around "Super!" and "Wow!" and a lot of other peppy words with exclamation points. It is, however, a lot better than if you can't finish. If you have to come back in a wheel chair, they'll give you a one-handed shoulder rub--a touchy-feely "Aw, gee"-- and say things like, "You'll get it next time, Gus." This is encouraging, unless your name isn't Gus.

FOOD

At various times, hospitals have touted their food as a reason to choose them over the competition. Some have even hired famous chefs to supervise the Food Services department. For medical students who are applying for internships, good food in the cafeteria is a small but positive selling point. In many cities, where security concerns permit, the elderly and others on fixed incomes have come to view the local hospital as a place where they can get a meal for a very reasonable price. If your hospital subscribes to the Planetree system, the chef comes around and the two of you have a confab about your food preferences. Undoubtedly, this is of great comfort when you are puking your guts out from chemotherapy or an anesthesia hangover.

As a patient, however, it doesn't matter how good the food is. Your goal as a post-op heart patient is to sample as little of the hospital food as possible. Once you are keeping food down without the technicolor yawn, you should feel well enough to work on your escape from the hospital. It's a good idea to get out before you can really taste anything. It is especially important that, while in the hospital, you not eat anything you have enjoyed in the past or are likely to want to eat in the near future. At least for a while, your brain will do an excellent job of associating anything you eat with the sights, sounds and smells of your hospital room and bed. For my first full post-op meal, a well-intentioned friend brought in a huge bowl of pasta packed with onions and garlic. I gagged down what I could. It was several years before I could eat anything with onions or garlic without feeling waves of nausea and disgust wash over me. Occasionally I can still hear the beep of a cardiac monitor when I taste garlic. It gives me the creeps.

After an abdominal surgery, such as an appendectomy, cholecystectomy (gallbladder removal), or abdominal aorta replacement, your gut doesn't start working for several days. Initially, either you are not hungry or a tad nauseated. If your nausea is severe or prolonged, there are a host of meds they can shoot into your IV to calm your stomach. If you are a smoker, smoking a cigarette post-op often will relieve your nausea. However, don't look for anyone to wheel you out of the CVICU to catch a smoke outside. Even before your NG tube is removed, you can start with sips and chips, if only to relieve the dryness in your mouth. That means sips of water and ice chips, not Dewar's and Doritos. Anything you swallow is simply sucked back up by your NG tube. If you put colorful dyes in the water or ice chips, you can create your own little rainbow in the suction canister on the wall. Once the NG tube is out, you can start advancing your diet. Cardiac bypass surgery doesn't affect your gut all that much, so you will usually have your NG tube pulled within the first twenty-four hours and start sips and chips immediately.

Once your NG tube is out, the diet order reads something to the effect of, "Clear liquids. Advance as tolerated." That means you will be given a tray with apple juice and Jell-O. If you can swallow them and keep them down, the next meal will be "full liquids", which means pudding and other soft slop. Next stop after that is regular food. Given that cholesterol probably played a role in landing that zipper on your chest in the first place, you can expect a "cardiac" diet, which means low cholesterol and low salt. Most patient food is pretty tasteless, and there's not a lot of wiggle room for tony continental gourmet dining. Generally speaking, once you are healthy enough to bitch about the food, it's time to go home.

YOUR BOWELS

To get out of the hospital, you have to be able to walk without requiring supplemental oxygen, you have to be able to eat without vomiting, you have to be able to urinate without a catheter, and you have to be able to poop. Postoperatively, several factors conspire to keep you constipated. First is the anesthesia, which tends to slow down the activity of your intestines. Second are the narcotics, like morphine and demerol, you receive to relieve post-op pain. Third is the relative lack of activity; you are bedridden or sitting in a chair for most of the time and get to walk for a few minutes a few times each day. Fourth is the possibility of having to use a bedpan. Hospitals have all sorts of things to help you go, from stool softeners to laxatives to rectal suppositories. If you are smart, you will start popping stool softeners as soon as you are taking clear liquids and drink as much water as you are permitted. If you are walking well and eating well and you can't go, the quickest way to start things up is a suppository, because it is inserted and works right at the action zone. Some people prefer oral laxatives, and I guarantee you nurses prefer administering meds via that route, but some laxatives can cause nausea and vomiting. Pick your poison. If all else fails, there is the enema. All parties concerned will hate that route.

Before you can be transferred to telemetry, you pretty much have to have all the lines and tubes out. There's the ET tube, to assist with breathing, which we already discussed. There's the NG tube, which should become unnecessary within twenty-four hours. When the NG comes out, you will gag, but after a few seconds you should be fine. The arterial line into the radial artery in your wrist, which is a handy dandy way to measure your blood pressure AND to obtain blood for lab tests, comes out by the time you are up and walking. Thereafter you get the standard blood pressure cuff, which is no big deal, but if you have blood tests ordered, usually to check your potassium level and kidney function, you'll be getting stuck with a needle. The internal jugular line in your neck will come out when you are no longer having any blood pressure issues or irregular rhythms.

Occasionally an old guy with a history of prostate problems will go home with a Foley catheter, to follow up with a urologist, but usually the Foley, which you have never let out of your sight, should come out within the first day or two. It hurts for a few seconds when the Foley comes out. It hurts way more if the balloon at the end of it, the thing that keeps the catheter from falling out onto the floor, isn't deflated first. Again, it's your dick, so don't take anyone's word that the balloon is down unless you see them cut the balloon port or suck out ten cc. of saline.

The tubes that really hurt coming out are the mediastinal drainage tubes. They are placed during surgery to allow fluids and blood to drain into a bag rather than sit in your chest and potentially become infected. Those typically exit your body below the solar plexus in your upper abdomen. They are often 24 to 36 French in size, which is BIG, because the smaller ones tend to clot up with blood and become blocked. When there is little or no drainage into the bag for twenty-four hours, it is time to pull them. When they are pulled, your abdominal muscles will do things you never thought they could. It feels like someone, say, Dr. No with his superstrong mechanical hands, reached into your abdomen and twisted your rectus abdominis, the thing that used to look like a six-pack. Your rectus will do an involuntary seismic spasm for more than a few seconds. Generally speaking, anything involuntary is bad, and this is no exception, but it does give you a new appreciation for belly dancers.

Some bypasses are done through a thoracotomy incision on the side or back of your chest, rather than a mediastinotomy on the front. For a thoracotomy, unless you have significant ongoing bleeding, you will typically have a much smaller chest tube, say a 19 French. When that comes out, the pain is extremely brief and nothing more than a slight twinge. That is, if the sutures holding it in place are cut first. If not, it's not going anywhere, or at least the part inside your chest isn't, and it will hurt a lot more. Make sure the tube removal person cuts the sutures first.

YOUR SQUASH

"Squash" is the term physicians commonly use to describe your brain and its level of function. Most likely that's because your brain can turn into mushy goo if it isn't properly protected. A typical sentence would be, "So his ticker's okay and his lungs are okay. How's the squash?" Expect your brain to feel like nothing for the first day or so--no ambition, no curiosity other than, "Where am I?" or "What happened?". Unless you've had a really hard life, you have just had the most physically traumatic experience since your birth. Your brain has been put to sleep for hours. All sorts of chemicals have been injected into your body. You probably couldn't muster the strength to swat a fly if your life depended on it. Visitors understand the physical weakness, but for some reason, if you aren't mentally ready to enter into a discussion of quantum mechanics, their alarm bells go off. "Nurse, call the doctor. Something's wrong. He's not making any sense!" After the nurse explains why you can't speak clearly and why your attention span can be measured in nanoseconds, they usually calm down.

Even if you suffer a serious case of pump head, your squash will improve every day. The first couple of days, visitors may come and go while you, aided by morphine, sleep for large chunks of time. Every time you wake up, you may have to be re-oriented as to where you are. Don't sweat it. Your brain knows what it has to do to keep you alive. With some stimulus from your nurse, you will be able to increase your physical and mental activity.

That one guy you hope won't come to visit always does. It's as if your surgeon gave him a call while you were being rolled into the CVICU. He's the one who comes armed with a quiver full of inane observations and stupid jokes. When you get a visit from Mr. Game show host/quizmaster, who feels like he has to entertain you and anybody else in your room, it is perfectly okay to pretend to be sleepy, even if you aren't. Otherwise you'll be answering jokey questions about how your Foley feels, how the food is, do you think the nurse is cute, etc. Odds are, after a few minutes of any visitors, given the jumbled state of your squash in combination with those much-needed doses of morphine, you really will be sleepy and won't have to fake it. Play the dopey patient as long as you can. Feel free to put your nemesis on the "No visitation" list. Your nurse will be glad to back you up. Her job gets much easier once the visitors go away, especially that guy.

If all goes well, there is no reason why you can't be free of all your lines except for a single peripheral IV, out of the CVICU, and onto telemetry within forty-eight to seventy-two hours. If, while in the CVICU, you haven't accomplished all of the requirements for discharge, you can work on them in the step-down unit.

References:

1. Morris, Douglas C., Clements, Stephen D., Jr., Pepper, John. "Management of the Patient after Cardiac Surgery." *Hurst's The Heart.* Ed. Valentin Fuster, Ed. Robert A. O'Rourke, Ed. Richard A. Walsh, Ed. Philip Poole-Wilson. New York: McGraw-Hill. 2008. 1519-25.

91. DISABILITY INSURANCE

Private disability insurance may seem like a luxury. When I first went to a financial advisor, somewhere in the early 90s, I was about forty years old and seemingly in good health. I could hike any of the peaks in Flagstaff without stopping, skied badly but without aches and pains either in my chest or any of my joints. The thought of being laid up for more than a day or two was ridiculous. Nevertheless, this financial advisor, Ron Oddo, who was older, wiser, and had seen more of life than I, got on this jag about my needing disability insurance. Blah blah blah. On and on. All I wanted was a place to park my retirement money so that it would be there in sufficient amounts when I got sick of working, in my 70s at the earliest. I couldn't conceive of retiring at sixty-five, let alone forty-five.

None of that meant a thing to Ron. In his very low key way, he kept hammering away at me to get a disability policy. I figured he would be getting a cut, but that didn't bother me. Finally, just to shut him up, I signed up for the maximum amount of benefits my income permitted. He reminded me to increase the monthly benefit amount whenever it was permitted by the insurance company. Because I was self-employed, I couldn't get as much insurance as someone making the same amount but employed by a company. I guess they figured a self-employed person is a riskier bet to keep paying the premiums. So instead of putting away a sizeable chunk of change each month, I was spending it on insurance premiums. There was absolutely no doubt that I'd never see one dime in benefits.

After about five years, I received a whopper of a check in the mail from the insurer. I had no idea what it was for. I called Ron. He told me, apparently for the second time, that if I didn't file a disability claim, I could expect an identical check every five years. Who knew? Had I read the policy, or listened to his description of the policy, I would have. I went on paying the premiums and getting the benefits increases with a lighter heart. It might be money down the drain, but at least I could look forward to some sort of return on my investment.

About twelve years later I began to have my heart problems. After my first surgery, I called the insurer, then sent them a ream of records, including my cath report, operative note, and discharge summary. Voilà! A check appeared within a week. As long as I kept them up to date and had my cardiologist complete a form every month or so, I would be maintained on short-term disability. As a bonus, as long as I was on disability, I wouldn't have to pay the monthly premiums either. I figured that I might get a monthly check for a while; another little benny to take the sting out of that money going "down the drain".

After my second surgery, the insurer said screw it and put me on long-term disability. They said that if my heart and my brain ever got back to normal, I could stop receiving checks, go back to work, and start paying my monthly premiums again, as if nothing had ever happened. You can say what you want about being on the dole, and I said all those things too, but without that disability policy, even with all my savings, I'd have been up Shit Creek without it.

Ron's still around, working to keep idiots like me from going broke. It's a full-time job. Do yourself a favor. Get a disability policy.

92. TEN THINGS YOU DON'T WANT TO HEAR WHEN YOU AWAKEN AFTER SURGERY

1. God, look at all that blood.
2. Heads I tell him, tails you do.
3. This fax says his insurance lapsed yesterday.
4. How was I supposed to know the Foley balloon was still inflated?
5. Are you sure? That doesn't look like any MRSA I've ever seen.
6. The surgeon said it was open and close. There was nothing he could do.
7. They said he'll be on the ventilator for at least a week.
8. How the hell are we going to reattach that?
9. Wow, I've never seen that rhythm before!
10. Clear!

93. S.F.N.

Nurses and their assistants come with all sorts of initials and titles: L.P.N. (if that even exists any more), C.N.A., R.N., M.S.R.N., N.P. No matter what the initials, degree, title or position, when something goes wrong, they are bound to be labeled with another title: S.F.N. Stupid Fucking Nurse. According to some physicians, more than you would think, when a patient under their care experiences an unexpected or annoying complication, the reflexive response is, "When in doubt, blame the nurse." The S.F.N. degree is usually conferred late at night, from one physician to another, over the telephone.

One night I was called up from the E.R. to the CVICU to see why a patient's heart rate had slowed down. After talking with the nurse on duty and examining the patient, I called his cardiologist and told him the temporary pacemaker he inserted earlier in the day had become dislodged.

"Stupid fucking nurses. I can't believe they fucked that up."

Wide awake and full of fun, I asked, "Well, if they're that fucking stupid, why wouldn't you expect them to fuck it up?" When you are checking out a patient problem in the middle of the night for a guy who's home in his comfy little bed, you can get away with a certain amount of sarcasm. You have him over a miniature barrel. All the while, I toyed with the temptation to put him on the speaker phone at the nurse's station. However, I figured the nurses had already heard his rant more than once. I only had to deal with him on special occasions like this one. They had to work with this guy on a daily basis.

After I reassured him that the patient would be fine until he saw him in the morning, he threw in a few more S.F.N. references, thanked me and hung up. I thought about critiquing his suture technique, which was the underlying problem. Amateurish and slovenly, it exemplified the skill set of a blind monkey. However, even at night, even when you play the role of the Good Samaritan, there is only so much you can get away with. This particular guy, by the way, liked to portray himself as the "Physician Friend of the Nurse." At least that was his self-ordained title during daylight.

Over the years I experienced at least a dozen actual S.F.N. references, and probably five times that many implied ones. Most were some variation of "Stupid Nurses." Interestingly, the ire was almost never focused on an individual. More often it was a condemnation of the entire nursing profession, meaning, I suppose, that every nurse within the nuclear blast zone of an untoward complication was indictable for the crime of being in the wrong place at the right time. And, of course, as irony would dictate, nine times out of ten, the complication was either unavoidable or pretty much the fault of the attending physician or his consultant.

Most women physicians tend to have closer professional relationships with nurses. Sometimes they're buddies. Thus they are far less likely to go to the S.F.N. card. Surprisingly, however, I've come across a few lady doctors who like the term as much as or more than their male counterparts. One female physician, whose patient developed severe internal bleeding hours after a surgical procedure, actually called the nurses on the ward "Stupid cunts."

I waited about ten seconds. " 'Stupid cunts.' Did you really just say that?"

"Of course not. Some of my best friends are nurses." Anytime you hear, "Why, some of my best friends are...", rest assured, you are dealing with a liar and a denier. As far as I know, that was a one-time-only performance.

Without regular reinforcement, situations fade from memory. Then something happens to remind you. The Ebola outbreak's arrival in the U.S. reminded me of the S.F.N. issue. Except at night, on the phone, out of earshot of the nursing staff, most negative references regarding nursing intelligence are subtler than the classic S.F.N. When two nurses from the institution soon-to-be formerly known as Texas

Health Presbyterian Hospital Dallas contracted Ebola, everyone wanted to know how that could happen. The current head of the CDC, Dr. Thomas Frieden, a specialist in Infectious Diseases and one of the pre-eminent figures in the field of public health, became the go-to guy for answers about anything and everything Ebola. Sporting a nice suit and an affable demeanor, he was omnipresent on the national news shows and particularly on the Sunday morning network news roundups.

At the end of one of his appearances, he had the option of closing with an investigatory, sleuthy statement, invoking an image of him in a trench coat with a magnifying glass, on the order of, "We continue to evaluate the Texas Health situation, and we will get to the bottom of this." Instead, he opts for something to the effect of, "Obviously, there was a breach of protocol somewhere in there and that's why those nurses contracted Ebola." In other words, "Those Stupid Fucking Nurses fucked up and brought this on themselves." Hoo Boy. All this on the world's largest speaker phone, without any prompting from anyone.

It has been reported by one news organization that when the E.R. doctor from New York developed symptoms of Ebola, he initially lied to the authorities about his activities in the city. First he told them he had self-quarantined in his Harlem apartment, presumably twanging away on his banjo. Unfortunately, an examination of his MetroCard and his credit card statement indicated a romp around several of the boroughs, including a trip to Gutter, which is alleged to be a bowling alley in Brooklyn, and The Meatball Shop, presumably a place in the Village where you buy meatballs. His gallivanting drew some criticism in the media, but even that was defended by the medical community. After all, he was doing exactly what the CDC recommended: taking his temperature, presumably twice daily, and living his normal life as long as he was free of symptoms. Even a long-time veteran of the Marburg epidemics and previous Ebola outbreaks weighed in, saying that the right thing to do is take your temperature twice daily. If you are deemed too irresponsible to do this on your own, you should expect twice daily visits from a county health department worker to take your temp for you.

Every time this E.R. physician is brought up in the media, there is a face shot of him, followed by a shot of him posing in his hazmat suit, presumably while he was volunteering in West Africa. Occasionally they throw in a shot of him with his girlfriend. Unlike the nurses at Texas Health, it appears he was supplied with the appropriate gear while caring for Ebola patients. If that is indeed the case, and if he followed the protocol, how on earth did he contract the virus? Given his alleged problems with the truth, you might expect to hear Dr. Frieden suggesting that the physician broke protocol at some point. Alas, Dr. Frieden has taken a powder; his opinions have been confined to Twitter. Given his loquacious tendencies in previous situations, it must be damn difficult to conjure up a juicy diatribe about S.F.N.s in only one hundred forty characters.

Clearly, even the most experienced of researchers and clinicians don't know everything there is to know about Ebola. Right now, the word is that Ebola cannot be contracted via airborne transmission. My Dean of Admissions at UVA, Ed Pullen, PhD, said on our first day of medical school, "50% of what you learn here in the next four years will be proven to be incorrect in your lifetime." This from a guy who specialized in anatomy and histology, meaning he had all the answers right in front of him, either macroscopically in a body part or a corpse, or microscopically on a glass slide. Less than forty years later, it seems he was spot on. If he bats only .500, then the diseases we encounter every day will be thought of far differently in the next twenty to forty years. For a disease like Ebola, which in the past has raised its head sporadically and, until now has always been self-limited, we probably know even a smaller portion of that whole story.

Isn't it just the slightest bit odd that of all of Thomas Eric Duncan's Dallas contacts, who stayed in the same apartment with him while he grew more symptomatic, not one took ill within their twenty-one day incubation period? As the patient grew sicker, it's highly unlikely that the family was looking at the CDC's website for guidance on isolation best practices. As far as we know, nobody has any natural immunity to Ebola, and there is no guarantee that contracting and surviving the illness confers any significant immunity. In addition, viruses don't follow rules, and they have been known to mutate at the most inopportune of times. So this twenty-one day incubation period that seems etched in stone might actually be etched in Play-Doh. One thing that you can count on: The more the experts assert that there is no chance of airborne transmission of Ebola, the more likely that a case will turn up with just such transmission. We are sometimes wrong, but we are never in doubt. It seems arrogant and just a tad condescending of the CDC or any other authoritative body to assert that following their guidelines will guarantee safety, and that anyone who does follow them and yet has the temerity to fall ill obviously screwed up.

Should all volunteers who go to West Africa be quarantined for twenty-one days? The U.S. military thinks so, even though their Commander-in-Chief says otherwise. Obviously, letting politicians set medical or public health standards is a bad idea; we can't expect them to decide whether they should do what is best for their constituents or whether they should do what they usually do. In a year or two, or five or ten, we'll know for sure what to do when it comes to Ebola contacts. For now, nobody has become ill when coming into casual contact with an Ebola-infected health care worker, so the CDC recommendations are probably as good a compromise as any. Then again, if the shoe rental guy at the Gutter starts exploding ass-first into a trashcan or Mr. Meatball starts vomiting blood into the bucket of sauce, hopefully the marinara and not the Alfredo, or the good doctor's girlfriend (Think she's a little nervous?) checks in with a temp of 103, all the while singing, "Stand By Your Man" to a banjo accompaniment, those guidelines might get ramped up a bit. Nonetheless, treating them like criminals is not going to help the situation one iota.

On the other hand, when it comes to the face of the U.S. Ebola situation, it's a toss-up between Chris Christie and Kaci Hickox for least likable. If Karma had any say in the matter, both of them would end up with Ebola, hospitalized together at Bellevue, playing gin rummy to while away the hours. The big winner in that scenario would be Silent Boyfriend of Hickox, who would have one last chance to escape a looming life of misery.

If we follow the advice of National Nurses United, we should "Stop Blaming Nurses. Stop Ebola." But nurses are such easy targets. And their representatives come off just a tad shrill to boot. What's an expert to do?

There is one other time-honored tenet. When all else fails, blame the patient.

94. ONE MAN'S MEAT

Simmons was working the walk-in clinic. The chart in the box said "Thomas Haskins, Korean War, non-service connected." It was thin. A first-timer. That told Simmons the guy had insurance through his employer or was already on Medicare. Most of the vets who obtained their health care in the private sector came to the VA for med refills, which cost three bucks per month. Occasionally a veteran showed up for a second opinion.

"Good Morning, Mr. Haskins. I'm Doctor Simmons. Come on in and have a seat while I look over your chart." They shook hands. He was thin, wiry, had the face of a smoker. Big Popeye forearms and hard, rough hands. Maybe a manual labor job with union benefits. Probably not a concert violinist. Simmons sat down behind his desk, opened the chart, and read the encounter sheet.

"It says here you've been diagnosed with gallbladder disease."

"Chronic collie something or other."

"Chronic cholecystitis?"

"That's what they say, Doc."

"Uh-huh. And who exactly is 'they'?"

"My doctor, Doctor Lewis."

"Doctor Mortimer Lewis? The general surgeon at Holy Sawbones Hospital?"

"Yup, that's the guy." Haskins coughed. It was harsh, raspy. Not just tobacco, Simmons thought. Something more. Asbestos?

"How did you end up seeing him?"

"I live up in Miami. I used to go to the mine hospital up there, but they closed that down about ten years ago. The local hospital nearby doesn't take the mine company insurance anymore, so my brother-in-law got me an appointment with an internist, Dr. Sargent. He did some tests, then he referred me to Dr. Lewis." Simmons looked at the second sheet in the chart, the personal information form. Sure enough, the guy was retired and still lived up near Globe.

"With all the retired miners up your way, I'm kind of surprised the mine company didn't work out some kind of deal with the local hospital."

Haskins laughed. "I'm not. The mine company works the same as the VA, Doc. Negative incentives. The VA uses waiting times to discourage us vets from getting our care here. The mine company signs all their contracts with doctors and hospitals down here or in Tucson. That way, you have to really want to see a doctor or else be sick as a dog to seek care."

Simmons thought, *Rough hands but a sharp mind.*

"What exactly did you do for the mining company, Mr. Haskins?"

"Oh, I started out down in the mineshaft when I was sixteen. Eventually I moved up to daylight, as a mechanic on the belt."

"Oh. Where'd you learn about the negative incentive business?"

Haskins laughed, then coughed. "My wife worked in the HR department before the operation closed down."

"Okay. Let me ask you something. I see here that you have both Medicare and private insurance from the copper mine. From what I can tell, whatever isn't covered by Medicare will be covered by your insurer."

"That sounds about right, Doc." He smiled like a man who was about to get a new Cadillac from the 50-50 raffle at church.

"So, since it wouldn't cost you a dime to have this surgery done at Holy Sawbones, and you had your entire workup done there, and you've got a surgeon there, why do you want to come here?"

"That should be pretty obvious, Doc."

"Enlighten me."

"The food's better here."

While Simmons had never been a big fan of hospital food, and Holy Sawbones resembled a poorly-run version of Hell, this was nonetheless a bit of a stunner. He'd been to eat a couple of times in the cafeteria; the food was perfectly acceptable. Perhaps the patient food was much worse than the cafeteria fare. He considered sending an anonymous tip to Diane Sawyer to go hide in a closet and see what was going on.

"Better food here than at Holy Sawbones?"

"Sure." He eyed Simmons, looking for signs of idiocy or lunacy.

"Why is that?"

"Jesus, Doc, they've got better cooks here."

"Better cooks. Really?"

His eyes took on a dreamy look. "Yup. Army cooks."

95. BUSINESSMAN'S LUNCH

"Good morning, Dr. Simmons," Jeannette the resident greeted him. They were standing in one of the offices reserved for the house staff teams, each of which consisted of two first-year interns and one second- or third-year medical resident. Chalkboards on three walls held lists of patient names and their locations in the hospital. Jeannette paged through her 3 x 5 cards and tallied them off against the names on the board. There looked to be about twenty cards, one for each patient, which meant the team was close to maxing out. New rules forbade an intern from carrying more than twelve patients at a time.

"Hi, Jeannette. We all set?"

"Yessir. Everybody's present and accounted for." Both interns, Dan and Dana, were on the desk phones. They seemed to do everything simultaneously. He wondered about the everything part. "They'll be ready to go in a few seconds." They both finished on the phones, grabbed their clipboards, and stood up.

Simmons thought, *How can they not be related? Other than Dan being a boy and Dana a girl, they look identical, including those moon faces, their names are almost identical, and they're heading for the same specialty. That's it. Moon twins.*

He awoke from his reverie. "How'd you guys do last night?"

"Not bad. A couple of early hits, then one guy with a history of lung cancer came in around 2 A.M. with bad pleuritic chest pain, among other things."

"Anyone fascinating?"

"He might be. He just went down to x-ray, so we'll see him at the end of rounds."

"Is he on heparin?"

"No. I don't think he needs it."

"So he's not going to die of a PE before we get to him?" The moon twins, behind their almost identical horn rims, ogled Jeannette, waiting to see if her head exploded.

"He better not, or I'll have to change my middle name to Stupenagel." She smiled.

"Yes, you will." *Progressing nicely, was Jeannette.* "Withholding therapy, though. Shows a lot of moxie." She flexed her biceps.

For the next forty-five minutes the team rounded on the new guys, the old guys, and decided who needed what done and who needed to go home, to the intermediate care ward, or to the nursing home. Nobody was going to the morgue. Not today. Not yet.

"Let's go see if Mr. Perkins is back from x-ray." Jeannette led the way to the last room on the left. No Mr. Perkins. It was almost noon and David's friend Mike from County was doing the noon conference on a Korean War Vet with classic myxedema. Jeannette walked up to the nursing desk. She looked a little worried when she returned.

"He came back from x-ray, but then he said he was going down to the lobby."

Simmons shrugged. "Probably going to have a pre-lunch smoke. Any IV's?"

"Just some antibiotics for a fever...."

"Well, I doubt he's getting antibiotics this time of day."

"...and a morphine drip." Her chin and her biceps sagged noticeably. Dan and Dana looked at each other, then at Jeannette, then at Simmons. The way they looked at each other reminded him of the weird-eyed kids in *Village of the Damned.*

"Morphine, eh? That should buy him a few packs of cigs on the street. Let's go find Pleuritic Perkins."

The lobby was lunchtime empty. No vets or visitors, just the receptionist. Simmons rarely came down to the lobby, but whenever he did, there she was, with her blonde bouffant and her high-necked dress in a bright primary color. Like a mannequin stationed there behind the desk, she never seemed to quite fit in. He had never heard her speak. He led the team over to her. Today it was royal blue with a white collar buttoned to the very top.

"Pardon me. My, that's a lovely dress. We're looking for a veteran who probably came down here for a smoke. With an IV pole. Jeannette, what does he look like?"

She turned to the receptionist, a little red-faced, David thought. "He's the one who's sweating on one side of his face."

Simmons did a double-take. "He's got a Horner's?"

The receptionist spoke up. Her voice was deep, calm, measured. "Yes, I saw him a few minutes ago." *Good voice for radio commercials,* he thought. She turned to Simmons. "What's a Horner's?"

"It's something you can get when you have lung cancer. It affects your nervous system and produces weird effects, but only on one side of the body."

Simmons went on. "Did you see where he went?" Wordlessly, the lady in blue pointed straight ahead. Through the glass doors, beyond the front circular driveway, and across Seventh St. She had surprisingly long arms and fingers. Simmons thought, *Marfan's syndrome?*

"He's in the Jag? With the IV pole?" She nodded. The twins and Jeannette stared at Simmons.

The two Ds spoke at the same time. "What's the Jag?"

The bouffant in blue said, "It's a Gentleman's Club." David regarded her with renewed interest. It had never occurred to him that she might have a past. *Those quiet ones.* She looked straight at him for an eternity. When he felt the heat rising in his cheeks, she smiled and looked down at her desk. *She's very comfortable making a man blush.*

"What's a Gentleman's Club?" came from the twins, in unison, of course.

Simmons said, "It's a nudie bar. What do you know, morphine at the Businessman's Lunch. First time for everything." After wishing the receptionist a pleasant day and promising to explain Horner's syndrome to her over dinner sometime, David led the team out. It was supposed to get to ninety, warm but not outlandish for mid-October. There was a cooling breeze blowing down Seventh Street from the north, and the quartet stood on the sidewalk enjoying it while waiting for the traffic to clear. About twenty yards to their right, a skinny brown guy with a Jethro Tull hat sat on the steel bench at the bus stop. Simmons decided to take the opportunity to enlighten his charges about history and life.

"See that guy?" The twins turned their heads in perfect harmony. Jeannette leaned around David to see. "He's what we call an orbiter."

Dan and Dana looked at David with wide eyes, then back at the brown man, as if they expected him to blast off at any minute and disappear into space like John Glenn. "VA patients, mostly psych guys, move around the country according to the seasons. I believe they were first described by a shrink from one of the Boston VAs. Mostly males from cold weather cities, they come to Phoenix or L.A. or Houston for the winter. I think I heard that particular guy is originally from Cleveland or Youngstown, somewhere in the steel belt for sure. Eventually, they get tired of the travel, which is not exactly first class on the Concorde, and stay in one place. Usually it's a warmer locale. A lot of them are homeless, so they tend to congregate around the VA."

The twins had lost interest in Simmons' tale and were writing little notations on their clipboards. Both were headed into Ophthalmology and were counting the days until their rotating internships were over. David estimated they'd both make excellent retinal specialists, which would require absolutely no personality, let alone bedside manner.

Inside the Jaguar No. 2, it was cool, dark and smelled like a flower bomb had just gone off. A pair of neckless fire plugs in tuxes stood inside the front door on either side of the foyer. One guy had hellacious acne, including throughout his flat top. Otherwise, they were indistinguishable.

Simmons spoke. "Hi. We're looking for an old guy in green pajamas and a green bathrobe. He probably came in a few minutes ago."

"Could you be more specific, Sir?" This from the clean-faced one. Simmons was momentarily taken aback, both by the clarity of his speech and by his question.

"How many guys are in here from the VA across the street?"

"Most weekdays, a number of gentlemen join us for the Businessman's Lunch."

"You let guys in green foam slippers in here to eat? They don't have any money for table dances."

"Everyone's welcome to the Businessman's Lunch, Doctor. It's always been a policy of the Jaguar No. 2."

"Look, we're making rounds, and we have to see everyone. I'm sure you don't want any customers dying in here." The tuxes looked at each other, then at Simmons, without the slightest bit of emotion. Perhaps guys dying in the Jag was no big deal. "From a narcotics overdose, that is." Again, not much panic on their part.

"There he is," Jeannette pointed, "over there at the far end of the stage."

"Still got the pump?" Simmons couldn't see the guy.

"Yes."

"Okay. Look, it'd be better for everyone if we just retrieve our patient. Won't take but a minute, I promise, and no fuss." The tuxes stepped aside and the four physicians went in. A woman well into her fifth decade was doing a very slow pole dance in front of a crowd of eight or so, all of them watching her with detached interest while eating sandwiches and potato chips. Off to the left sat a buffet table with more of the same. Most of the guys were sipping on drafts. Some had taken advantage of the two-for-one special. Nobody else was wearing the VA costume.

"So none of you have ever been in here before?"

Jeannette laughed. "Me? You must be joking. Have you, Dr. Simmons?"

"Once or twice. Research purposes only. Hi, Mr. Perkins, I'm Dr. Simmons." Perkins looked up at him, half his face dripping sweat, the other side bone dry, right down the middle, with the requisite droopy eyelid. A heater, most likely a hand-rolled Bugler from the VA canteen, hung from the wet side of his mouth.

"Can you guys come back later?" *By all means*, thought David, *just raise your hand when you want another sandwich.*

"Mr. Perkins, we just want to examine you, figure out what is causing your pain, and get you started on treatment."

"Not having any pain. I feel fine." He turned back to his baloney on white.

"You realize that the morphine in that IV pump is relieving your pain, and if we leave, we have to take it with us."

"What the fuck for?" Simmons seemed to have finally gotten his attention.

"The law says you can't have inpatient narcotics floating around an outpatient facility." David doubted the DEA thought much about strip joints when they defined "outpatient facility".

"I'll sign out AMA, then you can't touch me, and I'll go home and call my patient rep and my congressman." He stuck out his jaw defiantly. Dan and Dana were whispering to each other behind David, probably something about the one-sided waterfall of sweat coming off Perkins' chin.

"Tell you what, Mr. Perkins. How about we go back into that room, we check you out, and then you can come back and finish your Businessman's Lunch?"

"What the fuck I wanna go back there for?"

"Well, Sir, it's the dancers' dressing room." Perkins eyes lit up, at least the one on the sweaty side. *Gotcha.*

"Let's go!" The old vet was surprisingly nimble, and in no time he was up and heading to the back of the room, shoving his IV pole ahead. The four doctors followed behind.

Jeannette looked at David. "Are we really going to leave him here after we check him out?" She looked genuinely alarmed.

"Of course. A deal's a deal. Word gets around you backed out of a deal, you'll be shunned by the greater vet community, and that's never a good thing. He's going to be dead from that lung cancer soon, so he might as well have some fun. Besides, the bag of morphine on the pump is just about finished. He'll come back home and get a refill when he starts hurting again."

He turned to the moon twins. "Dan and Dana, try not to stare. It makes the girls uncomfortable."

96. ROUNDS

Rounds in the hospital are rarely as entertaining as that little adventure, nor do they usually require a road trip, but they are important. They are your one chance each day to plead your case for getting the hell out of the hospital. In the old days, doctors rounded whenever their office schedule permitted. That meant a busy GP might not see you until 8 at night. It wasn't uncommon for a physician to have patients at three or four hospitals. Nowadays, the emphasis on discharges early in the day means that your cardiologist, your hospitalist, and your heart surgeon will likely see you first thing in the morning. If your cardiologist has early caths or your heart surgeon has early cases in the O.R., it might be mid-morning before they get around.

The purpose of rounds after heart surgery is to make sure everything is going smoothly. By the time your doctor arrives for rounds, the night shift nurse has recorded her observations on a tape recorder; once your day shift nurse has listened to them, she will be heading your way. If you are experiencing some discomfort, it is a good idea to bring it up to the day shift nurse, rather than keeping it to yourself. First, if there is a real problem, the nurse can address it. If it's something serious, they either follow a protocol for treating it, talk to the doctor and get orders to treat, or page one of your doctors to rush in and evaluate you. Even doctors who like to run marathons don't like to hurry when they are in the hospital (It is considered undignified.), and running is frowned upon in hospitals anyway, so a running anybody usually means something bad has happened. It is always better to have a physician run past your room than into it.

Second, it is a bad idea to withhold information from your nurse, only to spill the beans when the doctors show up for rounds. Nobody likes surprises and nurses generally do not like to look like they don't know what is going on with their patients in front of the entire medical team. Likewise, if you have questions about your hospital stay, it is a good idea to bring them up with your nurse. Most of the time she can answer your question, and if she can't, let her bring it up with the physicians during rounds. Your nurse is your advocate and he or she will be spending far more time with you each day during post-op recovery than anyone else on the team. Do not piss off your chef, your lawyer, or your nurse. On the other hand, if you don't have an answer from her or she fails to mention your concerns during rounds, it is open season; fire away with your questions.

Rounds should be a low-key affair. If all is going well, there should be nothing new to see, no new diagnoses to make, i.e., everything boring and stable and progressing nicely. Remember, your entire hospital stay, from admission through surgery to discharge, is most likely to go smoothly if there is no disruption in the protocol. If rounds in your room involve any new findings, that pretty much constitutes a setback in your recovery. It's very unlikely that you will surprise your team of doctors with good news.

In a teaching hospital, depending on the setup, most likely you will go through rounds the same way you went through your admission and

H & P--third-year medical students, fourth-year medical students, interns, residents, then the whole crew with the cardiac surgery fellow and the cardiac surgeon. It is, once again, repetitive, but the greater the number of examiners, the better the chance that one of them will pick up any abnormality. If you're bored, feel free to ask questions like who cut you open, who harvested your saphenous vein, who bone-sawed your sternum, who did the bypasses, and who closed you up.

Surgeons have a penchant for pulling the dressings from wounds, poking around to make sure there isn't any unusual swelling or drainage, then leaving the wound exposed for the nurse to redress it. A smart nurse never changes the dressing on the wound until after rounds. It is no secret that one of the greatest risks for a postoperative wound infection depends on what bacteria are growing in the examiners' noses, as in staph aureus, MRSA and other heinous pathogens. It's one of the reasons everyone in an OR wears a mask and gloves. Thus, at least for the first forty-eight hours, nobody should look at, breathe on, or touch your exposed surgical wounds without a mask and gloves. They ought to wash their hands before and after examining you. Folks are wising up about this, but you will now and then run into someone who continues to miss the boat on infection prevention. Yes, it is intimidating to demand a doctor or nurse put on a mask or gloves, but look at it this way. Do you want to piss someone off with a reasonable request or do you want your sternum rotting away because of an infection? A plastic surgeon once put it this way. "You can do it the right way, or you can do it like a jerk." Don't let anybody act like a jerk around your wounds.

Should the nurse feel that a situation requires intervention of some sort, but the doctor does not, you might see the following on your chart: "Doctor aware, no orders given". Kiss of death. Sometimes the nurse is definitely a step ahead of the doctor, and something is very wrong. Sometimes the nurse is wrong. Sometimes it means she's just pissed. Best of all, sometimes there's a history between the two. You probably won't see this notation, as you probably won't be reviewing your chart unless something goes very wrong. Then there will be other people reviewing your chart. People on the M&M committee. People in a lawyer's office.

When it comes to being in your room for rounds, don't sweat it. After bypass surgery, your day consists of walking in the hall, lying in bed, or sitting up in a chair. You won't be unavailable when the doctors come around, unless, of course, you are off the floor getting an x-ray or some other procedure, in which case there is a complication and you aren't going home today anyway. It is considered poor form to be out in front of the hospital in a wheelchair smoking a cigarette. Bad for your heart and lungs, bad for your image ("Look at that old creep in pj's and slippers smoking over there.") and bad advertising for the hospital.

If you want to get out of the hospital as soon as possible (ASAP) after heart surgery, start whining to your doctor about the quality of the food. If a patient is complaining about the food, he is usually well enough to go home. Bitching about other aspects of your care is also helpful in determining that your presence is no longer required. This is not the same as family members or visitors bitching about the quality of your care. When that happens, the doctor usually unloads on the nurses and everybody pretty much hates you and your entire entourage. In general, if you have visitors who like to complain just for the sake of complaining, it's prudent to issue mouth-sized strips of duct tape for them to wear while they are visiting. Otherwise, you'll probably have to lean on that nurse's call button to get your pain meds, and let me tell you, leaning hurts.

97. TELEMETRY

Once all your tubes are removed, most likely you will be transferred to a step-down unit, so named because, in terms of intensity, it is one step down from the CVICU. You don't actually have to step down to get there. Very often it will be on a different floor than the O.R. and the CVICU, more likely a higher floor than a lower one, so you could call it a ride-up unit. Hopefully the elevator is working and you will be treated to a wheelchair ride, so it won't be a walk-up unit. You will be joined there by patients who have had various forms of cardiac surgery, MI's or any other illness or procedure where the patient has had irregular rhythms or is at risk for arrhythmias. The step-down unit is less expensive, the nursing care is less intensive, and the patients are more stable than in the CVICU.

These floors are usually known collectively as telemetry units. They are more likely to resemble any other hospital ward, but every patient has a set of EKG leads attached to them via sticky pads. At the other end of the lead wires will be a battery pack or some other power source for transmitting your rhythm to a monitor at the nurses' station. If an irregular rhythm occurs, an alarm sounds on the monitor, and a hard copy of the rhythm is printed out. If it's really bad, a nurse will come running and administer some type of anti-arrhythmic medication.

Arriving on the telemetry unit is similar to being released from solitary confinement at the big house into the general population. However, unlike prison, new arrivals are not greeted by the three-hundred-pound cyclops muttering "fresh meat". Hazing is frowned upon. There's no risk of getting shivved in the back. Theoretically. You don't have to shower with all the other guys.

Walking is a big part of the step-down unit experience. You'll be expected to get up and go walk either with assistance or on your own several times each day. This is particularly important. You must develop the energy and confidence to walk on your own because when you get out, your complete recovery will depend on how much time and effort you expend in walking. If you land on a particularly happy, energetic unit, the staff will be there at the end of the first couple of walks around the ward to congratulate you. Much like the Boy Scouts, some hospitals even give out walking merit badges.

By now you should be eating regular food. Unless they have put you on a fluid restriction because of congestive heart failure, drink as much water as you can comfortably tolerate. That will make everything work better and heal faster. Depending on infection control policies in your hospital, after about forty-eight to seventy-two hours post-op, your wounds may be open to the air. Don't expect the food to be any better. It's still "cardiac diet" for you. Console yourself with the knowledge that it's far better than a dialysis patient's diet, which contains no spring, summer or autumn colors, just winter in Siberia: gray and brown and white.

On the telemetry unit, you are usually allowed to wander freely. If something happens off the ward, the power unit often won't be able to send a signal to the central monitor, so if you leave the unit, for example to go get an x-ray, a nurse has to accompany you with a portable monitor. As long as you're being monitored on the telemetry unit, you'll have a saline lock--an IV catheter which does not require an IV bag or line--in the back of your hand. That way, if you require intravenous meds for an arrhythmia, they can be administered ASAP. Usually you cannot draw blood effectively through a lock, so you'll require a separate needle stick for any blood tests. After the third or fourth stick for labs, you'll start to miss that radial artery catheter.

On the telemetry unit you'll continue to have educational sessions with the nurse and a dietician, maybe a physical therapist. The goal is to enlighten you as to the causes of your heart disease and how to prevent recurrences of the events that landed you in the hospital in the first place. You'll learn about your blood pressure and your cholesterol levels. If you are diabetic, there will probably be some teaching about better control of your blood sugar. There will be instructions in taking your meds and possible side effects.

As these sessions are required by various monitoring agencies, you will probably be asked a question or two, and may have to sign off, stating that you have been instructed and understand. While this stuff is done primarily to satisfy requirements, it does help you to comprehend what's going on and what you can do to keep yourself alive and out of the hospital in the future. If all goes well, after a few days on telemetry, you can go home. In most centers, the average length of stay from surgery to discharge runs from five to seven days. That includes patients who are elderly, develop complications, or are weenies. If you are young, relatively healthy (except for the heart thing, of course) and motivated, you can be out the door in as little as two or three days after surgery. The sooner you bitch about the food, the mattress, the noise or the smells, the sooner your nurse will declare that you have reached "maximal hospital benefit" and load you into the circus clown cannon for your next stop, discharge home.

98. INFECTIONS

Infections are always one of the top five reasons patients go to see health care providers in the office, the urgent care center, and the E.R. Many patients are diagnosed with a URI, an upper respiratory infection, which is usually caused by a virus and best known to the public as the common cold. Others, usually women, suffer from a UTI, a urinary tract infection, better known as a bladder infection, which is usually caused a type of bacteria, E. coli. A third common cause for a visit is a wound infection. You cut your hand on a dirty piece of metal, you don't take care of it properly, and the cut eventually gets infected.

In the case of the common cold, unless you get sicker or die of complications from the unnecessary antibiotics, you get better with time. The bacterial pathogens in UTIs and wound infections are unremarkable and sensitive to first-line antibiotics. They usually resolve without further agony. All three of these types of infection cause millions of hours of lost work and end up costing the American economy upwards of $25 billion every year.

If you are in the hospital and become the unlucky recipient of a nosocomial, or hospital-acquired, infection, you are much more likely to be infected with a bacterium that is sometimes more aggressive, usually more persistent, and often resistant to multiple antibiotics. Hospital-acquired infections often involve bacteria which in the outside world are your basic ninety-pound weaklings. In the hospital, these normally wimpy germs are incubated and grown in the presence of the latest and strongest antibiotics; anything that survives such a hostile upbringing is going to be extremely difficult to kill. Conversely, they are much more likely to kill YOU. And, despite Aunt Tilly prattling on every time life kicked you in the ass, which made you want to kill HER, nosocomial infections that don't kill you don't necessarily make you stronger. You may emerge minus a limb or a large chunk of flesh or a functioning brain or, in the case of cardiac surgery, your breastbone. The whole breastbone. Just like that wishbone thing at Thanksgiving, except, instead of you and drunk Uncle Boris wishing and yanking, millions of evil bacteria are chewing on it and eventually your cardiac surgeon has to go in and pull it out. Permanently.

Except for doing the research and formulating new immunizations, preventive medicine is extremely boring. If you do your job well and prevent illnesses, there's never a great case or a weird complication of a disease. Nobody pats you on the back for preventing illnesses in your patients, and they sure don't--at least not yet--compensate you for a preventive job well done. Insurance companies don't like to reimburse for preventive measures. Drug companies rarely come up with a sexy new preventive medication that boosts their bottom line. The news media has an absolute horror of anything that prevents a catastrophe. Catastrophes boost readership and viewership. However, like Aunt Tilly said, an ounce of prevention is worth a pound of cure. Drug companies would love to be able to come up with an antidote to disease prevention that they could sell by the pound. Preventing nosocomial infections is especially boring. Ninety-nine per cent of it involves washing your hands.

A few years ago, for a couple of weeks I counted the number of times I washed my hands at work. On average, I would see between twenty and twenty-five patients in a twelve-hour shift. I would wash my hands before and after seeing each new patient. Most times I would see them or examine them at least once more before admission to the hospital or discharge home. Pretty consistently I would average between four and five hand washings per patient, which came to between eighty and one hundred twenty-five times per shift. Sounds excessive, but that's what everyone in the hospital should be doing. That and the gloves.

As researchers have demonstrated, you can transmit the common cold more effectively by shaking someone's hand than by sneezing on them. If you catch a cold just before or after heart surgery, at the least you will be coughing; that is going to hurt. So your nurse and doctor and anyone who comes into your room should wash their hands before they lay hands on you. They should put on a fresh pair of gloves as well. Insist on it. If someone refuses, ask the charge nurse to page the hospital infection control nurse. They love stuff like that.

Before we had methicillin-resistant staph aureus, a.k.a. MRSA, we had plain old staph aureus. It turns out that, when it comes to preventing your sternotomy wound from becoming infected with staph aureus, one of the most dangerous disease transmitters is your heart surgeon's nose. That is where we harbor staph. Ideally, everyone in the hospital would wear a mask at all times. That might float in the Orient, where people seem to view surgical masks as a fashion statement, but it'll probably never catch on here. Alternatively, it would be nice if every hospital staff member and visitor shoved a Q-tip dipped in mupirocin (Bactroban) cream up each nostril every morning. That would be costly, and eventually, we'd have Bactroban-resistant staph aureus to deal with. However, at least for the first forty-eight hours postop, anyone who examines or undresses your wounds on your chest or legs should be wearing a mask and gloves. Be on the lookout for nosepickers as well.

Another big area of infection prevention involves those tubes entering your body. Every day, ask your nurse and doctors if there are any catheters or IV lines that can be removed. Insisting on all of the above will really annoy everyone, but it will increase your chances of leaving the hospital without a nosocomial infection. In addition, everyone will be on the same wavelength when it comes to getting that annoying patient, a.k.a. you, out of the hospital ASAP. The longer you stay, the greater the risk of acquiring an infection, which will make you sick, add days to your stay, and add thousands of dollars to your bill.

99. INTERNISTS

An internist is basically a pediatrician for grownups. They treat just about any medical condition. They tend not do surgery, except maybe to make a few bucks assisting surgeons. They tend not to deliver babies. They tend not to treat children, although some of them do a residency in both internal medicine and pediatrics and often specialize in adolescent medicine.

I once spent an entire morning in lectures at an Internal Medicine conference. Well, actually, not the entire morning. It took only thirty minutes of the four hours of lectures to figure out that I didn't really care whether it was better to collect three or six samples to determine if your patient had blood in his stools. As one guy said while we were walking out, "How many angels do you need on the head of a pin to decide that your patient has colon cancer?" I asked him if he was an internist.

"No way. I'm an FP (family practitioner). I thought I was going to learn something new and helpful about occult G.I. bleeding, but that's not going to happen here." That pretty much sums up how Internal Medicine used to be. Back when I did the IM rodeo, in the early '80s, there were two separate subsets of Internal Medicine—academic and private practice. The academic guys did research, wrote articles—trust me, there were countless articles written and published in journals about the blood in the stool thing—and taught students and residents. The private practice guys saw patients and treated normal everyday medical problems. I went to an ivory tower med school. In the internal medicine department, the goal was not to train guys to go out and start private practices. It was to train guys to go do fellowships in some subspecialty like Cardiology or Hematology, and then go teach in an academic setting. Training private practitioners to take care of adults was the bailiwick of the Family Practice department.

It was a great time to be an internal medicine student, resident or attending. The private practice guys would find some patient with a weird set of symptoms or signs or lab tests or x-rays, and would admit him to the local hospital for a workup. When they failed to come up with a diagnosis, or when they came up with a diagnosis that required exotic treatment, they shipped the patient off to the local mecca (Every resident thought he was training at "The Mecca"), where the workup would begin anew, usually repeating every test and x-ray that had already been done at the private doc's office and at the other hospital (The other place was always referred to as "St. Elsewhere", hence the name of the TV series.), and then have every possible consultant see the patient, then come up with another boatload of tests and x-rays and whatever other procedure was new on the scene.

Sometimes, if the patient actually survived the daily bloodletting and radiation, the mecca would come up with a diagnosis. Not uncommonly, they would not. If they came up with a diagnosis, sometimes there was a treatment available. Not uncommonly, it was untreatable. If there was a treatment, sometimes the patient responded to the treatment. Not uncommonly, he did not. Sometimes the combo of workup and treatment killed the patient.

They would always say, when we were taking care of patients in medical school, "When you hear hoofbeats, think horses, not zebras. So that is how we got the term "Zebras" to describe a rare diagnosis. Make that rare squared. Problem is, when you are learning about medicine at "The Mecca", they are teaching you to find zebras. Zebras are cool. Horses are boring. If you are told to go into a corral full of horses and get a horse, well, other than getting kicked, stomped and bitten, you are probably going to be able to find a horse. When you are told to go into a corral full of horses and get a zebra, that is going to take a little more time. Or money. Or both. So when you went to "The Mecca", they were basically saying, "Get me a zebra. But if you can't find a zebra, then a five-legged horse will do." Again, very time-consuming or very expensive. Or both. The beauty of the system at that time was that the insurance companies paid for all the time you spent looking for that zebra. And if you FOUND the zebra, not only could you run around yelling, "I made the diagnosis! I am hot medical shit in a champagne glass!", you could also publish a case report. AND the attending or the consultant could get the patient into a study of this particular species of zebra. That meant money, fame, prestige, etc.

Then we got DRGs. Dianostic Related Groups. That happened in the early '80s. That was pretty much the beginning of widespread Managed Care. Kaiser Permanente began their managed care system in California in 1945, but when DRGs came along, it really made sense to manage the care of a patient or a large group of patients. Now, when a patient had a very strange set of symptoms or tests or x-rays, they could go to the hospital, but the insurance company would only pay a fixed amount, whether the patient was there for a day or ten days. The hospital and the doctor now had an incentive to get that guy out of there ASAP, BUT they could move him to another hospital and the payment wheel might, in some cases, start all over again. In some cases, The Mecca was also under the DRG gun to figure out what was going on with the patient ASAP. And THEN the insurance companies began to ratchet down the amount they would pay for a particular DRG.

Pretty soon, if you weren't a cost-effective hospital, you went out of business. AND, if you were not a cost-effective doctor, you were kicked out of health plans. The old guys I was training with back then really hated it, because here they are in their 50s or 60s or even 70s, when you are about as flexible as rebar, and they are being told to dramatically change the way they practice medicine. Adding insult to injury, the hospital is sending around NURSES, for Christ's sake, to tell them they have to get their patient out of the hospital within twenty-four hours, because he has reached his Maximum Hospital Benefit. A bunch of them retired, muttering that this was the end of the American Health Care System. Oh, look at that! That's what the guys my age in private practice are muttering about BO's Health Plan today as they retire. Some things never change. Mutter, mutter, mutter. Whenever you hear somebody muttering about how the little guy is getting screwed, it usually means he just found out he was one of the little guys.

Getting back to the DRGs. They drove workups out of the hospitals. The hospitals, even The Mecca, got paid less to go hunting zebras. So then they had to start admitting more horses. This was good for residents and students, because they saw more and more horses. Thus they would be better trained to find horses, which is what they'd most likely be doing in practice once they left The Mecca.

100. DISCHARGE

You're going home! Hopefully.

You've done all the right things, you've had a bit of luck, and now you are ready to head home. No hard feelings, but everyone is ready for you to go as well. Though there's a ton of paperwork involved, it is fun to admit and discharge patients on a regular basis. That means the hospital machine is functioning smoothly. A patient who hangs around on telemetry more than a couple of days starts to smell; he accumulates complications as well. You know you've been there too long when you've become acquainted with every nurse on the ward.

A typical discharge includes reams of paperwork. There will be instructions for wound care--your chest and leg incisions. You will also receive a paper with dietary recommendations and activity suggestions. Bear in mind that nobody at home will be shepherding you through your day the way the nurses did. Even if you've got a harem of wives, each in their color-coded tent, or a polygamous circle of state-assisted single-wides, it's still going to be up to you to make the effort necessary to recover to your full potential. In other words, you have to decide what to shovel into your face and when to get off your ass to take a walk. Although most patients feel a sense of relief at going home, a certain percentage will experience withdrawal with respect to the structure of the hospital routine. If you are one of those, the best way to get over your separation anxiety is to set up a rigid structure at home. Write out a schedule for sleep, meals, and exercise--nothing else really matters for the first week anyway--and, as far as your physical condition permits, stick to it.

Except for very rare circumstances, you will probably receive a couple of prescriptions as well. There will probably be one for an ACE inhibitor, perhaps a beta blocker, a platelet poison or two, and almost certainly a statin for your cholesterol. If you have someone who can fill them at your local pharmacy, good for you. Given your fragile status, you won't do well standing in line waiting for the guy in front of you to finish arguing with the pharmacist about the Vicodin refill that was "stolen". If you don't have anybody who can help, the hospital can probably send you home with a week's supply of each. They won't like it, but if you put on your most pathetic face, they'll cave.

Most hospitals won't let you go home alone or in a cab. They want someone to make sure you walk into your home alive. You could hire a baby sitter for an hour or so, but if this is your situation, give your nurse a heads-up at least a day before, so she can run it by your case manager or a hospital social worker or discharge planner. This is the sort of thing they do on a regular basis. Likewise, if you will need some help at home for a while, they can arrange something for you until you are back up to snuff. Just don't act too wimpy, or they'll ship you to the...

101. SNF

Pronounced "sniff", the Skilled Nursing Facility (SNF) is where you end up when you are not sick enough to be in the hospital but too sick or frail to go home. It sounds like a safe haven, and occasionally it is, but for the most part, it is not a desirable destination. If you have to go there, and, honestly, nobody chooses to go there, you want to make it a very short stay.

It's great if you can find a SNF that is purely a short-term rehab facility. Unfortunately, many SNFs take all comers. That includes people recovering from pneumonia, urinary tract infections or wound infections. It also includes long-term residents with head injuries or spinal injuries, some of whom have tracheostomies, are on ventilators, and have feeding tubes. There are a lot of infections floating around in those folks as well.

Placement in a SNF usually requires that you have need of an IV, often antibiotics. Other patients go there for physical, occupational or speech therapy. If you don't require any of these, you may end up in a less skilled situation, like a rehab place. Neither is terrific, but anytime you don't have an IV involved, you are less likely to meet your new worst enemy, MRSA.

102. OUTPATIENT REHAB

Congrats on getting out of the hospital in one piece!

Whereas your goal upon awakening from surgery was to get out of the hospital as quickly as possible, your goal now is to do whatever you can so that you never have to go back. Like the cards say, "Get well soon!"

Life at home will bear very little resemblance to life in the hospital. If that's not the case, your home life is disastrous; consider relocating. Unless you reside in an insane asylum, there should be much less noise, as there will be only one patient--you--and far fewer staff members. Most houses do not have a PA system, and beeping monitors would definitely be out of place. If you hear voices outside your door, it's probably not the night shift making their rounds; consider starting an antipsychotic medication.

Your home should smell much different than a hospital room. There may be some residual benzoin on your dressings, that cinnamon aroma, but it should not be overpowering. Nobody in your home should be experiencing a GI bleed.

Your sleep cycle will probably continue to be interrupted. Don't sweat it. If you do wake up at 2:00 AM, at least there won't be an oddly-featured individual of indeterminate gender bent over your bed, staring intently at you as if trying to decide which condiment would go best with your face. Avoid benzodiazepine sleeping medications. They're the ones whose chemical names end in -pam. Diazepam (Valium), flurazepam (Dalmane), alprazolam (Xanax), lorazepam (Ativan), midazolam (Versed), oxazepam (Serax), temazepam (Restoril), and zolpidem (Ambien) all belong to the class of drugs known as sedative-hypnotics or soporifics. If you take them every night for more than a few days, they will become a necessary part of your life. Once you develop a dependency on them, you will probably have to endure more sleepless nights; you are right back where you started, but probably a little worse off. If you have to use them, try to limit them to three times per week, and drop them after your second week home.

I was going to put psychological aspects of your early recovery in a separate chapter, but, if you are at all like me, you'd probably just skip over it.

Like those Vietnam vets who still walk point around the backyard with their M-16's all night long, waiting for Charlie to attack, you've been through a near-death experience, so a modicum of PTSD is not at all uncommon. Like most illnesses, PTSD comes in all sizes and shapes. A seemingly trivial life event can result in some degree of PTSD, anything from troubled sleep with weird dreams to mild anxiety, to flashbacks, to full blown hyperventilation syndrome, complete with shortness of breath, sweating, pains or numbness in your arms, chest pain, and lightheadedness. In short, an episode of PTSD associated with the recent trauma of your heart surgery can mimic a heart attack and send you right back to the E.R. courtesy of your local ambulance crew. How's that for a cruel twist of irony? Often PTSD resolves with nothing more than time and a return to your normal routine, but it's not uncommon for some patients to require long-term therapy and occasionally meds to send it packing. Great. More meds. If you get to the point where you are having suicidal thoughts, you will definitely require professional help pronto. It's time to call a suicide hotline or 911.

A dash of reactive depression can mar your early recovery too. Reactive depression is defined as mild to moderate depression following a stressful event. Even if your admission for heart surgery was planned far in advance and went as smooth as silk, the whole experience definitely qualifies as stressful. Most patients with reactive depression don't get to the stage where they think about suicide; they just feel more than the normal amount of grief. If, however, excessive sadness continues to interfere with your life, therapy is in order.

Although most experts differentiate reactive depression from endogenous depression, where your brain chemicals are absent or present in the wrong concentrations, there are those who feel that medications are warranted to get you up and going. Unless you spend a significant portion of your day curled up into a ball, moaning pathetically while rocking back and forth in your bed, you probably don't require anti-depressants.

Regarding emotional or psychological complications, your cardiologist and your cardiac surgeon may be the sweetest humans ever to walk the earth (doubtful), but they don't really want to hear about problems inside your head. If you are having problems with anger, anxiety or depression, talk to a friend or, better yet, contact your primary care provider. Your PCP can put you in touch with a therapist, which would probably be more beneficial than talking to Thor, your ex-Marine next door neighbor, whose solution to every problem in life is to "suck it up" or "shake it off". Those suggestions didn't work too well for him, which is why you never see him without a can of cheap beer in his hand.

Your narcotic pain reliever should be Percocet (oxycodone). Vicodin (hydrocodone) is much less potent; it's basically a wimpy-assed pain reliever, so patients end up taking more of them more often. That's why it's such a popular drug of abuse. Avoid long-acting narcotics, like oxycontin or MS Contin or methadone, as these can build up in your system and make you nuts. Most of the popular oral narcotics have some acetaminophen (Tylenol) in them. Taking too much of any of them can lead to acetaminophen toxicity, which, in its most extreme form, causes liver failure and death. Most likely you will find that taking some narcotic at your usual bedtime will be effective in sedating you and relieving your pain sufficiently to allow you at least four hours of sleep at a time. Get off the narcs as quickly as possible. Unless you continue to increase the dose, they usually aren't all that effective after a couple of days.

NSAID's like ibuprofen are probably better for long-term pain relief. While pain experts recommend taking them as often as stated on the bottle, the more you take, the more often you take them, and the longer you take them, the more likely you will run into side effects, especially GI upset, ulcers, and GI bleeding. If you are old or have any degree of kidney impairment, the meds will hang around in your system longer and do more damage to your GI tract, kidneys and maybe your heart than they would to young healthy people. Always take them after eating, in the lowest dose that provides pain relief. I found that a low dose of Tylenol in combination with a low dose of ibuprofen two or three times a day was pretty effective at taking the edge off my pain.

WALKING

At least for the first couple of weeks, the only exercise you really need is walking. However, you must do it every day, even on the days when you feel like shit. Pick the time of day when the temperature is closest to 70 degrees F. Wear loose clothing so it doesn't rub against your wounds. Start out walking up and down your street for five to ten minutes. Do it as often each day as you can tolerate. If you live in San Francisco, you have my sympathy. Walking up and down those hills fresh out of the hospital may indeed kill you. To avoid becoming permanently hunched over like an old crone, stand up as straight as you can. There should be some discomfort, a feeling of stretching in your sternal wound. The term surgeons use is "eyes on the horizon".

Not only is walking good for the recovery of your muscle tone and your cardiovascular status, but it also works to normalize your autonomic nervous system, which probably is still on the fritz. If you get tired, it is best to keep walking, even at a snail's pace; if you stop and stand still, there's a good chance blood will pool in your legs, you'll get lightheaded, and possibly pass out. If you absolutely can't go any farther without resting, the next best thing is to sit down. Get moving again after a minute or two, unless of course you are having chest pain or are short of breath. Bring your cell phone with you, in case you have to call 911 or a friend to come get you. While this all sounds incredibly stupid, there will be days when your energy level completely deserts you and it will be all you can do to walk a few minutes.

Your discharge meds should not have much effect on your walking. ACE inhibitors will tend to make you more orthostatic, but that effect is greatest when you start the drug or increase the dose, and gets less noticeable over time. As always, orthostasis is worst when standing still, and much less common while walking. Beta-blockers are usually prescribed in much lower doses than in the past. They tend to keep your heart rate from speeding up. Occasionally a patient with asthma will notice increased wheezing on these meds, especially when exercising; that deserves a call to your physician. Aspirin or Plavix, both of which thin your blood, probably won't affect your exercise tolerance much. Likewise, statins and other hypolipidemics have side effects, but impairing your ability to walk isn't one of them. If you start having pain in your muscles beyond what you would expect from walking, call your doctor, as statins can cause rhabdomyolysis, a breakdown in muscle. Avoid reading the PDR or medication package inserts for side effects. The power of suggestion is especially formidable when you are not feeling your best.

Remember that every automobile is your enemy, especially the BMWs driven by the youngish guy with the cell phone stuck to his ear and the hair plugs stuck in his scalp. Your thought process should be that you are absolutely invisible to anyone driving a car, and even if they do see you, they don't give a rat's ass whether you live or die. From years of experience, I can assure you they do not. When possible, walk along paths or sidewalks. When you cannot avoid crossing at an intersection, take your time, stay in the crosswalk, and never assume you can run to make it across a street before the oncoming traffic takes a shot at you.

FOOD

Start out light. Try to set some good habits from day 1. Drink lots of water unless you are on a fluid restriction. Adding a couple fiber capsules twice a day will help keep you from binding up. You don't want to be straining to take a crap. That hurts when you've got a new incision through skin, muscle and bone. Theoretically you could pop a stitch too.

If you are overweight--if you're not sure, look south towards your thrill hammer--try to eat three small meals daily. That means a meal that fits on a small plate, not the usual big one. No second helpings and no desserts. Whether or not you believe that carbs are the stuff of Satan, if you cut them out, it is almost impossible not to lose weight. You have my personal promise that you won't starve to death either.

Eliminate sugar. Right now it is the hot topic when it comes to your health in general and cardiovascular disease in particular. Despite all the hoopla, nobody really knows how the sugar story will play out ten years down the road. However, it is clear that sugar adds useless calories to your diet. So try your coffee or tea, your cereal, without it. If you must have sweetening, like in recipes, use some sort of artificial sweetener. No matter which kind, the less you use, the less likely you will get that nasty chemical aftertaste to ruin your day. If you have to have dessert, try one of those one hundred calorie things. Better yet, get used to fresh fruit as your go-to for dessert or a late-night snack

Eliminate salt. Odds are you're not one of those rare birds who needs added salt to keep your blood pressure up to normal. Even if your blood pressure is normal, no good comes from adding salt to your daily diet, especially if you are on medications, which undoubtedly you will be.

If you were intubated for any length of time, you may feel lung congestion for a week or two after you are extubated. Coughing up bloody crusted slop from your lungs hurts. Stand in a hot shower and let the water beat on your back. It tends to loosen things up; those bloody chunks will rise up from your bronchi to your throat, so that you can just spit them out. Sounds disgusting, but it is effective. Because you are probably on new medications and your autonomic nervous system still isn't operating at full speed, make sure you don't stand under the hot water so long that your blood vessels dilate and send you crashing into the bathtub in a dizzy swirl.

It's going to be a while before your sternal and leg wounds heal completely. My dermatologist recommended I open a vitamin E capsule and rub the goo into my wounds every day. Theoretically it aids in healing of your wounds. In addition, he prescribed mupirocin (Bactroban) ointment for my wounds, especially the ones south of my butt. You can use plain old over-the-counter bacitracin or triple antibiotic ointment instead. Any of these will keep your wounds soft while they heal, and they might prevent an infection as well. Some experts recommend daily doses of oral vitamin C to promote collagen production, and the application of zinc oxide, which speeds healing of acute or chronic wounds. Just to be on the safe side, be sure to check this out with your cardiac surgeon and your PCP before applying anything to your wounds.

References:

1. Graham, Ian, Ingram, Shirley, Fallon, Noeleen, Leong, Tora, Gormley, John, O'Doherty, Veronica, Maher, Vincent, Benson, Suzanne. "Rehabilitation of the Patient with Coronary Heart Disease." *Hurst's The Heart.* Ed. Valentin Fuster, Ed. Robert A. O'Rourke, Ed. Richard A. Walsh, Ed. Philip Poole-Wilson. New York: McGraw-Hill. 2008. 1529-43.

103. OFFICE FOLLOW-UP

There is no way you will confuse a cardiologist's office waiting room with an Obamacare pep rally. Occasionally there will be a young person with a history of childhood surgery for congenital heart disease who has outgrown the sliding board entrance to the pediatric cardiologist's office, but for the most part, the average age of a cardiology waiting room denizen is around seventy, a tribute to the medical profession and the pharmaceutical industry. Back in 1978, when *The House of God* was written, once a patient was diagnosed with congestive heart failure (CHF), he could be expected to live no more than ten years, usually less than five. Nowadays, CHF patients can sport fat juicy ankles for decades.

Likewise, in the 1970s the basic rule was, "If you make it to eighty-five years of age, there is no way you will die of cardiac disease." In addition, if you lived to eighty-five, you would probably live to be one hundred and die of cancer. Or pneumonia, the "old man's friend." Or old age. That implied that either you were going to have heart disease or you weren't. If you had it, you would not live to see eighty-five. If you didn't, that meant you had good genes and would never get heart disease. Now, thanks to the myriad of interventions and medications available, you can be diagnosed with heart disease at sixty-five, live well past eighty-five, and still die in your early nineties of heart disease.

When you follow up in the cardiologist's office after a hospitalization, you are expected to be either stable on your meds and/or doing well after your angioplasty or CABG. Remember, nobody likes a troublemaker. It is considered bad form to show up and admit you are feeling like shit. That means either more tests, a trial of a new medication or a dosage adjustment of an old one, or back to the hospital you go. Whatever you do, do not try to die in the cardiologist's office, especially the waiting room. It is embarrassing for you, lying there sucking air like a beached blowfish while the rest of the patients squirm in their chairs or lean over to take your last action photo. Worse yet, it screws up the office appointment schedule and necessitates the noisy arrival of a fire engine, meat wagon, and a dozen or so firemen and paramedics. Very messy.

When you show up for that first post-operative visit, it's a little more complicated than subsequent appointments. That's because the only links between your hospital stay and your office visit are you and your cardiologist. With the availability of hospitalists, nurse practitioners and physician assistants, there's a good chance your discharge medication prescriptions were written by someone other than your cardiologist. Those discharge med scripts are usually for a month or less, often with no refills available, so on your first visit someone has to rewrite them. Depending on how far behind the hospital's dictation service and medical records department are, your op note and discharge summary may or may not be available. So it's a tough go for all parties concerned. For a patient in his seventies or eighties, with or without a family member, it's much more difficult. Me, I was just happy to get on and off the scale and sit on the exam table before passing out.

On your first visit to the office, you will usually get an EKG. That's to make sure you didn't have an MI in the intervening week and to make sure your meds aren't causing some bizarre arrhythmia that may eventually lead to your untimely demise. Imagine that, surviving open-heart surgery, only to be felled by a diuretic or beta-blocker or ACE-inhibitor, some age-old drug that millions have taken safely. Still, it happens. Since you haven't yet established a routine regarding office visits, someone will probably draw your blood there as well, to make sure your kidneys are working okay, your electrolytes are within normal limits, and you are not too anemic. One of the staff will review your prescriptions to ensure that you are taking the correct meds and in the dosages prescribed.

When the doctor comes in, he'll check the discharge summary to make sure everything is kosher. Then he'll take your blood pressure, check your pulse, and listen to your heart and lungs. Everything should be okay; you can ask a few questions if you like. Once he cuts you loose, run like hell. Or at least stagger at top speed.

104. OFFICE FOLLOW-UP: CARDIAC SURGEON

When you follow up with the surgeon who invaded your body with a sharp knife, do not expect much. Don't bother bringing up annoying complaints about how you feel. When your wife brings out her two-page list of questions regarding your crummy appetite, your inadequate bowel output, your lack of interest in anything at all, gently remove it from her hands, tear it up, and drop it in the trash can. This saves the surgeon from repeating twenty or more times, "You should ask your cardiologist or primary care provider."

If you don't have any sutures that require removal, and there are no slabs of necrotic (dead) flesh dangling from your wound, the visit is pretty much a waste of everybody's time. Even a wound infection is better treated by your primary care provider. Barring any catastrophic complications, the cardiac surgeon's job essentially ends after the first twenty-four hours of post-op care. The follow-up visit with your cardiac surgeon is basically a matter of adhering to medical tradition, with just a dash of satisfying malpractice insurance requirements thrown in for spice. Since you have obviously made it past that time limit, you might want to thank him for a successful bypass, maybe bring him a box of chocolates or something. Though your favorite grandchild is an artistic genius, unless your surgeon is a pro-lifer, his day won't be any sunnier for your having presented him with one of her framed second grade crayon creations, even if it's titled "Thank you for saving Grandpa's life!". Medical office building dumpsters are chock full of such masterpieces.

105. PUMPHEAD

His name was Robert Waldman. His friends had called him Robbie all his life. He was able to work his way through his first name, but when Simmons asked him, "Robbie What?", he stared blankly, then looked down and pulled the blanket up under his chin. The air conditioning had the place nice and cool. While the pre-menopausal nurses wrapped themselves in sweaters and blankets, Simmons and his menopausal colleagues loved it that way. It kept him awake and alert; they cut way back on their sweat output.

"Mrs. Waldman, has this been getting better or worse since he was discharged?"

"The same. They told me he'd be fine in a couple of days, but it's been over a week. It's like living with an old man in a nursing home." She was a fine looking woman, probably in her late fifties, which put her about fifteen years younger than the patient.

"How long have you folks been married?"

"Seventeen years. I was forty and Robbie was fifty-six. God, he was dashing back then. He swept me off my feet at a cocktail party and in forty-eight hours we were lying on the beach in Monte Carlo." David looked back at Mr. Waldman. He was nodding off, a touch of drool sliding down his chin, clearly incapable of sweeping anything off of anything. The dash was gone, probably for good, and she knew it.

"Has he ever had this problem before?"

"Of course not. It was that damn bypass surgery that did this to him. I called his surgeon's office. They said he didn't need to be seen until next Tuesday. When I told them about the way Robbie's acting, they put me on hold, then gave me the number of some psychologist to call."

"How'd that go?"

"Oh, he's scheduled to go in and be tested on Monday."

"That sounds like a logical next step. That's only three days from now. May I ask why you brought him in tonight?"

"I was hoping you could give him something to wake him up. We have a reception to go to at Loews tomorrow night, and obviously he can't go like this."

"Wake him up. Hmm. Is he taking any pain meds or sleeping pills?"

"Are you kidding? Sleeping pills? All he does is sleep. The psychologist's office told me to stop giving him the oxycodone. He hasn't had any since yesterday morning. It hasn't made a bit of difference. Of course, that was probably a good idea, since he doesn't seem to have any pain. Even if he did, you wouldn't know it." She stood up and straightened out her dress. *My goodness,* Simmons thought. *You sure know how to take care of yourself, don't you?*

"I don't think anything is going to wake him up. The CT didn't show any signs of a stroke or bleed in his head, and his blood work is pretty much normal. It may be that he still has some residual oxycodone in his system, but I think this is going to be a problem for a while. Most likely he's got what they call "pumphead", which is damage to the brain associated with the bypass machine during surgery. The experts say that to get better, the brain has to grow new blood vessels over the next year or two. If the patient develops new blood vessels, the problem gets better. If that doesn't happen, often the problem persists for years or permanently. He's not the worst I've seen, but he's pretty bad. Usually these severe cases will improve to a certain degree, but I wouldn't count on him being the same guy he was prior to surgery."

She frowned, did some calculating in her head, then smiled at David.

"Could you do me a little favor, Dr. Simmons, is it?"

"Favor?" He could feel the charm exuding from her.

"Our housekeeper and cook are off the weekends, so it's just Robbie and me. Could you keep him here in the hospital or wherever until Sunday morning? I promise I'll pick him up by noon. It's just that I have this really special cocktail dress I bought just for this reception, and it seems such a shame to let it go to waste."

106. DOCTOR'S ORDERS

Things were going swimmingly in post-CABG clinic. The patients who came here had undergone bypass surgery in the past six weeks, either emergently at one of the local private hospitals or here at the San Diego VAMC on an elective basis. First they went to chest surgery clinic one week after discharge from the hospital, to have their chest and leg wounds checked. After that, they followed up at three weeks and six weeks in the cardiology division post-CABG clinic. If everything was going well, it was back to their primary care clinic in another month, with a three-month follow-up in routine cardiology clinic.

As the only physician in the clinic on this particular Friday afternoon, Simmons was running the show. Not the entire show, but the portion of the show that wasn't run by the nurses and the techs. All the cardiology docs had headed off to Atlanta for the annual American College of Cardiology conference. The meetings were a big deal, just slightly less important than the meals, drinks, and road trips to the Jaguar III. He'd already seen eight of the ten scheduled patients. No major complications, just a few medication adjustments, the nurses in the clinic treating him like a god because he'd volunteered to sub. Two more patients and his Friday was over. Simmons was feeling like a cardiologist. Angie the clinic charge nurse walked in.

"A patient named Robert Rizzell is outside. He wants to see a cardiologist today. Something about a complication from his surgery. He's quite agitated."

"Oh, that guy. Yeah, I know him. I saw him in walk-in clinic about a month ago." He'd come in complaining of dizziness and palpitations while working out. His resting EKG was normal so Simmons referred the martial arts instructor for an outpatient treadmill. Somehow they'd squeezed him in the next day. When he developed ST depressions at seven minutes and then passed out in V tach, it was off to the cath lab and then to surgery for a four-vessel CABG within another twenty-four hours, which might have been a record for the VA. Although he'd rather see him here than down in the trenches, there was one last ray of hope for a deflection. As the acting cardiologist, he felt the need to maintain the status quo. Keep the hordes at bay.

"I didn't see him on the clinic list for today." Subspecialty clinics were notorious for their rigidity. No appointment, no visit, no exceptions.

Angie wasn't the charge nurse in this plum department job for nothing. Ready for all contingencies, she countered. "He's on for his three-week checkup next Friday. Our other two scheduled appointments won't be showing up today. Mr. Hobson is back in the hospital, and Dan Ackerman couldn't get a ride with the DAV, so we're pretty much done for the day. You want to see him or not?" Simmons mulled this over a bit. No reason to deep six the goodwill he was building. He might need to squeeze in one of his lovable old WWI vets for a procedure in the future, and Angie had a long memory for favors and trespasses.

"Might as well get this over with. Give me a minute and send him in." David looked up at her from his desk chair. "He's nuts, you know."

"He's a nut with coronary disease. There's a difference."

"All right, but if you tell the cardiologists I let in an unscheduled patient, they'll hang me by my nuts from the flagpole out front. This is just between you and me."

"Agreed. It'll be better if we just see him and send him on his way. Otherwise I'm sure he'll head down to the LSU, and that would end up with a cardiology consult or admission." *The Life Support Unit. What a name for an emergency room. About the only thing on life support down there was the unit itself.*

"Does he look like he's having angina?"

"No, but he sure is fidgety out there. Rosalita the housekeeper is giving him the stink eye and praying in Spanish."

"Tell her to say a prayer for me."

"I'll get an EKG and bring him in."

Five minutes later, Rizzell barged into Simmons' newly adopted exam room. He was far less bulky than Simmons remembered, his head was tilted so far to the right his ear was practically lying on his shoulder, and he was whining some unintelligible jibberish. When he saw Simmons, his head lifted with surprise. Then he screamed and his head came back down on his shoulder.

"Oh my God, you're the doctor from the walk-in clinic. You're not a cardiologist!"

"I am today, pal. If you'd prefer, you can come back next week to see a real cardiologist."

"No! I can't wait. You gotta help me, Doc. My chest is killing me. Something's wrong where they cut me open. It feels like something's caught in there. I think they screwed something up." He climbed up on the exam table and screamed again. Simmons sighed. *As expected.*

"Mr. Rizzell, go ahead and unbutton your shirt." Angie came in and placed his chart and a new EKG on the desk. The op note and discharge summary had just arrived and weren't yet filed in the back of the chart. Other than the amazing speed of the workup and surgery, it all appeared pretty uneventful from start to finish. Simmons saw that the discharge instructions were a little peculiar. Rizzell had apparently asked the cardiac surgeon when he could start practicing his martial arts again. The instruction sheet specified that he was to wait at least three months. In the meantime, he was to stick to walking.

Simmons put down the summary and turned to look at the patient. His head was still leaning to the right, and he was moaning softly.

"Whatcha been up to, Mr. Rizzell?" He stepped directly in front of the patient.

"What do you mean?"

"I mean, what kind of physical activity have you been pursuing the past couple of weeks?"

"Well, you know, like the surgeons said, walking, no heavy lifting. That kind of thing." He tried to avert his eyes. He reminded David of an elevator operator in an old comedy, Huntz Hall maybe, popping his head around the door. *Going up?*

"It says something about no martial arts for three months. That ring a bell?" Simmons ran his hand lightly down Rizzell's sternotomy scar. Instead of a smooth vertical line, the incision zigzagged back and forth like a red Z. Where there should have been a slightly irregular but basically smooth ridge of bone, his breast bone was a maze of knots and overlaps.

"Aw, Doc, jeez, do something for me, will you? This is killing me."

"How long did you wait before you started punching and kicking?" Rizzell jerked his head up again, then screamed and set it back down to Position A. Simmons thought to himself, *This guy has really poor short-term memory. Either that or he likes the pain.*

"I didn't! Honest."

"Really? You couldn't wait, could you?" Simmons raised his eyebrows and waited.

"No, I couldn't! I can't believe this hurts so much. I felt fine last week. I started my routine, lifting some weights too. Oh, God. What can you do? Help me!"

"Well, I can give you some pain meds and then you can go to the Chest Surgery clinic Tuesday afternoon. Are they still seeing you?"

"No, they discharged me last Tuesday, said my wound looked good and I should be fine." *That was pretty quick work*, thought Simmons. *Screwing up a perfectly good sternotomy in ten days.* "Do you think they can fix this?"

"No, sir, I don't. Even if they reopened your sternum, which they won't, no matter how much they sand and scrape, you are going to be misshapen pretty much forever."

"Oh God, what have I done?" He looked over at David. "They won't reopen it?"

"Not a chance. Much greater risk of infection, and, like I said, it won't help. But you might as well go see them. Maybe they'll have some idea that will help a little."

"Thanks, Doc. I can't believe how stupid I am."

"I'm trying to get my head around it as well, Sir. Give me a minute to fill out the referral form and write you a script." Moments later, Simmons stood up and handed the paperwork to the former martial arts instructor.

"Good luck, Mr. Rizzell. Don't be too hard on yourself. Everybody screws up all the time. That's why I have a job."

They shook hands. As the patient shuffled out, Simmons thought, *Change the scenario a little here and there, and that could be me.*

107. TEN THINGS TO DO IF YOU THINK YOU ARE GOING TO DIE IN YOUR SLEEP

1) Don't leave any dirty dishes in the sink.
2) Leave all insurance policies and your will in plain sight.
3) Turn off the burglar alarm if you are alone in the house.
4) If your child is staying with you, teach him to call 911 if Dad won't wake up.
5) Leave written notes to loved ones.
6) Specify funeral wishes.
7) Do the 12-step thing: apologize to all whom you have offended.
8) Wear boxers to bed. No reason to ruin someone's day by finding you dead and naked, especially your kids.
9) Put away all sex toys and porn. Odds are, if you think you are going to die in the next eight hours, you might have trouble getting it up anyway.
10) Make a deal with anyone, including the devil, to stay alive until morning.

108. LONG TERM FOLLOW-UP

The long-term follow-up consists of office visits. Usually these are every month for a few months, then every three months for a year or so, then every six months. Count on getting your fasting lipid panel drawn, so your physician can go over your cholesterol levels with you and make any necessary changes in your meds. Likewise, if you are on meds that affect your kidneys, like ACE-inhibitors or diuretics, your renal function and electrolyte levels will be checked. Hopefully you can get your labs drawn a week or two before your appointment, so that he can discuss the results with you face-to-face. If not, then you'll have to get it done at your appointment or afterwards; your cardiologist will have to call you with the results and that is a pain in the ass for all concerned.

Every year or two, count on undergoing a nuclear treadmill stress test. The rationale for the nuke tread is that it can predict the likelihood of your developing angina or an MI. The party line is that if your nuke tread is normal, you should have a green light for the next two years. Even if you are running marathons twice a week without angina, there will be pressure on you to do the nuke tread.

"I want to keep an eye on things before something big develops." This assumes that a nuke tread can predict plaque rupture, which it can't. It does show areas of the heart that are ischemic during exercise. It doesn't pay for the whole Beemer, just the tires.

Every three to five years, expect an echocardiogram and a carotid study to be added to the to-do list. The echo is to look for valvular disease, ventricular performance and ventricular wall thickening. It gives the cardiologist a better idea of your cardiac output, the amount of blood pumped by your heart every minute, and your ejection fraction, the percentage of blood in your left ventricle that is pumped out with each contraction. Both of these measurements are indicators of how well your heart pump is working. There seems to be a consensus that the nuke tread does not do a good job of estimating either. Again, if you are very active, and are having no shortness of breath, most likely your EF and CO are doing just fine. Don't try to tell that to your doctor. Go with the flow. You are too old and lazy to try to swim upstream.

The carotid studies are non-invasive, basically ultrasounds of your carotid arteries. The idea is to make sure that the disease process that caused your heart problems, atherosclerosis, is not planning an assault on your brain as well. Carotid studies on a regular basis are important mainly because treating moderate disease is a lot easier than treating severe disease. If the disease becomes too severe before it is detected, you could end up with a stroke. It would be a shame to survive heart surgery only to end up wheelchair-bound or dead from a plaque and a clot in your neck or brain.

I once met a gastroenterologist. He was married to a rich girl and decided that he could afford an unusual arrangement. A sensible deal. If he recommended an upper endoscopy, a flexible sigmoidoscopy or a colonoscopy, and found nothing or found exactly what he expected, he would waive his fee. To his way of thinking, if the procedure didn't make a difference in the diagnosis and didn't change the treatment or the prognosis, it was superfluous and the patient shouldn't have to pay for it. If he found something unexpected or something that required further testing, he would charge the patient. Great idea. Then he got divorced from the rich girl and suddenly had to earn enough to pay for those pesky details of life, like a mortgage, car payment, taxes, stuff like that. Au revoir to free exotic vacations, the good life, and the sensible deal.

Assuming you don't have more angina or an MI and you don't drop dead, after a year or two you'll get used to the idea of being well again. Unless you're a worry wart, you'll stop fretting that your cardiologist will find something godawful when he sees you every six months or so. The office appointments will become less intimidating. Another year or so and they'll be a minor inconvenience. Even if your cardiologist gets bored with you, he won't divorce you. Once you have a chronic disease, you are in the system. It's like that Jean-Paul Sartre play, *Huis Clos*. No Exit. Everybody wants a piece of the pie that is you. You can decide to have your primary care doctor do your semi-annual blood work and office visit, then do the nuke tread and other tests with the cardiologist every couple of years. If you continue to follow-up regularly with your cardiologist, there will undoubtedly be some repetition of blood tests.

109. INTRODUCTION TO "ME"

I started this book with the idea that I would tell the story of my journey through the minefield of heart disease. Undoubtedly that would be fascinating to everyone, because, as we all know, our lives are so unusual and so very special. They say that everyone has one good novel in them. They do not say that everyone has one good life story in them. After about two years, when my brain finally started to function in a manner barely approaching my normal, I realized that my story, while good for about ten minutes of spellbinding bar chatter, would bore most of the earth's population to tears, should anyone be silly enough to start reading it. Nevertheless, you must do something with your free time.

I started out life with an adept left brain. What little I had in the way of right brain creativity didn't exactly get nurtured in the Catholic grade school system (conveyor belt). Nevertheless, I came out of my education with a knack for testing well, a faultless memory, and true skill at spitting back what I was taught. After my health travails, with much of my left brain lifetime skills reduced to below average, my right brain finally said, "Enough, let me out!" Somebody had to run my life.

No matter how hard your job, it is mostly a matter of showing up, doing what is expected of you, solving some problems, and going home. The framework is there; whether or not you succeed is often decided by how well you fit in. Creating, on the other hand, requires that you show up even when nobody makes you, nobody watches you, and, unless you create something special, nobody cares what you do. Nor will anybody pay you to do it.

I tried waiting for inspiration. Inspiration is something that comes to you when you are in absolutely no position to act upon it. In the end, I gave up on the self-motivation idea and hired a nun. Sister Mary Carpet-tack stands behind me. In her right hand she holds a three-sided brass ruler. Any time I stop typing, she gives me a whack. Across the back, occasionally across the side of my face and ear. Never, however, the moneymaker. No, that's not my face. My hands. I can't type with broken knuckles. That particular limitation really rankles her. For years, that was how she made her living.

"Hold out your hands, Francis." Old habits die hard.

My story is just an illustration of a few of the many things that can go awry in the course of diagnosing and treating heart disease. Longtimepractitioners of medicine know that those in the health care professions or their family members tend to have worse results than the general population. I used to think this was because health care providers treat other providers or their loved ones differently than normal patients. However, I now think that this kind of "special treatment" occurs only a small percentage of the time. Perhaps it's just karma. I do know one thing. If you toil in the land of patient care long enough, no matter how compassionate you may be, eventually you become a tad hardened to human suffering. There is nothing like your own personal illness to bring you back to earth. From my perspective, especially after having gone through the process, illness is a great equalizer. Everybody looks the same in a hospital gown. Well, almost.

Whether or not you agree with the way the medical system works here in the U.S., whether you love or hate the recent changes coming out of D.C., now more than ever, most of us have a fighting chance of surviving heart disease. We take a lot for granted here, things many people in other parts of the world would look on as nothing short of a miracle. Clean water. Easily accessible food. Indoor plumbing. A backyard safe from falling bombs. Air conditioning. An ambulance when you dial 911. While we Americans are all just a cough or a sneeze away from a heart transplant, that is far better than being just a cough or a sneeze away from death.

Okay, enough of the pontificating. The take-home message from this section is that I am not a tough guy. If I can get through it, so can you. I apologize in advance for any whining.

When I showed a couple of these "Me" chapters to my daughter, she read them and, too polite to offend, simply said, "I don't remember it that way."

Translation: "Dad, you're full of shit."

Nonetheless, this is how I remember it. I made notes along the way, not because I expected to use them, but because it was something to do, something that might benefit my hand, my eyes, and my brain. Because so much of this section was put together using random notes I made over the years, there may be a fair bit of redundancy. There's also a good chance that much of what I've written may be out of sequence or overlap time periods. Oh well. You want nice orderly sequences of days, weeks, months and years, buy a calendar.

I warn you in advance. Reading this upcoming section is like watching a car wreck in slow motion. With Neil Young's *Fuckin' Up* playing in the background.

110. ATTENTION, DUMBO PILOTS!

He sat in the middle. Not a muscle moved. His face, craggy but steely still, had the dry stiffness any botox addict would die for. Even when he spoke, only his lower jaw bone showed signs of life. The microphone, positioned perfectly, required not so much as a tilt of the head to intone his commands to the squadron of pilots.

In a way, my journey through the world of cardiac bypass surgery started around 1997, eight years before I was rolled into the O.R. My daughter was four. Since the time she was four years old, we'd been travelling, usually just the two of us, occasionally with relatives or friends. This was one of our first big FNF (Fun, Not Family) trips, to Disney World. We'd already done a two-dayer to Disneyland, where I learned she was destined to live life on the funny side of the street.

When you are a parent and still getting to know who your child will be, there are some moments, some days, where you see the first glimmer of a large portion of her personality. That was the trip to D-land. Half a dozen rides through "It's A Small World" (You mention that attraction and most adults just shake their heads, roll their eyes, and stick a finger in each ear), her head whipping around at each curve to see the new chorus of singers, was barely enough for either one of us. The best thing about Mickey's Toontown was that Minnie had her house and Mickey had his--just like Mom and Dad.

In between visits to the park, during toddler "nap" time, which is actually designed for the exhausted approaching-middle-aged parent, I got a peek at the real her. Bursts of energetic fun, running from wall to wall, all within the confines of an Anaheim hotel room. A two-hour wait time in the airport for a delayed flight home, most parents' nightmare, turned into endless giggle-filled runs down the long hallways between gates. As crazy as I was about my daughter before that trip, that's when she became my favorite person on earth.

If you have a flexible work schedule, the best thing about having pre-school-aged kids is that you can travel when nobody else with kids can. Our favorite times to travel during that period were early May and late October. The lines are shorter, there is breathing space, and the chance of your kid catching some bizarre virus is much smaller. Equally important, below a certain parallel, pretty much everywhere in the U.S. features nice weather during those two months. One exception is Phoenix, but we were leaving there anyway.

Before Orlando became synonymous with all things healthy and happy, a sizeable military population was stationed in the area. The smaller the city and the larger the military presence, the more influence soldiers' preferences will have on the entertainment available there. The passenger terminal at Rapid City, S.D. Regional Airport specialized in ads touting cheap motels with hot tubs in each room. Every poster featured a muscular young guy with a crew cut, undoubtedly on leave from Ellsworth AFB, chatting amiably with one (or two!) of the local talent in a steamy, apparently very hygienic jacuzzi. I was there with a few buddies for a federally-sponsored conference, I didn't have a crew cut, and I'm not much for amiable chatter. It was tempting, though.

Prior to the arrival of Disney, Orlando was a small urban oasis in the middle of thousands of acres of orange groves, golf courses and cattle ranches. In the mid-60s, we took a family vacation through Florida. At night the freeways in and around Orlando glowed with billboards offering table dances and lap dances at venues with exotic one-word names. Even at the age of ten, I knew enough not to ask my parents about that. When I brought it up for discussion at school a few months later, nobody at the cafeteria table had a clue. Of course, they weren't privy to the ads, the ones where you could almost smell the cheap perfume and feel tiny pink bubbles from the champagne spritzers going up your nose. As I described the scenery in detail, the class bully corps regarded me with something other than the usual predatory glares.

Once Disney came in, all that adult fun stuff went away. Clean as a whistle. Disney said, "You can Kissimmee my ass, U.S. military. You are out of here and so are your titty bar billboards."

Ninety-nine percent of any Disney operation is spotless, as are the employees. No beards unless you get to play Captain Hook. Even with my experience, there was no way in hell I could get an interview for toilet scrubber. Every employee exudes the party line: "Look at me, I'm young, perky and harmless." The first time I walked through the gate at Sea World in San Diego, a gull took a giant crap on my head. At D-world, the birds fly around gracefully, but they are forbidden to drop their bombs anywhere near the Magic Kingdom.

That's why I first noticed him. Compared to all the vice-free, fresh-faced youngsters working the park, the squadron leader and air traffic controller on "Dumbo the Flying Elephant", a scrawny ancient character with the hangdog mien of a seventh-decade sharecropper, stood out like a pustule on the tip of your nose. He offered no opportunity to verify his tooth count. Everything about him led me to expect that, after his shifts on "Dumbo", he had a favorite barstool to grace in air-conditioned luxury, firing up an unfiltered Camel and ordering up his usual--a shot of Four Roses neat with a beer back. He looked like an older, craggier version of John Carradine, how the actor would look at the age of one hundred twenty. How does a guy with his croaker of a voice and that scarred-up mug get to run a ride for kids looking to have fun? He had to be Walt's uncle.

At the beginning of the ride, once all the parents had buckled in their kids and wedged themselves in, he started his spiel in a voice as steely as grade 75 rebar.

"Attention, Dumbo Pilots! Prepare to take off." All the kids grabbed the throttle and looked to him. I looked too. There he was, sitting on a canvas chair in the middle of the apparatus, our very own air traffic controller. I expected him to fall over dead at any moment. The ride started and he kept up the chatter. "Time to elevate, Dumbo Pilots." On and on it went. From time to time as we went round and round and up and down, you could imagine some semblance of control over the elephant. Probably an illusion, but intermittent reinforcement is the strongest.

That morning, while getting ready in the room for a day at D-world, we decided that, instead of the usual six high half-side ponytails or two high pigs or some other combination of hair stylings co-designed by a clueless fortyish male and a four-year-old little girl, we would let her hair just hang out. There was a lot of it, and large numbers of clips or bands were usually required to keep it under control. While she worked the throttle to go up and down--it seemed to me the thing worked only when it was in her hands, never in mine--all business in heeding the granite-faced old geezer's commands, her hair aloft behind her a good foot or so, her face exuded pure freedom and joy.

Wouldn't she have a blast riding in a convertible? Top down, of course. Put that on the list.

We made it through every attraction designed for the under-forty-eight inch crowd. We spent a day at Blizzard Beach, the best-ever water park for little kids and overly-protective dads. Toward the end of our last day, we had to decide on our last ride before heading home. What will it be? I should have known.

"Dumbo." Of course. We'd already flown three or four sorties aboard the cheerfully determined pink elephant, but I liked how seriously she took the responsibility of piloting me safely through the air. In my optimistic illusory world, that bode well for her future behind the wheel. We headed over. It was late in the day, and most of the little kids still left in the Magic Kingdom were asleep in their strollers or crying. We got on right away.

"Buckle my seat belt. Roger. 10-9-8-7-6-5-4-3-2-1."

For the first time, there was no sign of the old guy. I hoped that after a long day he was having a good time unwinding at the corner tappy. His replacement, a hyperactive twenty-something with high hopes for a career in the entertainment industry, bubbled over with enthusiasm. His long-winded spiel went on and on and on. As our most excellent flight ended, my captain brought us back down to earth, nailing the landing.

On the way out, I asked, "Are you glad we flew Dumbo for our last ride?"

"It was pretty good. What happened to the real air traffic control man?" That wasn't exactly how it came out. On our first night at D-world, after her maiden solo flight, we'd talked about Saint Ronald the Reagan and PATCO. She'd grasped the concept, but getting the job title right was going to take some more work.

I thought about the old guy, where he would be right now. That wouldn't cut it.

"He probably had to go home to play with his puppy. Why?"

"He's better than the new man."

111. THE GODS SMILE

On a Sunday in February, 2003, we drove my nine year-old maroon, bottom-of-the-line Pathfinder down to the Phoenix Art Museum. February in Phoenix is pretty much the reason people move to Phoenix in the first place. It was Family Sunday, a time for upscale attractive parents and kids in color-coordinated outfits to explore art together and create masterpieces in fun, happy-faced workshops. Quality family time. Never mind the grumpy dads wandering in concentric circles to get extra bars on their cell phones or the kids wishing they could be making history in the video arcade at the mall. We were meeting friends and arting. Whether it was Paint on Pottery or playing together with watercolors at home, my unease with the idea of creating anything artsy was usually soothed by watching my daughter transform lumps of nothing into works of beauty. Needless to say, like most of her good qualities, she got that from her mother.

I parked my jalopy, with its manual locks and window cranks, between a newish Lexus sedan and a Jag convertible bearing a temporary tag as proof that one lucky boy had picked up his toy just two days before. It was a teaching opportunity for my little girl.

"So how long has that car been on the road?"

"I don't know." She gave me that look, the one that said, *Can't you take time out from being weird on Family Sunday?*

"See those numbers there? That's when this tag expires. What's the date?"

"It says 03-23-03. March 23, 2003."

"Right. These temporary tags are good for 30 days here. It can be different in other states. So when was the tag issued?"

"February 23."

"Only 28 days in February this year."

She thought for two seconds. "February 21. That's only two days old."

"Good job." We walk across the parking lot to the front door of the museum. I'm congratulating myself on being the greatest teacher since Socrates; she's thinking that the word "hemlock" has a nice ring to it.

We spent a couple of hours dodging crowds and doing a little painting with our friends, and then headed out in the late afternoon. We had visions of hot dogs and hamburgers sizzling on the grill and hanging out in the backyard. Nice lazy, fun Sunday.

When you lose your auto in a parking lot due to amnesia, invariably you find it in the last place you look. In this situation, it is best to start at one end and work the rows in a methodical manner. It helps to have the electric door clicker that makes the horn beep and the lights flash. Perhaps. Sometimes the process involves crying, which can help get you a ride in the Security guy's golf cart in the airport parking garage. Usually it involves having to schlep a load of suitcases and a kid or two from floor to floor of said garage because you forgot to write down the parking level, its jungle animal symbol, and the number of the space. When in doubt, ask your four-year old. She usually remembers that you parked on the orangutan level. Or, as she puts it, "the orange monkey at the zoo that tried to steal my binky and then peed on me."

When your loss is the result of theft, the simplest path is to call the police and, after finding out that they don't care, call someone for a ride. The trick is knowing which scenario, theft or amnesia, applies to you. I was lucky, but not well-equipped. All I had was a key. The parking lot was small. Fortunately, I distinctly remembered the Lexus and the Jag; where there had once been an aging beater of an SUV, there was now a big fat empty space. It might as well have had one of those signs on a pole. "Reserved for ugly old boxy car on Family Sunday. All other vehicles will be left untouched." I thought to myself, *Who the fuck steals a crappy old Pathfinder and leaves behind a new Jag and a new Lexus?* I got the answer from my insurance company the next day: any thief who doesn't want to screw around with a car alarm. *Oh.*

Things got better. Par for the course with Americans, any foreign language I had learned in high school and college deteriorated over the years in perfect proportion to my dreams of living half the year in Europe and half in the U.S. You can walk into any hotel sundry store in the Caribbean and find a sixteen-year-old working there who speaks six languages fluently. When was the last time we had a President who could converse in French or Chinese or Italian or Russian or German beyond, "Ich bin ein Berliner"? Despite having lived in Phoenix for over fifteen years at the time, I had never delved into the Spanish language. When I called the cab company for a ride and reached a very nice young man for whom English was not quite his second language, I knew there were more challenges ahead before we reached home. I resolved to check on my biorhythm later that night.

Needless to say, it took about three calls and a little over an hour before we were driven home in a big yellow taxi. We had a good laugh about the stolen car, and I called the next day to report it to the police.

I considered calling Sunday evening, but the thought of an APB out on my vehicle on the Sabbath just didn't sit right with me. I would have felt guilty with half of Phoenix PD and all of the Arizona Highway Patrol engaged in a tense dragnet, the requisite roadblocks on all the major highways out of the city, on the lookout for my Pathfinder.

Monday was always a day off for me, so I spent a portion of it reporting the car theft of the millennium to the Phoenix Police Department and my insurance company. The insurance guy was much more interested than the police in the details of the heist, so I spent a half hour or so chatting with him. The take-home message? If my car remained missing for twenty-eight days, they would total it and send me a check, amount to be specified later. With one hundred twenty thousand miles on the odometer, I was hoping for ten percent of the original eighteen grand purchase price. After hanging up, I fished out a calendar and a Sharpie.

The call came from the police on the twenty-seventh day. My car had been tracked down in Laveen, about twenty miles south and west of me. It is not the sexiest part of town, unless you get turned on by animal husbandry and the attendant aromas. I asked the police officer how they'd found it.

"We went to the center of the square mile of Laveen that was blacked out when your vehicle hit a utility pole." I was a little disappointed. I figured it could have been used as the getaway vehicle from the scene of an armored car robbery, or perhaps some famous local politician had done a Nelson Rockefeller while "dictating" to his "personal assistant" at the drive-in. Oh well. I hung up and called the insurance guy. He was ecstatic to hear that the car had been found. I suspect ecstatic was pretty much the way he went through his work day. Whatever he was taking, at this point he was much happier than I. He promised to go see the car at the impound lot the very next day. I told him to take his time. Perhaps an off-season haboob would intervene and carry it off.

"Maybe we can fix it up for you!" I hung up.

As promised, the very next day he called with bad news.

"I'm afraid it's totaled." I tried to maintain my serious funeral voice. He had a question for me. "Other than a bunch of fast food wrappers on the floor, the only thing in the car was a new box of condoms. Do you want me to send them to you?"

The check arrived within two weeks. Ten grand. I was stunned. The next time my daughter was over, I showed it to her.

"What kind of car should we get? Another SUV?"

It took her all of ten seconds to decide. "Let's get a convertible. A red one." Suddenly I remembered our trip to D-world and Dumbo Pilots. Sold.

I did much more research than I'd done in buying all my previous vehicles combined. Nobody I knew at the time had any good stories about American autos, so I focused on foreign. I needed a back seat, in case my daughter had to lie down to sleep on one of our road trips. I wanted fast and powerful, but not a gas guzzler. In the end, I settled on a red Mercedes CLK 430, my first eight-cylinder vehicle in over twenty years. It took almost a month to find one, but as I drove it off the dealer lot, a rather curvaceous bombshell driving in looked at me, looked at the car, and said, "You look terrific in that sexy car." Probably a set-up by the salesman, but I didn't care.

One last detail. About a week after I picked up my new red convertible, a letter arrived from the local power company. Included was an invoice. It seems I owed them some money. The letter explained that it cost them fifty grand (night and weekend differential included) to repair the utility pole and restore power. Slightly panicked, I called right away. I was directed to a guy who could have made a good living doing voiceovers for Ben Stein.

Much like a confident hunter who has just winged his trophy buck with a hundred rounds from an AK-47, this guy was in no hurry. He read the entire letter aloud, while I read along silently. Then he asked me when he could expect the cashier's check. Or, if I preferred, he supposed he could accept a credit card number over the phone. I did my best, but at that last part, delivered in that monotone, I finally cracked up and had to pretend to cough for about thirty seconds. He waited patiently.

"The car was stolen." I gave him the date.

"Mmm-Hmmmmmmm. Well, I'm sure you reported it to the police?"

"Of course. The next day."

"Mmm-Hmmmmmmm. So of course you have the police report number?"

"Yes. It'll take just a minute or two. Will you hold?"

"Mmm-Hmmmmmmm."

I am the world's worst when it comes to keeping records of any sort, and far worse when it comes to finding something I've "filed away for safekeeping." I am very good at finding things a year or two after I've stopped looking for them. Miraculously, it took only about five minutes to locate the record number. I grabbed the phone.

"Hello, are you still there?"

"Mmm-Hmmmmmmm." I started laughing again, this time not bothering to cough cover. This guy wasn't going anywhere. I read him the number.

"Mmm-Hmmmmmmm. Well, this should be the last time you hear from me."

"Oh, okay, thanks."

"Unless you're lying."

112. CLOONEY AND CHUCK

At long last, more than eight years after our Dumbo adventure, we were making a getaway in our convertible. We'd rented ragtops on vacations from time to time, and there'd been little trips to San Diego in the Benz, but this was the real thing. A road trip for two weeks up and down the coast. A chance to explore one of the most scenic slashes of America together. Hopefully we'd return closer, like the Griswolds but without all the angst. Or the dead aunt.

In June, I'd seen a guy die from a stroke. Young guy, maybe fifty-five. At the age of fifty, fifty-five still looks young. When I was nine years old, my grandparents, in their early fifties, looked ancient. I started taking an aspirin a day in early July. I figured that it wouldn't prevent me from dying from everything, but it might keep me from ending up a hemiplegic drooler.

We set out from Phoenix mid-afternoon on Friday the twenty-ninth of July. The plan was to wend our way north to Neah Bay, Washington to see friends from Oklahoma who were living up there. It doesn't matter what time of the year, the trip across I-10 from Phoenix to L.A. on a Friday always feels like a death march. It's the universe preparing you for actually driving in L.A., which is even worse. A little under four hundred miles from my door to Hermosa Beach, given the posted speed limits, the trans-desert journey should, according to Google maps, take less than six hours. Sure. It took us over 8 hours. We checked in at around 11:30 that night and didn't wake up until about 9 the next morning. Late start but fine with me. I had about eight hours of driving ahead of me, but I figured traffic would be much lighter on Saturday than during the week. Francis the Naive.

After breakfast and check-out, I got the brilliant idea of purchasing a laptop for the trip. I'd always relied on a desktop, and the thought of crashing head first into the new (barely twenty years old) technology of the portable computer was a tad unnerving. Before leaving Phoenix, feeling not quite ready to make such a bold leap, I actually considered bringing my desktop and monitor on the trip. I saw myself writing a travel diary along the way every night after Ari fell asleep.

Uncharacteristically, I realized how silly that would be before trying to load the desktop apparatus into the trunk. There was a Costco along our intended route. It didn't require getting onto a freeway.

We ended up in a parking lot the size of the Pacific Ocean. Miles of cars, miles of stores, pretty much any big box retailer you can imagine. In front of Costco, the lot was mostly vacant. We started to get out of the car when I noticed a young couple sprinting from the Trader Joe's nearby. They stood out not because they were strikingly attractive and exuded affluence, but because they were running. People in Southern California don't run, at least not in upscale resort casual attire in a parking lot. They run in festive athletic outfits in Santa Monica. The woman was setting the pace in spiky heels. The guy, just a few steps behind, was fiddling around with the top of a wine bottle. They jumped into a 3-series Beemer ragtop; clearly she was the motivating force in the relationship, outlegging her male-model companion and taking command of the driver's seat.

At 10:30 on a Saturday morning, anyone running to a car with a bottle of wine is either picking up their contribution to a wine-tasting brunch, shoplifiting, or in serious need of a drink. I imagined the first option, some tony affair overlooking the Pacific.

"They're probably late for brunch at Clooney's."

"What's Clooney's?"

"George Clooney's house on the beach somewhere around here, I think Malibu, up north."

"The actor?"

"Not just an actor. He makes his living acting in movies, but his real job is ruling the universe." At this last morsel of make-believe, my daughter smiled and shook her head a little. She knew where this was headed. I was off the rails. On a normal busy work day, she'd distract me by staring intently into the distance as if a major event was about to begin. However, as I'd told her on the way over the night before, this was a big vacation trip. "Anything goes. We let the red convertible take us wherever we want, whenever we want. For the next two weeks, nobody gets to tell us what to do."

"The Hand of Clooney is a subtle but powerful force that makes all things happen just so. It's karma, it's zen, it's all the good things wrapped up in one." Now I was on a roll, pilfering jingle phrases from my youth. She waited patiently for me to build to a crescendo, which is just one of the reasons I loved her as a one-girl audience. I reworked a verse from a cheesy TV detective show called "Hawaiian Eye", featuring Robert Conrad, Connie Stevens, and Poncie Ponce, the token native Hawaiian guy in a porkpie hat and Hilo Hattie shirt.

"You cannot stray from, you can't run away from, the Hand of Cloo-oo-oo-ooney." She rolled her eyes, more at the painful sound of my voice than the obscure concept behind it.

"Honey, we are coming to a point in time when there will be but one time zone. Clooney Standard Time."

She started to say something to egg me on, but our two sprinters interrupted her. She pointed. "They're running again."

Sure enough, Page and Andrew--while waiting, we'd come up with suitably charming monikers--were out of the Beemer and bolting back to TJ's. It was time for us to make our move. A team of seasoned gumshoes, we strolled nonchalantly over to the storefront window. While commenting on the beautiful flower arrangements displayed outside, we took turns stealing surreptitious glances through the big front window. Eventually we abandoned all pretense and peered in, hands cupped to block the reflection, groveling for info like two hungry street urchins drooling outside a medieval banquet.

After a few minutes we saw them get into a checkout line. Between them, they steered two carts filled with three cases each. Pretty soon the subjects of our recon mission came barreling out with their treasure trove. They were even better-looking up close. I read the label. "Charles Shaw". Now the wedding thing seemed more likely. Besides, if Clooney wanted anything, from a diamond tiara for his latest conquest to six cases of champagne from Trader Joe's, all he'd have to do is clap his hands together once and visualize. As for the wine, the name was familiar, but I couldn't remember why. I figured it was probably cheap champagne for the big toast. They bolted across the lot, put the top down, and loaded cases into the trunk and back seat. Then they screamed away.

Still mystified, we walked in. I should say, I was mystified. My daughter wandered over to check out the indoor flower section. TJ's lacks the tween gossip and fashion mags so prominent in Safeway checkout lines. The clerk who'd helped the pretty couple had an empty line.

"Excuse me."

"Yes, sir?" He was an affable curly-haired twenty-something proudly wearing the official TJ vest loaded down with pins, patches and stickers from all his favorite nonprofits. Rescue dogs, climate change, Greenpeace, Vegans Seeking the Death Penalty for Butchers.

"That couple that just left with all the Charles Shaw. First they bought a bottle and ran to their car with it, then they came back for six cases. What's up with that?"

He gave me his friendliest smile, all organic and safe. "Oh, we received a big order of Two Buck Chuck after closing last night. You should have been here an hour ago. Folks buy a bottle and go to their cars to taste it. If it's really good, they'll buy a few cases. I had one lady this morning who bought ten. If it's bad, I mean, not terrific, we'll end up selling it by the bottle and it will take a couple of weeks. When it's a good batch, the word gets around fast. For sure, by the time we close today all one-hundred cases will be gone." He pointed toward the back of the store. "If you want some, it's back in the wine section but sort of off by itself near the cheese case. Better get it now while you still can."

Southern California. Hoo boy. We left the store, sans Chuck, bought a laptop, then drove thirty miles in two and one-half hours on the 405. We started out with the top down, but after a half-hour, even with hats on, we were frying. The traffic was so slow I didn't have to pull off to raise the roof. Six lanes in each direction, no construction, no accidents, just sheer overwhelming volume, all on a Saturday morning in July. Our adventure had begun.

113. ITS UGLY HEAD

"We're here."

"Hooray, Dad!"

"Go ahead, say it." At the age of three, she'd come up with a phrase of praise for those rare occasions when, against all odds, I actually got something right.

"I'm so proud of you. I knew you could do it."

"Thank you. Let's unload our stuff and go check in."

Our trip began with an escape in a red convertible from the monsoon season of Phoenix on a Friday afternoon in late July. After a soul-sapping couple of hours getting up close and personal with a Saturday morning L.A. traffic jam, I witnessed something I'd been looking forward to since our first trip to Disney World eight years earlier. With the top down, my little girl sat next to me in the passenger seat, without a care in the world, soaking up the sun and the breeze. We spent a few perfect days on the road, taking our time. A stop in Lake Tahoe, exploring small towns, enjoying the greenery and scenery of the Pacific Northwest.

The Pacific Northwest is the seasonal mirror image of Phoenix. In the world of organic chemistry, the term is enantiomer. Phoenix is at its greenest in the winter, when the rains of November and December, particularly during the winters of el Nino, give birth to long-hibernating desert flora, which you can enjoy in sunny warm weather. In summer, other than vincas and basil, everything exposed to the merciless sun dries up and dies. In combination with the relentless heat, that brown sameness is what drives legions of annoying Zonies from their air-conditioned homes, like a Yahweh-commanded plague of locusts, to invade any and all destinations on the West Coast, from Soldatna to San Diego.

A postcard of summertime Portland might make you think the city stays green all year round, what with the ubiquitous conifers and all that winter rain. Up on Mount Hood, where evergreens dominate, that's the way it is. In town, however, during the winter, if you open your eyes, you realize how many deciduous trees make their home in the Rose City, particularly down by the Willamette. That's one of the reasons the views of Mt. Hood from Portland are so terrific during the winter. You are looking through bare trees. It gets pretty grey. On the upside, it's usually raining, so most pedestrians tend to walk with their heads down. Once summer arrives, usually after the Rose Festival in June, everything is leafy and green. Couple that with moderate temperatures, low humidity, a surprising paucity of mosquitoes, and relatively little rainfall, and you can understand why folks are willing to suffer through nine months of depressing grey drear. For sheer beauty and user-friendliness, no other American city can beat it. Savor the smell of the river. Take a ride on the MAX light rail out to the International Rose Test Garden in Washington Park to have a laugh at the names of the new varieties. Hike in Macleay Park, where I took my angry dog Melissa to chase squirrels.

We had just reached the Rose City on our trek north. It was Friday afternoon at rush hour, and I was relieved to be settling in for three nights before getting back on the road. Never overly crowded, the city is full of sights and activities; between its walkability, especially downtown in the Southwest and Northwest districts, and a world class mass transit system, it's an easy place to explore. Ari's Mom was born and raised in the Quad Cities--Milwaukie, Oak Grove, Jennings Lodge and Gladstone. The two of them had been up a few times to see family and friends. I spent four years there in the early 80s during my residency, kept in touch with a few friends who still lived there, and had nothing but good memories. This was our first trip to Portland together. The whole idea of a road trip is to see new places, but it would be nice to take a time out from our adventure in a town we both considered something of a second home.

We had a reservation at the Embassy Suites downtown. Built by local mover and shaker Philip Gevurtz, it opened in 1912 as the Multnomah Hotel. It's listed on the National Register of Historic Places and has hosted Charles Lindbergh, Rudolph Valentino, Jack Benny, Bing Crosby, Jimmy Stewart, and every president from Teddy Roosevelt to Milhous. The pictures online just scream "swanky". While it might not match the Benson for ornate styling, every room's a suite, and there are free cocktails in the evening and, more importantly, free breakfasts in the morning. In the summer, Portland is one hungry town, and finding a place to eat breakfast on the weekends often entails a wait of an hour or more.

We found the parking garage across Pine Street from the hotel. After stretching our legs, we pulled Ari's suitcase and a cooler from the back seat. Then I opened the trunk and lifted my suitcase out. As I leaned forward to place it on the ground, a tearing pain shot through my upper back. Since the age of sixteen, I've lived with chronic low back pain, probably from carrying the weight of the world on my shoulders. This was different. It wasn't the usual muscle spasm just north of my butt. An inquisitive grizzly was tearing away pesky flesh to get a peek at the inside of my left shoulder blade.

In medicine, you hear it all the time. "Pain doesn't kill you." It occurred to me that this one probably wouldn't kill me either, but it was piggybacking on something that could. For a nanosecond or two, I was no longer in that parking lot on a Friday afternoon. I was nowhere. I didn't actually see the Reaper, and no, there was no white light at the end of a tunnel, but somewhere inside me there was nothingness, a lack of life.

After a few seconds it softened into a pressurized steady flow of painfully hot water; Old Faithful erupting from my left upper back into my neck. It didn't radiate anywhere else. I could breathe, I didn't sweat or feel like passing out. I stayed bent over.

"What's the matter, Dad?" Ari is a sweet and caring girl; she can sniff out suffering like a bloodhound. Until her first year in college, when she eventually figured out that the world was full of chronic victims who would take delight in sucking the life out of her, I thought she might end up an empath, absorbing everyone else's self-inflicted pain.

"Just my back, Sweetie." She knew well Dad's propensity for throwing his back out. It had accompanied us on a couple of our vacation trips together over the years; suitcases were usually involved. "I think this will go away if I just wait a few seconds."

I straightened up slowly. For some reason, I put both my hands on my hips and walked in a small circle. It seemed the right thing to do. Ari waited patiently. After about five minutes, the pain eased and disappeared. I put the small cooler on my suitcase and we rolled our luggage out of the garage and across the street. I put it all out of my mind and looked forward to a fun weekend. For starters, a shower and a freebie Embassy Suites cocktail sounded pretty good.

114. SHI SHI

The drive from Portland up to Neah Bay on the Makah reservation is about three hundred miles and takes six hours. We wanted to get off I-5 as soon as possible, so at Longview we cut over to the 101. The drive along the coast is easier, prettier, and I wanted Ari to see the Grays Harbor area. Possibly the wettest tri-cities area on the face of the earth, Aberdeen, Hoquiam and Cosmopolis, a small town that sounds big, average over ninety inches of rain per year.

At one point, her Mom and I had considered settling in Aberdeen. She wanted to return to the Northwest, and this would leave her a mere three-hour drive from her family and friends in Portland. A private practice was looking for another internist. We spent the night before the interview in a local motel. While loading my suitcase the following morning, I threw my back out, which meant an entire day of interviewing and touring in supragluteal agony. Every position change was excruciating. I considered the possibility of doing the whole day in a golf cart, so I wouldn't have to stand up. From the age of sixteen, my back has always been correct when it was time to make a significant life decision. Back pain at the start of an interview day meant only one thing--this job was not for me. To ignore that portended a life of lumbosacral misery.

We spent a few hours talking with a couple of the internists. One of them fancied himself the second coming of William Osler; nothing more fascinating than a guy who takes himself and every aspect of his life way too seriously. After fifteen minutes with him, I was ready to suck on a tailpipe. The other guy seemed like a better fit for me, but he clearly didn't enjoy working with his partner. The medical group's administrator was a nice guy who spent most of our time together bragging about his success in the stock market. Back then, in the late 1980s, the markets were flying and everyone was a stock picking genius. Then, in 1989, thanks to Charles Keating and his ilk, the savings and loans went belly up; geniuses morphed into genies, disappearing into thin air.

After talking to most of the big fish in the very small pond, we toured around with a local realtor lady, looking at potential homes. The clincher on the deal was her comment that, of course, we would want to buy a house up on one of the hills rather than down in the flatlands.

"Oh, why is that?"

"Because it floods down below almost every year."

Rain is a different creature in the Southwest than it is in the Pacific Northwest. If you walk up some of the less-travelled areas of Phoenix's Squaw Peak in the rain, especially in the summer, pretty soon you will see little tadpoles and guppy-like creatures floating down the hill in the runoff. Perhaps during the endless dry spells they live in a state of dessication, or, if you are a sci-fi buff, suspended animation. A few days later, if there is still some standing water at the base of the peak, small but mature amphibians will be swimming around. When I've mentioned this to experts in the field of amphibia or rain or both, they eyeball me oddly, then back away slowly, careful not to make any sudden moves. My dog saw them though. On our way up a rivulet, she stuck her front paw into the downhill current. Dozens of fishy swimmers flitted around her on their way down to the next eddy. She looked up at me with her *Did you see that?* face, a mixture of pride, amusement and fascination.

A week or more after a healthy Southwest rain, ocotillo will start to sprout new leaves. A few days later, the peaks burst forth with brilliant emerald rye grass shoots--only in the winter, excess seeds blown there from winter lawns--and native desert plants. A single good rainstorm will blanket any exposed area in green for a couple of weeks. Then it all dries up and turns any of a number of shades of brown.

Especially in urban areas, nothing in the Southwest does more damage than water. Rain runs off the hard-baked earth and asphalt, overwhelming storm drains and causing flash floods on streets and in arroyos. No matter how much infrastructure is added to handle torrential floods, somewhere downstream somebody will be featured on the six o'clock news, standing knee-deep in brown water in the middle of what was the living room. Now it's the mud room. Flat roofs, usually constructed of polyurethane foam on less than a ten-degree pitch, often provide unwelcome little surprises when the weather changes; once the rain hits, you find the inevitable leaks that have developed unnoticed during prolonged dry spells. Shake roofs, through which you can see the sunny blue sky during dry weather, swell up almost immediately with the first few drops of dusty Southwest cloud sweat.

Everyone loves a grey day or two in the Southwest, and on the first day of rainy weather after a dry spell, all you hear are variations of, "Thank goodness for the rain. We really need it." After a day or two, despite the magnificent scents in the air as new life explodes, Phoenicians are tired of it. By the third day, you can see the depression setting in. "Will the sun ever shine again?" After twenty-five years here, I have to admit I get a little edgy after four days of clouds with some rain mixed in.

In the Pacific Northwest, rain is omnipresent. Driving through an extremely wet area like the Olympic Peninsula, you can't help but notice the visceral quality of the green. It doesn't just exist, it dominates, almost like a cancer obliterating every other cell around it through the sheer excess of its growth. You can feel the greenery demanding the rain to fall. And that's without ingesting any magic mushrooms. People can be depressed, seasonally affected to be sure, but they are always ready for the rain. Roofs don't leak, floods occur only after huge amounts of rainfall, even the snowmelt ends up where it's supposed to. God help you if you have a flat roof.

Although you can expect only an inch and a half of rain during the average Olympic Peninsula August, it drizzled or poured the entire trip up to Neah Bay. But it was green and we were still grooving on the green. My daughter, who doesn't miss a thing, looked around as we drove through the Grays Harbor area. I suspect she was deep in thanks that we had not settled there. I was reminded of that billboard you see when you're stuck in traffic, the one with the arrow pointing to some godawful apartments a stone's throw from the interstate, the one that says, "If you lived here, you'd be home by now." That's when you think to yourself, *If I lived here, I'd jump in front of this traffic.* I snapped out of my reverie and voiced the observation that this far north in the summer, at least sunset comes late in the day.

"What good is a late sunset if it's raining?" Touché, Kid.

Once you leave the 101, well before it turns east to Port Angeles, you head northwest through the forests along the Strait of San Juan de Fuca, which separates the Olympic Peninsula from Vancouver Island. There is a "dry" side to the Olympic Peninsula, but this ain't it. Seals consider this area too wet for habitation. Perfect for anything to do with lumber and fishing; logging trucks blasting their way east and south, rows of totems for sale in parking lots alongside stretched smoked salmon filets.

If Alfred Hitchcock had wanted to make a terrifying sequel to *The Birds*, the Makah reservation would have been a good choice. Hills packed with dark, foreboding evergreens look down disapprovingly on stretches of empty grey sand. Even in summer, odds are that you will arrive to an overcast sky. You know the sun is up there, but you don't know exactly where. Shacks and lonely beaches accompany you on the right. To the left stand the occasional food market, bait store, church and government buildings. All that's missing is the rib frame of Ahab's abandoned ship alongside the skeletal remains of a sperm whale. Your best bet on catching a glimpse of the sun is right at sunrise, before it is swallowed up by the seemingly omnipresent cloud cover. Don't bother looking for a sundial.

The Makah tribe's history is one of working the land and sea for their survival. Prior to the arrival of the white man, they occupied a parcel of land in the shape of an isosceles triangle whose peak sat at the northwesternmost tip of the Olympic Peninsula at Neah Bay. They had summer homes and winter homes. So intertwined was their culture with life on the sea that they developed more than a half dozen different styles of canoe, including one model designed specifically to train children to ride the water. Although the Makah were known to be tireless paddlers, they also enjoyed more leisurely water travel when the winds allowed. Most of their canoe designs included sails. Not a bad life, fishing, sailing, trading, lumbering, hunting sea otters, and building cedar log homes, complete with the mother-in-law house. Theirs was the life that Microsoft millionaires dream of, on their private islands in the San Juans, eighty miles to the east.

Long before the arrival of MS-DOS, the well-intentioned white man brought the usual assortment of febrile contagious diseases like smallpox and measles, which decimated the population. Economically speaking, the worst thing they brought was an afebrile disease in the form of legal documents, which decimated their land holdings. In a strange twist of fortune, probably because at the time cedar was considered more valuable than sashimi, Mr. Paleface stole the inland forests and left the Makah to suffer with oceanfront and straitfront land. While it was still a crapbox deal, the Sioux and pretty much any other non-oil Native American tribe would give their eye teeth for the reservation to which the Makah were consigned. We arrived in late afternoon. Even with the top up, our red convertible drew wide-eyed stares from the little kids.

You don't often see an Air Force Station without a runway, but that is exactly what was constructed at Neah Bay. In 1950, fearing invasion during the looming Korean War and the omnipresent Cold War, the Air Force built permanent radar stations across the northern tier of the U.S. The goal was to have an impenetrable net of detection for any Commies piloting nuke-laden long-range bombers. Given the strategic location of the Makah Reservation, straight across the Pacific from the Kamchatka peninsula of Russia, Neah Bay was chosen as one of the original twenty-eight.

When I think of military installations in the U.S., Pensacola, Virginia Beach and San Diego come to mind. Unlike the Navy, who usually end up within spitting distance of a beach, most Air Force bases are located in godforsaken locales like Minot, North Dakota, Wichita Falls, Texas, or Thule, Greenland. Every so often they get one right. No matter where they are, however, the base commander and his seconds-in-command tend to land in nice digs, courtesy of the U.S. of A. At Neah Bay, the flyboys commandeered a bluff overlooking the area and plopped down a few houses for the local top brass. When the USAF presence disappeared in 1988, somehow the Indian Health Service was able to scoop them up. Leslie, who has always managed to find a scenic domicile in each of his postings, scored a winner once again.

He and his wife Charlotte lived in one of the houses on the bluff. At sunset, Vancouver Island gleamed in the distance. One of those things I wanted my daughter to experience before she became a teenager was tent camping, including the setup and all the associated facets of life in a campground. It wasn't long before she was outcamping her instructor. Les and Charlotte were kind enough to pitch a tent in their backyard for our stay. After a fantastic Pacific NW barbecue, when the clouds deigned to part, we took in the constellations, so much more brilliant than in any metropolitan area. Down below the bluff, the Waatch River gurgled its way southwest to Makah Bay and the Pacific.

My back pain of a few days ago returned once during the night. I was sleeping on my stomach. The medical term for the position is "prone". When it hit, there was none of the initial tearing pain, just the hot pressure under my left scapula. I turned over on my right side and it disappeared in a few minutes; it was gone so quickly and seemed to respond to the change in position, so I immediately forgot about it. A light drizzle in the middle of the night left the air damp and fragrant. We awakened just before dawn to an eerie amber glow. While seabirds screamed, the rising sun transformed coarse dark fog on the strait into a soft golden pelt.

After breakfast the four of us tossed our day packs into the back of their SUV and drove south. We skirted the west coast of the reservation along Makah Bay until we reached the end of Shi Shi Beach Rd. Shi Shi Beach itself, a good hundred feet or so below the road and parking lot, was undoubtedly at one time a favorite summer spot for the Makah. Now it is one of many spectacular beaches within Olympic National Park, off the reservation. The hike from the parking lot includes a short walk over a foot bridge with rope handrails, very primitive, which my daughter especially liked. We descended from the bluffs down a winding sandy path into the fog. After you trip over the first tree root or feel your hiking boots being sucked off your feet by a mud bog, you begin to pay more attention to the trail. Rope lines placed here and there add to the feeling of exploring some recently discovered rough territory.

Shi Shi beach is not like anyplace else. You can see the Pacific to the west and Point of the Arches at the far southern end of the beach, but the base of the cliffs behind you are completely invisible until the fog burns off later in the morning. We moseyed south along the water, talking, exploring, searching the tide pools, looking for odd sea life. There was a half-hearted treasure hunt for geoducks and razor clams, just so we could say we did it. The entire two-plus-mile stretch of beach was all ours. From that quiet, relaxed couple of hours came the best photo I've ever taken. My daughter, holding a starfish in her hand, with a huge grin of satisfaction. The message on her face, beaming into the camera, "Look what I found!" My friend Leslie peering over her shoulder, with a goofy smile, like they're sharing some inside joke. That moment was the last and best record of the time before I was forced to acknowledge that I'd have to do something about this pain of mine.

In late morning, on our return trip up the beach, I realized how clueless I had been about our solitude. As the sun heated up the air, we could watch the fog lift straight up the face of the cliff. Dozens of tents appeared at the base, and actual human beings emerged, starting campfires and cleaning up their gear. In a burst of non-humbuggery, the great and powerful Oz had thrown back the curtain on a live performance.

For the previous five years, I had devoted more time and effort to aerobic exercise than at any other time in my life. Three or four times per week, I spent a couple of hours at the local fitness club, working with free weights, various weight machines, and a forty-five-minute workout on the elliptical, most of that at the maximum inclination. At least three days a week I was running outside, three miles at an eight-minute per mile pace. In addition to that, whenever I could, I was hiking the hills in the Squaw Peak recreation area or riding my road bike for an hour. I'd never be confused with an exercise enthusiast, but for a fifty-year-old with a life, I was doing pretty well. I didn't think much of the idea of running up and down hills, but it was no trouble at all climbing any peak trail in Phoenix or Flagstaff at a healthy clip without having to stop to rest.

While we climbed the trail up from Shi Shi Beach to the cliffs, I thought about a hike I'd done with Les a few years back. While living the miserable life of a Kansas flatlander, he visited me in Phoenix. It was a work trip for him, but he managed to wrangle a day off, so we drove up to Flagstaff. My favorite hike up that way is Kendrick Peak, a 4 1/2 mile trail that rises from 7700 feet at the trailhead to 10,300 at the summit. I was getting up there at least once a month to do that hike or one of the others in the area, so it was nothing more than routine for me by then. At that stage of life, Leslie was fairly active, but not at that altitude. I could tell it was hard work for him, but he ground it out like a trooper.

About a quarter mile from the top, he hit the altitude wall. All of a sudden he complained of a headache and lightheadedness, and seemed a tad confused. He sounded short of breath, but he wasn't gasping. We went back down the trail maybe twenty-five yards and his symptoms resolved. Being a plucky Okie, as well as a proud Cherokee, he tried to ascend again. His symptoms returned at exactly the same spot. I was up for repeating the experiment a few more times, just to rule out coincidence, but he got bored with feeling sick, so we went back down.

For whatever reason, I began to worry that something like that would happen to me on this hike. The rope handholds that had seemed so quaint on the way down were now my lifelines. Like some old prospector, I ended up bent forward at the waist while climbing, so that my upper torso was parallel to the slope. By the time I got to the top, I was sucking gas. I don't know if I resembled the emphysematic Marlboro Man inhaling an oxygen tank, but I sure felt that way. That same pain came back over my left shoulder blade, and I felt a little sweaty. I had to walk around in circles, pushing my hands down on my hips for about five minutes before everything felt okay again. I was embarrassed for having kept everyone waiting; they pretended to have a conversation about the weather.

Now that shortness of breath was added to the symptom menu, I knew it was more likely that this pain might be coming from my heart, but I convinced myself that it was a result of my posture, rather than the exertion. We walked back to their vehicle and climbed in. Exhausted, I nodded off for a half hour, then awoke feeling absolutely normal. Ari kept an eye on me. We spent a few hours playing at Sol Duc hot springs, where, to reassure myself as much as everyone else that I was just fine, I jackassed around as the pool clown. The rest of the afternoon was pain-free.

Our perfect day ended with an excellent meal and one of their full-bodied Willamette Valley pinots back up on the bluff. Drizzle came and went. Sometime in the middle of the night, an owl hooted for about an hour outside our tent. He woke me up, but my daughter slept like a child unburdened by care.

Years before, while entertaining the Dyes at my home in Phoenix, an owl landed in a palm tree and started his hoot routine. Charlotte, a Sioux, told me that the owl brings death. I tried to make a joke of it until I realized she wasn't kidding.

"I've heard they're hard on rodents."

She gave me a look. "I'm talking about people." Hard to snap off a comeback to that.

Who am I to label as superstition a centuries-old belief held by an entire culture? It didn't sound any stranger than a dead carpenter rolling a massive boulder aside on a spring Sunday morning so he could escape his burial cave and go hunting for brightly dyed hard-boiled eggs.

I didn't mention my strigine visitor the next morning. We bid adieu and headed back down the Olympic Peninsula, gliding through rainfall with the top up. I was glad we had made the trek north, but it would be good to see the sun again. Hopefully the sunshine would burn away all the outdoor gloom and the worry inside my head.

115. A CHANGE IN PLANS

After bidding adieu to Leslie, Charlotte and the Makahs, we sped south. Our goal was to get to my sister and brother-in-law's place in

Anaheim Hills in three days, spend two nights with them, then head home to Phoenix on Sunday.

Ari and I were both in the mood to make tracks south. Even with our nice layovers in Portland and Neah Bay, ten days on the road was a lot. A couple of girls can talk nonstop through a two-week road trip and the time would fly by. By comparison, especially when I'm driving, I'm not much of a conversationalist. When we started our road trip, it was with the expectation that we'd enjoy some rain along the way. "Some rain" has a different meaning for Phoenicians than for Oregon webfeet. Our fascination with grey skies and windshield wipers had ebbed; we wanted to enjoy summer sunshine that doesn't cause spontaneous combustion the way it does in Phoenix. Relentless mist and drizzle accompanied us as we retraced our way along the 101 through the Olympic Peninsula. Once back on I-5 above Centralia, the sun came out and we got to travel a while with the top down. Along the way, we saw our share of greenery, which looked better with the sun shining through it.

By the end of the first day, we had covered the four hundred miles to Eugene, a college town dedicated to three things: Ducks football, coffee and Birkenstocks. Sometimes, when you blow out a Birkie, the coffee leaves you listless, and the Ducks do not receive an invite to the big dance, or it's just too rainy to walk, you are almost obligated to purloin the nearest automobile. According to the National Insurance Crime Bureau, the Eugene-Springfield metro area usually leads the state of Oregon in car thefts and often occupies a proud position in the top fifty nationwide.

As one of the Tzu boys, I think it was Sun, put it, "The general who wins the battle makes many calculations in his temple before the battle is fought." Translation: Fortune favors the prepared man. Armed with the car theft data, I found a motel where we could park right outside the room. This time I was ready. The anti-theft alarm light blinked reassuringly from the dash and I slept like a baby. In a strange twist of fate, an old maroon Pathfinder was parked two doors down. No car alarm. I checked. It was still there the next morning.

Ari has been a leading actress since grade school, and we attended stage productions whenever we could. I wanted to take her to Ashland, Oregon to see a play. One section of town, Elizabethan in design, is the permanent home of the annual Oregon Shakespeare Festival; there is the usual assortment of fools, minstrels and big turkey legs for the enjoyment of visitors. Because I have real issues planning any further than the length of my nose, by the time I called for tickets, all the shows were sold out. Frank M. Procrastinator. So we went to plan B. Entertainment that didn't include a long drive from the I-5.

Jacksonville is a restored mining town down near Medford. It's named for Jackson Creek, the site of one of the earliest placer gold claims in the area. It's okay for adults who like to pick over antiques; Harley AARPers love to roar into town. For kids who are not into panning for gold, there is the old-timey drug store where they make old-timey ice cream sodas at the old-timey counter. If you don't belong to one of those demographics, it's a bit of a yawner.

Gold Hill, however, is home to the Oregon Vortex. If you've been to Sedona, you may have hiked to some of the four (or six, or eleven, depending on the expert) major vortices in the area. Once you get close, they are easy to find. Just follow the red rock cairns, those personalized, whimsical piles of stones ostensibly built to mark the way, but actually nothing more than self-congratulatory eyesores constructed in defiance of the two laws of wilderness hiking: Take nothing but pictures, leave nothing but footprints. Anyway, the vortices (Excuse me. In Sedona the plural of vortex is vortexes, but then again, in Sedona, McDonald's arches aren't golden, they're teal.) are supposed to be centers of beneficial energy and you are pretty much supposed to visit, meditate and heal. It's your basic spa experience without the bathrobes and the cucumber slices on your eyelids. So soothing, so regenerative.

There's no way you could mistake the Oregon Vortex for a healing place. HQ for the OV site is the House of Mystery. What I meant to say is "The World Famous House of Mystery". Anything with the words "World Famous" in its title is sure to be cheesy as hell and absolutely not to be missed. If you want healing energy, head sixty-five miles northeast to Crater Lake, the remnant of the last eruption of Mount Mazama. It's knee-deep in mysticism and misty enough to hide Wizard Island on a regular basis. The World Famous House of Mystery is a goofy illusory sideshow worthy of P.T. Barnum. According to the lore, long before the white man settled the Rogue River Valley in Southern Oregon, local Indians could not get their horses to go near the site of the House of Mystery and thus named it "Forbidden Ground", or something to that effect in the Takelma language. Around the turn of the century, the House itself was built by a mining company as an assay office and later used as a storage area.

No "scientific" mystery can thrive without the lifelong dedication of the requisite Wacky Professor. In this case, his name was John Litster, and he hailed from Scotland. That would be the same Scotland where they've been able to keep the Loch Ness Monster hoax going for over fourteen centuries. He opened the place in 1930 and spent the next three decades conducting "experiments" on the "whirlpool of force" concentrated in that area. Visitors are unable to stand up straight; rather, they incline toward the magnetic north pole. The usual rules of perspective are reversed, so that things that incline away from you look taller than things that incline toward you. It's enough to make Count Floyd wiggle his palms and warn, "Oooooh, Skeddy." Must-see stuff. Ari came away from it wearing her eyes-peeled, thinking-really-hard look, struggling to come to grips with all the eerie "facts" she learned. Trying to keep a straight face, I bit the inside of my mouth. Even with all the inclining and mystery, I didn't experience any of that back pain.

We decided to forsake making good time and got off the I-5. We'd already driven that route through northern California on the way up, and figured the 101 would be far more pleasant and adventurous. Somewhere around the Oregon-California border we passed a town for sale. The whole shebang. Although there didn't seem to be any oceanfront acreage, it's southwestern orientation at the mouth of a creek promised striking sunset scenery. This place had "If I were king" written all over it. We spent a few miles discussing how I'd look in a postmaster's uniform.

The 101 is plenty scenic, but we wanted more Pacific seascapes. At Leggett we skipped over to the coast on Rt. 1, a winding two-lane that lets you stop at any number of bluffs and beaches and gawk wistfully at the ocean. It takes much longer to get anywhere, but, surrounded by all that beauty, you really don't care. That took us all the way down through Marin County. It was a bright sunny afternoon when we rejoined the 101 in Sausalito. When we came around one of the last curves before the Golden Gate Bridge, up ahead it looked as if we were heading for a wall of rain. I had to pull over illegally to put the top up.

On the bridge, the wind blew and rain slanted down on us to the point where I could barely see the taillights of the semi in front of me. I learned later that the drainage on that bridge is pretty efficient, but between the buckets of rain and the wind blowing from the right side, we hydroplaned toward the guardrail a couple of times. Other vehicles were invisible until they roared by, drowning us in a giant wave of water. When we reached Lincoln Blvd., I relaxed enough to look in the rearview; a curtain of black rain blew sideways up on the bridge. *Hmm, none of that pain. I guess it isn't just stress-related.* Perhaps some of those poor souls labeled as jumpers were actually ejected from their cars by the wind and rain howling through the Golden Gate strait.

It is not unusual for severe storms to blow through the Golden Gate. In 1951 the bridge was closed for a several hours when seventy mph winds caused it to flutter. As frightening as the drive was in the blinding rain, it was probably better to not be able to see what was going on around us. At least there wasn't any fluttering. Once out of the San Francisco metropolis, we drove long miles up and down deathly dark hills to get to Half Moon Bay.

The next morning, it was sunny, breezy and perfect for top-down driving. We followed Route 1 along the coast for a while, then jumped on the 101 around Salinas. Driving through Gonzales, right along the highway, we saw ranchland being taken over by vineyards.

"Do cows eat grapes?"

In Paso Robles, we happened upon a funeral procession for Chris Kanton, a firefighter, extreme sports enthusiast and apparently quite the character from the Paso Robles area, who, according to a couple of folks on the street, fell off the back of the fire engine on his way to a fire. Not exactly. Turns out his Riverside County fire engine was en route to a call in the midst of severe storms and flooding when the engine rolled down an embankment and he was killed. A couple dozen fire companies from all the surrounding communities, in a surprising variety of colors you didn't think could adorn an engine, sounded their sirens and rumbled through town at lunch time. People on the street were laughing while they reminisced about his various antics on the slopes and on his motorcycle. They teared up while recounting his efforts on behalf of his friends, family, and the community. Only the good die young and only when it's their day to die.

At some funerals, especially the ones for children and those who die suddenly, everyone cries their eyes out. Some funerals are poorly attended, because the people who knew the deceased are most likely celebrating in a bar, exchanging high-fives and thinking, *Good riddance to the number one asshole in town*. Any time your mourners are laughing and crying at the same time, you've done a good job and you will be sorely missed, not forgotten. That's what Chris Kanton got: crowds, laughs and tears. We all hope that's what we get. Unfortunately, none of us will be around to find out.

For a Friday afternoon, we made good time on our way to L.A. That is, until we actually got to within one hundred miles of L.A. At Santa Barbara, our luck ran out. The speedometer just kept going lower and lower. Just past Ventura, well before entering L.A. proper, we hit the wall.

There's a lot of fun to be had in Los Angeles. The beach is theoretically free; everything else costs a ton of money, but you can visit Hollywood, see concerts and sporting events on any given night, dine in fabulous venues, and drive past celebrities' homes in Malibu, Brentwood and Bel Air. Like at Alice's Restaurant, you can get anything you want in California.

If you are stuck on a freeway in L.A. at rush hour--it's always rush hour--and you don't have to be anywhere for the next five hours, watching the other drivers can entertain you enough to take your mind off the traffic. If, however, you have a dinner engagement in Anaheim that requires you to drive through the entire length of L.A. from north to south on a Friday afternoon, you might as well be crawling on your hands and knees around the nine circles of hell. Bumper to bumper misery for sixty miles. I remember thinking, *Well, the traffic must be pretty light in New York City right now, because every fucking car in the United States is on this freeway, going my way.* We plodded along for hours. For me, Anaheim qualifies as a destination only if you are heading for a rendezvous with Mickey and Minnie. My sister and brother-in-law were serving a one-year sentence there for a job.

When we finally arrived, I promised Ari I would never drive her anywhere near L.A. again. My sister came out to greet us. We all hugged.

"You guys are staying until Sunday, right?" I was popping the trunk; just before I bent over to take out a suitcase, I stopped.

"There's been a change in plans."

116. PAYBACK IS A BITCH

After I delivered the news that we wouldn't be staying until Sunday, I bent over to pull a suitcase out of the trunk. As I was setting it down on the ground, I had another bout of pain. Again, none of the tearing agony, just that hot pressure in my shoulder blade. This time I didn't let on. I finished unpacking the car, locked up, and wheeled my suitcase and the cooler up the driveway. The pain lasted about five minutes and wasn't as severe as the previous episodes. By the time I reached the front door, it was gone.

Before you reach adulthood, if you are lucky, you have a mother who smacks you back into line when you deviate. A married guy has a woman in the house, the one with the title of "wife", who stands ready to help him make good choices. When he makes a wrong turn, there she is, guiding him, with whatever means necessary, back on to the desired route.

A single guy, on the other hand, has the opportunity to make bad choices on a regular basis, with no wife to overrule his knuckleheaded decisions, nobody to reroute him away from a joyride on the Freeway of Folly. It goes like this. First comes the opportunity to make a good choice. It's pretty straightforward. *This choice is good.* Then the universe, or a red guy with horns and a pitchfork, throws the single guy bad options by the fistful. You've seen him on Pinto's shoulder in *Animal House,* advising him on his next move with Clorette. At this point, the smart move is to retreat back to the original good decision, put Clorette in a shopping cart and push her home. On a computer, you would push the ESC button until you've extracted yourself from yet another self-inflicted quandary. The single guy, however, remains undaunted. There is the easy way, the good choice, the simple decision that makes sense and leaves all interested parties with big fat satisfied smiles on their faces. Mr. Bachelor, however, likes simple only when it involves food. Make that food and beer. Okay, food, beer and sex. *Anyone can make a good choice. Time for me to reinvent the wheel. Let's consider all these other options.*

In this case, the bad choice meant dropping my daughter off with her Mom a day early. I talked it over with Ari, feeling awful as I did so. I'm not real clear on what a cad is, but I felt like one. She seemed fine with the change in plans, so she called her Mom. They both were up for it. *It's been a long trip, and I'm not much of a conversationalist. She's ready to go home and spend an extra weekend day with her Mom, make up for the quality girly-chat time she's missed out on for the past two weeks.* I could use that as an excuse.

After laboring for years to get more time with her, I couldn't believe I was doing this. Pulling strings of night shifts so I could spend unfettered quality time with her. Making every effort to be there for the milestones, the special moments. If you're married and you duck out of a ballgame, a play, a recital, the reliable wife is always there to cover for you. If you're single, there's usually nobody to cover for you. It's enough to keep a guy from getting divorced. Or at least it should be.

Why was I changing the plan? For the worst possible reason, that's why. When asked, I'd agreed to accompany a woman I was dating to a party. For reasons I forget, it was supposed to be an important one. Looking back on it, I knew it was a stupid, shallow, self-defeating move. Nonetheless, I did it. What a guy. Not only was I stiffing my kid, but I'd made a commitment to stay with my sister and brother-in-law. *They're really busy and could use some down time without having to entertain us.* There. Another excuse.

From the moment I made the decision, I knew I was doing the wrong thing. For a long time a fair number of people have thought of me as a goofball, unpredictable and unreliable. They didn't know how hard I'd worked to be the best Dad ever, hands-on and dependable. Here I was, confirming their impression, flushing my efforts down the toilet, sinking to the level of others' expectations. In the great scheme of things, I guess one day more or less after two-weeks together doesn't seem like such a big deal. If that's the case, why does it still sting like a bitch ten years later?

I couldn't believe I was giving up precious time with the most important person in my world for the sake of going to a party. Sometime on that Friday evening, I decided the best thing to do would be to go back to the original itinerary, but by then Ari was already planning to spend the extra day with her Mom, and I knew if I changed plans again, that would only make things worse. So I consoled myself with the thought that, as a father, I was making the worst decision ever. On the other hand, I'd had at least one episode of pain every day the past week, some while lying prone in bed. I had this unshakeable premonition that something bad was coming my way, and I wanted to distance my daughter from whatever lurked in the near future.

We had a great evening with my sister's family. After two weeks on the road, I could tell Ari was ready to be home, and I felt a little better about turning her over to her Mom a day early. I have always been a big believer in doing one's best or suffering the karma konsequences. I fully realized that this was not my best, but it would probably work out okay. Nonetheless, I knew I had something coming for this latest bad choice.

The ride home the next day was uneventful and went all too quickly. Ari said she wanted to go straight to her Mom's rather than stop at my place and then have to drive again. I hadn't let on about the episodes of pain I'd been having since we left Neah Bay. I was concerned that it might worsen or become constant, but it wasn't going to do either of us any good for her to be worrying about me. She had a couple of weeks left before school started, and she and her Mom were going away for a week or so. I figured that if the pain recurred, I could get it taken care of by the time she returned. If it didn't return, so much the better. I dropped her off, we told each other how much fun the road trip had been, exchanged, "Love you's" and I hugged her and left.

Once home, I unpacked my bag and did some laundry. In the midst of rushing around getting things done, I had a bad episode of pain. It lasted a good ten minutes and I was short of breath. Once again, I felt better walking in a circle around the center island in my kitchen. When you hear the word "island" in association with a kitchen, you usually think, "Pretty nice kitchen." My island was covered with avocado formica, straight out of the early '70s. Even worse, it was, and still is, paired with an avocado refrigerator. I still haven't located the part of my brain that deals with interior design.

The party that night turned out to be the fiftieth for a friend of my date's, down where most of them lived, about twenty miles from my place. The birthday boy and his wife had rented a suite and a couple of rooms for the guests. I thought about getting a room as well, but I was sick of hotel rooms. The pain episode that day shook me and I thought I would probably do best by coming home. I didn't want to die in some strange room. To top it off, I was feeling even guiltier about abandoning Ari, and I had visions of her needing me in the middle of the night for some emergency.

By the time we arrived, everyone was pretty well into the drinks. They had all checked in around 4:00, started at the hotel pool, then headed to the rooms when the sun went down. Just as we arrived at the suite, I started having pain, so I excused myself and went into one of the bathrooms. The pain lasted about ten minutes. I had been taking an enteric-coated aspirin at bedtime for about the past two years, so I popped one right then. Then I came out and started sampling the wines.

We left after about four hours. I had a little nagging soreness in my left shoulder blade, but it was different than the pain I'd been having, duller, more of a throb from overuse. My heart was pounding harder and faster than normal. I thought again about getting a room, but I figured if I were going to die, I'd rather do it in my own bed. I never even thought about a cab, as I didn't think I'd had that much to drink. It was a little over five miles from the hotel to my date's house.

About halfway there, the pain returned. This was a bad one. It went up into the back of my neck. I felt sweaty and thought I was going to pass out. This was the first time I'd experienced it while driving, so I pulled onto a side street. As I was getting ready to park, I reached for my cell phone. I think I had some vague idea of calling an ambulance, or at least a cab. With the sweaty palms and all, and feeling lightheaded, of course I dropped my phone down between the seat and the center console. I put the car in park and went diving for the phone.

After what seemed like five minutes, I finally got my hand around the phone. My date was talking about something, but she sounded like she was talking from inside a plastic bag. My pain suddenly lessened, but I was still dizzy. I brought the phone up to see the keypad, and there in my rearview were those blue and red flashing lights. The first thing I thought was, *Well, dumbass, this is what you get for being a bad parent and a bad citizen.* Karma comes a calling in a police car.

Considering some lingering palpitations and mild dizziness, I thought I did fairly well on the sobriety maneuvers, but the police officer disagreed. After about an hour doing the breathalyzer, which settled the debate in his favor, and fingerprinting and photos in the DUI van, I was sent home. I woke up the next morning, wondering if any of it had really happened. The citation verified that yes, it had really happened.

Feeling like a complete loser, I retrieved my car and drove home. All day Sunday I looked forward to work on Monday. Routine is a refuge when things spin out of control. In college, whenever a girl broke up with me, and there were plenty of those, I would clean our disgusting kitchen from floor to ceiling.

My plan was to work my shifts for the coming week, see how I did, and, if the pain recurred, I could always get an EKG on the spot. Sooner or later, the cause of this pain thing would reveal itself.

117. THE IDES OF AUGUST, 2005

After two weeks off, I was ready to get back to work. To make up for the time off, I had a bunch of shifts scheduled for my first week back. My energy wasn't all that good, but I was optimistic that I wouldn't have any more episodes of the pain and dizziness I'd experienced over the past ten days. My daughter was with her Mom for the week, so I had time to schedule a consultation with a lawyer. I figured that unless he thought I had a good reason to go to trial, I would plead no contest and get things over with as quickly and as cheaply as possible. What little research I did before going to see him indicated that, since this was a straightforward DUI, not extreme or aggravated, I would be sentenced to ten days in the tents, with nine of those days suspended. There would be several months of classes, AA meetings, and fines. Lots of fines.

The attorney pointed out that I had not been driving when the police encountered me. I didn't think that made much difference, but, of course, he felt otherwise. There was some provision working against me, in that even though I was not driving, I had been in actual physical control of the vehicle at the time of the arrest. Apparently, merely being in possession of car keys anywhere near your vehicle meant you were considered to be in control of the vehicle. Like any rube on the midway, I bought into the illusion he conjured up. I forked over some money and went home. I wasn't optimistic, but the trial would be a good five months off. A multitude of things, such as the diagnosis of some fatal illness causing my pain, could occur before then, and I figured nothing could be gained by fretting over its possible outcome. Nevertheless, for the first time in my life, I began waking up in the middle of the night and couldn't go back to sleep for an hour or more. Big surprise.

Rather than start a workup of my shoulder pain, which would disrupt a big stretch of shifts I was scheduled to work, I put off seeing a physician. I was pain-free, doing my job and working out every other day at the fitness club. I put on my optimist's hat, which doubles as my wait-and-see hat, and let things take their course.

Naturally, as soon as my life began to get busier again, the pain returned. I was hoping it was angina, but it sure wasn't acting that way. Sometimes it was exertional, sometimes not. Usually it lasted only five minutes or so, with a little shortness of breath thrown in, but I had no further sweats or dizziness. About the only time it was even remotely predictable was when I was bent over at the waist, doing something strenuous with my arms. More often than not, lifting and pushing heavy things that were waist-high or lower would bring it on. At home I always slept on my side, so it never woke me up. Nor did it ever come on while sitting up and reading, eating or typing. I had it narrowed down to atypical angina, pancreatic cancer or some spinal cord tumor. The latter two were long shots, but pancreatic cancer can present with mid-back pain, as can any spinal cord disorder. I was hoping for a cardiac cause, because, of the three, that was by far the least likely to kill me or leave me paralyzed. Providing I actually did something about it, that is. After my first episode of pain while lifting weights, I gave up going to the gym.

118. WELCOME TO HEART DISEASE

For the last week of August and the first few days of September, I spent most of my time at work either having pain or anticipating it. It seemed that everything I did in the E.R. involved exerting myself while bent forward. I found that if I climbed stairs perfectly upright, I could move at a fair pace and not experience any discomfort. If I ran up the stairs bent forward, the pain was almost inevitable. Trying to avoid situations where the pain was likely to come on was slowing me down at work, and I was already way too slow. A few days before Labor Day, while positioning a young woman for a spinal tap, the pain came on again. She was cooperative, slender, and slid around easily on the trauma room table; in other words, it was a piece of cake to get her set up. Nonetheless, just bending forward at the waist to move her and ascertain my landmarks gave me pain that took more than ten minutes to resolve, one of the longest episodes so far. It finally sank in that, sooner or later, while hustling upstairs to run a code or deliver a baby, I was going to be stopped in my tracks by the pain, and that would cost a life, either mine or someone else's. By the end of the first week of September, I figured it was time to do something about it.

I thought about my options, and on the Friday before Labor Day, called Frank Surdakowski's office to schedule a stress test for the following week. My rationale was that I might as well start with the diagnosis that was fixable. I was hoping for an abnormal stress test, an abnormal cath showing a big fat solitary lesion, a stent, and back to work. That is how things are supposed to work these days.

Labor Day weekend went surprisingly smoothly. On Tuesday I dropped my daughter off at school and drove over to Frank's office. It was right across the street from the hospital. I have always been partial to guys who could walk from their office to the ER or the OR or the ICU in a minute or two. It bespoke loyalty to that particular institution. To my way of thinking, those docs were usually going to make the trip more reliably and much more quickly than a guy with his office a couple of miles away. Other than to run across the street for the occasional cardiac arrest, I hadn't really been to many of the local private practice guys' offices. I considered that a good thing. In the back of my mind, I wondered who was working the ER that day. Hopefully someone who would run across the street for my code.

I checked in at his office and sat for a few minutes before they called me back to the treadmill room.

Frank shook my hand. "What are you doing here?"

"Back pain."

That earned me, "Back pain. We don't do back pain."

"Yeah, I know. I'm hoping though."

"All right, let's get this thing over with." I had picked Frank for a few reasons. First, I've never had a bad experience with a guy named Frank. Second, he was as cynical as I. Third, when he came to the ER, sometimes he was in a crabby mood, but after a few wisecracks, he usually left laughing. There are crabby guys who are not good clinicians, and there are really nice guys who are excellent physicians. In general, though, you are more likely to get good care from a crab than a sweetheart. From what I had heard, Frank had as good a pair of hands in the cath lab as anyone in the city, and his judgment was considered sound. In other words, he was not one of those cath jocks who would squirt dye into a dead guy. I'd never considered that to be good form, cathing a guy without a pulse. Unless, of course, that guy happens to be me.

They started me off with a resting echocardiogram. Basically an ultrasound of your heart, it evaluates each of the four intra-cardiac valves. More importantly for someone with chest pain, it looks at the wall motion of the cardiac muscle, to see if there is any previous damage, say from a heart attack, as well as the thickness of the muscle. Thickening of the myocardium is most commonly caused by longstanding high blood pressure, but there are some congenital diseases that can progress in adulthood and lead to muscle thickening and chest pain.

My resting echo was completely normal. Now he was starting to get irritated. His opinion of my cardiac diagnostic skills in the ER was so-so. Every so often I nutted an obscure or unlikely diagnosis, but in general I was known as an excessive worrier and a grade A sieve when it came to admitting patients with chest pain. I've had clown cars full of guys come down to the ER and tell me I was full of shit with regards to my admitting diagnosis, and rightly so. On a hand that had tangled with a high-speed saw blade I could count the number of times someone stopped by to tell me I got one right. Boo-hoo. Poor me.

While I was lying on the table, the echo tech did my resting EKG. He handed it to Frank, who looked at it, looked at him, looked at me, shook his head, and said, "It's normal." Well, I thought, that's a start. You don't usually go into these things hoping for a bad outcome, but the idea of rotting away from metastatic cancer or being confined to a wheelchair with an inoperable spinal cord tumor had me pulling for my heart. Hoping for heart disease. A fairly pathetic way to start a day.

I stood up and the tech strapped on the harness. With all the gear on, it's hard not to feel like a cross between Uncle Safety, the school crossing guard, and the tin woodsman without his oil can. I stepped up onto the treadmill, and with the push of a button, it started rolling. Assuming you are in even the slightest bit of shape, the trickiest part of taking a treadmill stress test is pacing yourself. In the beginning, you are walking on a level surface at a very slow pace. For people with really short legs, it can require a normal pace. For anyone else, you tend to move in slow motion. Too fast or two long a pace and you can end up stepping up into the front of the machine. At this point, I was feeling fine and the EKG tracing wasn't showing any ST changes.

The other thing you have to resist on a Bruce protocol, especially in the early stages, is the tendency to become bored. If that happens and you lose your concentration, there is a good chance you'll slow down too much and exit off the back like Wile E. Coyote. The guys running the tests understand this, so they ask you way too many questions to keep you focused. It's a big deal when three minutes elapse and you move on to the next stage, which means an increase in both the speed and the degree of incline. You get questions about symptoms, like chest pain, shortness of breath, lightheadedness. Your blood pressure gets checked and recorded. Sometimes a 12-lead EKG is spit out. A cheerleader with curly blond hair, big tits and pompoms doing back flips would be a nice distraction. In lieu of that, Frank posed a series of questions to obtain a more thorough description of the pain.

"Now where is this chest pain?'

"Under my left scapula. Inside it."

"Does it radiate?" He wasn't talking about radiation, as in the nucular type, but about whether I could feel the pain extending to any other body part.

"Not really, sort of ends up on the left side of my neck, in the back."

"Is it predictable?" I'd never heard that one before. I made a note to start using it in my workups.

"Not at first. Now more so."

"Oh. What brings it on?"

"Position changes, usually when I bend forward. The worst one was last week. I was bent over, moving this woman into position for an LP."

"We're doing this for positional back pain?" Pain brought on by change in position was pretty much guaranteed to not be cardiac in origin. If our roles were reversed, I'd be equally skeptical. I just kept walking while he stewed over this last bit of information.

The first and second stages went pretty much as planned. No chest pain, no shortness of breath, no changes on the monitor or the 12-leads. I could feel the steam building up between Frank's ears, but I thought, what the hell, might as well see how far I could go. Given my exercise routine of the previous five years, I had hopes of Stage 5 or beyond. My heart rate wasn't going up much, and, unless symptoms develop, it is pointless to stop until you reach your heart rate goal, so I figured that even if Frank blew a gasket, he had no reason to stop me prematurely.

As Stage 3 began, with increased speed and incline, I found myself bending forward a little. About a minute into it, I felt that rush of hot water in my mid-back, just above the left kidney. I said, "Here it comes. That pain's starting." To my right, the tech looked at the monitor, then looked over at Frank and shook his head. If I were having the same pain and there were no EKG changes, that would more or less confirm that the pain was not caused by my heart, and he could have the satisfaction of telling me I was full of shit. I kept going, mulling over the ramifications. Frank walked around behind the treadmill to stand beside his tech.

"Got something." It was Frank. "Gee, look at that." He looked up at me. "Are you having any pain?"

"You mean, am I still having pain?" I gave him a look, partly because I don't like it when people don't listen and partly because there was nothing he could do about it. It is considered bad form to verbally abuse a patient who is experiencing cardiac pain. I gave ground a little with "Yeah, still the same pain."

"Okay, we're going to stop. As soon as you stop walking, I want you to lie down on the table here." I did as I was told. Frank gave me a nitroglycerin tablet. As I was putting it into my mouth, he said, "Put it under your tongue." I thought about giving him another look, but just let it go. I'd never enjoyed taking care of physicians, especially the ones who wanted to run the show, and I don't imagine he was all that thrilled with this turn of events.

The tech printed out a 12-lead while Frank took my blood pressure. As soon as he was done, the tech started working the echo probe over my chest. Frank handed me the 12-lead. There was plenty of ST depression to go around. After about five minutes, Frank said, "No sign of any ventricular dysfunction." That meant that despite the anginal symptoms correlating with the EKG changes, my pump was still working normally. By this time my pain was gone. The tech ran another 12-lead. All the ST changes had resolved.

"I want to admit you to the hospital right now. We'll go to the cath lab first thing in the morning."

I thought about how I'd botched the end of my road trip with Ari. "I can't do that. My daughter is with me tonight. How about tomorrow morning first thing?" We argued back and forth a bit, and then agreed that if I had any pain, I would call 911. He gave me a bottle of nitro, I got dressed, and left. I stopped at the E.R. to see Ute, the lady who ran our group, and let her know that I'd be going into the hospital. I had a few shifts scheduled over the next week. Normally, if I knew in advance that I was going to be unavailable to do a scheduled shift, I'd call the other docs and make a trade. Because I didn't think I was in the mood to negotiate, I asked her if she would do it for me. Once she got over the shock of hearing that I was having heart problems, gracious as ever, she agreed.

Now that I knew for sure that I had a coronary cause for my pain, I was relieved and started planning the next few days. Undoubtedly Frank would stent me and I'd be back at work within seven days. I drove home to go over my will and find the words to explain all this to my daughter when I picked her up at school. I didn't want to mislead her, but I didn't want her wearing her worried face either.

119. THE CATHETERIA

As I was driving over to her school, I realized that Ari and I were less than six weeks out from departing on our best road trip ever. So much had happened since then. Now, not quite thirteen years old, she was about to learn that her Dad, who ran beside her in the mornings, took her camping and skiing and chopped mesquite logs for the fireplace, had significant heart disease. No matter how things went on the morrow, I knew that life would never be the same. I just wanted to stick around until she graduated from high school, six years off. In the end, I put that out of mind and concentrated on having some quality time with her. I picked her up, took her over to her Mom's house, and the three of us talked for a while. All things considered, I went home at peace.

That night, I didn't have any chest pain. Sleep came in short bursts, filled with bizarre nightmares from which I awakened drenched in sweat. Most of the scary stuff involved bloody slime eels chewing their way out of my chest. Overall, I felt relief that there was a cardiac cause for my pain. Pretty much any diagnosis sounded better than a crab devouring my pancreas or a blob taking over my spinal cord. Nevertheless, despite good odds, I knew that anything could happen in the cath lab.

I got a ride to the hospital early the next morning. When I was a kid, I developed a reputation for blowing lunch whenever I rode in the back seat. As an adult, I was still an uneasy passenger. In the space of nine minutes over a three-and-one-half-mile trip, we hit the curb twice. Visions of an ambulance ride to the E.R. while strapped to a backboard didn't bring on any angina. By the time I arrived at the hospital at 6:30 A.M., I was scared shitless and grateful that there hadn't been a wreck. On the bright side, my worries about the impending procedure had evaporated.

Word got around that I was going to be admitted to the hospital. A few of the night shift people from the ER stopped by to wish me luck. I'd done a stretch of about five years strictly on nights. The night shift staff are a terrific group of people, but working night shifts while the rest of the world sleeps in their comfy beds sucks. Still, I envied them as they left to go home. After the usual paperwork and wallet biopsy, I went over to have blood drawn and get an EKG. Right now I was feeling apprehensive but otherwise okay. As long as everyone stuck to my script this would end happily. I was curious to find out why I had suddenly developed this weird pain a month earlier and kept having it. My EKG the previous day had shown no evidence of an MI, and I hadn't dropped dead yet.

After a short wait in the cath lab waiting room, the process got started. I traded my clothes for a hospital gown. When I was a kid, they had this show on TV called "Queen For A Day". The host was a Man-Tan aficionado named Jack Bailey, who could switch emotions from overly chipper cheerleader to sincere, handkerchief-proffering comforter in the blink of an eye. At the end of each show, after the tally of the applause meter readings, the tension was broken by the coronation of the Queen. While gushing tears to the strains of "Pomp and Circumstance", she was wrapped in this red velvet robe which for some reason I called a gown. I've been to a few snooty affairs where women wore ballroom gowns, most of which were festooned with yards of ghoulish ribbons, bows and pleats. Ditto for wedding gowns. I've worn an academic gown (for those of you who never graduated, it is the lower portion of the "cap and gown" ensemble) on three occasions.

None of these had an opening in the back. When it comes to hospitals, for some reason it is more acceptable to exhibit partial posterior nudity than partial frontal nudity. A gown with an opening in the back makes sense if you are undergoing a procedure involving your back or your butt. I, however, was not anticipating any ass time in the cath lab. I started to speculate on this concept with my pre-cath nurse; she gave me a smile and ignored my babblings.

I got on a gurney, and one of the staff put in an IV. I have great veins, or at least I did before all this began, so, other than the time I let a nervous nursing student practice her IV skills on me, nobody's ever had to stick me twice. A couple more folks from around the hospital stopped by the waiting area to say hello and wish me luck. After I was wheeled into the cath lab, the supervisor and more cath lab staff came in to ask if I needed anything. I wasn't feeling giddy with excitement about being there, but, on the bright side, if I wound up as a case number at the monthly morbidity and mortality conference, there shouldn't be any confusion when it came to identifying my corpse. I looked around at the staff who would be in the cath lab with me. I had at least a couple of allies. When you are about to undergo a potentially life-threatening procedure, especially for the first time, it's comforting to know who's in your corner.

Speaking of comfort, the cath table feels about as soft and cozy as a slab of flagstone. The surface has to be firm and inflexible, yet, because film cassettes go underneath, it can't inhibit the passage of x-rays. You can put small pillows here and there, and if you are cold they can throw on a warm blanket, which invariably produces an "Ah", but the table is still hard. It is known far and wide that I have no butt, so that is where I felt the table the most. I comforted myself with the knowledge that, even if Frank performed an angioplasty or two, I'd be in there for no more than a couple of hours, so I wasn't going to develop bedsores. Besides, once the action started, I sure wouldn't be thinking about a sore butt. Focusing on relaxing every muscle in my body, I nodded off for a few minutes.

There's a lot of preparation before the procedure itself begins, and the conversations in the lab reflect that. Meds have to be loaded in syringes, the catheters have to be unwrapped, and everything has to end up on the Mayo stand. There are all sorts of medical instruments known as Mayo this or Mayo that. None of them, not even the Mayo enema, has anything to do with mayonnaise. They were all devised or improved by someone at the Mayo Clinic. The Mayo stand is the gold standard for holding instruments during a procedure, from a simple laceration repair to exotic brain surgery. Everything that goes into a cath is sterilized, and the staff that stands nearest the cath table is gowned, masked and gloved. Once everything is in place, they page the cardiologist.

Frank walks in. While getting all gowned and gloved up, he begins with the warmup chit-chat.

"Hi, Frank, how are you doing?"

"I'm good." Then I ask the bigger question. "How about you?" The way I see it, it's very important for the guy holding the knife or the needle to be having a good day. It's going to be a good day for the guy lying on the table only if he's still alive and anatomically intact at the end of it, and that depends mostly on the guy who's standing over him.

"I'm okay. Any chest pain since the treadmill?"

"No, I had a good night." He starts palpating for my right femoral pulse, down in the crease of my groin. I've felt thousands of groins for a pulse, but I'm not wild about a guy doing it to me. To take my mind off of that, I review the arrangement of the various structures in there. NAVEL. From the side to the middle, it's Nerve, Artery, VEin, Ligament. You are supposed to find the artery by feeling for a pulse. Sometimes you find the artery when you stick a needle into what you think is the vein. Arterial blood, which has been oxygenated in the lungs and pumped into the arterial system by the left ventricle of the heart, is fairly bright red and comes out in impressive spurts. Theoretically, by measuring the height of those spurts, you can determine someone's systolic blood pressure. Of course, by the time you measure it and do the calculations, most likely the height of the spurt is dropping, and the patient is in need of a blood transfusion or two. Venous blood, which is returning to the heart to be oxygenated, tends to be darker and flows more slowly and evenly. For most heart caths, you want a catheter in the artery and nowhere else. First some lidocaine, which burns initially, to numb up the skin and subcutaneous tissue, then the needles for the catheter.

"How are you doing?"

"Little sore."

"Still? How about some MS (morphine sulfate) and Versed?" This combo, or some other narcotic and benzodiazepine, is one of the combos used during procedures for conscious sedation, also commonly known as "twilight anesthesia". Theoretically it allows you to stay awake and answer questions, but I've used it to knock people out when I had to reduce a dislocation, and I can tell you, there's no way they could have answered any questions with that stuff on board. It doesn't last very long in your system. Like a stand-up hypnotist routine in a comedy club, after he snaps his fingers, you awaken remembering nothing. Nothing about the procedure, that is. I wasn't ready for that. As long as I didn't act like a dick or squirm around like a fart in a skillet, I'd get to choose.

So I asked, "How about more lidocaine instead?"

"Sure." He pumped more of the clear liquid into my skin and soft tissues. This time there was no burn, just dull numbness. From here on out, I would feel pressure but no pain. Frank picked up a catheter with a needle protruding from the tip and stuck me with it in the groin. There was a slight crackling noise. Judging by the looks the staff were giving each other, everybody had heard it.

I asked, "What was that?"

"You've got a lot of calcium in your artery." Arterial walls are supposed to be flexible and relatively soft, like a rubber band. Significant concentrations of calcium in the walls of an artery make it more like an eggshell. If the concentration is high enough, you can actually see the outline of blood vessels on a standard x-ray. That rarely goes along with good health or a good prognosis. For me, it meant that any cholesterol plaques in my coronary arteries were likely to be calcified. That made everything from here on out more difficult and more dangerous. I did my best to absorb this latest informational gem without getting all panicky.

The primary purpose of the cath is to identify lesions in the coronary arteries. Usually these are cholesterol plaques that have caused narrowing of the lumen of the artery. During the cath, the cardiologist threads a catheter (thus the name) from the insertion point in the femoral artery up through the aorta into the heart. From there he works the catheter into position so that dye can be injected into the various coronary arteries. Usually there are three: the left anterior descending (LAD) and the circumflex come off of the left main, which is really just a stump. The right has its own origin. Occasionally there is a fourth, known as an intermedius or a diagonal, with its own origin.

Frank did the coronaries, which took about ten minutes total. If you are heading for bypass surgery, some cardiologists routinely cath the left internal mammary artery, which is the graft of choice for an LAD or circumflex lesion. Unlike the coronary arteries, when the LIMA is injected with dye, you may feel a burn across your shoulder and down into the left side of your chest. Then he shot a load of dye into my left ventricle, to see how well the major pumping chamber of the heart sent arterial blood throughout my body. I'm not sure "shot a load" is the best term to describe a ventriculogram, but you get the idea.

I asked, "Are you doing a Swan too?" Sometimes, when the cardiologist is evaluating narrowing of the aortic valve (aortic stenosis) or high pressures in the pulmonary arteries (pulmonary hypertension), he'll insert a catheter into the femoral vein as well. You run the venous catheter, sometimes called a Swan-Ganz catheter, up the femoral vein, through the vena cava (the venous equivalent of the aorta), into the right chambers of the heart and out into the pulmonary arteries. From there you can measure pulmonary capillary wedge pressures ("the wedge") and determine cardiac output. The latter allows you to measure the degree of narrowing of the valves on the left side of the heart. I asked this just to take my mind off the calcium issue.

"No, don't need to." He looked up at the films on the monitor, which was positioned for him at eye-level and across the table, to my left.

"Okay, here's what we have." He pointed at the monitor. There was a static film of my coronaries filled with dye. Because of the angle, I could see the lower portion of my heart best. There were several areas of minor narrowing down there.

"Just those down there?"

Frank looked at me. "No. Up there." He pointed to the upper portion of my heart, near the origin of the LAD.

I tilted my head so that I could see. "That flap?" Halfway down the left main, there was a flipper-looking thing sticking out at an angle, obscuring a good ninety-five percent of the lumen. It reminded me of that age-old complaint, "You never put the seat down". All of a sudden my mouth felt a little on the dry side.

"You ruptured a plaque in your left main." *I did that? I didn't mean to.* It isn't all that common a finding. You almost never see it in a cath. It does, however, show up in autopsy reports.

"Oh. You're going to stent that?" My mouth was now way beyond "a little on the dry side".

"I'm done. There's nothing I can do with that. You're going to the O.R. today. As in now."

"You can't put a stent in there?" That came out a tad plaintive.

"That plaque is unstable. If it breaks off during the angioplasty, it'll lodge a little further down and that will be that. You need a bypass."

Suddenly it dawned on me. That tearing pain in that parking garage in Portland a month ago must have been the initial rupture of the plaque. You can say what you want about aspirin, how the studies have shown that for the general population, the risks--G.I. bleeds, bleeds in the brain--outweigh the benefits. Maybe so. I like to think that, had I not been taking aspirin regularly when that plaque ruptured, a big fat clot of platelets would have formed around that flipper and I'd have died on the spot, right in front of my daughter. Then I realized that it could have completely obstructed my left main at any time during our trip in the red convertible. The road trip of my dreams ends up killing me, and maybe my little girl too.

I'd kept it together pretty well the whole time mostly by thinking this would all be over in a day or so. Now somebody was deviating from my script. I realized I'd be in the hospital for my daughter's birthday, and I started to choke up. Other than at sappy movies and during bad allergy seasons, I'm pretty good at controlling my tear ducts.

Fortunately, a very nice nurse came over and told me, "It's okay to let it out." I thought, *No it's not.* That was the end of that.

There's no crying in the cath lab.

120. ON THE SLAB

Before I got to enjoy the CABG procedure, a bunch of calls had to be made. Given the now clearly recognized fact that I had an unstable ruptured plaque in about the worst place possible, my impending surgery was designated an "emergency". The irony of that was not lost on me. Here I'd been driving up and down the West Coast, then walking and working with this flipper in my left main for over a month, and now suddenly it was an emergency. I understood the liability issue, but the temptation to get dressed and go home for a few days was pretty attractive. After all, if the toilet seat hadn't opened up permanently, there must be something, a sticky hinge, maybe a wedge of some kind lodged up at the base of the flap, that was keeping the artery partially open.

Once Frank had explained the significance of what I was seeing on the cath film, I understood why the pain came on more often when I was bent forward. I was thinking now that continuing my daily dose of aspirin to prevent any clots around the ruptured plaque would give everybody time to think things through more clearly. One of the Frank's partners was doing a few laser procedures to open coronary arteries. Someone might come up with a way to balloon and stent the plaque. I knew I'd already pushed my luck to the far reaches of probability, but I also knew that, in general, elective surgery almost always turned out better than its emergent counterpart. If nothing else, I could get the first time slot in a few days when everybody was fresh and the operating room was spiffy clean.

The problem with having an "emergency" anything is that, except in the Emergency Department, there isn't anybody standing around with nothing to do, twiddling their collective thumbs, until an emergency arrives. Even in an E.D., you might arrive with an emergency when no bed is available. Every so often you have to treat a guy with major life-threatening conditions in the OB-GYN room, the one with the stirrup table, usually reserved for women who require pelvic exams. Every E.R. doc has sewn up a laceration in a hallway rather than wait three or four hours for a bed to open up. It's not M.A.S.H., but you make do.

That holds especially true for the operating room. Time in the O.R. is almost always the most expensive time you can buy in a hospital. When you go in for surgery, a major part of your bill is rent for the O.R. space. Before we got to all the discount plans conjured up by hospitals and insurance companies, you paid for O.R. time in fifteen-minute blocks. There were busy hospitals with pricing power that actually charged by the minute. Obviously, that worked in favor of the fastest, most experienced surgeons. They were able to get in and get out more quickly than their less experienced, slower colleagues, so their cost for a given procedure would be lower. Faster surgeons are also good for patients. The greatest risk factor for intraoperative infections is the skin-to-skin time, the period from the time of the initial incision with the aseptic scalpel to the time of the placement of the last suture closing the surgical wound; the faster your surgeon, the lower your chances of acquiring an infection.

Surgeons like to operate as early in the morning as possible, and the guys with pull usually get the first slots in each operating room schedule. This means you know exactly when you are starting. Your operating room was cleaned and stocked at the end of the day before and rechecked an hour or so before your scheduled cutting time. Your patient has already been prepped in the pre-op waiting area. The starting time for every procedure after the first slot is listed on the big board as "TF", to follow. After each procedure, the room has to be thoroughly cleaned, all the equipment restocked, and the patient brought in from the pre-op waiting area. In the best of circumstances, where everybody does their job and there are no complications, it'll be at least a half-hour before you slice into skin. If for some reason the previous surgery in the room turned into a "dirty" case, involving bowel or infected tissue or excessive bleeding, turnaround time could easily exceed an hour. Meanwhile, everybody's waiting.

I waited on a gurney in the cath lab until they were ready for me in the O.R. It might have been almost an hour, but for me it raced by. Several co-workers stopped by to wish me luck. A friend of mine, a respiratory therapist who spent a fair portion of his workday in the E.R., came by with a pretty young girl.

"Hi, how are you doing?"

"Okay. I'll be better when they take me in and knock me out."

"Speaking of which, this is Julie."

"Hello, Julie."

"She's an RT student, just started her clinicals here this week. She hasn't started any radial art lines yet. If you wouldn't mind, it would be a great experience for her to start your art line."

"Okay by me. I'll be out cold, so, sure."

"I was thinking it'd be a better experience if she did it here, before you go under." Julie looked at him in alarm.

I asked, "Are you serious?"

He laughed. "Nah, I'm just screwing with you. Good luck in there." He shook my hand and walked away. I'm not sure who was more relieved, Julie or I. It kept me from thinking about the near death experience I was about to undergo. By this time I was done feeling sorry for myself. I wanted this over with, so the sooner they put me out the better. At that point I would have given anything in the world to hug my daughter for a nanosecond.

They contacted the surgeon I requested, Casey Huston. As luck would have it, he was the only guy available at that point in time, so that worked out perfectly. It took a while to find a cardiac anesthesiologist, a perfusionist, and a surgical assistant. The cardiac surgeon or the assistant, often a general surgeon, harvests the saphenous vein from one or both legs. Back in the 70s and 80s, obtaining a saphenous vein required a long incision down the medial aspect of the leg, from your groin to your ankle. Nowadays the standard is a couple of tiny incisions at the top and bottom. A scope is rammed through under the skin, the vein is freed up, ligated (tied with suture material) at each end, cut free and pulled out with the scope. This method is faster, cleaner, and pretty much does away with post-op and long-term infections. I'd taken care of more than a few guys with the long scars who ended up gobbling penicillin every day for the rest of their lives. I didn't know either the anesthesiologist or the surgical assistant. Didn't care, either.

Once the O.R. was available and everyone was ready, I was wheeled into the room. I had a flash of the surgery scene in *All That Jazz*. A bunch of people helped me slide onto the operating table, but none of them were Ben Vereen singing "Bye Bye Life". I took that as a good sign. The surgeon walked in and said "Hi", the anesthesiologist injected something into my IV, and I ceased to exist. From wide awake to pure nothing in less than a second.

121. BACK TO LIFE

My memory of the five days I spent in the hospital recovering from surgery is pretty much a blur, partly because my memory in general has been shit canned, but also because the whole time I felt like I was lost in a fog in Half Moon Bay. I didn't have enough going on upstairs to realize that this was abnormal, let alone whether it was temporary or permanent. About the only abstract thought I had the entire time in the CVICU was something I call "Duh". Everything else was primitive brain, visceral, as in "I got to pee." or "My leg hurts." Some visitors opined that it might be residual from the anesthesia. I didn't really care. At the time, neither they nor I considered the pumphead syndrome. At least I didn't. If they did, they were kind enough to keep it to themselves. So bear with me. I didn't start making notes until I was discharged. While the notes were nothing to write home about, they were of some help in keeping things straight in my mind.

All of a sudden, I'm alive again. Although I can't see, move or talk, I do hear a couple of beeps, the sound of a ventilator triggering, and voices. One voice is giving a report to another voice. It takes a while before I realize they are talking about me. Not really anxious to wake up yet, I lie there listening. I have a vague understanding that I went somewhere for a while, someplace dissociated from life.

In my second year of college, I met the high school friend of a woman I fancied. He looked every bit the part of an uninteresting nerd; I was just learning that appearances were often if not always deceiving. This guy was into the study of mind control. He devoured every slice of information he could get his hands on about using more of his brain. He told me that every night he programmed his brain to dream about something specific. Our mutual friend, the girl, asked him what he wanted to dream about most nights.

He just shook his head and said, "Oh, lots of different things." Ha! I knew the answer to that one. The same thing every twenty-year-old guy wants to dream about. Sex. Ever since, I have tried to follow his simple instructions. Think about one thing and one thing only just before you get into bed. Unless there is something going on in my life that causes me particular concern, it usually works.

As they wheeled me into the O.R., I was mulling over the grotesque possibility of my having a heart attack and dying on the road, my daughter riding shotgun in the red convertible. While unconscious during surgery, I must have managed a dream to that effect, because, when I regained consciousness in the CVICU, my first instinct was to look over to my right to see how Ari was doing. Unfortunately, I couldn't see. I was aware that I couldn't move my legs. *Well, I'm paralyzed from the waist down, but at least I'm alive.* That thought lasted all of two seconds. At the same time, I remembered heading for open heart surgery. Combined with the lack of feeling in my legs, my next thought was that I'd have to go home in a wheelchair.

All of a sudden, every part of my body was working. None of it was under my control, but things were moving. Something was blowing large volumes of air into me at regular intervals and my lungs weren't enjoying it at all. I coughed, or tried to, and realized there was a giant plug in my windpipe. My head and legs came up involuntarily; my arms tried to, but something held them down. A new, more annoying beeping noise began sounding over to my right. Then I started inhaling on my own; I have no idea why. The beeping noise ceased. Invisible voices around my head chatted back and forth. The next thing I knew, something was being pulled out of my throat. I coughed and gagged. A different something was shoved into my mouth: someone was suctioning my upper airway. After they were finished sucking all the air out of my lungs, or so it felt, that irritating object was removed and a different irritating object was placed into each of my nostrils. Now I could feel air flowing into my nose. A voice from above me said to take deep slow breaths. I still couldn't see. A voice inside me said, "You're not blind, idiot. Open your eyes." So I did.

At first, everything was blurry. By the time I was able to focus, there were only a few people in the room. A couple of nurses were working on the various lines coming out of my body. I could hear someone doing something at the foot of the bed, but it was too much effort to raise my head and look. I lost interest and fell back to sleep.

The only other memory of that first day must have occurred several hours later. When I woke up, my room was pitch black. My brain made the connection and told me it was night time. Down past the foot of the bed, I could see enough by the glow of the nursing station to figure out which room I was in. *First one on the right, the corner room. Right by the door to the unit. Escaping from here will be a cinch. Maybe later.*

Suddenly a huge moon face appeared right in front of me. It floated there, less than a foot from my face. It wore the puzzled but disinterested look of a hungry alien, trying to decide which part of my face to chew off first. Terrified, I tried to scream, but nothing came out.

Then I was gone again. The next day I asked around about who had been in my room that night, even described its massive face and the way it floated in mid-air, but nobody came up with a name. My nurse suggested that I had been dreaming. *Yeah, right.* My face was intact, though.

The next morning, I was awakened by my day shift nurse. The clock on the wall said 7:15, so I figured she'd just finished getting report from the night nurse. She wrote down my vitals, asked me a few questions and left. I drifted back to sleep. When she returned, I could tell it was go time. As in, things were going to go away.

First to go was my Foley catheter. In college, I volunteered for a research study. Someone in the medical school was studying a new ADH inhibitor. ADH (anti-diuretic hormone) helps your kidneys hold on to water, so an ADH inhibitor prevents your kidneys from retaining water. The commonest ADH inhibitor, the only one you can buy without a prescription, is ethanol, a.k.a. booze. Now you know why you wet your pants when you pass out from drinking like a fish. A really attractive young nurse, who would be working with me for the day, explained that she'd be putting a catheter into my bladder. I thought, *Through my dick?* As I recall, that part of the deal went unmentioned until I was in the hospital bed and had signed my life away for the day.

Happily for all concerned, especially me, my prostate was nice and small; the catheter slid in without a hitch. If there was any pain, I didn't notice it, mainly because I was doing my best to avoid a trip to Bonerville. When you're twenty, not getting it all that much, and a woman, any woman, is holding your dick, even with latex gloves on, not getting a hard-on requires serious concentration. *One hundred, ninety-nine, ninety-eight....*

The catheter stayed in for about eight hours. During the first four hours, the baseline period, the catheter was clamped for fifty-five minutes each hour, during which time urine was prevented from LEAVING, then unclamped for five so it could empty. I could feel my bladder swelling, but it was tolerable. At the end of four hours, they injected me with this new experimental ADH inhibitor. That's when things got interesting. The protocol remained the same as in the baseline period.

The first hour was not too bad, but I dumped about twice the volume of urine. The next three hours, my urine output kept increasing. Based upon my bladder agony from minute 30 to minute 55 each hour, this new drug was doing a terrific job. Think of the worst pee urge you've ever had and multiply it by ten. By minute 54 in my last hour, it was all

I could do to keep from unclamping the Foley myself. As soon as she deflated the balloon and pulled it out, I was up and heading for the door. All thoughts of asking her out were gone.

For my troubles I think I received a hundred bucks, by far my biggest payday ever. Better still, I had a slightly embellished story to tell my friends when I bought a round of beers. More ADH inhibitors, down the hatch.

During my career, I'd put in well over a hundred Foleys, some easy, some not so easy. While draining someone's bladder can relieve incredible misery, nobody ever said, "Hey, that felt really good." Nobody ever got a hard-on either. I'd removed a few as well. Most times they wouldn't say anything, they just exhaled deeply. Mine had been put in after I was anesthetized, in the O.R. I was a little apprehensive about having it removed, so, as my nurse worked, I kept a close eye on the proceedings. I relaxed when I saw her suck out ten cc. of saline from the balloon port with a syringe. That meant the balloon at the tip of the catheter, in my bladder, was deflated. Right after that, she pulled the catheter out. There was a little stinging for a second or two, then everything was AOK.

Next to go was my radial artery catheter, which was placed in the O.R. for monitoring my blood pressure. It was also a reliable, painless source for obtaining blood samples. On the up side, removing it meant there weren't any concerns about my blood pressure. On the other hand, if I needed any blood tests, I'd be getting stuck each time.

Pretty soon it was time for me to get moving. I'd never written routine orders for a bypass patient, so I really had no idea what to expect the first post-op day. I figured I'd be up in a chair, then maybe do a little walking the next day. Uh-uh.

As soon as she was done removing stuff from my body, my nurse hit the bed control button. Up went my head. I felt a little lightheaded for about five seconds. I looked over at the monitor. At first my heart rate went up about ten beats per minute, then settled back down. She asked me how I felt. When I replied that everything was okay, she helped me swing my legs around and over the side of the bed. *Oh, the dangle.* That went better; soon I was standing while she recorded orthostatics. A moment of lightheadedness passed. Next thing I knew, we were headed out the door, she pushing an IV pole while I stumbled along behind a wheelchair, feeling like a demented eighty-year-old nursing home gomer taking his daily walk around the facility. My right leg, bandaged from groin to ankle, hurt some, my chest not much at all. I was weak as a kitten. I wasn't having any shortness of breath, but breathing wasn't easy.

I'd never before been an adult patient, certainly not after major surgery. I'd heard stories of physicians trying to run the show from their hospital beds. Generally speaking, nurses don't get much of a kick out of a patient telling her what to do and how to do it. Not a problem here. That first day, I couldn't have run a damn thing.

By the end of my first full day, I was already bored but too sluggish to do much about it. Now that I could urinate without a catheter, I knew that to get out of the hospital, there were three more things I'd have to be able to do on my own: walk, eat, and poop. I also knew all too well that the longer you stay in the hospital, even on a clean unit like the CVICU, the greater the chance you'd end up with an infection. Not just an infection, a nosocomial infection. Nosocomial infections, the ones you catch after you are admitted to the hospital, are the ones that involve the really nasty bugs, the ones that swallow most antibiotics and spit them out in a fit of laughter. The last thing I wanted was to languish in a bed with pus draining out of my leg or sternal wound, or a case of necrotizing pneumonia, or a MRSA- infested bedsore. So, beginning on post-op day #2, I forced myself to walk the loop as many times a day as I could. The nurse was obligated to get me up at least once or twice on the day shift, and once on nights. I grabbed anyone I could, from a nurse's aide to visitors, to help me navigate the hallway. After a couple of days, I was able to go on my own. It wasn't easy, and at the end I felt like I'd need an entire day to rest up before my next walk, but it helped with the other two requirements. Between the risk of blood clots and passing out from orthostatic hypotension, bed rest can kill you.

Anyone who complains about hospital food probably doesn't need to be in the hospital. I ate the jello, the broth, the pudding, all that slop. None of it tasted like anything, good or bad. I had no appetite, I just ate when they told me to. It went down and stayed down, that's all that mattered. In the outside world, some people eat to live, some live to eat. When you're a patient, you eat to get out of the hospital. Once that mission is accomplished, you can reward yourself with a good meal at home.

The five-hour surgery had required the administration of lots of IV fluids and a number of blood transfusions. That's probably why I received intravenous diuretics the first couple of days, to get rid of "excess" fluid. I knew I was dry because my urine kept getting darker and darker. Right after I got my daily injection I'd urinate a ton, which is why you give them, but then I'd barely produce any more urine until the next dose. When you are dehydrated, it's a lot harder to take a crap. I finally pointed this out to my docs, and they got rid of the diuretics. Within a day I felt better when I stood up, and the color of my urine gradually retreated from burnt umber back to lemonade.

The rest of my stay blurred along at a snail's pace. A couple things still stand out, though. I had a matched set of mediastinal tubes, big 30 or 35 French hoses placed right behind my sternum during surgery. They exited through puncture wounds in my upper abdomen, and were connected to a drainage collection system. Once the drainage, first bloody, then serosanguineous (thin and reddish) was reduced to almost nothing, it was time to pull them out. I dreaded that for a couple of reasons. One was the memory from medical school, the first time I saw a chest tube of any kind removed. A noted TCV surgeon yanked a mediastinal tube from a patient of his. Half the tube came out, the other half remained inside the patient's chest. It seems the tube got caught on one of the sternal wires and ripped in half. He double-timed it out of the room, leaving his TCV surgery fellow to explain to the patient the concept of reopening her chest. First impressions like that tend to stick with you.

The other reason for my apprehension was that I knew it was going to hurt. I'd inserted dozens of chest tubes into patients in the E.R. and the ICU, mostly on the side, below their armpits. I'd pulled a few as well. Just yanking one out through the intercostal muscles, the muscles between their ribs, caused considerable muscle spasms in some patients. Mine were going to come out through my upper abdominal muscles. I've never been much of an aficionado of sit ups or crunches, whatever they are, but my abs were okay. Hidden, but okay. When removal time arrived, my nurse cut the sutures holding them in place. She did a nice job of yanking them simultaneously; both came out intact. For a nanosecond, I thought, *Hey, that wasn't so bad.* The next thing I knew, my abs were rolling like waves in a mid-Atlantic squall, ten times worse than my worst-ever muscle cramps. Though the pain lasted only a minute, it scarred me for life. I can't even watch the belly dancer scene in *From Russia With Love* without getting a stomach ache.

Speaking of muscles. Like I mentioned before, I was arguably in the best shape of my life when all this started. While nobody would ever describe me as buff, and I had a small donut that hid my belly button and my abs, in scrubs I looked fit and trim. At least, I thought I did. The first couple days, when I was still peeing in a urinal bottle and had no desire to take a crap, I'd catch a vague reflection in the glass doors around the nursing station as I walked by. It wasn't until I stood in the bathroom, staring at myself in the mirror, that I realized how scrawny I'd become. I undid the top tie on my gown and pulled it down.

Someone had robbed every strand of muscle from my chest, shoulders and upper arms. I was down to skin and bone. And flab. I'd heard that patients in long surgical procedures often lost a fair bit of muscle mass. One surgical nutrition specialist told me that protein stores, especially skeletal muscle, simply melt away, moved elsewhere to assist the healing process. It doesn't do a thing to your fat stores, though, at least not the ones you can see in the mirror. Skin and subcutaneous fat hung on me like a saggy drape. My chest was shaved. My bones stuck out everywhere. The word "ghoulish" came to mind, like Marley's ghost. I tied my gown back up immediately, afraid that if I looked too closely, I'd be able to see right through my chest.

I shuffled out of the bathroom and picked up my bedside chart. Between my admission to the hospital and my second post-op day, my weight had dropped from my usual 174 to 151. During the rest of my hospital stay, it remained right around there. Had I not seen the evidence in the bathroom mirror, I'd have guessed it was fluid loss from the diuretics. It was definitely muscle loss.

Most surgeons like to keep dressings on for at least twenty-four hours, some for forty-eight. I had one down the middle of my chest, covering my sternotomy wound. There were a couple of long ones covering the medial aspect (inside) of my right leg, from mid-thigh to my ankle. I was curious about the latter. It looked strangely similar to the ones patients received back in the '80s. When my nurse took off the dressing, I was horrified. I had a wound running the entire length of my leg. Over the years, I'd treated a number of patients with recurrent strep cellulitis (skin infection) of their saphenous vein harvest site. Eventually they ended up taking penicillin or some other antibiotic daily for the rest of their lives. I had visions of flesh-eating strep devouring my leg, leaving a puddle of tissue glop on the floor and me with a stump. 1980 technique in 2005. When I asked around, the word I got was that my surgery was such an emergency that there wasn't time to do it right. I was pissed off for a minute or two, then went to acceptance mode. Nothing to do about it anyway.

I'm well aware that physicians and their families often have worse outcomes than the general population. Maybe in the long run it's best if the staff doesn't know who you are. Since I was up in the CVICU seeing patients or responding to codes on a regular basis, that wasn't likely. One good thing did come from my being on staff, though. On the third post-op day the head nurse asked me if I wanted to stay in the CVICU until discharge rather than move out to telemetry.

"Can I?"

"I think we can arrange it."

"You bet." I still wasn't thinking very clearly, but I knew the staff, who preferred to care for patients who were acutely ill and not winding down their stay in the hospital, would be chomping at the bit to get rid of me. On telemetry, probably because the beds are more plentiful and less expensive than in the units, there is less urgency in sending people home. If the change in plans bugged the crap out of Frank, so much the better. Sooner rather than later, everyone on the health care team would grow sick of my mug and we'd all be on the same page: time for me to go home.

Now that the goal of getting out looked attainable, I kicked it into high gear, relatively speaking, for my walks. I was now shuffling along as fast as your average seventy-year-old nursing home gome, leaving the eighty-year-olds to eat my dust. I ate everything, drank tons of fluids, and finally cranked out a mini-poop. Next day I was out the door. I remember being wheeled out to the pickup area in the parking lot thinking, *My last day as a patient. How sweet it is.*

122. ADRIFT

My first day home, after I was dropped off, it was all I could do to stagger into the house and collapse on the sofa. I wasn't feeling much pain in my chest wound, just a dull ache in my sternum. The saphenous vein harvest site on my right leg, the retro gift from the '80s, hurt enough to wake me up at night. My breathing was nowhere near normal, but it didn't hurt to breathe, and as long as I didn't try anything stupid, my lungs weren't an issue. Looking in the mirror was painful. My hair had gone from salt-and-pepper to pure white in less than a week. By far the worst feeling was weakness. I was down at least twenty pounds from my pre-op weight. Nobody's ever associated my physique with the word "cut". Now I looked more like an octogenarian finishing a long course of chemo and radiation for some cancer chewing on me from the inside out.

I was a little anxious as well. Most of the time, if something were to go wrong, I was on my own. Anxiety consumes an awful lot of energy. The best thing about the weakness and fatigue was that I had no energy to spare, so any anxiety was limited to a minute or two. My brain was dull as a runcible spoon, I assumed from the anesthesia and five days in the hospital. While I had heard of and seen cases of pumphead over the years, I didn't even consider the possibility that I might have it. Even attempting to figure that one out was beyond my capacity.

The housing construction boom was in full swing. Three McMansions were being built on my street. Sunrise in mid-September was around 6:15. Usually the birds in my neighborhood start their singing exactly fifteen minutes before sunrise; for the next six months, I never heard the birds over the sounds of the construction across the street. Promptly at 5:45 AM, accompanied by a boom box at full volume, a crew of ten would rev up saws, drills and hammers.

On the one hand, it pissed me off, because I was waking up in the middle of the night for an hour or two. I'd get back to sleep around 3:30 or 4:00, then get serenaded awake by the sounds of a mariachi band. On the other hand, the daily high temps still hovered in the mid-100s; waking up early allowed me to go for my walk before it got too hot. Groggy from being up for a couple of hours in the middle of the night, I'd crawl out of bed, dangle for about ten minutes until everything stopped spinning, and get dressed.

Over the years I have received, or, even more pathetically, purchased a number of Hawaiian shirts that can best be described as garish. None of those really classy numbers you see on politicians and news anchors in the islands. Were mine any classier, they would have come with a dimmer switch. And a trash bag. Most of them were already two sizes too big. At this point, a good twenty pounds below my usual weight, everything hung on me. The looseness of the Hawaiians allowed me to walk without the shirt scraping my chest hair stubble or irritating my sternal wound. In the mirror, I looked like a skeleton in a moo-moo. When I walked by the construction crew, they would stop what they were doing and stare at me as if I were some gaunt agent of death come to take them to the afterworld. Occasionally, one of them would look down at the ground and make the sign of the cross.

I started by walking to the end of my street and back. Although I am the founder of the Cul-de-Sac Club of America and editor-in-chief of Cul-de-Sac Magazine, a journal dedicated to the documentation and promotion of the cul-de-sac lifestyle, the truth requires me to confess to living, not on a cul-de-sac, but on a dead end. Just like that guy who backs a '78 rust-accented Fiesta out of his garage, bidding adieu to walls festooned with posters of speedy new Ferraris, I am a fraud. Up to the end of the street and back is about two hundred yards. By the time I returned to my driveway, I was gasping an agnostic prayer of thanks that it was downhill to the front door. I collapsed on the sofa before I fell down, and stayed there for a good hour.

I did the dead end walk for a couple of days. By the end of the first week, I was able to circle the block, about a half-mile. I considered doing the route twice a day, but just thinking about it wore me out. There were inclines involved. I felt even slight rises on my walks. A stiff breeze slowed me down, my moo-moo fluttering like a luffed jib in the wind. At any challenge, I would stop and rest. If a landscape wall appeared, I would sit on that for a few minutes. Pushing myself beyond my low limits left me absolutely exhausted. I knew that walking was the right thing to do, but I couldn't wait to sit down at the end of my fifteen-minute stroll. People stared at me. At first I thought it was the shirts. Eventually it occurred to me that I looked like a cadaver come back to life. Lazarus minus the Jesus-centric fanfare.

I stuck to well-protected streets and sidewalks. I soon realized that cars and even loud trucks could come up behind me without my noticing it. When they passed, I'd just about jump out of my skin. It wasn't that I couldn't hear them. The noise just didn't register. Same thing for some visual cues. I'd look straight at something and not notice it. It took me a couple of weeks to realize that I was completely invisible to drivers. I've always been a big walker and got by with just basic awareness of traffic around me. Now, even with the white walking man on the stoplight beckoning me to cross in complete safety, I made sure that not one car was anywhere near me before I ventured off of the corner. It felt like I was walking in midtown Manhattan at rush hour. Caveat ambulator.

Some chronic pedestrians like to confront cars in a crosswalk, dare them to run them down, maybe collect a few bucks, courtesy of PITLA. Not me. I don't go for Pyrrhic victories, especially if they conclude with me in a hospital bed, external fixators screwed into my shattered bones, just counting the seconds until that big floaty clot in my thigh decides to take a Carnival cruise north to lodge in a pulmonary artery, the Alaska of my thorax.

At least in Phoenix, every community has its share of The Walkers. I'm not talking about either end of the walking bell curve, the leathery homeless with shopping carts or the retired senior couples in their matching pastel running suits. There are silent, skinny people traveling the sidewalks of most neighborhoods, sunup to sundown, looking neither left nor right.

There's a guy who does this most days around where I live. I've been keeping an eye on him for twenty years. He started out really well-built, good-looking, and well-kept. Over the past two decades, he has lost some weight, tends to wear the same clothes for days at a time, and, eschewing any form of headgear, has acquired a craggy, leathery look to his face. Except in the bitterly cold Phoenix winters, he walks all day without a shirt. No water bottle either. A few times a year he carries a plastic white supermarket shopping bag. If you approach him he usually crosses to the other side of the street as if he'd been planning to do that all along. Occasionally he would let me walk by him. He lives with a perpetual sun squint, so you can't see his eyes. He never gives evidence of noticing you, but he does. Most folks, especially people in cars, don't notice The Walkers, because they blend in. The good ones always time their street crossings, even at a corner where they have the right of way. They prefer invisibility.

Hunger was a distant memory. I ate, partly because it was something to do to pass the hours in the day, partly because I knew I was supposed to. I focused on drinking liquids, namely water. Even that was going to become problematic. There was no way I could lift a five-gallon jug into place, and unfiltered Phoenix tap water is slightly less palatable than Hanford waste.

The first few weeks after my surgery, I don't think I had a single coherent thought. Even as events were occurring, they became forgotten blurs. I now recollect that time as floating through space; had I truly been able to float, life would have been much easier. Soon after I left the hospital, one of my oldest friends, Bill, came down from Portland. He stayed for a week. I'm not sure what he thought he would have to do for me, but it turned out that his biggest job was reorienting me on a regular basis. Most days I took a nap in the afternoon. I'd wake up, come out of my bedroom, and be stunned to find him sitting in the living room. For a few minutes I couldn't remember why he was there or when he'd arrived. Then again, most mornings I woke up not knowing my own name or where I was. I know I drove us out in my car a couple times, and I made sure the drive was five minutes or less. Any longer than that, there was a good chance I'd forget where I was headed. If he told me it was time to do something, depending on how much energy was required, I could do it.

Because Bill's an excellent cook and I am a serviceable sous-chef, we cooked most evenings. He'd tell me what to do, which wasn't anything new when it came to us cooking together. I could handle step-by-step instructions, but if he told me to do something complex, like "Make the salad", I'd be completely flummoxed. I could not figure out step 1. Brain inertia. I'd just stand there until he asked where my salad bowl was. Prior to my surgery, I had gradually become pretty good at feeling when a steak or a slab of fish was ready to come off the grill. After the surgery, that timing skill was gone. I overcooked or undercooked everything. Although I've improved over the years, it's still a guessing game, not a confident decision.

After Bill returned to Portland, I stopped driving for a few weeks. Without him there to navigate and keep me oriented, I lost the confidence to get places safely. I tried once to get to my bank. Things went well until I had to make some turns. Suddenly I was completely lost, less than a mile from my home. I sat in my car in a parking lot for about ten minutes before I could figure out how to get home. I had to forget about the bank. For some of my early follow-up appointments I took the bus.

By the third week, I was able to walk the half-mile to the supermarket. If I had a list of things I needed--usually there were about ten things I needed, but when I wrote my list, I could only think of maybe four--I could find them, pay for them, and walk home with them, stopping at least twice along the way to rest. Carrying four items in a plastic bag was hard work. Without a list, not only could I not remember what I wanted, most likely I'd get out the door and not be able to remember why I was outside. I felt like my brain had been replaced by a ball of fog, but I couldn't think clearly enough to know how dense I was. After I started doing the walk to the supermarket, I realized that people were no longer staring at me. Maybe it was the shopping bags. I lost touch with everything moving around me, as if I were invisible. That was somewhat comforting. Occasionally I would get an e-mail from someone I knew, asking me if I were okay. They'd seen me on the street, thought they recognized me, but weren't sure.

I talked with her mother about Ari coming over after school for a few hours each day. It meant she'd have to pick her up from school, drive her to my place, then come by later to take her home. Thankfully, she agreed. She ran the idea past Ari.

"I don't think I can cook for him, but I guess I could make him a sandwich or something." When her Mom told me that, I laughed, then broke down and cried. Breaking bread with those you love. A brief emotional event with long-lasting symbolic importance.

I didn't feel capable of managing any emergencies that might arise, so overnights were out for the time being. I was tickled to be able to spend time with her, but on more than one occasion, once she was there, I had no idea how she had arrived. Sometimes I'd ask her why she was there, sometimes I'd ask her what day of the week it was. If I'd been thinking more clearly, I would have recognized how frightening this all was for her, and I might have asked her Mom to stop bringing her over. When you are adrift in the sea, you will grab onto anything that resembles safety, regardless of whom it hurts. There were days when she went out to her Mom's car to go home where I thought that I was seeing her for the last time ever. I wasn't even capable of sadness, just standing there outside my front door watching her and thinking, *Where's she going? I guess I won't see her anymore. I wonder why.* I would wave goodbye, then go inside and think, *Now what do I do?*

When she was gone, it was as if I stopped existing until she returned the next day. As uncomfortable as I'm sure it was for her, seeing her once-vibrant Dad reduced to a dumb old skinny guy, it was absolutely the only time of the day I awaited with any emotion.

Weekends were interminable. I had no interest in anything; even if I had, the energy bin was empty. Over the years, I have lived through periods when I was very social, and other times when I lived a fairly solitary life. Now I was neither. I didn't feel as if I had a place on earth. A stranger in a strange land.

Reading has always been one of my passions. Fiction, magazines, the occasional historical piece. Suffering through yet another badly-written medical journal article. Now I could barely stand to look at pictures in Rolling Stone. Nothing sank in, most things just irritated my brain. My rate of retention hovered between zero and nothing. Television and radio weren't any better. I'd put a CD on the stereo, sit out back watching the sunset, and not hear a note of music.

After three or four weeks at home, some of me was moving in the right direction. I was walking more, at least a mile twice a day. I was eating, not because of hunger, just because it was something to do to kill time. A glass of wine or a beer made my heart pound for hours, a little faster but a lot harder. I did a little swimming in the pool, which helped my upper body loosen up. Again to kill time, I started doing little chores around the property. I was working at regaining my physical health, but mostly it was a matter of waiting for things to get better. Time healing the wounds and all that.

Mentally I wasn't making much progress. If someone asked me a question, or if I tried to remember something, I could feel information moving slowly from deep inside my brain. Like a worm taking its own sweet time winding its way through Swiss cheese, the factoid made its way out to my cerebral cortex. On a good day it took fifteen minutes to come up with an answer; sometimes the information I'd wanted at noon arrived in the middle of the night, rousing me from a fitful sleep, or even a day or two later.

When times are hard, you find out who has your back and who doesn't. I was lucky to have friends, mostly from work, come over and visit from time to time. Some of them drove me places, a few came over and cooked for me or brought me lunch. Though I was a lousy host, it was nice to have company. When they told me what was going on at the hospital, I felt hopeful that eventually I'd be heading back to work. For the first time in my adult life, after twenty-five years of caring for patients and helping to save lives, I knew how it felt to be contributing nothing to society.

123. TUSSLES WITH HYPNOS

Even though I had bounced back and forth between twelve-hour day and night shifts for fifteen years, I never had any trouble getting to sleep or staying there. Some of my colleagues over the years had significant insomnia when they returned to day shifts or normal life after a few consecutive night shifts. Not me. When I worked nights, the trick to getting back on a day schedule on my days off was to get to sleep early in the evening. If I stayed up past 10 P.M., I was wide awake until 2:00 or 3:00 in the morning. Getting up at the crack of dawn with my daughter after three hours of sleep left me in a fog the rest of the day.

When I arrived home from the hospital after surgery, I was weak and lazy, but not sleepy. It was nearly impossible to pursue any activity for more than ten minutes without having to sit or lie down. Having been used to manual labor around the house and property on a daily basis, as well as working out in the gym several times per week, this new level of inactivity took away the driving force behind my successful sleeping habits. Consequently, I never felt sleepy, just foggy. I attributed that brain haze to the anesthesia. When you are truly dull-witted, you are too dull-witted to know how dull-witted you are.

Now sleep was problematic. No matter what time I went to bed, it would take an hour or more to fall asleep. Invariably I would awaken at 2 A.M. feeling neither clear-headed nor well-rested. For the first few nights I just lay there, usually until 5 A.M. or so, whereupon I would fall back to sleep for an hour until the construction crew showed up across the street. I tried reading, which in the past could put me out in minutes, but, no matter how light the subject matter, I just couldn't concentrate; that pissed me off enough that I gave up reading for almost a year.

After a few days of that, when I'd awaken in the middle of the night, I'd get up, stagger to the sofa, and watch TV. Then I could fall asleep for a few hours on the couch and wake up somewhat refreshed. I realized I was sliding down the slope to mental numbness and stupidity, but that felt better than staying awake all night.

Although by about the second day home I was no longer in need of Percocets for pain relief, I tended to take one-half tablet at bedtime. It was probably the reason I could get four hours of sleep at a time. After a few days, I learned to take one-half at 2 A.M., and I could sleep until the construction guys across the street woke me up. Pretty soon I was able to cut out the bedtime dose. For the next couple of weeks I did that, then realized that Percocet really wasn't designed to help me sleep and I cut it out altogether. To this day, I still awaken almost every night at 2:00 A.M.. Now I can concentrate enough to read and be back asleep in a half-hour.

Whether because of my foggy brain or because I truly worried about it, I went to bed every night for the next year or so assuming I would die in my sleep. In my barely functional but fully delusional mind, it made sense. After all, the twin brother of Hypnos, the Greek god of sleep, is Thanatos, the god of death. Normally a naked sleeper, I took to wearing boxers to bed, especially the nights my daughter stayed over. I had recurring nightmares that she would be the one to find me dead in bed. She and I were standing next to my bed, looking down at my corpse. I didn't want her to have to discover me dead and naked.

124. REALITY CHECK

Seeing myself in the mirror once I arrived home, I was surprised they didn't want me to follow up in the office the next day. Scrawny and white-haired, all I needed was a pole up my ass to do time as a scarecrow that could have frightened, or at least creeped out, peregrine falcons. Fortunately, I had a whole week to make myself look presentable in society, not just on the street but in a waiting room, face to face with real humans.

One week later, the mirror mirror on the wall concluded that I was still too wraithlike to pass for a living human. Prior to my surgery, I routinely sprinted up four flights of steps to deliver a baby, no problems breathing when I got there. Today my friend Bill and I gladly took the elevator up to the third floor of Frank's office building. I was in such bad shape I actually felt worse leaving the elevator than entering it, as if I'd just hand-cranked it up to the third floor.

I had only been in this office once, for the stress echo that had started me down the path. That time the waiting room had been almost empty, and I looked like a normal healthy middle-aged guy coming in to get his blood pressure checked. This time, when I walked in, there were a dozen or so people sitting in chairs, and a couple standing at the reception window signing in. I must have smelled like death because, as I entered, every head came up to look at me. Some stared, some looked down at their laps, not wanting to incur the attention of the Grim Reaper.

I walked over to get in line, but after all of a half-minute, light-headed and weak, I had to sit down and rest. I must have looked as bad as I felt, because I caught several looks of alarm, as if they were worried that I was going to die right then and there. A natural-born people pleaser, normally I would have given them a valorous smile and a thumbs-up. Now I felt too crappy to bother.

When I finally got checked in, I collapsed back in a chair next to Bill. Despite having worked in the medical profession for almost thirty years, I had very little experience in private medical practice offices. Most of my time was spent in E.R.s. Prior to that, I worked in hospital-based settings, with a few years of government clinics thrown in. My only long-term office experiences were in my Dad's pediatric office and at the veterinarian's clinic. In both these places, the caregivers were usually eyeballing each other and comparing notes, while the patients were sniffing each other's butts or crying because they pooped their diapers. Even with the crying kids, there's a general feeling of "glad to be here." There was a lot of noise and activity. In a cardiology office, not much happens. Muffled conversations between patient and spouse or patient and daughter, interrupted by the occasional discussion between the receptionist and the invariably deaf patient about the insurance status. Nobody seems happy to be there.

The routine in medical offices and clinics has always been for the nurse to call out a patient's name at the doorway leading from the waiting room to the exam rooms in the back. You stand up and follow them back, where they get your vital signs, take a brief history, and check your med list. Nowadays, some places have medical assistants that fulfill that duty.

When Frank's nurse Maryann called me, she said, "Doctor Price." That got everyone staring at me again. I could feel the whispers.

"That old scrawny guy's a doctor?"

I appreciated Maryann's gesture. Made me feel that someday I would feel strong enough to return to practice. On the other hand, I have never been one to favor the spotlight. I like to keep a low profile, stay out of trouble as much as I can (Ironic, eh?), so it was a bit uncomfortable. I stood up, got lightheaded, and promptly sat down so I wouldn't fall down. That jolted my sternotomy enough to make me cough, which made the incision hurt even more. I thought, *Jesus H. Christ, even the simplest activity has become a giant hurdle.* Bill looked at me and asked if I was okay. I nodded and said, "I think so." I took a few deep breaths and stood up again. I remembered to get moving right away, before my entire blood supply surrendered to gravity and ended up south of my knees. After a few stagger steps, I was on my way.

One thing about cardiology offices. There aren't any mirrors on the wall because nobody wants to see if they look as bad as they feel. You want mirrors on the walls, head for a plastic surgery office suite. When you walk into a cardiology office, no matter how bad you look, there's always some other patient who looks worse. So, despite the stares in the waiting room, which were basically because I looked like an escapee from a concentration camp, I felt like I blended in for the first time since my discharge. Old guys were getting loaded into wheelchairs, other guys were sitting on exam tables waiting for their doctor to come in, some missing a leg, some with obvious permanent impairments from a stroke. That I could walk in under my own steam made me feel comparatively good.

Working in an E.R. for so long, seeing so much death and disability, you cope with it by thinking that it can't happen to you. If you think, *There, but for the grace of God, go I* every time you see something tragic, you won't be able to get through a shift. So you distance yourself from the patient population. Not intentional, just a survival mechanism. I saw illness and death every day at work, and dealt with it efficiently and effectively. But when it came to illness and death in family and friends, I was as uncomfortable with it as anyone in the general population, sometimes more so. And it wasn't just me. If a co-worker should come in and tell the rest of the staff about some horrible illness that had befallen a loved one, we'd all look at her in disbelief, thinking, *How could the father of one of our own contract a PATIENT illness? That's not supposed to happen.* It's as if there is a giant chain-link fence separating the rest of the world, particularly patients, from the staff.

Maryann checked me in and ran an EKG to make sure I hadn't suffered an MI since my discharge. She told me it was normal and I felt oddly relieved that something I hadn't even considered as a possibility had not come to pass. I thought, *How desperate is that?*

"Francis will be with you in a few minutes. You take care now." I thanked her as she left. I tried to sit back up, got dizzy and nauseated, and lay back down. A minute later I tried again, this time more slowly. A little transient lightheadedness, but no nausea, so I stayed up, sitting on the exam table, dangling my legs. In some part of my brain I understood that I was supposed to be thinking of something, but I couldn't remember what it was and I didn't care.

After a few minutes, Frank walked in. I was struck by the feeling that, compared to me, he was full of energy. I wondered what it would feel like to walk that fast, with no worries about tipping over.

We shook hands and exchanged greetings. He checked my blood pressure, then listened to my heart and lungs.

"What are you doing these days?" I gave him a brief rundown of my daily activities. That took all of about twenty words and thirty seconds.

Miraculously, all the hospital dictations were in my office chart, which had fattened up nicely since my first visit for the stress echo. He ran through them, found the discharge summary, and reviewed my discharge meds with me. I told him how orthostatic I was, and he decreased the dose of my beta blocker. I told him that one of my friends, a cardiologist, told me that most bypass patients come out of the hospital on an ACE inhibitor. Why not me?

"Your blood pressure was already low. If I have to pick one or the other, I'd rather have you on a beta blocker." It sounded good to me. I wondered how it would feel to stand up and not worry about passing out, the way it used to be. A slow moment of dread, thinking that maybe nothing will never be the way it used to be.

As I got up to leave, I posed my last question to Frank. "How long will this bypass last?"

I figured he would say, "Oh, about twenty years or so," then laugh and tell me not to worry. Instead, he said, "Oh, probably about five years or so, then you'll need something else done."

That took a few seconds to sink in. "Something else like what? Another bypass?"

"I can't say for sure, but most likely you will need something. I really don't know what we'll be able to do for you." I didn't yet realize what he'd already figured out, probably at the time of the cath: something was not quite right about my illness, not quite the normal CAD that gets put on hold for a couple of decades by a CABG.

I walked in feeling like warmed-over shit but hoping that things would gradually get better over the next few weeks. Now I was thinking, *Five years? All this for five more years? What kind of a deal is that?* Then it occurred to me, *Well, five years would get me to the beginning of Ari's senior year in high school. At least then she'll be able to drive.* I had a vision of her driving the red convertible to school on a sunny, crisp November day in Phoenix. Top down, of course.

I shoved my prescriptions into a pocket, settled up at the exit window, got scheduled for two weeks hence, and headed out into the still-hot late September sun. Thoroughly deflated, I thought, *Five years. I'd better get my ass up and get going. Time's a wastin'.*

125. NEEDLESS WORRY

I was scheduled to see my cardiac surgeon, Dr. Huston, in his office a couple of weeks after discharge from the hospital. From my experience in medical school, I knew that surgical follow-up consisted primarily of looking at the wound, making sure the organs underlying the wound were normal in terms of location and function, and discharging you from the surgeon's care. In other words, as long as everything looked good, not a big deal.

A few days before my visit, I noticed some drainage from my sternotomy wound. First clear, then a little cloudy and bloody. The term is serosanguineous. Sometimes it merely means that a collection of sterile fluid is gradually wending its way to drainage. It can either drain inward, drain outward, tunnel under the skin and exit somewhere else, or stay put where it is. Drainage externally is the preferred route. If it stays in one place, either it is reabsorbed by your body, it attracts calcium and hardens into a nodule, or it gets infected. You might ask how that is possible, given that the procedure was done under the most sterile conditions imaginable and the wound has been sealed since you left the O.R. Beats me. Apparently there is at least one bacterium in the fluid collection. It can sit there unnoticed, slowly replicating, from a few days to a decade or more, until there is a critical mass of bacteria. At this point it draws the attention of your immune system. To the rescue come all sorts of white blood cells and immunoglobulins to fight the good fight. Those white blood cells are the ones who turn a serous or serosanguineous fluid into a purulent exudate, also known as pus.

So even though this drainage was scanty and not particularly threatening, I knew it could turn into something really nasty. In addition, the skin around the site of the drainage was redder than the rest of the wound, and it was tender when I pushed on it. I had visions of a gloved hand reaching inside my chest and pulling out a half-rotted, pus-dripping sternum. Dr. Huston looked at it, suggested I put some warm compresses on it, and follow up with my primary care provider. Obviously, he didn't think it was anything to worry about. To his credit, he didn't knee-jerk and put me on two weeks of Keflex. I didn't have a PCP, so I asked him to swab it and send the sample for a culture, to see if any bacteria grew out. When it turned out that he didn't have any culturettes around the office, he wrote a prescription for me to go to the hospital lab and have it done there.

He listened to my heart and lungs and told me everything looked pretty much normal from his perspective. He reiterated "Eyes on the horizon." I was discharged from his care, with the proviso that I should follow up with my cardiologist. We shook hands and I got up to go. By this time, thanks to the lower dose of beta-blocker, I was able to stand up without keeling over. On my way out, I thought of one more thing.

"Do you know why I have this full-length scar on my leg?"

"Yes, I saw that. I think it was because your case was such an emergency."

"Oh, okay." I left thinking that I'd endured that back pain for a month, then still ended up as an emergency. Nonetheless, I was happy to be moving on. One more small step in the right direction.

A few days later I called the hospital lab to check on the culture of my chest wall drainage. The initial gram stain showed very few white blood cells and no bacteria. The culture was reported out as "No Growth". Best news I could hope for, and I didn't have to take antibiotics. As usual, the surgeon, the one with the experience, was right, and I, the worrier, was wrong. With that concern out of the way, I looked forward to gaining some weight, getting a little stronger and a lot clearer in the head, and getting back to work.

126. LITTLE STEPS FORWARD, BIG STEP BACK

I'd been a good boy. For the better part of two months I walked every day, gradually increasing the distance from once around the block to a little over two miles. It took me a good hour, but when I returned home, I wasn't ready to collapse. Increasing my speed or walking up a good incline still left me a little short of breath, but I didn't have to stop. I was finally to the point where I didn't expect to have that shoulder pain if I exerted myself or bent forward. In fact, I had forgotten what that angina felt like. My brain was doing its job in that respect: in other areas, not so good. My short-term memory was gradually improving, but was still far below what I thought I needed to be able to work a twelve-hour shift in the ER. Despite being far from one hundred percent in all these areas, I had confidence that things would continue to improve. Not quite bulletproof, but I felt like my body could stop a slow-moving nerf ball without falling over.

The month of November began with a notice in the mail about a pretrial hearing, scheduled for mid-December. A day or two later, I received a letter from my attorney's office, stating that they would "keep me posted". Soon after came another note, advising me that one of the staff would attend the hearing, so it was not necessary for me to show up. Six weeks hence held as much relevance as the next millennium. My horizon was hours, not days or weeks, so I stayed focused on sleeping, walking, and putting out the trash. Not what you'd consider big picture items, but at least they fit my limited skill set.

My wounds, both the sternotomy and my retro 80s right saphenous vein harvest site, were healing nicely, to the point where they no longer itched or drained. I was making a point of keeping my head up and stretching the top of my chest scar, which had contracted a bit. The one on my leg threatened to hatch a keloid, one of those big bulbous knots you see from time to time on a scar, but I was rubbing vitamin E on everything twice a day. With the improvement in my wounds, the Hawaiian shirts were back in the closet. Festive skeleton had been replaced by successful gastric bypass patient. I could walk around the nearby park unnoticed by the people with their kids and dogs. Comfortable anonymity.

I hadn't felt hungry since surgery. I still weighed in the low 150s, a good twenty pounds below my pre-op weight. Eating went pretty well in the late afternoons and evenings, but each day started with dread; anywhere from four to six hours of nausea, dry heaves, and the occasional technicolor yawn, starring last night's meal. It was pretty much daily morning sickness, only two or three times as long, and without the urgent hunger that usually follows for a pregnant woman. As you may remember, one of the teleological explanations for morning sickness is that pregnant women vomit first thing in the morning to empty their stomachs of bacteria and viruses that end up there during the night, especially TB. I didn't know what was brewing in my gut.

The weather in Phoenix had cooled nicely; it was still warm in the sun, but the heat didn't sap me the way it had in September. Nights out back were incredibly pleasant. I was just getting to the point that I felt well enough to have my daughter stay overnight. That is, I was just getting to the point where I thought I might die in my sleep, rather than knowing that I would.

I had a little scare on another front. A black spot had shown up on my left great toenail in July. Since the nail is transparent, anything under it in the nail bed will appear as a dark spot. The differential diagnosis, the list of most likely causes, includes trauma, like dropping a brick on your toe, and malignant melanoma. If it is due to trauma, the dark spot, usually dried blood trapped under the nail, will often move toward the tip of your toe or finger. If it doesn't move at all, and a dermatologist can't tell whether it's dried blood, there's an obligation to biopsy it. That requires removing all or part of the nail and digging the black lesion out of the nail bed. Once the nail is removed, sometimes the clump of dried blood will simply fall off and the diagnosis is obvious. Then, because there was no disruption of the nail bed, the nail will grow back normally.

I wasn't exactly on a hot streak, so "simple" was not an option. My dermatologist removed half the nail; there was no nice flat slab of dried blood that fluttered away in the wind, so it was on to the nail bed biopsy. It suddenly occurred to me that I'd gone through one life-threatening illness, and yet I might succumb to another. That didn't keep me awake that night, but the post-op throbbing after the lidocaine wore off sure did. A couple of days later the pathology report came back with no signs of malignancy; the presumptive diagnosis was trauma. I filed that away and moved on. In some small part of my brain, I was shocked at how little I felt about the whole thing.

I still had no interest in sex. Not that you needed to know. For the first time since the age of ten, I couldn't get it up, but even if I had, I was too weak to do anything about it. And even if I were able to do something about it, I hadn't come across any women who wanted to get it on with a gaunt old man with white hair.

Drinking even a glass of red wine gave me pounding palpitations a few hours later. They were a little faster than my usual heart rate, and there was no pain associated with them. It just felt like my heart wanted to do the Alien wiggle dance and jump out of my chest.

Most importantly, I had gone almost two months without a single episode of angina. I was able to walk without dyspnea. I could roll the trashcans out to the curb. I could barely lift a five-gallon water bottle high enough to place it on the dispenser, and then I did need to collapse on the sofa. Ute, the incredibly patient lady who ran our physicians group office and made up the work schedule each month, was putting me on for twelve shifts in the month of December. If there was ever a German woman, complete with accent, who could absolutely destroy our American presupposition about the stern Prussian frau, it was Ute. I was nervous about returning to work, where one fuckup on my part could result in a patient complication or death. I wouldn't be doing any of the critical care stuff, which meant I would not have to run up several flights of stairs to a code or a delivery, but I would be expected to handle a full load each shift, which meant twenty to thirty patients over twelve hours. I was worried about my energy level more than my heart. Most of all, I was worried about my squash.

Although I lived every day within a giant ball of fog, my mind was starting to clear, to the point that I could recognize on some level how poorly my brain was functioning. My short-term memory and recent recall were still shot. My cognitive skills, which had normally run like a sprint car, now slugged along like a tandem bike with flat tires going uphill against a headwind. The former King of Trivial Pursuit could barely read the cards, let alone come up with an answer. That information earthworm, the one delivering answers to my cerebral cortex, was still doing his slow crawl.

In our modern society, there is this notion that you must be happy every moment of every day, and if you aren't, you are depressed. If sad days intermingle with happy ones, you must be bipolar. Back when there were only tricyclics and a few other equally unpleasant antidepressants available, very few depressed people went looking for a cure for their depression. The meds took forever to work, and the side effects often made depression seem like a cakewalk. Truly bipolar patients, a.k.a. manic depressives, were prescribed ECT (electroconvulsive therapy, a.k.a. shock treatment) or lithium. You'd have to be way beyond crazy to go back to your shrink and politely ask for more of those. Now we have a slew of meds that are easy to take, make us feel better, and make a ton of money for the drug companies who manufacture and market them. No doubt it is just coincidental that the diagnosis of bipolar disorder has skyrocketed.

I had a ton of sensible friends in and out of the medical field who have ridden the normal roller coaster that is called "life". They understood that when shit happens to you, you are supposed to feel bad for a while, then eventually you get over it. That period of time varies from event to event and from individual to individual, but I think it's safe to say that in the case of devastating medical mishaps, that period of time is more than a week or two. Reactive depression is normal. I had a few acquaintances in the mental health field who, on at least one occasion, told me I was depressed and I should be on meds for same. All I could say was, "Huh?" When I think back on that time, I find it hilarious that they could confuse mental dullness with depression. One even said that I was displaying vegetative signs of depression. I remember thinking, *Have you seen me with my shirt off?* I wasn't depressed, just sagging.

Mid-morning one day in early November I was bringing in the ubiquitous blue recycle dumpster on wheels. Half the twenty yards from the curb is downhill, the rest is perfectly flat. I got the dumpster back into its resting place without a hitch. I turned and started over to a spigot to turn on an irrigation hose. Suddenly, for the first time in two months, that same warm welling-up feeling crept over my left scapula. It was a half-minute or so before I realized I was having pain. At first I thought it was just a cramp in my shoulder. I rotated my shoulder back and forth to no avail. Half in disbelief and half in a panic,

I thought to myself, *Ah, shit.* Other than during my tread echo, this was the first time I'd had angina that I truly knew what was going on. I kept walking, first up to the end of my driveway, then in a small circle. It never became unbearable, I didn't sweat, and my breathing was fine. After about five minutes, it went away.

About two hours later, I was washing and drying some dishes. I bent forward and the pain returned, identical to what had happened earlier. *All that fucking work for the past two months down the drain.* I took it easy the rest of the day. I had another bout of the pain during my morning walk the next day. Around 9 A.M. I called and left a voice message for Maryann, Frank's nurse. I knew this information would not be well-received.

A short time later, Maryann returned my call. She said, "Hold on for Francis."

"Hi, Frank. What's up?"

"Hi, Frank. I started having that same pain again yesterday."

There was a pause of about five seconds. I could visualize Frank mulling this over. Then he said, "I find that hard to believe." A vision of Maxwell Smart saying, "Would you believe...?" came and went. *Yup, here we go again.* Again, if our roles were reversed, I'd be doubting him too. In one study from the 1990s, less than two percent of LIMA grafts became blocked within ten days of surgery. Another study showed that, two years after surgery, about eighty percent of vein grafts were still open. The odds of one of mine closing, especially the big one, the one that had taken away all my pain, were exceedingly low.

"Well, it's definitely the same pain. Same location, exertional, positional, no dyspnea, no sweats, no radiation." I waited while he thought. He didn't need any more details.

"Did you take a nitro for it?"

"Nah, it's only lasting five minutes. If I take a nitro, I'll be flat on my back for thirty."

"All right. I'll set you up for a nuclear treadmill tomorrow. Maryann will call you back in a while with the time and instructions." I could tell he didn't want to believe me, but he remembered the first treadmill. I felt like I had failed him and everyone else. Later, I called and talked with my daughter after school. That evening, getting ready for bed, I wasn't sure if I wanted to wake up the next morning. There was no way I was headed for good news.

127. NUCULARNESS

This time the treadmill was downstairs in the nuclear medicine suite. I discovered this after I climbed the stairs to the third floor main office, short of breath but feeling no pain. Because this was more of a follow-up treadmill than a first-timer, one of their nurse practitioners would supervise the procedure. As far as I knew, the NPs never came to the hospital. Once I checked in, however, I did remember coming over to code a guy who was post-op and collapsed during a nuke tread. He did not, shall we say, do well. That did nothing to allay my anxiety.

Because of the radioactive isotopes, which are delivered to order every morning, nuclear treadmill testing areas are often located ideally in the basement, away from prying eyes, or, alternatively, on the ground floor. If you expect to hear humming or buzzing or woo-wooing or some other creepy sci-fi sounds, you'd be disappointed. Maybe Muzak, which after a while can creep you out too. The lights don't glow a weird color and they don't flicker eerily every so often. There's no distinctive smell, specifically no odor of burning flesh. The whole place is safer than your average Safeway, but the "Nucular" sign on the door occasionally causes a commotion among the local halfwits.

Nuclear treadmills take far longer than either the standard or the stress echo. Depending on the number scheduled for that session, you can be there anywhere from two and one-half to four hours. Interspersed with frequent walks to the back and brief periods under the scanning camera and an even briefer stretch on the treadmill, are long spells in the waiting room. It is as much an exercise in boredom as it is a diagnostic study. You can't eat or take your meds until near the end. I brought a couple of mindless magazines and spent most of my waiting time thumbing through them looking at the pictures. Like I said, my brain wasn't what you would call functional.

This was my first time doing a nuke tread. I met the tech, a guy named Shad. He was terrific. Unlike a lot of the techs, who act like they'd rather be attending a dirty diaper symposium, he was friendly, intelligent, empathetic but objective. In other words, he did the job, made you feel good, and didn't take anything personally. Unflappable. By the end of the day, I wished he'd been the only staff member I'd dealt with.

After I checked in and waited a bit, he called me back and stuck a saline lock in a nice big vein in my hand. He went over the rules and the plan of action. I still wasn't absorbing much, forgetting almost everything immediately, including his name once, and I told him so. "Don't worry, just go where I tell you and I'll take care of the rest. We'll get you through this." My kind of guy. Keep it simple. I went out front and waited while he stuck IVs in the other two patients. Both were older guys who looked to be in congestive heart failure. I hoped there wouldn't be a code that morning. I wanted to get in and get out, and someone trying to die usually screwed up the schedule. It wasn't until the next day that I realized that if someone coded, I might be of some assistance in resuscitating him. I was thinking less and less from the perspective of a health care provider.

After a while, I went back, got the injection of the Cardiolite, waited some more, then lay in the scanner while the resting images were obtained. Then back to the waiting room again for a while. The worst thing for me about all the prelim steps and all the waiting was knowing that, after busting my ass on the treadmill, I was going to be rewarded with more angina. No matter what Frank thought, or hoped, to my way of thinking I was experiencing angina, which meant something recently went awry in my coronaries. Typically, when somebody has unstable angina, you go straight to a cath. It is not considered good form to have a guy drop dead on your treadmill. If he's going to drop dead, you would much rather it be in the cath lab or in the O.R., where, at least in theory, you can do something about it. Your health insurance company would prefer it happen at home, away from prying, intervening health care personnel. Case closed, no further intervention necessary. No high-tech equipment required. Just a shovel.

After Shad (Boy, I sure hope I got his name right.) had toiled to get everybody pretty much at the same stage in the process, I was called back to the treadmill room. The nurse practitioner took my baseline vitals. Shad loaded the harness onto me and put on all the stickies. My baseline EKG looked essentially normal, which meant I probably had not suffered a heart attack before, during, or since my bypass.

It's weird to know that you are participating in something that will certainly cause you pain and possibly permanent damage or death. While there is a measure of comfort in knowing that there are medical personnel on hand and you have a nice patent saline lock through which they can push lifesaving meds, it is even weirder to think that they are intent on causing you to have pain. When I went in for my first treadmill, I didn't know what I had. Now I did. It made me a little hesitant to push myself. Nevertheless, I got through stages I and II in okay shape. I felt weak and my breathing was strained.

A little into stage III and the feeling started crawling up my left shoulder blade. I said, "Here it comes." Shad had me describe it and wrote down my responses. The nurse practitioner was watching the EKG tracings on the monitor. I looked over. Nothing so far. I kept going. Suddenly the pain increased about tenfold. Although there was none of the tearing feeling I'd initially experienced in Portland, this was by far the worst pain I'd ever had. I felt like I was going to pass out, and I have no idea how I kept my legs moving. I thought, *Fuck me, I'm going to die.* I actually visualized some schmuck presenting my case at the monthly morbidity and mortality report. Then I realized that if I didn't die in the hospital, I wouldn't even be a hospital statistic. At this point my ST segments had dropped through the floor. Somebody stopped the treadmill, and the next thing I knew I was sitting on the table, wanting to lie down. Honest to God, the nurse practitioner turns to me, all panicky, looks at me, and yells, "Are you having pain?" I thought, *Oh shit, am I in a room with someone who has never witnessed a positive treadmill test?* Next thing I know, I am lying down, a nitro tablet under my tongue. After about five minutes the pain had deceased by about half and I thought, *Hey, I might get out of here alive!*

The rest of my time there was a blur. I don't remember the final scanning session, although I know it took place. By the time everything was done, I was scared shitless but pain-free. I think they talked to Frank, and in the end I was allowed to leave.

On my way home, I imagined a stand-up scenario:

"I've got good news and bad news. Which one do you want first?"

"Um..."

"Never mind, they're both the same."

I was going in for my second cath.

128. BYE-BYE, BYPASS

I didn't sleep well that night. Having my angina return when it did was unsettling. Most bypass grafts that fail do so either in the first week or years later. Once again I was way off the bell curve. I took comfort in the fact that despite my weird presentation initially and now this odd complication, I was still alive. Clearly my day to die had not yet arrived, but my experience during the nuke tread had scared the shit out of me. All night long I kept having short dreams about coding the post-op guy years before. I was the coder, doing CPR and giving orders for cardiac meds. When I looked down, the guy I was working on was me. The little movie had me playing two roles. Just like the Patty Duke show.

I talked with my daughter on the phone, told her I was going in for a day or so, and that I didn't expect anything more than an angioplasty and a stent. Of course, I'd thought that the last time and ended up with a couple of scars to remind me not to assume.

Lucky for me, I was scheduled first that day. By 7 A.M. I was checked in, had the blood work and EKG done, and was being wheeled in to the cath lab. There wasn't as much fanfare in the hallway this time, and I was grateful for that. I felt I had failed everyone, showing up here after only two months out, a parolee who screwed up and winds up back in the slammer. They say love makes the world go round. Maybe, but if love slinks back to the dugout, Catholic guilt is always on deck, ready to step up to the plate.

On the other hand, having just undergone this procedure a mere two months prior, and knowing there was pretty much no way I'd be going back to surgery this soon, I felt comfortable lying there. The crew was more or less the same as last time. Everything rolled along smoothly. I figured that one graft had clotted or narrowed and could be reopened with a balloon and a stent. Undoubtedly, Frank was hoping the same thing. I suspect he was getting a little tired of working on the right side of my groin.

Surprisingly, the dye injections were more uncomfortable than before. The injection of my right coronary artery, which supplies blood to the inferior portion of my heart, produced pain in my upper abdomen and a little nausea. Before he shot the LIMA, he warned me that I would feel discomfort. There was a burning in my shoulder and upper chest. When he was done, Frank went over the films with me while I was still on the table.

"You have three new areas of stenosis." *What?!* He pointed them out. Each one was just distal to where a graft had been sewn in to a coronary artery. The term was "post-anastomotic stenosis". At the time I wondered if that was a normal process a couple months after bypass grafts are placed. So few patients undergo a cath two months post-op, I doubted anyone knew for sure. None of them looked bad enough to me to be causing my recurrence of angina. The fact that my discomfort was in the same area and had the same characteristics as my pre-op angina made me think that the problem was again centered on my left main. That toilet seat was still stuck partially open. I asked Frank about that.

"Well, the LIMA that runs to your LAD is wide open. The fourth area of concern is the jump graft between the LAD and the diagonal to your intermediate. It's blocked."

"That same pain from just the intermediate? Any idea why he didn't run a separate graft from the aorta to that?"

"I don't know. I wasn't there. Doesn't matter now."

"Can you open that with a balloon?"

"No. To get to it, I'd have to go through that left main lesion. If that breaks off during the procedure, you'll infarct your intermediate, your LAD, or worse. There's no way to get to it via the LIMA either."

"So I need another bypass?" Once again, my expectations flushed down the toilet.

"No, we'll angioplasty those three and see how you feel."

"Okay. Now?"

"No, not now. I want to talk to one of my partners, show him the films, see if he can maybe laser that ruptured plaque out of the way. Then we don't have to worry about the jump graft. I'm also going to talk with Brady. Either way, we'll be doing something next week."

I went home to think about this latest development. I'd been working here at John C. Lincoln for over five years. I wasn't up on everything happening in the hospital, but given all the time I'd spent taking care of heart patients in the ER and in the units, if anyone was performing laser treatments on coronary lesions on a regular basis, I'd have heard something about it. I didn't know much about the state of laser treatment in Phoenix, but I knew if I were going to have it, I wanted somebody with a long track record in the procedure. As in somebody who had done a hundred or more, say at the Cleveland Clinic or Stanford or Mass General.

So far, other than my screaming nurse practitioner friend, everyone who had laid a hand on me was more than experienced in what they were doing. In addition, I doubted that it was commonplace anywhere to laser an unstable plaque in a left main. I wasn't going to rock the boat, but I wasn't real excited. And I didn't think angioplasties on a bunch of lesions was going to do anything for my angina if that intermediate artery remained poorly perfused. I started thinking that a second surgery was inevitable. All the misery and healing for the past two months down the drain.

I spent the rest of that day doing mundane stuff to keep my mind off the laser thing. The next morning, I got a call from Frank.

"We took a look at your films. Nobody thinks it would be safe to laser the big plaque." *Thank you, God.* "Surgery isn't much of an option at this point either. I'll balloon the other three and see how you feel. Are you okay with that?" *Yeah, buddy.* Anything that didn't involve the laser thing was AOK with me. Still...

"You think that'll help?"

"I don't want those stenoses to worsen. As far as helping with your pain, I hope so. If it doesn't, we'll talk about what else we can do."

"Okay. See you next week."

"First thing. Good-bye."

Angioplasty. Another new experience. Then again, it's what I'd expected the first time around. I did my best to avoid running down all the complications that could occur.

129. MORE BAD NEWS

Once again, now for the third time, Frank was messing with the right side of my groin. I took a weak stab at lightening the mood.

"You down there messing with my groin again. It's not about the cath anymore, is it?" I got a halfhearted "Hmmph" out of him. I had another one-liner ready, but decided not to push my luck. He was already sick of screwing around with my skinny calcified vessels. He couldn't get back at me in the E.R., at least not until I returned to work, but he was wielding a number of long thin needles, with real sharp points, and he was the one controlling the lidocaine.

Running in the various sheaths and catheters went well. They did the dye shoot. There were three areas of narrowing, each one just a few millimeters downstream from where a bypass graft had been sewn in. I'd been thinking about that the night before. It was highly unlikely that each one had developed a tiny clot at the same place. Likewise, the odds against cholesterol deposits setting up shop within two months in three different places were astronomical. For me it came down to two possibilities. The first was that this was nothing more than a typical post-op occurrence; manipulation of the coronary artery caused temporary narrowing, which would resolve in time. Arguing against that was data that did not show that sort of finding in patients undergoing repeat caths soon after bypass surgery. No doubt Frank had experience in that area, and he didn't think much of that theory when I brought it up.

The other possibility was that this whole cardiac event was the result of some subtle inflammatory process going on in my heart. There are a lot of smart people, both in cardiology and infectious diseases, who believe that infection, which causes inflammation, is an important cause of coronary artery disease and MI, especially in patients who don't have the usual risk factors. Infectious agents with the strongest links to coronary disease include chlamydia pneumoniae, cytomegalovirus, herpes simplex, Helicobacter pylori, and periodontitis (gum infections) Maybe I had something like that going on. Frank did check some labs. One of them, the CRP (C-reactive protein), a measure of inflammation in your body, was elevated.

The staff was mostly the same as for my previous two caths. I was starting to think of the cath lab as a second home. The procedure went smoothly. I imagined it would take far longer than a regular cath, but Frank was done in no time. When it comes to any medical or surgical procedure, nothing beats experience, confidence, and good hands. He located the stenoses, ballooned them up and placed a stent in each one. I didn't have angina during any of the angioplasties, not even when the balloon was fully inflated and the coronary artery was completely occluded for a short time. I figured that about clinched it; none of these lesions were responsible for the return of my angina. My angina. Now I was owning it.

After he finished up the last of the three, I asked Frank, "Have you figured out a way to get to that jump graft?"

"No. Even if I could, it's so tortuous I doubt it would stay open. See that?" He pointed to the screen. The jump graft, from my LAD to my intermediate, took a ninety degree turn near its origin. No doubt the vein graft had looked fine when it was first sewn in. Time and tension had caused a kink that prevented blood and dye from moving through.

"So I just go home and see how I do?" I was hoping he'd say yes. The first time you operate on any part of the human body, there are nice clean landmarks and tissue planes separate cleanly. Any subsequent foray into the same area is much more difficult. Scarring makes the landscape more difficult to navigate. Those nice clean tissue planes are gone, and bleeding is more of a problem. A CABG re-do, especially a repeat sternotomy, is far more difficult than the first time around. The last thing I wanted was to stay in the hospital, undergo a second CABG, and start the rehab process all over again. I just wanted to go home and do my best, get back to some sort of limited routine.

"You stay here overnight, then you go home and see how you do."

That was fair. I was wheeled over to the CVICU and settled into a room. The overnight stay was dictated by the fact that I still had the sheath in my femoral artery. For some reason, it is considered bad form to send a patient home with a catheter sticking out of his groin. If one or more of the lesions re-stenosed or became occluded by a blood clot, Frank could go right back in and drip in a clot-buster or reopen the artery with a balloon. Since you can't turn over with that sheath in place, and since I don't ever sleep on my back, it made for a long night.

Early in the morning I had a repeat EKG. Then my nurse pulled the sheath and put in some plug material. Putting the plug in hurts, a heavy pressure. There was a clamp on there for a while. When the day shift nurse took it off, everything looked good, and I got out of there. One of the nurses from the cath lab took pity on me and dropped me off at home. I wanted nothing more than to rest, get up the next morning and resume my restricted lifestyle. I was disappointed about that jump graft, the only one that mattered, but grateful to get out of the hospital alive once more.

130. RESTARTING AGAIN

The day after my discharge, after a theoretically curative procedure, or at least one that would take away my angina, I was feeling like I'd jumped from one limbo to another. Prior to the return of my pain, I was worried about going back to work. The plan was for me to start doing shifts in December. My head was still foggy, and I found it impossible to concentrate on any reading material for more than about fifteen minutes. I couldn't remember what I'd done five minutes earlier, and I spent much of my day looking for stuff I had misplaced. Given that the cause of my pain had not been corrected, Frank told me to cool my jets and not go back to work in December. I called Ute and gave her the bad news. The December schedule was already in circulation, and once again my partners were going to have to suck up my shifts. I felt like a complete loser, but there was a side of me that knew I would do a terrible job. I had a nightmare of patients disintegrating into grey slime while I was examining them.

As soon as I got home, I began walking and puttering around the house. Between my mile-long walk and putting out the trash, I had three or four episodes of that pain. It was the usual, and went away in about five to ten minutes. The first episode really surprised me, as I was walking on level ground at a moderate pace. After that, I guess I just accepted that my pain was, for the foreseeable future, back to stay. By the end of the first week home, I knew that the angioplasties may have prevented future complications, but they had done nothing to alleviate my angina. On the other hand, Frank's procedure kept me out of the O.R. for a while. For that I was grateful.

Frank told me to start a bunch of vitamins. It was becoming clear that I had some inflammatory process going on in my vessels. We talked about the possibility of starting corticosteroids, namely Prednisone, but he wasn't convinced that it would help, and the downside of high-dose steroids would make my life that much more difficult.

I also started Plavix. At first I bled excessively from every nick. A styptic pencil was useless for shaving cuts. It would be over a year before that calmed down a little. In the meantime, I was going through cotton balls by the family-sized bags.

131. HAPPY HOLIDAYS!

By December 1, I was glad I wasn't going back to work. Part of it was fear, part was my lack of energy, and part was the recurrent back pain. I did my best to limit my efforts, sticking to walking and light chores around the house. Nevertheless, I was having three or four anginal attacks every day. I read everything I could find on the power of positive thinking, and promised Ute I would work a dozen shifts in January. She was a little hesitant to rely on me, but a lot of the other docs wanted time off. If I didn't work, either someone was going to get stiffed on their vacation requests or the group would have to hire temps. I owed everyone big time for covering for me for four months. I figured somehow I'd get through a month of shifts. If it didn't kill me, it might make me stronger, right?

December sailed by. I slept better, my brain felt a little stronger. My short-term memory and recent recall were still in the tank, but I could string together sentences better and could follow the plots of mindless page-turners and TV movies. My co-workers continued to help out whenever I needed something. As a big believer in self-reliance, I am not much for asking for help. At this point in my life, I had no choice but to rely on others for virtually everything.

Somewhere in there, I saw a neuropsychologist for an evaluation of my memory. Something still wasn't right. He tested me. Simple written and oral exams, which normally I would have flown through with flying colors, slowed me down to a mental crawl. Apparently what I felt didn't translate to the results. He advised me that my long-term and short-term memory were adequate. He didn't have an explanation for my symptoms. He did say that my memory was probably better than average before my surgery, so "normal" for me might be different than normal for the general population. Some mention was made of pumphead and PTSD, and, of course, ADD. I was concerned that if I did go back to work, I would overlook an important detail or forget a critical piece of information in the history and physical. Worse yet, I'd forget what to do during a code and someone would be irreparably harmed or would die. I decided to follow that silly aphorism which is probably the best life advice you can give:

Hope for the best, prepare for the worst.

I had a big scare on my legal issue as well. In early November I received a notice of a preliminary hearing scheduled for mid-December. My attorney told me that he or one of his associates would attend; it was pointless for me to go. Apparently he completely forgot about it, because nobody showed up. During the holidays, while I was spending time with my daughter, I received a letter stating that, because my legal team and I were no-shows at the hearing, an arrest warrant had been issued for me. Technically, I was now a fugitive from the law. When I called my attorney, he said he'd take care of it. I didn't know what that meant; all I knew was that there was a chance that some officer of the law might show up on Christmas Day and haul me away in handcuffs. Karma was teaching me a lesson. All I could do was my best and keep my fingers crossed. I kept thinking that if I'd gone with my instincts and pleaded no contest for my fuckup, I wouldn't have to worry about others fucking up on my behalf. Just before he hung up, my attorney assured me that my case was solid. Right.

About a week later, I received a notice that my pretrial hearing had been rescheduled for mid-January. Again came a letter from my attorney's office promising to "keep me posted". Two days later I had to post bail so that I wouldn't be arrested. The hits just kept on coming.

No matter what happened in January when I returned to work, I wanted to make sure our Christmas was as normal as possible. My daughter was back to staying with me overnight again. That felt good, something of a return to our normal lives. Somehow I wrestled a Christmas tree from the tree lot into my truck and then home. Setting it up took most of a day rather than the usual twenty minutes. Pure stubbornness egged me on. The exertion, when added to frustration with my weakness, caused me a couple of bad anginal attacks, but by the time I fell asleep, it was more or less upright in the stand. I tied a rope from its top to an old eye screw in the ceiling to make sure it didn't fall over while I slept. Had I awakened to find it lying on its side on the floor and had to start all over again, I doubt I'd have even tried.

An invitation to a holiday party arrived in the mail. The couple throwing the bash didn't live far from me, so I decided to take a cab over and back. It was nice to see so many people from the hospital. Everyone inquired as to how I was doing. While I don't usually like much attention in a crowd, it felt self-indulgently good to be worried over.

The best line of the evening came from one of the TCV surgeons, a guy who always did the right job in a low-key manner. No fanfare, just wry Southern humor. He commented that he'd seen my cath films and described my situation as a "ticking time bomb". I had heard that some in the hospital doubted that I was as sick as I claimed, so that felt good to hear. I was telling him and another guy how amazed I was by all the help I'd been receiving from my friends from work.

Without cracking a smile, he said, "You don't have as many friends as you think you have." *O-kay*. Just the opposite of all those social media e-mails.

"Frank, you have more Zuckerface friends than you think!"

After I stopped laughing, I thought to myself, *Not as many friends as I think? Probably not, but the ones I have are better than I could hope for.*

I'd been dressing up on Christmas Eve since Ari was about three. At first it was just to deliver a special present to her at her Mom's house. After a year or two, I figured, *If I'm all dressed up, I might as well make several stops, rather than just one.* Word got around, and soon I was making between four and six house calls every Christmas Eve. The biggest reception ever was a few years earlier at the home of one of my co-workers. Expecting a family of three, I walked into a house of twenty people, about half of them little kids. There was a roaring fire and the temperature inside must have been close to eighty, which made me feel like passing out. I've had a lifelong case of stage fright, but, maybe because of the disguise, I nailed the entrance, performance and exit in front of a packed house. It made me feel good, and I like to think that at least some of those kids will never forget that live visit from Santa on Christmas Eve. Some of the toddlers, who screamed their heads off, probably still have nightmares about the fat guy in the red suit.

Now I felt weak as a kitten and my driving skills were virtually nonexistent, but I had the urge to do something for others, especially those who had helped me so much in the previous four months. I contacted some of my regulars and ended up with four stops. Every part of the evening took three times as long as normal. When I finally finished putting on my costume, my bedroom mirror framed a droopy red stick; the garb and I sagged like a candle after a week outside in the Phoenix summer sun.

"Mommy, Santa looks like warmed-over dog poop."

It was slow going, driving in the right lane, well below the speed limit. At one point I was passed by a Mormon missionary on his bicycle. During my first stop I had to lean against my car--the red convertible, of course--and wait out an attack of angina. As far as I know, nobody noticed me in the dark, sucking gas, hoping for the pain to pass. Luckily for Santa, everyone wanted him to sit down and rest from his long, weary travels (out of the car, up the walk, and into the living room), during which time I was able to catch my breath and regain my strength. I came out of each house thankful that I hadn't dropped dead in front of Little Bobby. I got through the night and crashed on my bed, still in my Santa suit, for eight hours of uninterrupted shuteye. That was the best night of sleep since my surgery. Don't tell the yard apes, but it was a good thing I didn't really have to fly all over the world that night.

As per our custom for years, Ari and I spent Christmas Day together. It wasn't the usual joyous occasion of the past, but we had a nice time for a couple of days. Having survived everything thus far, I felt I was probably going to make it to the New Year. I am not much for religion, but a couple days later, when she left to spend time with her Mom, I said a prayer of thanks that we'd shared that time at the holidays. At least while she was with me, I had hope that going back to work in January would be a good thing, not a bad one. With a child in your life, there is always hope.

132. POP GOES THE BUBBLE

If you are at a cocktail party and your dentist host starts doling out stock tips along with the canapes, urging you to buy, smart investors make an urgent call to their brokers. It's time to sell everything. I'm the one who puts in a buy order.

For most of the country, the bubble burst and the Great Recession began in December, 2007. Arizona historically has led the nation into and out of recessions. Our housing industry ran like a record-setting pyramid scheme, which it was, from 2002 through most of 2005. Investors bought up houses by the dozens--mostly new construction out in the remotest suburbs, but anything with a front door was a hot item--and "flipped" them at a considerable profit to the next wave of buyers, who then did the same thing. By mid-2005, if you wanted to buy a house, your agent would log on to the MLS at 12:01 A.M., find a new listing, call you to confirm, then call the seller and offer anywhere from $10,000 to $25,000 more than the asking price. By 8:00 A.M., virtually every new listing had been sold. First-time buyers who owned poorly constructed stuccos out in the boonies were doubling their money in less than a year. Like every bubble before and every bubble to come, the dumbest buyers, the ones at the bottom of the pyramid, are the ones holding the deed when the engine grinds to a halt. By the fourth quarter of 2005, prices were ridiculously high.

In March of 2006, a film called *The Secret* was released. By then, we in Phoenix knew that there was at least a temporary setback in the rolling thunder that was the local economy. Other than a few formerly fast-growing locales (California, Florida and Las Vegas, which were seeing the coming storm), the rest of the country was blissfully unaware that the bubble was already bursting in the construction sector and would soon spread to the rest of the economy. *The Secret* came along at just the right time, to delude viewers and, in November of that year, readers, into believing that to get what you wanted, especially more money, you just had to want it really badly. Right up until November of 2007, *The Secret* fueled the fire of refinancing and buying houses you couldn't afford. It was perfectly okay for homeowners to suck the "equity" out of their homes. If you wanted a big screen TV, go ahead, refi and get it. Same for motorcycles, boats, boob jobs. After all, if you keep wanting stuff, including first and second mortgage payments, you're gonna get 'em. Incidentally, the film and book versions of *The Secret* grossed over $300 million between 2006 and the end of 2009. So it did work, at least for somebody.

It wasn't an entirely new idea. There was a book written way back in 1910 called *The Science of Getting Rich*. Rumor has it that the author of *The Secret* read it before she started writing her bestseller. I went to a Tony Robbins symposium in the early 2000s where a guy who billed himself as "The World's Greatest Salesman" gave a speech on how to get what you want. A dapper little guy in a shiny suit, he claimed that to get what you wanted most in the world, all you had to do was write it down on a piece of paper, put the paper in your pocket and look at it every day. That way your mind will focus on what it is you want. The more often you look at the paper and concentrate, the faster you'll get what you want. The underlying principle behind all of these methods for getting what you want was "The Law of Attraction." In *The Science of Getting Rich*, it is called "The Certain Way of Thinking". Apparently the universe is just waiting for you to decide what it is you want and how badly you want it. All you have to do is think really hard, and presumably work a little, attract to you everything you will need to get what you want, and you'll get it. To get what she wanted, Rhonda Byrne wrote the book version of *The Secret* and sold almost twenty million copies. That's a lot of thinking and attracting.

After *The Science of Getting Rich* came out in 1910, the U.S. experienced eight major recessions, including the Great Depression, over the next thirty years. After *The Secret* arrived on the scene, the U.S. experienced the most severe recession since the Great Depression. Coincidence?

During the '90s and the first five years of the new millennium, I fancied myself a stock investor. In fact, during the '90s, I considered myself a stock savant. I read *Barron's* cover to cover, got up early to catch Mark Haines on Squawk Box, listened to Cramer, subscribed to *Motley Fool* (mainly because my daughter thought their silly jester hats were funny), subscribed to a couple of stock newsletters, read the Peter Lynch books, did all the things savvy investors recommend. All these sources were spot-on in their recommendations. It was virtually impossible to lose money in the market during the '90s, so I did well. I did have the troublesome habit of missing the sell signs and sticking with a stock just a tad too long, which usually cost me a small chunk of profits.

When the dot-com bubble burst in 2000, I felt safe because I'd looked on the whole dot-com thing as a scam. What I didn't recognize was how much business the big tech companies were getting from the dot-coms. A small detail, but that cost me and many of my not-too-smart brethren a penny or two. Oddly enough, it also kicked all the big stock market gurus in the ass as well. The geniuses seemed to lose their touch in picking winners during the ensuing bear market. Go figure.

After that burn job, I took a couple years off. From 2003 through 2005 I invested more cautiously and did okay. That real estate market sure looked good. An acquaintance of mine, a real estate agent, bragged about how well the industry was doing, especially in the areas of flipping houses and investing in rental property. In December, 2005, in the midst of my cardiac woes, I got it into my head that buying a rental home would be a great idea. Clearly, my head was the worst place in the world to formulate plans of any kind, especially the kind with long-term implications, but once I believe something, all the evidence to the contrary becomes background noise.

After meeting this realtor, my daughter told me she didn't trust her. *Silly child*, I thought. I'd been reassured by a realtor that buying real estate, through her of course, was a can't-lose investment. Just like having an insurance salesman advise you to buy more life insurance.

How could anything go wrong?

Renting would become a success in the coming years, but only in areas that weren't relying on the housing pyramid. I bought a place right smack in the center of the construction boom, miles from anything else. Once the construction ceased, so did the rental market fueled by construction workers. I owned an overpriced rental in a ghost town.

The housing bubble in Phoenix officially ended in December, 2005, days after I purchased my rental. The official story? The smart investors saw that prices had peaked and there would be no more wiggle room to make a profit in the flipping business. The real story? Word got around that I'd entered the real estate investment market; once they heard that, the savvy investors were off to the next hot market, leaving me and my slow-footed peers without a chair when the music stopped.

133. OUT WITH THE OLD, IN WITH THE NEW

Obviously I made it to the New Year.

It was 2006. 2004 had been a terrific year, and the first two-thirds of 2005 as well. The last four months of 2005 felt like I was no longer me. Nothing dramatically changed over New Year's; I was still having angina three or four times every day. It was almost always predictable. Emotional stress was the most reliable trigger. My biggest worry was what would happen to my daughter if I dropped dead. Thinking about that would get my heart racing and I'd get a little sweaty and then I'd feel that pain come up over my shoulder. In terms of exertional angina, the stents seemed to help somewhat, as it took more physical effort to bring on the pain than before they were placed. Nonetheless, I still felt weak and short of breath with the angina.

The folks at work had scrambled and covered my shifts in September and again in December. I felt like I'd let them down, and even though I knew I was in suboptimal shape to work twelve-hour shifts, there was no way I was going to ask them to cover for me in January. I figured this was pretty much where I'd be for the foreseeable future, so I might as well give it a go. My brain was still foggy, and concentration was next to impossible. Ute kept me off the critical care service as much as possible so I wouldn't have to go running to codes or deliver babies upstairs. Toward the end of the month I had a couple of shifts on CC, but I figured by then I'd either be dead or better.

My first shift everyone welcomed me back, then kept a fearful eye on me at all times. I got a lot of "Are you okay?" questions, all of which I responded to with an affirmative lie. When I went to see a patient, instead of listening and relying on my memory when it came time to dictate, I wrote down every word. Each history and physical took much longer than normal, but all that writing distracted me from dwelling on how crappy I felt. It was painful to make a decision other than the basic workup for the patient's chief complaint. Figuring out disposition--discharge or admission--was about as easy as climbing Mt. Everest barefoot and naked. My eye for lining up wound edges was faulty, and I didn't want to start over after the second or third layer, so I stayed away from attempting what would normally be my favorite procedure, complex facial laceration repairs.

I started to notice some weird flashes at the periphery of my vision, especially when moving. Walking was a challenge; in a doorway or narrow hallway, I had to put out my hands because I felt like I was going to hit the sides. While driving, I kept mistaking these side flashes for oncoming cars, so the four-mile trip from the hospital to my house took twice the usual ten minutes. I tried it for a couple of shifts, then gave up driving and took the bus. Walking to the bus stop had its problems as well. After twelve hours of work, walking in the cold (cold for Phoenix, anyway) at night invariably triggered one good anginal attack. A couple of times, when I had to rush to catch the bus, the driver looked at me with alarm. Evidently their ideal public transit system customer was not a skinny guy with white hair, pale, sweaty and gasping for breath.

In the middle of the month my attorney or one of his designates showed up for the pretrial hearing. At least I assume it went that way, because I didn't receive another arrest warrant in the mail. One morning I received a call telling me that my trial was scheduled for mid-February. Other than a dull dread, something that might happen one month hence left me with no feeling whatsoever. I was beginning to accept emotional numbness as my new norm.

Remarkably, I got through the month without any overt screw-ups. Nobody bitched about how slowly I worked, at least not that I heard about. Towards the end of my penultimate shift at the end of the third week of January, I had to go up to the second floor to see a patient in the CVICU. I was able to take care of the problem, but I bumped into the charge nurse. Apparently I didn't look too great--I'd had my usual anginal episodes and it was time to go home and collapse on the sofa until I could make it to bed. She looked me up and down.

"How are you doing?"

"Not great. I don't have the stamina for twelve-hour shifts yet."

"You look tired. Are you having pain?"

"Not right now, but yeah, a few times each shift. Some of it is worry, some of it just simple exertion."

Talking with her made me realize that I would never get through another month of shifts if something didn't change dramatically. I felt like hot shit in a champagne glass. Minus the hot. Minus the champagne glass. The next day, on my last shift of the month, I got a call in the E.R. from Frank.

"How are you doing?"

"Not as well as I expected."

"Yeah. Elsie stopped me this morning, said you looked pale and sweaty upstairs yesterday. She considered putting you into a bed in the unit. Still having that pain?"

"Yeah." Admitting that made me feel like a failure. Again. Somehow I thought I could overcome my anatomy, heroically control my coronary blood flow, labor on through discomfort and fatigue. That line of thinking comes from working in an E.R. for years, helping to snatch victims from the jaws of death despite being physically exhausted and mentally depleted. Some look at that as arrogance. I think of it as confidence borne of experience. In this case, however, it was nothing more than blind, misplaced optimism.

"I think it may be time to consider a re-do on that bypass." While I didn't look forward to starting anew, I was so sick of being sick that it didn't sound nearly as dreadful as it would have a month prior, when I was home and could limit my exertion. I realized it was either fix the problem or remain incapacitated, waiting for the big one for the rest of my life. "You're on the cath lab schedule tomorrow morning, to follow the first case."

He'd taken the decision out of my hands. What a relief. All I could say was, "Okay."

"All right. See you then." I knew he wasn't looking forward to this any more than I was. Neither one of us is a member of the touchy-feely school of medicine. If he'd been standing in front of me, though, I would have hugged him in gratitude.

"Frank?"

"Yeah?"

"Thanks."

"You're welcome. Bye."

134. ONCE MORE, WITH FEELING

I went in and talked to Ute after Frank hung up. I was going to screw up her schedule for the month of February, maybe longer. This would make at least the third time in five months that she would have to re-do the entire shift schedule with almost no notice. When she saw me coming, she knew something was up. It would have felt better if she'd screamed at me or thrown something. She just dove in and went to work after wishing me well.

Prior to my surgery, I had been pretty good about seeing the patient, writing down my orders, too many orders, and getting out of the nurse's way. In almost every ER, there is at least one doctor, physician's assistant or nurse practitioner who monopolizes nurses' time. They have nurses running around doing tons of useless shit. Usually these are the ones who shout out a lot of verbal orders, rather than writing them down and handing them to the unit secretary. I guess you could be charitable and say it's because they are disorganized. I tend to think it's more an attention-seeking behavior. It is a real pain in the ass to work alongside them; the stuff you need done, just basic stuff, gets shoved to the back burner by the squeaky wheel. The squeaky wheel also tends to think of him/herself as "the friend to the nurses". I knew if I kept working the way I felt, I would head in that direction, not because I wanted the attention, but because I kept forgetting to write stuff down and I didn't have the energy to go find the chart and write what I'd suddenly remembered. Of course, the stuff I forgot to write down was the important stuff, the stuff that made a difference in the quality of care of the patient.

It was getting to the point where the trip to the cath lab was becoming part of my activities of daily living. I had become a familiar face in the waiting area, and not in a good way. I checked in, went upstairs, got into my gown and had my blood drawn and saline lock inserted. I believe Frank knew, and I certainly knew, what the cath would show. Pretty much what the dye shots had shown after the angioplasty. It was virtually certain that I was headed for a second CABG surgery. I wasn't looking forward to the rehab process all over again, although in February the weather in Phoenix is absolutely delightful and perfect for walking outdoors. Nonetheless, I was excited this time, as I believed I was headed toward a more permanent resolution of my angina. It was hard to imagine, but somehow I hoped that in a month or two I would awaken one day with my usual energy and gratitude for life. I felt like I had been treading water in a cesspool for the past five months. I was looking forward to getting on with my life.

He started the conversation. "Good morning, Frank." Once again, the right side of my groin. No jokes this time. Everyone was sick of this routine.

"Hi, Frank, how are you?"

"Good. You ready?" *Ready?* It sounded like one of those Outer Limits episodes where the human is about to blast off to live on a world full of snot-covered cannibals.

"Yeah, I am."

Everything went smoothly. In some ways, this was the best of the four caths, because, unlike the first one, I knew I was going to end up in surgery, and unlike the second and third, there was a good chance that what was planned was really going to help. There were no surprises. The stented vessels were all patent, the popsicle stick was still evident in my left main, and the jump graft was still closed. Probably one of the few times in cath history where there was a glaring defect that couldn't be remedied on the spot and yet everyone in the room, standing and lying down, was pleased with the findings.

"Well, looks pretty much like what we expected." Frank pointed out the salient features to me after he had finished up. No matter how many times I tried, it was never easy to orient myself to the cath films while I was lying down. I guess that's why nobody reads films in a hammock.

"Yeah, I'm good with that. We're talking about a re-do bypass, right?"

"Looks like it."

"Who's going to do it?"

"You got to pick last time. This time I pick." He gave me a significant look. I chose my first surgeon because he knew his stuff and, from what I knew, had a solid reputation. Apparently he was not on the top of Frank's list, but, to his credit, he never said a negative word. I imagine somewhere during this ordeal he'd wished he'd opened his mouth. "I'll call Brady, see if he's around. I'm sure he won't want to go today, but stick around just in case." I thought, *Well, this is going to mess up my busy schedule, but all right, just this once.* In truth, I was in what my uncle, a general surgeon, referred to as "Colostomy Reversal Mode".

"You can call a patient at 2 A.M. and tell them to be at the hospital in fifteen minutes because you're going to take down their colostomy, and I guarantee you they'll be there in ten." If Brady were to tell me he was going to do the bypass surgery right now blindfolded with one hand tied behind his back, that was AOK with me.

"Okay." I was wheeled out to wait on my gurney in the holding area. I tried to recall what Kevin Brady looked like. I think our paths had crossed once in six years working at JCL. Other than for new patients and chest trauma patients, if you see a heart surgeon examining a patient in the E.R., odds are that something's gone wrong. So I saw that as a good sign. On the other hand, if somebody had walked by dressed in green, I would have seen that as a good sign. I was grasping at omens. I wondered what constituted a good omen in Oman.

I dozed off. Suddenly I was awakened by, "Hi, Frank." Brady stood alongside my gurney, smiling and completely at ease. We shook hands.

"I took a look at your films. I can do a small incision laterally, put in one or two grafts, and be done inside two hours. I do most of my bypasses off-pump, and this certainly won't require a pump."

"So I won't need a sternotomy this time around."

"No. I'll be placing two grafts, and both are more accessible using a left posterolateral approach."

"This will be a thoracotomy, what do you call it, a MIDCAB?"

"Right. Minimally Invasive Direct Coronary Artery Bypass. I'll make a two- to three-inch incision between your ribs, and work from there." Anytime I hear anything involving the word "mini" or a derivation of that, my antennae go up. However, he seemed so self-assured that I actually found myself looking forward to getting it over with. I mean, how bad can a small thoracotomy hurt?

"Any chance you can harvest the saphenous vein endoscopically?"

He looked at my right leg and laughed. "I haven't seen a harvest scar like that in a decade or more."

"Nice, eh? They told me they had to do it open because it was an emergency."

He laughed again. "I'll have the saphenous out with a scope in ten minutes, tops. The endoscopic route is much faster and cleaner than an open incision." He pointed to my left knee and ankle. "You'll have a tiny scar here and here. How about we do this next week?" *Gee, I don't know. Let me consult my calendar.* That was it. No bemoaning my mini-tragedy, bad luck, whatever. I liked that. Time to move on to success. Nothing but confidence. "Any questions?"

"The last time around, the worst thing was those thirty-twos, the mediastinal tubes."

"Not this time. I'll use a single nineteen French on the side. It will come out painlessly. See you in a few days." We shook hands, he left, I had my saline lock pulled, got dressed, and headed home for one more talk with my daughter, hopefully the last one involving the words "heart surgery". I only wished that he'd operated right then and there.

135. BACK INTO THE FRAY

I spent the next few evenings reading, sitting out back watching the sunset and walking around the neighborhood. I figured it would be a while before I could walk without feeling like a bag of crap. I was just getting to the point that reading a page-turner or a magazine was not a chore. My retention, however, was still pretty much room temp. The next day I puttered around the property, doing some menial tasks, pretending I was accomplishing something. The day before surgery, in the late afternoon, I drove over to my daughter's Mom's place to let them know what was going on and to get a hug from my daughter. I gave them the news in the living room.

"You can't catch a break, can you?" This from Ari's Mom. I thought, *I caught the biggest break possible last August when I didn't drop dead driving across the Golden Gate with Ari in the car, so I'm good on the break thing.* My daughter had her eyebrows up, her go-to move when she was worried or scared but didn't want to let on.

"This should be the last go-round for a while, anyway." I held my daughter for a long moment, then got out of there before I choked up. I told her I'd see her in five days.

That evening, a couple of friends from work stopped by to wish me luck. It was nice to have people who cared what happened to me. Cared enough to come by and take one last look. On the other hand, I was aware that, as routine as a CABG has been for the past three decades, I could still end up a cardiac cripple, stroked out, brain dead, or plain dead. The first time around had been such a rush job that I had no time to worry. This time I had plenty of time to worry. I knew what I was getting into in terms of the rehab and healing process. From Kevin Brady's perspective, this would be a breeze. Pain was a minor concern. Having been around surgeons for years, I wasn't so sure, and in my line of work you tended to see the FUBAR cases, not the routine successes. I tried to focus solely on getting up in the morning and going to the hospital.

I had the routine down for getting my house ready. The first surgery I was out in five days; I was shooting for three this time around. Even when going in for the caths and the angioplasty I had to plan on complications necessitating a hospital stay of up to a week. Taking care of everything that needed taking care of took about a half-hour. In the winter in Arizona, backyard pools are open but idiot-proof. My houseplants would survive a week or more without watering. The families of rock squirrels that ruled my property were all laying low, occasionally emerging from their luxurious digs in my outbuildings for a sunbath and family forage fest. I was already feeling better, thinking that the future looked brighter than it had since early November. Given that I was heading into possibly my last day on earth, I slept pretty well.

A John Frankenheimer film, *Seconds,* came out in 1966. The plot consists of an old businessman who hates his life; he is offered a new one by "The Company". After massive surgery, he emerges as Rock Hudson. At first his new life is terrific--parties in his Malibu beach home, et cetera. After a while, however, he requests that "The Company" put him back into his old life and body. As the movie closes, the surgeons are putting him down...permanently. Rumor has it the film so frightened Brian Wilson that he refused to go to a movie theater for fifteen years.

Before awakening to the alarm, my last dream had me going back into the O.R. Instead of performing the bypass, Dr. Brady pulled my heart out, dropped it in the trashcan-on-wheels, stapled my chest closed, and said, "Next case." Not exactly admission requirements for entrance into the Optimist Club.

Brady's office had called to let me know I was going first, so it was NPO P MN, nothing to eat or drink after midnight. No reason to get up early and enjoy a cup of coffee, so I was in bed until 5:00 A.M. My ride arrived promptly at 5:30, and by 5:45 I was back in the admitting office, signing the forms and shelling out another grand to grease the wheels. I stopped in the ER to say hi to some of my night shift co-workers. I did it so they wouldn't have to come find me to wish me luck, but when you are heading into a dreaded procedure, it is nice to have something to anticipate on the other side. I imagined I would be back to work within a month. I made plans to get together with a couple of friends three weeks hence.

When I was eleven years old, a guy in a white Floyd jacket discovered twelve cavities in my mouth. There was some kind of barter deal between my stepfather and the dentist, so I went in on Saturdays to have them filled. He chose to do one per week for twelve weeks. For the first six weeks, I made sure we had something planned for the afternoon or evening after my dental visit. It reassured me that I would live through the procedure. For a clueless eleven year-old, it wasn't a bad survival plan. After about the sixth week, I had the pain figured out and didn't worry about getting through it all.

Upstairs I went through the routine for the fifth time. My veins were still holding up just fine, and the saline lock went in without trouble. The anesthesiologist came by, went through the questions, looked me over, did the A through G thing, and pronounced me fit for surgery. The nurse and an aide wheeled me into the OR. Dr. Brady said "Hi," I slid over onto the table, and, with the push of a syringe, the anesthesiologist sent me off to Nowhereville once more.

136. THERE'S A TROCAR IN MY BACK

In general, anytime you hear a medical term that begins with "mini", you'd be well-advised to run the other way at high speed. When I was an intern, someone came up with the concept of a "mini-code". These were patients who, if they tried to die, wanted any and all resuscitative maneuvers short of shocking their heart or intubating them and putting them on a ventilator. For the most part, these were chronically ill patients whose lifestyle included admissions to the hospital on a weekly to monthly basis. One look at these folks and, if you are sane, you'd say, "If I ever get to be that bad, please put me out of my misery."

That is, until the Reaper is gently rapping at your door. Once he crooks his gnarled, nicotine-stained finger at you to follow him into the afterworld, it's a whole different ballgame. Anyway, this mini-code thing caught on like wildfire. Suddenly everyone was a mini-code. It gave the appearance of trying to resuscitate a patient who had no business being resuscitated without really running the risk of prolonging said patient's life inappropriately. Families of very old or very chronically ill patients could feel good about "doing something" for their loved ones without involving the defibrillator or the ventilator.

Invariably, if someone has a cardiac or pulmonary arrest, meaning their heart stops or their breathing stops, the first thing you do is shock them while someone is intubating them. You would think that a mini-anything would remove some of the final steps, to shorten the process or the product. However, rather than removing the final steps, in a mini-code you are removing the first two steps. So you skip the truly lifesaving stuff and move on to drugs, fluids, ancillary shit like that. A fellow intern and I got called to a mini-code on a longtime dialysis patient who was having an upper GI bleed from the latest NSAID, something called Zomax. Sounds pretty powerful, eh? Zomax! Everybody and their uncle was taking this stuff, including more than a handful of the lifers, the folks who'd been on dialysis since the time of its inception. Anyway, this dialysis guy with no legs and not much in the way of arms is puking up blood by the bucketful. We get there and he's thrashing around on his back like a big tick, obviously choking to death on the blood. Normally I would have placed an ET tube down into his trachea and inflated the cuff, to prevent any more blood from backwashing into his lungs and drowning him. But I can't because he's a mini-code.

One of the nurses tries to shove an NG tube through his nose into his stomach so that we can suck out the blood. That really gets him agitated, so then he tries to sit up and fight us all off. Numerous staff members are trying to hold him down. In a moment of pure clarity, the other intern finally says, "Let him up. If he sits up, his blood pressure will drop and he'll pass out." Everyone looks at each other, they collectively shrug, and let him go. Up he goes, then down he goes. No longer flailing about, comfortably passed out, he is much more amenable to having his life saved. The NG tube goes in and everything gradually comes under control. We take off to go finish our workups. As we're walking out, I observe that everything would have been neater, cleaner, and less torturous for the guy if we'd been able to shoot him full of a paralytic and intubate him.

My friend turns to me and says, "Man, don't ever let nobody mini-code me." I later learned that nothing "mini" ever goes as planned.

This time around, I was to undergo a MIDCAB procedure, short for Minimally Invasive Direct Coronary Artery Bypass. As Dr. Brady explained it, he would make a two-inch incision on the left side of my chest, go between two ribs, and place a couple of bypass grafts. Mini. By comparison, the sternotomy scar from my first surgery measured eight inches in length, and that involved sawing my breastbone down the middle. So, even though I'm undergoing a thoracotomy, which means an incision into my thorax and through that godawfully sensitive parietal pleura, it should be a small entry wound and I'll just breeze through my recovery. Of course.

At least in the old days, when you ordered up a tube thoracostomy (chest tube) tray, you received a sterile tray full of instruments, towels, vaseline gauze, suture material, a selection of chest tubes in various sizes and colors, and a trocar. A what? A trocar.

Imagine you are a lonely but dedicated shepherd, herding your sheep in the clover or thistle or peat or gorse or wherever it is you herd sheep in Scotland. Suddenly, one of your sheep falls over on his side and doesn't get up. You walk over, with your shepherd's staff of course, and inspect the fallen ovine. You reach into your shepherd's cloak and pull out a steel instrument shaped like a giant sharpened pencil. You bend over and shove this pencil, this trocar, through the wool, through the skin, into the sheep's distended stomach. An explosion of green slime and putrid gas immediately erupts from the wound and envelops you. The sheep jumps up, or approximates a jump, and waddles off to eat more whatever. You wipe off your face and hands, de-slop the trocar, and return it to your cloak. That is a trocar. A giant metal pencil used to poke holes in things. This also explains why so many shepherds are lonely. Green slime and putrid gas.

You request a tube thoracostomy tray when somebody's pleural space, the space between the lung and the chest wall, is full of blood (hemothorax), air (pneumothorax), fluid (hydrothorax) or pus (No, not a pusothorax. An empyema. If you didn't know what it was, and you heard "empyema", you'd probably imagine some kind of yummy Mexican dessert.). First, using an aseptic scalpel, you make an incision somewhere on the chest wall. Then you insert a shiny metal hemostat, a Kelly clamp, into the wound and spread the tissues, including the parietal pleura, the lining around the lung. This hurts far more than you can imagine. Then you insert the business end of the rubber chest tube into the incision, between two ribs, into the pleural space, suture it to the skin so it doesn't fall out or get yanked, and hook the exposed end up to a wall suction unit. Whatever is in there is sucked out. Depending on the circumstances, the tube remains in place, sucking out the stuff that doesn't belong there, for two to however many days. For some reason, somebody came up with the idea that, rather than just make an incision with an aseptic scalpel and widen the hole by inserting and spreading a hemostat, it might occasionally be fun to shove the giant steel pencil, the trocar, through the skin, through the intercostal (between the ribs) muscles and through the parietal pleura into the pleural space, then thread the chest tube over or around the trocar, then remove the trocar. Despite having placed dozens of chest tubes, I have never felt the need to use a trocar, I have never seen one used, but I will say that while it is fine for decompressing a sheep rumen distended by the bloat, it lacks a certain je ne sais quoi, a certain finesse, when it comes to entering a human chest cavity.

Back to me. I awaken in my old room in the CVICU. Even though I don't smell any burning flesh, apparently the surgical team has misplaced a red-hot sharp something on the final instrument count, because it feels like it's still sticking into my back. Only a trocar could cause that sharp searing pain in the left side of my chest. I can't reach back there to pull it out. I've broken my share of bones, sustained far too many knuckleheaded injuries over the years, but nothing, not even after my first surgery, ever came close to the pain I feel when I awaken from anesthesia. In a cruel twist of fate, the universe's love of irony, this sharp pain is located in almost exactly the same position as my angina.

Let's review. As we discussed in the chapter on atypical chest pain, pleurisy is an illness characterized by sharp, penetrating chest pain worsened by coughing, sneezing or breathing. No matter who you are, pleurisy novice or lifelong pleurisy swami, your initial reaction to the onset of that pain is to breathe very rapidly, very shallowly. This, of course, makes you blow off carbon dioxide. You become lightheaded, your hands and feet spasm, and with any luck, much like the background hyperventilator on the Zombies' "Time of the Season", you pass out. If you listen to the song closely, you can hear the guy taking a break every so often. After a pause of a few bars, he wakes up, his hands unspaz, and he starts up again.

Nurses who are familiar with post-op pleuritic chest pain know that the only way to treat this is to have the patient breathe in through his nose and out through his mouth. You just can't breathe that rapidly when you inhale through your nose. It slows down your respiratory rate. Oh, and a big push of morphine helps too. I am still intubated and on the ventilator, so the breathing exercise is less effective. The morphine works just fine, however. I nod off. It is a long night. Both asleep and awake, the dream persists; I bob along just beneath the surface of a hazy sea. The good news is that apparently I can breathe underwater. When I wake up for the oncoming day shift nurse, I start to wonder why they haven't extubated me yet. I'm getting enough of something IV to allow me to breathe with the ventilator, not fight it. Fighting it just leads to coughing; when you are freshly post-op from a thoracotomy, coughing hurts.

Pretty soon the respiratory therapist walks in.

"Hi. I have to do some weaning parameters on you, see if we can get you extubated this morning." I nod my head. For some reason, this triggers the ventilator alarm. The sound gets me all agitated, I cough a couple times, and the really bad pain returns to my left shoulder blade. It takes a minute or two for everything to sort out.

"Okay. I'm going to take you off the ventilator so I can see how your tidal volume and minute volume look. Nice slow breaths, not too deep." Once the vent is off, I try a little too hard and my shoulder blade and ribs erupt in pain. Eventually I get into a smooth rhythm. It still hurts to breathe, but not as bad as when I cough. Somewhere in my foggy brain I tell myself I passed that part.

"Okay, now we're going to measure your NIF (Negative Inspiratory Force)." I've been involved with extubation protocols on enough patients to know that nobody likes the NIF. Once they're extubated, that's the first thing they complain about. The consensus is that breathing during the NIF measurement feels like you have a plastic bag shoved down your windpipe into your lungs. That doesn't come near to describing the discomfort. It's more like trying to inhale around a chunk of concrete wedged into your ET tube. No matter how hard you try, nothing comes into your lungs. To add to the fun, your respiratory therapist yells at you to "inhale, deeper, harder. Go go go go go".

Prior to this, whenever I'd see a healthy patient fail the NIF, I'd think, *You could have done better, but you didn't make the effort.* Never again. You are trying to inhale air that simply isn't there. I know I'm not suffocating, but it sure feels like I am. It hurts like hell to try to breathe, that incision back there is killing me, but I know that if I give up, I may stay on the ventilator, intubated, for another twelve or twenty-four hours. After endless sucking, I give up. That's what the NIF is. You sucking at sucking.

"Good job." He makes some notes on the clipboard, then looks at me. "Ready to get the tube out?" I'm too worn out and in too much pain to nod, but it doesn't matter. He's not really asking me for an opinion. My nurse appears on the other side of the bed. She is holding a set of nasal prongs and a suction catheter. The R.T. attaches a syringe to the cuff port of the tube and pulls on the plunger. For some reason, I expect it to fill with blood, but all that comes out is clear air. Next thing I know the tube is coming out, followed by a trail of fire engine red and maroon snot. Before I can start coughing, the sucker is in my mouth. The suction tube fills with dark blood. My nurse sticks nasal prongs into my nostrils and wraps the tubing around the back of my head and neck. While I cough, I think, *This sure was easier the last time, when I was half-asleep.*

Pretty soon I fall asleep again. This time there are no dreams of breathing underwater. When I wake up, Dr. Brady is standing next to my bed.

I rasp out the words, "Is there a trocar sticking out of my back?" Morphine tends to loosen one's tongue.

He smiles empathetically. "Hurts a bit, eh? Well, I have to say, things didn't go exactly as planned." That sounds like an "Oops". You never say "Oops" in the O.R. Even patients who are theoretically anesthetized and hanging out in Vanishedville have a nasty habit of remembering that word later on. As they say in the business, the eighth cranial nerve--the one that allows you to hear--never goes to sleep. So something went awry. At least I'm awake, lying in bed and there's no white light coming my way. I do my best to scan my body. All parts present and accounted for.

"They weren't kidding. You really do have small-caliber coronary vessels." Somewhat better than your urologist expressing his surprise at how small your dick is, but not exactly a point of pride.

"As a matter of fact, it was so difficult to graft onto them I had to enlarge the incision a bit." *So much for "mini".* "And your intercostal spaces are so small I had to cut through two or your ribs." Small vessels, big incision, broken ribs.

"Were you able to open up the diagonal and the intermediate?"

"Of course. Two grafts, short and sweet. No twists." Sometime later, I forget how, I find out that the procedure wasn't quite as short as he'd expected, either. On the bright side, he and his team had pulled me through; it still wasn't my day to die.

"So I can get up and start walking right away?"

"Certainly."

"Good. No offense, but I'd really like to be out of here in three days."
My nurse is standing next to him. Poker-faced, but somehow I can tell
she's thinking, *This wuss? Yeah, right.* Good. Now I have a goal: to
prove her wrong.

"That shouldn't be a problem. See you later." I began feeling invincible.
Unfortunately, I hadn't taken into account a new obstacle: post-op
pain. After all, chest discomfort had been the least of my limitations
the last time around.

All gung ho and feeling pretty tough, I start the walking regimen.
That's when it dawns on me. *She might be right. My ribs are killing me.*
After my first surgery, the limiting factor in my recovery was an
overall sense of weakness and my dull brain. This time around, I have
to cope with both of those and this new post-thoracotomy pain.
Actually, three different kinds of pain, all centered just below my left
shoulder blade.

First, there's the pain from the incision. It's decidedly different than
the incisional pain I felt after my sternotomy. This time it burns,
tingles, like your hand feels when it "falls asleep". Unlike the sleepy
hand, this doesn't wake up after a few seconds. Fortunately, it's minor
compared to the other ones.

Next, just a little deeper, there's the rib pain. Anyone who's ever
broken a rib knows that feeling: a dull constant ache punctuated by
sharp exacerbations, usually when you turn your torso, lift the arm on
that side, roll over in bed or, worst of all, cough. Even better, that
sharp crescendo of pain is accompanied by a nice crackling sound--
like the rib is breaking again--as the broken ends rub against each
other or irritate the surrounding intercostal muscles. Bones don't have
any nerves inside them, so the bones themselves don't hurt. The
periosteum, the connective tissue surrounding every bone in your
body, does contain nerves. That's why a bony contusion (bruise) can
hurt as much or more than a broken bone. The intercostal muscles can
also generate pain. As a bonus, underneath each rib is an intercostal
artery, vein and nerve. No doubt at least one of mine was cut when Dr.
Brady had to bisect a couple of ribs to get better exposure.

Much worse than the incisional or rib pain is the pleuritic pain. Except
for a sternotomy, if you want to get anywhere in the chest, you have to
enter the pleural space. The pleural space is the gap between the
parietal pleura, which lines the inside of your chest wall, and the
visceral pleura, which is attached to the outer surface of your lungs. So

to operate in the chest or just stick a chest tube in for drainage, you have to cut into and through the parietal pleura. Apparently the parietal pleura, a tough sheet of tissue, is loaded with sensory nerves.

Ask anyone who has ever suffered from pleurisy, inflammation of the pleura. When it is caused by a specific virus, usually Coxsackie B, the common term is "The Devil's Grippe" because it feels like Satan is sticking a pitchfork into your chest just to see how much you can take. It is an intense, squeezing pain unlike anything you've ever experienced. In my case it was completely unpredictable; sometimes a cough would set it off, sometimes the slightest movement would leave me gasping. Sometimes it would wake me out of a sound sleep. I'd think, *Somebody snuck in and shoved that trocar back in.* Surprisingly, a couple of times my chest tube inadvertently got bumped without causing any of that pain. After the first few times, I learned to breathe in through my nose and out through my mouth. It didn't make that awful pain go away, but it kept me from making all the other pain varieties worse.

Nonetheless, my nurses put me on the fast track. Visitors came and went, usually when I was in a deep morphine sleep, resting up from a walk. As Dr. Brady had promised, that nineteen French chest tube slid out without one iota of discomfort. Three days after the surgery, I was rolling out to the parking lot again, miserable from the pain but anxious to move on.

137. S.O.S.D.D.

I feel lucky to have survived yet again; counting all the caths, this last surgery is my sixth invasive procedure in less than five months. My first move when I get in the door is to fall on the couch and sleep for hours. I wake up disoriented in the dark, not knowing where I am. I have no recollection of my recent surgery. Then I sit up. Immediately, all those different types of pain in my back remind me. *Oh, that's right.* After lying in one position for so long, every movement hurts. I twist my body one way, then the other, hoping for relief. Finally, I stand up. After walking around for a minute or so, the pleuritic pain and the rib pain ease. Left with only the incisional burning, I am a happy guy. I fix myself something to eat, then fall asleep sitting out back, watching the stars ignore me.

Next morning, right on schedule, I wake up to the chirping of the birds. Fifteen minutes later, the sun comes up just south of Squaw Peak. Time to get moving. I lace on some tennis shoes--I can tell it's going to be a rough fortnight, because every time I bend forward or over, the severed end of my ribs grate against each other in a most unpleasant way--and head out for my first walk. Trying to pull on a t-shirt makes me feel like I'm being crammed into a turtle shell lined with trocars, so it's back to the moo-moos.

The best time of the year to do anything outdoors in Phoenix is late autumn through early spring. Lows from the high thirties to the mid-fifties. I have to dig out a jacket for my walk, as my usual winter wear, a sweatshirt, just won't work. Maybe it's me, but I don't sense the stares from passersby. Either the jacket adds the illusion of avoirdupois or I'm just old news. I make it about halfway around the block, then have to sit and suck gas. For whatever reason, in the hospital it wasn't obvious how much this thoracotomy would affect my breathing. Humans can't really remember how bad a certain pain is until it returns, probably a protective mechanism afforded by the brain. Anyway, I think I feel worse than the last time, but the experience of getting through it once before makes me less apprehensive. No fear of the unknown this time around. Within a week I am getting around the block with minimal dyspnea. Best of all, I can get out three times a day without worrying that the summer heat will turn me into a pale puddle of slime.

By the end of the week after my first surgery, I barely noticed the pain from my chest incision, a sternotomy about eight inches long. My leg wound, about twenty inches long, was far more painful and irritating. This time, the saphenous vein harvest site consists of two half-inch wounds, one just medial to my knee and one just above my ankle on the left leg. Neither one causes me the slightest discomfort. This time, the chest wound, a thoracotomy, is another matter entirely. Though only four inches in length, starting just behind and below my left armpit and angling up and back toward my neck, it causes me all sorts of pain from day one. Starting on the outside and working inward, there are four separate types of pain associated with my wound. First, the skin and subcutaneous tissues, including the superficial muscles, cause a constant low-level ache and burn. I figure the burn part comes from the severed intercostal nerves in that area. This pain does very nicely with either the Percocet or ibuprofen. After a few days, as long as I take the eight hundred mg. of ibuprofen four times daily, it bothers me only when I try to turn over in bed. Of course, taking that much ibuprofen or any other NSAID that often for an extended period of time, even on a full stomach, will exact its revenge on your GI tract.

The second pain occurs when the severed ends of my ribs rub against each other. It hurts, but it's the weird dull grating sound that really bothers me. It too is a problem in bed at night, but also causes me to come up short when I bend over or try to lift something. I still have some laxity of my rib cage up front on the left from my first surgery. Every so often the two rib abnormalities combine to give me unbelievable muscle spasms on the left side of my abdomen and chest. They last a minute or so, a nice reminder of those fat honking mediastinal tubes from my first surgical go-round.

Third is the pleuritic pain, an angry response by my pleura to the surgical violation of its integrity. It is much sharper and much deeper than the first two types of pain; not content to limit itself to the area of the incision, it envelops the entire left side of my thorax. It is bad enough at rest, but when I take a breath or move my upper body in any way, it is excruciating. My pleura has only one rule: Don't Mess. Violate the rule, and suffering will follow. Fortunately, it only shows up on occasion, but when it does, nothing helps. Nothing, that is, except to do what my nurse told me to do. Breathe in through my nose and out through my mouth. There is no way to fuck up the technique. Eventually, you will have to slow your breathing down. After a minute or so of that, the pain usually subsides enough for it to be tolerable. Occasionally it will stick around for longer, doling out misery until it gets bored with me and goes away.

About a week into my stay at home, I develop a new pain, an intense sharp ache that would come on while sitting down. It feels like the red hot poker treatment from down below up into the tip of my left shoulder. I chalk it up to referred pain from the invasion of my pleura. It comes on every couple of days and lasts a good half-hour. It is by far the worst of all my pains. Meds, my special breathing technique, changing position, taking a walk, nothing makes it better or worse. It's just there, unaffected by anything, its dead shark eyes persistently gnawing away, dwarfing my baseline discomfort.

Given these other pains, all at or near my left scapula, I can't tell if I am experiencing any of my customary angina. I conclude that I'm not and leave it at that. I am hurting so badly so often from the other pains that I prefer not to know.

Surrounded by all this pain, it is somehow comforting to know that, as promised, Dr. Brady had performed the second surgery off-pump. Something, however, possibly the anesthesia combined with increased need for morphine early on, did a number on my brain. I can't tell if I'm as bad as after the first surgery, but it's perfectly obvious to me that I'm really slow. Probably it's a little better this time around, because I can remember how Ari gets to my house and I realize how boring a conversationalist I am. I have the hardest time remembering who just called or what I just did. I hope it's just the anesthesia, not a little stroke. In the end, does it matter?

Sleep continues to be sporadic. Part of it is the accumulation of various pains. Part of it is the recurrent dream. I am being wheeled out after my second bypass surgery. I'm not sure how I know which surgery, but I do. Just as I am about to be wheeled into the CVICU, a voice on the PA system tells me to come back to the O.R. for another bypass. Back I go. The dream continues thusly, out of the O.R., then back in, again and again. It feels like I'm on a gerbil wheel. No, it's more like being on a conveyor belt, a pile of dirty restaurant dishes heading in to be steam cleaned. Somewhere in my brain, I guess I am thinking, *I'll just go on having bypasses every few months, until some endpoint is reached; maybe they run out of veins, or suture material.* The wakeup is always in a swirl of sweaty sheets, accompanied by pain.

My vision is a mess. I don't bother reading much because none of it sinks in. Whenever I'm moving, whether traveling in a car or just walking around the block, everything flashes by on either side, leaving trails like headlights in a time-lapse photo. If I'm going fast, the visual problems make me lightheaded. I try driving around the block. No dice.

When she was in pre-school and kindergarten, my daughter was fascinated by buses. There were two kinds: school bus, which was yellow, and city bus, which was white. None of her schools ever transported their students via bus. Anytime we travelled to a place with good mass transit, we made it a point to ride the light rail or the bus at least once. With this new eye and brain development, I have several choices: have someone else take her to school, take a cab, or take the bus. For me, the obvious choice is the bus. Though Phoenix is no Portland or Seattle when it comes to mass transit, not even New York or D.C., if you live near the center of town, the service is pretty good. So we start riding the bus. I figure it will be a matter of a few weeks at most before my head clears up. Hopefully my eyes will too.

At first, Ari is tickled. She sees new kinds of people, gets to put the money in the machine, get the transfer ticket, all that. We get to talk on the walk to and from the bus stops. After a while, her friends' parents see us, stop, and offer us a ride. I decline, figuring I need the walk, the exercise will do her good too, and it would be embarrassing for her to get into someone else's car with her sick old dad. Her sick old dad who makes pathetic grunting noises whenever he bends forward. I stick to my guns for over a month before I go to see my ophthalmologist.

"Everything checks out okay with your eyes. If this persists, even though I see no obvious signs of a stroke, you might want to check in with a neurologist." Thoughts of MRI's, CT's, angiograms and EEG's bring me nothing but dread. I go home resolved to start driving her to school the next week and hope for the best.

Besides camping, one of the things I wanted Ari to experience as a kid was skiing. Our first trip, a Saturday afternoon in Flagstaff, ended up with her sliding down the hill between my legs in a blinding snowstorm. A couple years later, at the age of five or so, we started taking a trip at least once a year. Though she never got hooked on it, she could get down most hills without difficulty. Now her seventh-grade class is going on a trip to Purgatory. Or should I say, what used to be called Purgatory. City big shots always know what's best for everyone else in town. According to a local, the Durango elite decided that the name "Purgatory" implied something to do with Satan; this was certainly the reason that not enough God-fearing skiers were coming to town. They changed the name of the ski area to Durango Mountain. When I heard this story, I thought, *You weirdos, I'll never ski there again.* Then again, my source for that story wasn't all that big on the truth.

When Ari tells me about the ski trip, which is scheduled over President's Day weekend, I can't imagine surviving more than a minute at that altitude, not to mention the cold. Her Mom can't go, though, so I think, *What the hell, I don't want my kid going as one of the orphans, with some other parent responsible for her.* She is one of the few kids in her school with divorced parents, and sometimes that has been a problem, explaining to her friends why we don't all live together. The least I can do is show up when she needs me. I pack way too many warm clothes, my meds, and we head up north.

Fortunately, most of her buddies are equally as proficient as Ari or slightly less so. She skis all day with the group, then we get together at night. The weather is accommodating, mostly sunny with the occasional snowfall. I can walk a good twenty feet or so without having to stop to catch my breath or wait for one of my pains to subside. When I can take a deep breath, there's the fresh cold pine air, lightly scented with fires from the restaurants and condos. We get through the trip intact. When I get home, I realize that I no longer have a fear of dropping dead in an awkward situation, especially in front of Ari; I am down to nightly premonitions of dying in my sleep. The trip is the first time I have been of real service to my daughter since September. That feels good.

My trial is scheduled to start later in the week. But first...

138. FINALLY, SOME GOOD NEWS

It was a week or two after discharge. My incision, ribs and pleura still hurt like hell. I'd jettisoned the Percocets after a day or two in favor of large doses of ibuprofen. My stomach was complaining, but the pain relief was much better. I was still producing large chunks of dried bloody snot in the shower. The steady flow of warm water on my back, so reassuringly different than my anginal pains back there, loosened them up in my lungs and windpipe, and I was able to let them slide out without coughing in agony. Ugly stuff, to be sure, but with them went the tightness in my bronchi. All in all, I thought things were going as well as could be expected.

Time for the surgical follow-up visit. Dr. Brady was his usual confident, professional, upbeat self. He was the kind of guy who could say, "Frank, it looks like I'm going to have to take your head off for a few seconds, but it'll feel much better when I reattach it," and you'd be okay with that. We shook hands and he took a look at my wound. Behind me I heard him remove an instrument from its sterilized paper and cellophane package. It is a very distinctive sound. Then there was the sound of snipping.

"I'm removing some necrotic (dead) tissue from your wound. I hope it's not too painful." That's when I made a startling discovery. Despite all the pain from back there, he wasn't hurting me a bit.

"I can't feel a thing. It's completely numb."

"Oh. That's good. There. All done." I was still marveling over the lack of sensation. I put my shirt on and turned to go.

"Can I ask you a question?"

He smiled. "Sure."

"After my last surgery, Frank said I'd need to have something else done in about five years, but he wasn't sure what that would be. How long will it be before I need something else done?"

"Well, he was right. You did need something else done. But that's done now." *Good point, Doc.*

"I expect you're good for twenty years or so. Come back and see me then."

Despite feeling weak and hurting the worst ever and knowing I had a long way to go in terms of recovery, I left feeling optimistic, the first time since November.

Like the guy from the power company, I hoped he wasn't lying.

139. TRIAL BY JURY

In case you are wondering, yes, it is terrifying to be tried by a jury of your peers. Even if the worst punishment is a fine and community service, being in the same room with twelve people who sit in judgment of you is a most powerless feeling, something short of watching your child suffer.

I went in to the trial resigned to my guilt. Starting with my attorney's screw-up in December that resulted in an arrest warrant being issued, every interaction with him left me feeling lower and lower. After every phone call or office visit, I thought it best to just plead no contest, take the punishment, and not waste anyone's time. At our last meeting before the day of trial, I said as much. He countered with the idea that my case was strong, simply because I wasn't driving when I was arrested. I had plenty of time on my hands and not much to do, so I figured I might as well have my day in court. There was nobody up on the gallows tying a hangman's noose, but I didn't have any optimistic wild cards up my sleeve.

During jury selection, only one of the pool showed any interest in being there, and he was eliminated during voir dire. The rest of the jury pool looked like they'd rather be shoveling dog shit pro bono in hell. I once had a job shoveling dog shit on the weekends. It was by no means my worst job ever, but then again, the weather was pretty nice and I was getting paid minimum wage. My attorney's performance during jury selection did nothing to bolster my spirits. I spent a fair bit of time trying to get comfortable without letting my back touch the chair. After a while, I noticed that most of the jury was watching me, so I quit wiggling around.

The arresting officer came on first. Guided by the assistant D.A., he walked the jury through the events of the night. I had no problem with what he said. On cross examination by my attorney, however, he confabulated a bit on some of the details. I didn't say anything because the crux of the case was that I was not driving when he encountered me, and anyway, it was basically my word against his on the performance of the sobriety exercises. My attorney asked reasonable questions, but his bumbling made me want to crawl under the table.

At best, he seemed ill-prepared, but that had pretty much been my impression the previous couple of weeks. I remember thinking, *I wonder how long it's been since he actually tried a case.* I was embarrassed for him, but I also hoped his efforts wouldn't end up pissing off the judge and jury. As I tried to sleep that night, visions of them sentencing me to ten years at hard labor to compensate for their pain and suffering danced wildly around my head.

The next day, when I got up to take the stand, I got one of those horrific shoulder pains. That left me short of breath, to the point that I took an overly long time to get to the witness stand. I'd thought about renting an oxygen tank just in case, but I figured the jury, who wouldn't know of my recent surgery, would suspect acting on my part. They were already tired of the whole legal process, I could see it in their eyes.

In response to my attorney's questions, I told the story of my entire day. I included the part about parking the car and turning it off to call a cab or an ambulance, dropping my phone, all that. It was obvious by the looks on their faces that the jury was not buying the distinction between driving a car and being in actual physical control of it. I was cross-examined by the A.D.A, the attorneys gave their closing summations, and the jury left to deliberate. I felt there was no chance of an acquittal; the best I could hope for was a reduced sentence. Exuding magnanimity, my lawyer took me to lunch.

At least the jury was prompt. They returned soon after lunch with a verdict. Guilty. The judge sentenced me to ten days in jail, all but one day suspended. She asked me when I wanted to serve my time. I wanted to get it over with as quickly as possible, so I opted for the following week, after my usual days with my daughter. I was also ordered to attend a one-on-one substance abuse counseling session, which would take less than an hour. And pay fines and fees.

Jail. Three weeks after open heart surgery. I shook hands with my attorney, glad to be rid of him forever, and took the bus home. It was white. City bus.

140. INTO THE TENTS--BRIEFLY

Tent City is located down in southwest Phoenix, next to one of the county jails. In the early 1990s, Sheriff Joe Arpaio said he would not release any inmates due to overcrowding. He found some surplus military tents, built a couple of block structures, and started housing non-violent inmates there in 1993. This was the start of his fame as

"The Toughest Sheriff in America". Over the years he's added green bologna to the menu and issued pink underwear so the inmates won't be tempted to steal them when they are released. There have been reality shows, countless interviews, and famous deputies--Steven Seagal and Shaquille O'Neal. He's been re-elected five times, all the while running possibly the most inept (hundreds of allegations of sex crimes, many perpetrated against children, left uninvestigated) and costly (successful lawsuits by numerous inmates, their survivors, and federal prosecutors, well over $100 million in settlements, judgments and legal fees) law enforcement agency in the country. He knows exactly how to stir up racial and ethnic fears among the leathery Sun City white folks who vote in droves.

I feel lucky to be doing my time in February. When I arrive on a sunny morning, it is fifty-five degrees, expected to get to the mid-seventies. It's snowbird season, although this particular part of town is not high on the birds' "must see" list. You line up for roll call, drop off your possessions, and head into a holding cell. There are less than a dozen of us sitting on the floor up against the walls all the way around the room. To relieve the pain from my surgery, I get up from time to time and walk a little. Here you have time to get to know each other's stories. We are all "kick outs", the name given to inmates who are here for twenty-four hours; the vast majority of kick outs are for simple DUI's. All of us were arrested at night. Among the Phoenix police there is a common practice of stopping drivers for "chirping" their tires as they pull out of a parking lot at night, especially if there is a bar nearby. Several of the guys were arrested for doing just that. And yes, we are all guys. The women have a separate intake area. I'm not expecting any conjugal visits.

After introductions and story-telling, the discussion rolls around to Joe Arpaio. According to urban legend, at least on this particular morning, it is common knowledge that he can't travel to California because he has outstanding warrants for failure to appear in court. The story is that he's been arrested in California eight times for DUI, but never went to trial. There's probably no more truth to this rumor than to any of the others; whatever makes you feel better in this miserable situation. I don't contribute. I know he's sitting somewhere, reveling in the certainty that we are talking about him.

Soon we are joined by a dozen other guys. Unlike our original crew, these guys are more seasoned, the kind of guy you could expect to say, "I can do nine months in the tents standing on my head." I get the feeling that none of them are kick outs. They sit down, relaxed, unlike us nervous rookies. Some of them know each other from somewhere, probably here. Nobody has the look of violence about them. Maybe ran afoul of the child support system, got caught dealing weed, boosted the wrong car, broke into one too many homes. The holding cell is starting to get crowded, too crowded for me to walk back and forth without bumping into guys. The last thing I want is to come into physical contact with anyone or to let on that I am hurting. The way I feel now, I couldn't fend off a one-legged cat. This crowd looks pretty tame, but I certainly don't want to be known as the most vulnerable member of the tribe. Frank the Gimp, everyone's bitch.

Pretty soon the guard who placed us in the holding cell takes off. He's replaced by a little guy who thinks it's hilarious to stick his face up to the grill in the door and say stupid shit. Apparently he's softening us up before we head for the big house. Short stature, bad teeth and low IQ. Probably the first of those is the only reason he was rejected for duty at Abu Ghraib. On the other hand, I've got normal stature, good teeth, and an allegedly high IQ. Every year, Charlie Whitebread, a former professor at UVA's law school, impressed on his first-year students the importance of obeying the law.

"When the green door slams shut, make sure you are on the OUTSIDE."

Despite my advantages, the little fucker is on the outside and I'm on the inside. So who's the dumbass here?

If he's at all typical of the guard mentality in the tents, the next twenty-four hours are going to be awful. From what I have heard, one of the cornerstones of the Arpaio jail experience--he is fond of describing Tent City as a "concentration camp"--is an extended stay in the holding cell, so crowded that nobody can even sit down. There are reports that he has kept a roomful of inmates locked in there for days at a time, claiming that their accommodations aren't ready yet. Luckily for us, we have only twenty-four hours; if he detains us for too long on any one ride, we'll be deprived of some other bizarre experience in his amusement park.

After a while, it's time to make the walk to the tents. First however, we have to be shackled in pairs, at the wrists and ankles. Shorty informs us that this is necessary so that we don't try to escape. Right. He knows it's bullshit, he knows we know, and that's how he gets his jollies. I get joined at the wrist and ankle with one of my kick out compadres. We discuss the silliness of the whole situation, both of us thinking, *Never again with this crap.*

Once out in the sunshine, we squint like survivors of a mine collapse. They line us up and march us from the intake building to the tent area.

I'm surprised Arpaio doesn't have a staff photographer snapping pix to sell to us later, like a jail-themed costume dinner cruise. We walk the fifty or so yards, then get checked in through the cyclone fence gate. There is a concrete building that houses the bathrooms, guard offices and kitchen. To the south sit the rows of tents, old canvas on poles, with dozens of bunks in each.

Inside the fence, we get a run-down of the schedule for meals, basic rules and regulations, and assignments to individual tents. The guards here don't seem to have the same intellectual limitations as Shorty. After the speech, the chief guard asks if anyone has any weapons or meds on them. I raise my hand. He comes over, takes me aside, and asks me what I have.

"Nitroglycerine." He gives me a look, trying to decide if I'm being funny. "I just had heart surgery, and I'm supposed to take it if I get chest pain."

"Oh, okay. Listen, I'm going to have to search you. I want you to turn around and face the fence." I comply. "Now, put your hands up on the fence, spread your legs, and step back. Good." Just like in the movies. He searches me, finds the little bottle of nitro in my pocket, then lets me turn around. No drama, just a guy doing his job, hoping everything goes according to plan. The way he handles the whole thing, matter-of-factly, makes me think I might get through this day after all.

"I'll log this in at the office. If you need any, come to the window over there and one of the deputies will get you your medication. You can go grab your bunk now."

I thank him and leave. Most of our kick out crew is in the same tent. I grab a couple of blankets, the usual hospital/institutional type, and throw them on an upper bunk. It looks like this one tent is used primarily for the DUIs. There are fans, not much else. In February, it is hard to remember how hot it gets in the summer, but again I am thankful I'm not going to find out about life in the tents when it's one-ten in the shade. I've heard that temperatures have been recorded as high as one hundred forty on the blacktop here in July. I start to wonder about the thermometers that go that high; not wanting to worsen my mindset, I shake that thought off and wander the premises. Walking feels good. It's about seventy degrees out; I can feel through my shoes that the ground is a good ten degrees warmer.

Adjacent to the tent area is a horse corral. Sheriff Joe considers himself a friend of the four-legged. Aside from illegal sweeps for illegal aliens, his favorite television ops involve rescuing animals that have been neglected by their owners. Given who he is, it's probably nothing more than an attempt to get animal lovers to vote for him. Several stables around town house horses used by his mounted posse. I'm not sure if the horses stabled here are active or retired. About a dozen older inmates care for the horses. Rumor has it that to draw this duty you have to be experienced with horses. It's considered a plum job among the long-timers here. Probably draws the envy of the other inmates, if only because it gives you something to do during the day. The corral smells faintly like horse shit, but the predominant aroma around the tents is pot.

After walking for a half-hour, I take a seat inside one of the tents. During the day, the canvas sides are rolled up and tied, so the tent becomes a canopy. There is a television on, with some sports news show playing. A dozen or so young guys are watching. All of a sudden, two of them get into some sort of argument in Spanish. Everyone else watches, waiting to see if it escalates. Not me. With visions of Walking Boss aiming his rifle at the troublemakers from a guard tower, I am up and out of there so quickly I feel a cracking in my back. *Great, I just tore the healing muscles or ribs again.* I walk for a while until things settle down, but the pain never retreats to what I was beginning to accept as normal.

The major occupation in Tent City is waiting. Most guys spend their time talking and hanging out. Absolutely nothing goes on there. Even through my mental fog, the lack of productivity boggles the mind. A month or two in this place would have to permanently propel your IQ at least ten points in the wrong direction. I listen to guys talking in groups. The kick outs are still recounting their tales of DUI-dom. Some of the older guys who know each other talk about mutual friends, most of whom are in jail somewhere else. Not much laughing, not much emotion of any kind. Everyone seems shut down, which is probably for the best. Contemplating life inside the fence is depressing.

Around 4:00 P.M., a voice on the PA system heralds the arrival of supper. Carts full of trays are wheeled out from the direction of the toilets. Sheriff Joe made a lot of news when he announced he would be serving surplus food to the inmates, including green bologna. In truth, numerous other law enforcement agencies have purchased surplus food for their inmates for years. I wander over to eyeball the dinner fare. Something brown, something white, something green. Three slimy puddles on the tray. If the green stuff is bologna, either it's spent way too much time in the sun or it's made the acquaintance of a blender. Plastic sporks are available. There are tanks full of fluid which probably is intended for drinking. The chronic guys pick up trays; the kick outs take one look, make a joke or two, and wander away. For me, it wouldn't matter if they were handing out lobster tails. I figure starving is better than food poisoning. The latter would require a trip to the toilets, and that is not on my itinerary.

Around sunset the tent sides are untied and rolled down. I routinely sleep on the ground in my backyard during the winter, so I'm thinking tonight will be a breeze. Around 8:00 P.M. I grab another couple of blankets, climb into my bunk, and fall asleep. Since the second surgery, I've been sleeping exclusively on my right side. Any other position and my ribs start to ache. It's colder than I expected. I should have brought an air mattress and one of my good sleeping bags, but it would have been hard to conceal them down the front of my pants.

After what seems like a half-hour of sleep, the loudspeaker starts blaring names. I'd heard that they try to disrupt your inner clock as much as possible. About twenty names into the list, I hear mine. *Wow, I'm getting out early!* I have forgotten the stories about the discharge process. It's about midnight when I walk up to the gate and join the crowd. I recognize most of my kick out buddies. After roll call, the guard opens the gate and we retrace our walk back to the intake building. No handcuffs or leg irons this time. Still no photographer for a sayonara snapshot.

We are herded into the holding cell; it looks and smells like the one we occupied that morning, but who can tell? There are about two dozen of us in here. I sit down in a corner and nod off. Next thing I know, there are voices and the door opens.

About twenty guys in prison stripes walk in. One of my kick out colleagues whispers to me that these are guys from the jail building. Although they all look pretty docile, apparently they were judged too dangerous or whatever for the tents. Clearly they've spent a lot of time together. The conversations are about family, plans for the weekend, job prospects. In a weird way, it reminds me of high school bus trips with sports teams.

The smell in the room changes noticeably for the worse. In my career, I've worked in all sorts of institutions, undressed and examined the homeless, lifted my share of corpses. The aromas of bodies and their fluids don't bother me in the least. None of that comes close to the funk these guys bring in with them. I fight back wave after wave of nausea. Finally, my olfactory nerve accustoms itself to the smell, and I can objectively evaluate it. It smells like these guys have been sleeping in the same clothes for weeks. There's not a lot of B.O., so presumably they could take showers, but then had to put on the same prison garb.

This is the first time in almost eighteen hours that my curiosity has been stirred in the least. And it's about how guys smell.

More guys are admitted into the holding cell. At this point, it's so crowded that those of us seated on the ground have to stand up. It's either that or get stepped on. I find a way to get wedged up against the wall without hurting my ribs. The dimly lit hours drag by. At times I feel like I'm going to pass out from standing in one place for so long. That brings on more nausea, but there's no way I'm going to bring any attention to myself. I lean against the wall and try to do multiplication tables in my head. When that gets boring, I begin an assessment of my situation.

IQ in the 140's, all A's through grade school, scholarship to a prep school, first in class at said prep school, National Merit Finalist, accepted by Stanford, wait-listed at Yale, Echols Scholar at UVA, first one admitted to med school class at UVA, Most Valuable Intern, board certified for life in internal medicine, and now hanging out here with scores of guys who never encountered even one of my opportunities. Nicely done, Frank. Such a creative way to fuck up.

While it's still dark outside, a new guard arrives. Like the morning guy, this one's short, stupid and cruel. She's also female. Now I'm definitely thinking about Abu Ghraib. Same stupid jokes about being in jail, and how's everyone feeling, standing in a room with one air vent which doubles as the tiny grilled viewing port in the door. It's everything I can do to keep from rushing over to the door to get some air. I start to hyperventilate, but fortunately, that stirs up a mother of an attack of pleuritic pain; the in-through-the-nose-and-out-through-the-mouth routine brings me right back to earth. I pass the time visualizing our guard bending forward in front of a speeding train and getting her head ripped off. I rationalize my situation thusly: I may be on the inside and she may be on the outside, but in a few hours I'll be free and she'll still be working in this shit hole.

When daylight finally arrives, we get marched out to the discharge area. They make us line up and stand at attention while our names are called. One woman in uniform, taller than most of the guys and clearly the most attractive woman I've seen in a while, keeps looking at me with just the slightest hint of a smile playing around her lips. She smells good too, soap and water. She stands right in front of me, no more than a foot away, while she gives us the rundown on where to pick up our possessions. I muster up what will have to pass for an attractive neutral look. I fear that if I smile, I'll get taken down for assault. For the first time in months, since my first surgery in fact, my dick starts to stir. A woman in uniform. All that's missing is a pizza and a six-pack. I consider saying something, but instead go with the sane option and leave her with my most charming smile. As I walk out, I think to myself, *She must have a thing for bony, flabby old guys with white hair.*

Outside the intake building, a number of guys beeline it for their cars. I'd considered driving, but I didn't trust myself not to get lost or get in a wreck. I have a pocket full of quarters for the bus ride home. It is another beautiful morning, and I suck in the fresh air on the walk to the bus stop.

The first bus, the one that would take me eight miles north, shows up within a minute. There are a couple other guys waiting, guys who weren't in my group. They have the look of the ones who'd been in longer, either in the tents or the jail building, but they're not wearing stripes and they don't stink. I don't recognize them from the holding cell, but that means nothing. I take it as a good sign that my brain is already erasing the last twenty-four hours from my memory banks. When we get on the bus, the rest of the riders, the ones who didn't spend the night in jail, give us the eye. I sit down and look out the window, never making eye contact during the fifteen-minute ride.

While waiting for the second bus, I keep an eye in the direction of the jail. I worry that someone will come get me and take me back for the remaining nine days. That feeling must be a thousand times worse for a guy who's been inside for a long time. To pass the time, I fantasize that the guard with the nice hair and the trace of a smile will drive by and pick me up.

When I get home, I throw all my clothes in the trash. They never smelled like that before. I consider burning them, but it's a no-burn day, and the last thing I want is another encounter with law enforcement. Besides, I'm on a roll, and I'd probably just fuck that up too. Then I jump into the pool. The pool thermometer says fifty-six degrees. It makes my heart flutter, but it doesn't paralyze my limbs the way an unplanned dip in the Box Canyon of the Rio Grande did twenty years earlier. Then I stand in the hot shower for about ten minutes. It doesn't remove the self- loathing, but it's a step. I do my best to clean up the house, say a prayer of thanks for getting through twenty-four hours with tolerable pain, and put the whole experience out of mind. The whole Arpaio circus has some screwy sideshows to it, but it is a deterrent. No more a deterrent than any other short stay in a jail, just a lot weirder. Nobody in his right mind would ever go through that twice. Just like in the movies.

"You'll never take me alive. I can't go back there."

141. NEW BUMPS IN THE ROAD

I was thinking that once I'd finished my brief stint in the tents, life would return to some semblance of normal. Not by a long shot. March and April were chock full of fun DUI-related activities. There was an eight-hour session of Traffic Survival School. There was attendance at one AA meeting. There was a series of eight weekly group counseling sessions for substance abuse. That assignment I actually enjoyed-- some of the folks there had taken very interesting paths to arrive there with me, and the lady who ran the program was a good moderator. Of all the parts involved in going through the DUI process, I'd have to say the group sessions were the most memorable and the most insightful for me.

In early March, the city notified the state Board of Medical Examiners of my DUI. That triggered a whole new cascade of activities. I was interviewed by an addictionologist. Although it's a long word, I think you can figure out what he does. I think he'd been an E.R. doc as well, had gone through rehab and recovery years ago, the route many take to addictionology. Nice guy, easy to talk to, good at what he did. I took the bus across town and back to see him; at this point in time, I was petrified of being involved in a motor vehicle accident. I even had a dream of a cab driver launching his taxi, with me in the back seat, over a bridge and down into the Grand Canyon. A modified *Thelma and Louise.* In the dream, I checked to make sure my seat belt was fastened, then taped a bag of marshmallows to my forehead to soften the landing. A hefty platter of fatalism seasoned lightly with optimistic futility.

There were more forms to be completed and letters to be sent, giving my side of the story. In the future, when the investigation was concluded, there would be a hearing before the board. The whole time, I had the foreboding that, dead or alive, I'd probably never practice medicine again. This concept, like everything else going on around me, left me feeling absolutely nothing. While some parts of my brain were working a little better, the emotional numbness was far worse than after my first surgery. Since the pump wasn't involved the second time around, I figured either the anesthesia had done a number on my remaining brain cells or I'd had a little stroke while on the table. I remembered Frank telling me in November that he thought I had some inflammatory thing going on in my vessels. It was a long time before I related that possibility to what was happening, or better yet, what was not happening, in my squash.

Around the middle of April, I started having "spells". The first one occurred one night at a local blues club. I was sitting talking with a guy I'd just met. While waiting for the headliner to come on stage, we shared stories of concerts we'd attended in the 70s. I was talking. The next thing I knew, he was staring at me.

"Are you okay?"

"Sure. Why?"

"You were talking and all of a sudden you stopped and just stared." I had no idea what he was talking about, but I couldn't remember what we were discussing. Just then the band walked on stage and that was that.

About ten days later, I was sitting out back watching the stars. It was getting close to my bedtime, around 9:00. I watched a shooting star arc its way across the sky, southwest to northeast, same as always, to disappear near the summit of Squaw Peak. The next thing I knew, the glass of water I'd been holding was lying in my lap. I felt my shorts. Wet and cold, not warm. Now the previous episode made sense. I knew something was up; I also knew I hadn't peed my pants.

There were a couple more similar episodes at night over the next month or so. Brief loss of consciousness, but no shaking--my muscles didn't hurt--or tongue biting. I figured I was experiencing absence seizures--no aura, short-lived, no confusion afterward--but it's pretty rare for them to start when you're fifty. Maybe complex partial seizures, but the lack of accompanying symptoms didn't seem to fit.

The good news is that they always occurred at night, right around my usual bedtime. I stopped driving at night and went to bed earlier. That first year I had some wild dreams, so maybe one or two of these spells occurred while I was asleep. Since then, I've had some weird experiences, almost always when I've stayed up too late at night two nights in a row. Of course, like everything else, "late" is relative. For me, anything past 9:00 P.M. is uncharted territory. I just put this new complication down to gradually maturing scar tissue from brain damage during my time on the pump. I also got to bed early.

As the pains from my surgery gradually resolved, I realized I was having attacks of angina again. Unlike the ones before each of my surgical procedures, bending forward during exertion sometimes made them come on, but mostly it was when I found myself lifting something heavy overhead. That didn't happen much the first few months. My friend Al the cardiologist had warned me not to lift weights, not even light ones, for at least six months after my original sternotomy. Not a problem. That time limit expired a little more than a month after my thoracotomy.

These anginal pains were mild and brief, lasting only five minutes. They were in the same location, deep inside my left shoulder blade, which, ironically, was where all my post-op pain had been centered after the thoracotomy in January. Emotional stress seemed to bring them on more easily, so I figured at least some part of it was in my head. Anyway, they made me stop doing what I was doing for a few minutes, but they never got severe, so I decided I'd live with them until it was time to do something, whatever and whenever that is.

My friends and co-workers continued to support me, coming over to visit, bringing lunch, taking me out for dinner, helping with my transportation needs. When you work with them every day, it's very easy to take the caring attitude of nurses and doctors for granted. Obviously I'd lucked into a vein of precious gems. I knew I didn't deserve their kindness toward me, but I sure appreciated it.

Before I got sick, it wasn't uncommon for a bunch of us to go out after a day shift, have a drink, and commiserate about the day and conditions in general. That was one of the best things about working where I did. Good people, not afraid to verbalize their feelings to one another, but not whiners either. Once I became ill, they were kind enough to include me in these after-work sessions. It took a while, but gradually I realized I was traveling in a different orbit than the one I'd occupied most of my adult life.

When the conversation got around to the department heads, there was general agreement that dealing with them was the least lovable aspect of the job. Safely ensconced on the dole, with nobody to answer to, I began thinking, *You don't have to put up with that crap. You should quit. Even though you've been working in the same place for fifteen years, you can get a job anywhere. No big deal.*

As impractical and totally screwed-up as my thoughts were, as long as they remained just thoughts, they weren't doing anyone any harm. I'd come home and obsess about the injustices my friends and co-workers were suffering. That would have been fine, but then I had to take it one step more. One evening I gave voice to the thoughts in my head. They looked at me as if I were crazy. It finally dawned on me that, yes, they did have to take that shit, just like me and everyone else in the working world. And yes, my thinking that everyone had my "freedom" was indeed crazy.

That didn't make me pull away, but it made me realize that my situation, at least at present, was completely abnormal. After a while I saw that I was developing a cold numbness that separated me from everyone else on earth. I'd never felt so alone, but in a strange way, I felt that I deserved it. If I couldn't produce, function as a member of a team, I didn't have a place in society. Somewhere inside me, I felt I didn't deserve the love and companionship of other human beings. I hoped my daughter didn't come to the same conclusion about me. She was my last connection to humanity.

Talk about dumping your mess on someone else.

142. BOMEX

In Arizona, you must renew your license to practice medicine on an annual basis. In the renewal packet is a list of the Board's requirements. In the event of an arrest or conviction, you are required to notify the Board within a certain number of days. If you bothered to read that and the other rules and regulations included in the packet, you would know this. Perhaps the worst individual in the history of medicine when it comes to reading rules and regulations, I checked all the boxes, sent in the check, and received my license renewal year after year. The informational portion of the packet, the stuff I was supposed to read before checking and signing and sending, went into a file I labeled "To Be Read". If I were honest with myself, it would have read "To Be Ignored".

The Board of Medical Examiners does not like it when you don't volunteer information. I had a phone interview during which the investigator brought up an arrest from about ten or twelve years prior. I'd gone to a local restaurant and had two drafts while I ate and watched a Suns game for two hours. On my way home, I came around a corner, swerved to avoid a rodent, and got pulled over. After all was said and done, I was arrested for a DUI. I thought there was no way I was over the limit, but kept my mouth shut. What started out as a DUI ended up as weaving over the line; the breathalyzers in the Phoenix PD DUI vans were out of whack, significantly exaggerating the blood alcohol level. No credit for not killing the rodent.

I found out that I was also being charged by the board for patient endangerment. That one didn't sound right, so I asked which patients were endangered. I was told that any time a physician was arrested, the patient endangerment charge was thrown in as a bonus. *Okay, your ball, your game, your rules.* I understood the rules: If you fuck up, don't expect karma, or anybody else for that matter, to reward you with a surprise party.

In June 2006, I signed an Interim Consent Agreement for Practice Restriction. The first time through I didn't comprehend what it entailed. My attention span was virtually nil, and multiple re-reads of the document didn't make it any clearer. I think the takeaway was that I couldn't practice medicine for the time being. From my perspective, it didn't matter anyway. I couldn't fathom going back to take care of sick, complicated patients anytime soon. I re-read the letter a little while ago. It turns out my license was restricted because the Board recognized that my medical condition precluded my practicing medicine on live human beings. In retrospect, I couldn't agree more.

When my annual medical license renewal packet arrived in July 2006, I wasn't sure what to do with it. I called the office of the Board and spoke to the very nice lady who ran the place. I understood her to say that I should wait to hear from the Board before renewing.
In December, 2006, four months after I should have renewed, I received a letter from the board stating that, because I hadn't renewed, my license had expired. Huh? However, it went on to say, because a license can't expire during an ongoing investigation, my license was merely suspended. Double Huh. Even reading it now, I don't understand the distinction. Back then, having not practiced for almost a year, I scratched my head and filed it away.

In April 2007, I received a notice to appear before the Board a month hence. The letter stated that I could bring an attorney with me if I wanted to. *Just what I need, another attorney. That should simplify things.* My sole issue concerned the patient endangerment charge, but from conversations I had with various representatives of the Board, it was clear that they'd never remove that one. That charge put their personal stamp on the whole deal; not only was I a bad citizen, but a bad doctor as well. I might not agree with that, but it wasn't my call. The whole time I was going through the process, I was pretty sure I'd never go back to practicing medicine anyway. I could have just refused to participate and turned in my license right then and there, but I figured whatever they dished out, I had it coming, and ducking the hearing seemed a tad cowardly. Anyway, I had about a month to decide what I wanted to do. A couple of phone calls in the following days made my decision much easier.

143. NUMBER, PLEASE?

There were only a couple of weeks until my scheduled appearance before the Board of Medical Examiners. I had the twenty-four hours in Tent City in my rearview mirror and was finished with all the classes required by the conviction. My brain was still a pile of mush, and, despite doing all the things the experts recommended for improving my memory, I still felt unable to retain information, events, faces, names. What stuck and what didn't was a flip of the coin. It seemed that the more important or relevant a piece of information, the more likely I was to forget it. I had no idea whether I'd ever practice medicine again. I did grasp that I was in no shape to go back to caring for critically ill patients in the E.R. or the units. I'd begun to realize that something was looking out for me; things weren't going as planned, but they were going. I left decisions about my future up to the universe.

Just about ten days before my hearing, in the middle of the afternoon, I received a phone call. The voice wasn't familiar, but her name was. I had met her and her husband a few months prior at a quasi-hospital function. He was a physician on the hospital staff, but we'd never worked together on a case, and I'd never seen him in the E.R. When we met, she and I talked about golf and the Desert Botanical Garden. Other than that she was involved with a few charities around town, I didn't know much about her. After inquiring about my health, she asked me if I'd mind writing her a prescription.

Rather than just hang up on her, I asked, "Prescription for what?"

"Oh, just some Ambien. My doctor is on vacation and I have to travel overseas."

My first thought was, *How did she get my home phone number? Oh yeah, that's right, it's in the book.* Then I thought, *Boy, did you call the wrong guy.* I can remember writing only one prescription for someone as a favor. A nurse at one of the hospitals where I'd worked about seven years earlier asked for a prescription for her child. Apparently the kid suffered from frequent ear infections and they always resolved with one particular antibiotic. There was some problem getting in to see the pediatrician, so I wrote what she asked. About a week later she confronted me and threatened to sue me; the kid had developed a rash and blah, blah, blah. After that, I refused to write prescriptions for anyone without a chart and a documented exam. Staff members in hospitals are accustomed to getting docs to write scripts for them or their families, usually antibiotics, so I was christened "Dr. No". That's not the only reason they thought of me as a butthole, but it was a big one. Eventually, they stopped asking me to do what most docs do routinely.

So now I have this woman, some doctor's wife, hitting me up for controlled substances. I thought about calling her husband, or notifying her physician, but I thought, *Aw hell, just let it go.* I told her I never prescribed meds outside of the E.R. She persisted a little and then hung up. I stood there for a minute with the phone in my hand. Even if my brain were working normally, none of that would have made any sense. I hung up and went back to working on whatever pointless task I'd chosen for the day.

A few days later I was doing some house cleaning when the phone rang. It was on the weekend, probably Saturday. I was waiting for my daily dose of morning sickness to clear so that I could eat. A very attractive voice said hello and introduced herself. I thought to myself, *Man, what did I do to become so popular with the lady callers?* Her name was unfamiliar to me. She said she was thinking of starting a charity to provide health care to the underserved. Would I be willing to write prescriptions for their patients? Just like that.

"I'm not in a good place mentally to be taking care of patients right now. As a matter of fact, I'm retired on disability for the foreseeable future."

"Yes, so I heard. We wouldn't need you to examine patients, just write prescriptions." *Uh-oh.* I was just starting to believe that a simple job in a clinic might be a first step back to practicing medicine. If it didn't work out, I could walk away with little or no harm done. This didn't have the ring of "strictly on the up and up" to it.

I lied, "Well, I could write scripts, I guess, but I don't have a DEA number anymore." In order to prescribe controlled substances of any kind, you have to have a number from the Drug Enforcement Agency. No DEA number means no narcs, no Ambien, no Valium, no fun drugs. My DEA number was good through the end of the year. There was the matter of my expired, nay, suspended license.

"Oh. Well, could you get one?" Like I thought, she wasn't after me to write for ampicillin or blood pressure meds. I wondered about the identities of these "underserved patients".

"No, I don't think that would be a good idea. How about a ballpark figure on the salary?" After a few more minutes of chit-chat, she hung up. She was vague on the pay issue, but it sounded like I'd be paid for each prescription I wrote. I thought about it for a minute or so, then realized my nausea had passed, so I made lunch. *Maybe I should talk on the phone every morning.*

Later that afternoon, I mused over the two calls. At first I tried to figure out whether they were related or just random chance. There had to be some link between the two, unless the second caller had connections to the hospital. It wasn't like my retirement was front page news. Then I realized it didn't matter either way, as there was no chance of my getting involved. I had enough to worry about without landing in the middle of some drug-prescribing mess.

After a day or so, I came to the conclusion that, given my lack of judgment and a longstanding love affair with co-dependency, sooner or later someone would convince me to "help them out". Sure as shit, I'd end up as the fall guy. Life was simple, a tad boring perhaps, but I could do without that kind of excitement.

People wonder why I don't like to talk on the phone.

144. BEFORE THE BOARD

When I received the letter with the date of my appearance before the Board, I was filled with dread at having to be judged yet again by my peers. Countering that was a sense that, once the hearing was over, I could get on with my life, whatever that was to be.

Immediately after the two drug solicitation phone calls, I decided to remove myself from consideration for any other "job opportunities". I wasn't working as a physician, I didn't think I'd be working any time soon, and keeping up with the requirements of holding a license to practice medicine would have been senseless. When it was time to renew my registration with the DEA, I let it lapse, so there was no way I could write prescriptions for controlled substances.

The night before my hearing, I was firmly in the corner of retiring for the foreseeable future and letting my license lapse. The next morning, however, while getting dressed, I flip-flopped again and decided that, depending on what the Board ruled, I'd hang onto my license to practice medicine in Arizona for at least another year. That is, if the "suspended" status could be changed to "inactive".

The Board has nice, relatively new digs out in Scottsdale. Ironically, until a few years prior, they were headquartered a ten-minute walk from my home. Because my appearance was scheduled after the morning rush hour, I decided to drive over, rather than mess with the public transit system. There wasn't much traffic; good thing, because a massive attack of vertigo, my first ever, hit me two-thirds of the way over. It started with a familiar sensation. As I drove, it felt like movie images were flashing by on either side of my head. I'd experienced that for almost a year after my surgeries, so it didn't worry me. The next thing I knew, the road was moving side to side. I felt like I was spinning around like a top. Fortunately, I was able to pull into a gas station and park the car without hitting anything.

I dry-heaved a couple of times into a plastic bag, which I carried with me wherever I went, then reclined my seat back as far down as possible. Despite the air conditioning blowing full-force, my face and clothes were drenched in sweat. No chest or back pain, no numbness or weakness in my arms or legs. That was all good. I wasn't hyperventilating. I wasn't sure what to do next, so I did nothing, just lay there with my eyes closed for a good five minutes. Once vertigo strikes, it usually sticks around for hours or days; I started thinking about how I was going to get home feeling the way I did. To my surprise, the nausea left, then the spinning, and my face stopped dripping. Ten minutes later, I still felt shaky but well enough to try driving. I considered calling the Board secretary and telling her I was too sick to appear, but I'd been dreading this day for long enough that I didn't want to postpone it and start all over.

When I arrived at the Board offices, there was a vacant parking spot right in front of the glass doors. After opening my car door, I bent forward, pretending to adjust my shoe. I wanted to see if moving my head would cause the vertigo again. Staggering out of my car into a Board hearing probably wouldn't do much for my case. Everything seemed okay. I had no idea what had caused the vertigo, nor why it had resolved so quickly. I put on my sport coat, which covered the wet spots nicely, tightened my tie, grabbed some gum, and walked in, a little shaky but able to walk a straight line. At least it felt like I was.

Inside I checked in and took a seat in the waiting area. The receptionist told me I was on deck. Ironically, the doc ahead of me was there for repeated abuse of his prescribing privileges, among other transgressions. I thought to myself, *How many times does the universe have to send you a warning before you get it through your thick skull that it's time? The phone calls, the vertigo, now this guy ahead of you showing what's in store for you if you don't pull the trigger.* That's when I decided to retire, at least for a while, until I was in better shape to practice. The way I was feeling right then, I couldn't have dressed myself, let alone taken care of a sick patient.

When I was called into the hearing room, I passed by the prescription guy in the hallway. He didn't look happy or sad, just kind of shell-shocked. I walked down to a table and sat down. There were other chairs there, I guess in case I brought along a lawyer or two. The members of the Board sat up on a low stage behind a row of desks or a table, I forget which. Each one had a name tag in front.

Someone up there read the story of my offenses. There was the DUI, the previous arrest, not informing the Board about either, and the patient endangerment charge. I thought about challenging the latter, but realized it would be fruitless and meaningless. When the reading was done, I had the opportunity to make a statement. I told them I'd made a series of bad choices and I regretted them all. I kept it short and sweet. I was feeling a little lightheaded and wanted to be done with this and out the door before anything else happened inside my head.

One or two Board members asked me questions. One crabby old fuck decided to get his licks in. He made a sarcastic reference to my "bad choices" statement, which was fine by me, but then ended up with some gibberish that went right over my head. The other Board members looked down at their papers. Obviously, they were used to this. He struck me as a back shooter. I looked at him, wondering if a response was expected. The Executive Director, a lawyer I think, broke the silence. He said the Board would make a decision. I didn't want to interrupt him, but I was starting to feel a little queasy again, and I wanted out before I had to resort to my spare barf bag.

"Sir, I've decided that I'm not going to practice medicine any more. My medical condition hasn't improved enough for me to return to work any time soon. I don't know what effect that will have on your decision, but I thought you should know."

Apparently I caught them by surprise. The norm was for a doctor to do anything he could to keep his license. I'd heard of guys going for six months or more to rehab facilities, paying all sorts of fines, being on probation for five years. I was still worried that one of my grafts would clot off and I'd suffer a fatal MI. I certainly didn't want to leave town, only to drop dead far away from home, getting rehabbed for a job to which I'd probably never return. My only goal in life was to spend as much quality time as possible with my daughter. Once I'd told them that, I felt an enormous rush of relief. I couldn't believe it had been such a difficult decision. I was finally done with all the legal consequences of my bad choices.

The Executive Director looked around at the rest of the Board members, then told me again that they would decide and inform me at a later date. I thanked him, got up, and walked out. I thought everything was done.

If anything was said at the May 2007 hearing about my failure to renew, it sure didn't sink in. In July 2007, I received a letter from the Board requesting my presence at another hearing in August. I sent a letter to the Board outlining my history and my understanding of the license issue. I apologized and said I wouldn't be able to attend, as my daughter and I would be out of town for my birthday. The Board decided on a letter of reprimand.

If you look me up on the AZ Board of Medical Examiners website, you will see that my license expired on December 21, 2006. My letter of reprimand, however, states that my license expired upon the resolution of my case, on August 10, 2007, two years and five days after the plaque in my left main ruptured in that parking garage in Portland. The outcome, that I would probably never practice medicine again, was expected. In terms of my license, "expired" sounded better than "cancelled" or "revoked" or "suspended"; the fact that I'd apparently screwed up again bothered me for months. I was beginning to think I'd never do anything worthwhile again. On the other hand, I was amazed that I had survived to see my daughter graduate from eighth grade. As is human nature, I started bargaining for another four years. Sticking around for her graduating from high school and heading off to college seemed like a worthy goal.

Over the years I have come face-to-face with a handful of physicians who had to go before the Board. While some of them were pretty matter-of-fact about their experiences, a few complained that the Board was out to get them or overly punitive for their offenses. I didn't see any of that, just a bunch of physicians and members of the community doing a job with little reward but plenty of second-guessing, both by the medical profession and the public at large. Overall, I feel that I got a fair shake from them.

145. ESCAPE BY A HAIR

If you were born an ugly boy, you can find solace in the fact that, no matter how long your parents let your hair grow, odds are you won't be mistaken for a girl. If, however, they haven't had a haircut by the age of two, cute little boys, especially blonds and kids with curly hair, can make a casual observer scratch his head in gender wonder. Such was the case with my nephew in San Diego. His twin sister, a redhead with the personality to match, would never be mistaken for anything other than a princess.

Their second birthday was approaching. The kid had beautiful blonde hair, wavy to mildly curly. Although he wore your basic toddler boy gear, you could see strangers speculating in their heads, especially if they saw him from behind. I arrived on a Friday afternoon. Apparently the discussion had been taking place all week. He had a subtle look of terror smeared across his freckles. The event was tentatively scheduled to take place the following morning. He verbalized the universal question posed to parents on every new adventure involving professional adults.

"Does it hurt?" He looked at me. I resolved to let the four of them work out the details. In certain situations, my sense of humor does not help defuse tension. Make that most situations. I peeled the edges of the beer bottle label with my thumbnail and feigned hearing loss.

"No, Aaron, it won't hurt. Right, Dad?" This from his mother, my sister.

"No, absolutely not. No pain at all." As nervous as the little guy was, his dad was even more so. Aaron picked up on that, now less convinced than ever of the safety of the impending procedure. Despite my non-involvement resolve, I could see this going sideways, making for a long night for all concerned.

"Tell you what, Aaron." His head swiveled my way. "I'll get my hair cut while you're getting yours, okay?" Uncle Frank to the rescue. My sister jumped up, grabbed my empty beer bottle and fished me out a fresh one.

As she sat down, my sister said, "That's great, Uncle Frank! Hear that, Aaron? Uncle Frank will get a haircut too, just to show you how easy it is." She was sounding a little shrill.

"You will?"

"Sure," I said. " You'll be doing me a favor. I was hoping I'd have someone to get their hair cut with me so I wouldn't be lonely. But it's very important that you have a good night's sleep before a haircut, especially your first. So if we're going to do this, you have to sleep tonight, okay?"

"Okay." We shook hands.

The next morning, after my usual dry heaves, I headed down for some coffee. They had this world-class coffee maker, an Italian forerunner of the Keurig system, that nobody seemed to know how to operate. Neither one of them drank coffee on a regular basis back then; they'd bought this chunk of steel and oak because they'd seen one at some rich guy's place in San Francisco during a Raiders' weekend. Half the time I ended up driving to Starbuck's for an Americano. I was about three months out from my second bypass surgery, still weighing in at a whopping one hundred fifty-two pounds of skin, bone and flab. A good day meant I dry-heaved a half-dozen times around 6 A.M., and liquids were tolerable by 8. Bad days I'd be lucky to eat or drink anything before noon. Pretty much accepting this as the new normal, I'd given up the idea of ending up old and fat; neither seemed attainable.

Aaron was excited. His folks had been giving him the specifics on the barbershop experience. Courtesy of his dad, he developed more of a fascination with the trappings than with the procedure itself. He wanted to know how the drape stayed on around his neck. There was some concern about choking. We headed out, Ray and Aaron and I, to the local clip joint franchise. I was already looking forward to an Americano at the coffee shop next door before the haircut. If that stayed down and I didn't start to blow last night's dinner during my time in the chair, some kind of Arnold Palmer would be waiting for me afterwards. With any luck, meaning I didn't puke on my barber and Aaron wasn't strangled by his, we'd all celebrate with lunch on the beach in Del Mar.

We were in luck. There were four doting young Latinas working that day, and the place was empty. The sleek little gazelle of the crew, a thirtyish woman named Dee, sat me in a chair and did the clipper thing. At the time, my head was crowned by a snow-white version of a crew cut, which took all of ten minutes to trim to virtual nothingness.

To my right, the other three young ladies, all of large proportions, were fussing over Aaron. I could barely see his little yellow head. Surrounded by six huge tracts of land, no doubt taking in the exotic aromas of three different perfumes, his eyes were glazed over. One of the ladies rubbed his shoulders, one stood right in front of him cooing his name and chatting with him, and the third snipped away with her shears. Long fine strands of blonde hair cascaded to the floor. After a bit, one of the other ladies went to work on the left side of his dome. Ray was jumping around, making like Shecky the emcee at a bar mitzvah, snapping endless photos of Aaron in Boobie Heaven.

I stayed in my chair until he was done. The coffee had gone down well, but no sooner had Dee finished my haircut than I began to feel a little queasy and weak. That happened from time to time, whether I ate or drank or not. Usually it would resolve in five minutes or so. This time, however, it stayed. I told Ray I had to go lie down at home. Aaron couldn't stop talking about his new experience. Getting up from the barber chair, I almost passed out. I made it home without getting sick, fell into bed, and slept for two hours.

A couple months later, on a trip to New York and Boston to scout out colleges with my daughter, I'd undergone another haircut in Cambridge Square. The young guy who performed the procedure was a surgeon with his clippers. Again I'd felt queasy for a few days afterwards.

Now, four months after Aaron's first haircut, still nauseated, weak and forgetful, I returned to San Diego for a few days. Each week following my last haircut I had felt perhaps a tiny bit better. No weight gain, but no loss either. There had apparently been a family discussion before I arrived. Aaron was excited.

"Uncle Frank, can we get our hair cut tomorrow? You and me?" No fear this time. I think he was looking forward to another trip to Breastonia.

I almost said, "Sure", but something inside made me hold back. Instead, I came up with, "Aaron, I'll go with you and sit next to you; I haven't decided whether to get my hair cut this time." Normally my hair grows very quickly, but after two months, it was all of an inch long. In four months, Aaron's had grown at least three. "I think my hair stopped growing! I might have to wait a few months." He gave me a funny look, betrayed, like I'd spilled the beans about the secret handshake, but took the news like a trooper.

As it turned out, the next morning the same delightful young ladies were in attendance and remembered him. "Ooh, Aaron's back!". His worried look melted away as they escorted him to the chair. They went to work right away, enveloping him just as before. The sleek gazelle, Dee, fetching in an orange and black outfit, was there as well. She had a customer in her chair when we arrived, but she graced me with her dazzling smile while I waited my turn. At first Aaron gave me a funny look when he saw me sitting in one of the waiting room chairs. After I offered him a thumbs-up and a smile, he seemed satisfied.

Dee finished with her customer in about five minutes. I stood up and walked over to her chair. Before I sat down, I noticed her state license on the wall next to the big mirror. Over fifty with rapidly deteriorating reading vision, I couldn't make out much of the print. However, I could see that both her first and last name were more than three letters. She walked over to me.

"Nice to see you again. We were all very excited when we heard that Aaron was coming in today." She looked over at the ladies working on my nephew and said something in Spanish. They all giggled. Then Dee pulled out a drape to put on me.

"I can't read your license. Is Dee your real name?"

"That's what everyone calls me. I'm Dee Hernandez." She stuck out her hand and we shook.

"I'm Frank Price."

"Nice to meet you, Frank Price." She picked up her scissors and comb. "Would you like anything special today, Frank Price?"

I thought, *Boy, would I.* For some reason, I asked, "Is Dee short for Delores?"

"No. Guess again."

I thought for a few seconds. "Deena?"

"Deena? No!" She laughed and took the certificate off the wall and handed it to me.

There it was. Not Delores and not Deena either. I jumped out of the chair and handed her back her license.

"Dee, please accept my apology. I don't feel too well. We'll have to do this another time." I pulled off the apron and headed for the door. I looked back briefly. She had a hurt look on her face, but then she smiled and winked at me.

"See you again, Frank Price."

"Yes. Perhaps you will, Delilah."

146. CHANGES FOR THE BETTER

Still the skinniest Santa, I made it through the 2006 holidays. Just before Thanksgiving I found out Ari would be staying with me for the month of February while her mom did a stretch at Harvard. At the end of 2005, in possibly the dumbassest financial move ever, after a five-vessel bypass and three stents, I talked myself into the notion that I could be a rental investor. I believed that purchasing a stucco shitbox 90 minutes away and renting it to itinerant construction workers would be the beginning of a new career. My daughter, all of thirteen years old at the time, warned me that the real estate lady I was working with, a "friend", was not to be trusted. Naturally, I ignored her this time and every time she gave me sound financial and life experience advice. If you are going to fuck up on a regular basis, it is mandatory that you ignore any and all warning signs the universe or its designees sends your way. After the first renter moved out three months in arrears, my next tenant, a one-hundred-thirty-pound bucket of slime with a bad attitude, moved in and promptly started making meth in the garage, where he, his skank girlfriend and their four pit bulls ended up living when all the utilities were cut off for non-payment. Judging by the burn marks and the bleach bottles that littered the garage floor, they kept themselves warm by sleeping next to their sterno meth stove. I didn't want to think about where they were doing their toilet time; hopefully it was at the Burger King a half-mile away. After the mandated ninety-day grace period, they were evicted the last week of January, 2007. I researched suspicious house fires on the internet. Not many went unsolved.

I resolved to make our month together most excellent. During her school day, I would be making daily ninety-mile round trips out to the rental to clean up burned food, unclog plumbing, repaint everything, and then arrange for housecleaners and rug specialists to remove all evidence of the animals, and their pit bulls too. Just about a year out from my last bypass surgery, I still had that dark, cold, hollow numbness inside me, filled, warmed and lit only when my favorite person in the world was within sight. A month of full-time Ari in the house was more than I could hope for. We had been back to our usual overnight schedule for about eight months or so, and, at least from my perspective, it was going as well as I dared hope. I was still a dud to be around, but my girl was a trooper and proved to be a big help with chores.

Each month since I had eluded Delilah I felt a little stronger. I was still having anginal pain up by my left shoulder blade three or four times a day, but it didn't leave me with that hopelessly weak feeling I'd had before the second bypass. The other multiple surgical pains had mostly disappeared. I was doing more manual labor around the property. Driving was not quite as frightening, but I still had visual difficulties, so I walked, rode my bike, or took the bus whenever possible. My memory and ability to concentrate weren't much better; the disability insurance carrier had determined that I was permanently unemployable in the E.R. I could find no evidence to the contrary. On the positive side, my hair was back to growing normally. I was now sporting three-inch white strands. Reminiscent of Andy Warhol, but without his classic rugged good looks.

I started growing a beard my senior year in college. It pretty much followed the accelerated pube schedule. By December it was full and dark. In photos, which consisted of student IDs and my Franklin Mint summer employee card, I looked years older, i.e., older than twelve, and a good one-and-one-half stone heavier, which would put me right about one hundred thirty pounds. I kept the beard through my first year of medical school, then made a habit of shaving it off each summer. At the end of my second year, just after I had shaved it off, I was invited to an ex-girlfriend's wedding. I would not have gone, but a very cute friend of hers needed a ride, so I thought, *Why not?* After all this was the Culpeper Baptist social event of the year. After the ceremony, it was either go through the receiving line or climb out a church window. I came up to kiss the bride, the groom eyeing me the whole time.

She looked at me funny. "Oh, you shaved off your beard."

"Yeah. What do you think?" Never ask an ex-anything how she thinks you look.

"You should grow it right back. You don't look good at all without it."

"Oh."

So I kept the beard another twenty-plus years. Didn't even shave it in the summer. Finally, after more than two decades, it all went gray, so it all went away. I ran into her a few years after that.

"Thank God you got rid of that awful beard. That thing was so ugly." She said this in a nice way.

"You told me at your wedding I looked awful without it." So clueless.

"I just said that so girls wouldn't be attracted to you. Don't you know that sixty percent of the women in the United States prefer a man with no facial hair at all, eighty percent with no beard?" I do now.

The head of gray hair I sported in the early 2000s before my surgery was not a bad look. Somewhere in there I was mistaken for Mark Harmon by a Phoenix restaurateur, who said he'd met me--I mean Mark--in California years ago. His folie-a-douze was shared by his wife and about ten other diners. I was pleasantly shocked for a minute or two. For the price of a round of drinks, I autographed one of his menus. It's not a good idea to burst the bubble of someone who is preparing your food. My date apparently could not see the resemblance.

"Don't you want to be able to say you spent the night with Mark Harmon?"

"Good night, Mark."

At the beginning of 2007, my Andy Warhol was pure white, but as it grew, the new stuff was more of my usual salt and pepper. In Phoenix, winter is the only time you can lie out in the sun without serious risk of spontaneous combustion. On a few January afternoons I spent half an hour napping out back mostly naked in a chaise longue. There still wasn't much besides skin, bones and flab, but the pasty translucent look was beginning to disappear behind a pigmented surface layer. Not much progress had been made on the dry heave front. I was still spending fifteen to thirty minutes hanging out in the bathroom every morning. When Ari stayed over, weather permitting, I'd get up extra early and do my hurling outside so she wouldn't hear me. It was rare that I could eat breakfast with her, but I'd hang out at the table, talking, doing crossword puzzles, hoping to avoid a dash to the bathroom before I took her to school.

Dinner was a different story. Although I no longer experienced hunger, most nights I could eat pretty well without feeling sick afterwards. Ari became a good little salad chef and enjoyed prepping the various ingredients before we cooked Chinese in a wok out back. Towards the end of our first week together in February, I got weighed at a doctor's appointment. I was two pounds heavier than at a previous six-month checkup, the first demonstrable weight gain since my initial bypass surgery almost eighteen months earlier.

By the end of the month, I was no longer heaving and I could eat breakfast with my little cure every morning. Despite my continuing angina, I no longer dreaded getting up in the morning to face a new day. The rental house, one of thousands out in the hinterland-turned-boomtown-turned-bustville, drifted from my consciousness into the hazy miasma of short sale. If only I'd listened to my teenaged sage. If only. Lucky for her, she has always been smart enough to listen to her gut. And ignore me.

147. FRANK THE BUILDER

In my darkest hours, usually the middle of the night, all through 2006, my greatest fear had been that I wouldn't live to see my daughter graduate from eighth grade. Despite Dr. Brady's statement that I wouldn't need any additional procedures for twenty years, I was unable to envision my place on earth for even the near future. I made all sorts of deals, perhaps in my head, perhaps aloud; my perception of reality was so scrambled I usually couldn't tell the difference. I begged of whoever was listening, I didn't care who, to just let me live through the end of May, 2007. According to a number of reliable individuals, I keep getting better-looking, so it was probably the devil who answered my prayers. The Dorian Gray day of reckoning will not be pretty. Look for a trocar-worthy event--green slime and putrid gas.

Ari's graduation from eighth grade went perfectly. Everybody attended, her Mom had a terrific reception in her home, and I got to talk with people I hadn't seen since our divorce. Although these were the friends her Mom got to keep in the breakup, everyone was very cordial towards me. I was finally gaining weight, but I still looked frail enough to evoke a nice chunk of pity. That night, at home, I thought to myself, *Well, I made it. Now what?*

My appetite almost back to normal, I was gaining a little weight. My exercise consisted almost entirely of walking three miles a day and taking care of the landscaping chores around the property. I tried getting back into lifting light weights, but that only brought on angina. Besides, the whole idea of getting stronger and building muscles just for the sake of looking better seemed ridiculously shallow. I figured I'd look like I was eighty until I was eighty, so what was the point? I was starting to take an interest in women again, but I still felt empty inside, and I hadn't the energy to disguise that with a more attractive outside. So I kept walking. It got me out of the house and I derived some pleasure in watching normal people go about their daily lives.

I tried working on my brain, as that had always been my most productive organ. Women said they found intelligent men to be sexy and interesting, so I followed the advice of friends and family. For about a year I did at least two newspaper crossword puzzles every day, including the tough ones on the weekend. I tried reading all sorts of books designed to improve your memory, but, even after a third reading, the abstract concepts were impossible to comprehend, let alone retain. I even read medical journal articles, hoping they would electrify the cognitive portion of my brain. Nothing stuck. Again, I realized that improving my memory merely for the sake of improving my memory was a pretty silly idea. I didn't really need a better memory. In fact, I was expected to have a poor recent memory. After all, that's why I was retired on permanent disability.

So here I am in the summer of 2007, about a year and a half out from my last surgery, with a worthless brain and a worthless body. Had it not been for my daughter, I would have been hard-pressed to come up with a reason for living. Even with her I was little more than the guy who cooked dinner for her, took walks with her at night, came to support her at her games, and took her on trips. I was abjectly disappointed in myself and, rightly or wrongly, imagined that she felt the same disappointment in me. It was time to do something valuable, admirable, courageous, perhaps even noble. It had to be something worthwhile, something with a benefit beyond just the performance of the task itself, something that would improve both my mind and body, an achievement reflective of the Athenian ideals. Something creative, something constructive. But what could it be? It took me a week to figure out what to do: I'll put an addition onto Ari's room.

By the time I bought our house in the early 1990s, it had suffered the indignation of life as a rental for over a decade. All the 1940s knotty pine tongue and groove paneling had been covered with two or three coats of paint. There was dirty grey industrial berber carpeting throughout most of the house. It took almost a year, but I gutted Ari's room, repaneled the walls, built a bunk bed complete with sliding board, and had saltillo tile installed. What had once been a dark and depressing cave was now a small but bright bedroom suitable for a little girl. Then I went on to clean up the rest of the house. After removing, stripping, varnishing and reinstalling the paneling, a chore that took another year and a half, I was satisfied with the result. Adobe, tile and wood; rustic but serviceable.

Now, ten years later, I decided to add on a study and a bathroom to her bedroom. Having grown up in a succession of single bathroom homes, I didn't mind sharing. Apparently teenage girls don't particularly like using Dad's bathroom. I figured a new addition would kill two birds with one stone: a new place for Ari to hang out and a physical and mental challenge for me. I needed something to do with my mind and my body.

I won't bore you with all the details of that three-year process; that will be better served with, yes, another book. One thing I will say: along the way I learned a thing or two about me and about life. I came out of it with better energy, a somewhat better-functioning mind, and a few regrets. Initially, my plan was to hire an architect, then hire a general contractor to supervise the project. My job would be to watch, learn, and pay.

My first mistake was to hire an architect. Architects have no connection to a construction project. They are artists. You give them information, they draw a picture, you suggest some changes, they suggest some changes, and then they have someone in the office draw up the plans. At least that's how my architect experience went. In the end, I had plans for a four hundred square foot addition, single story with a deck on top. Twenty pages of plans. I thought that was a lot, but he assured me it was the standard size for a project of this magnitude.

Next I looked around for a general contractor. The final plans were approved by the city in August of 2008. By now, the entire country is well aware that the bubble has burst, particularly in the construction industry. Absolutely nobody is building anything. Nobody, not even the scavenger investors, have started buying up the foreclosures. Except for a few isolated pockets of ongoing prosperity, approximately one hundred percent of construction guys are unemployed. Phoenix is not one of those isolated pockets of prosperity. I expect that, given the situation, it should be relatively easy to find a general contractor who's hungry for work.

One of the first things I learned about the construction business is that even when times are bad, nobody wants to work for less than they were making when times were good. A few subcontractors are busting their asses to make ends meet, cutting their hourly wage and making up for it with volume. However, most of the contractors I found had no interest in working for any less than what they were charging during the height of the construction boom. Some were charging more, because they had moved into the high-end remodel business, specializing in overhauling second homes for the one percenters. Those who were willing to cut deals in these hard economic times took one look at the twenty pages of plans and ran the other way.

I decided, *Okay, screw them, I'll be the GC myself.* I had no idea how to read blueprints, had very little construction experience, and could barely plan a meal for two. Nonetheless, I figured it would be a challenge, and, after all, that's what I was looking for. I interviewed dozens of masonry guys, framers, plumbers, electricians. Same story. They'd rather sit on their asses at home than work for a lower wage. I decided there were some things I'd need a lot of time and a ton of experience to do adequately, things like plumbing, block work, slab pouring, drywall, electrical work. For those, I was going to have to pay top dollar. The rest, like framing and finish work, I could do myself. I had time, some strength, and the Internet. Over the years I'd specialized in doing two-man jobs solo; I enjoyed the challenge of using physics instead of two sets of hands.

For the first time since the beginning of my cardiac adventure, I had a long-term purpose in life beyond staying alive to see my daughter graduate from high school. To achieve the latter, it doesn't matter what time you get up in the morning, as long as you're still alive when you fall asleep that night. When you have a project, or, more commonly, a job, minutes matter. I found myself developing a routine. I learned what all the funny symbols on the blueprints meant. I learned that if you want to find a good block man, pile up a few cinder blocks out by the street next to your driveway. The first load got stolen. The next pile netted me a block master. It's a good thing Angie's List has so many subs in their files. Again, most of them were scared off by the copious fucking plans. I learned later that the architect's intern had drawn them up, his first attempt at planning out a project. I vowed that for my next project, should the opportunity arise, I'd find an ancient draftsman in a nursing home, tell him what I wanted, and pay him under the table.

The project took me the allotted two years plus a six-month grace period. Some of the time involved waiting for subs to show up, but most of it involved my doing something the wrong way, then having to take it apart and re-do it the right way. Much of that I attribute to mis-reading the plans, but, as the city building inspector put it, "I didn't know you could build a three-story bank in this part of town." One day, when he wasn't rushed, he took a look at all twenty pages, then estimated that my project could have been planned out in seven. I hope the architect intern got an "A" for his efforts. No. What I meant to say is, I hope he got an "F" for all my wasted efforts.

At this point, my angina qualified as "stable". I could perform plenty of strenuous tasks. Walking three miles at a twenty minute per mile pace was no problem. My back pain triggers were lifting heavy objects overhead and emotionally tense situations. Fortunately, the two stimuli rarely occurred at the same time. My biggest challenge was figuring a way to get the ceiling joists, which were twenty-foot-long 2 x 12's, up into the joist hangers without having to hoist them over my head. I'll reveal the secret in my book on remodeling for the novice.

During the project, on an average day, I experienced three or four episodes of my usual pain. They never lasted more than five minutes, and they were never more than mild. I was growing more comfortable with them, so the anxiety component was essentially eliminated. Most importantly, however, I was getting better at avoiding angina. Toward the end, I was able to feel it coming on, stop what I was doing, concentrate on something pleasant, walk around a bit, and actually prevent the anginal attack. I did a little research on that, and didn't find much in the peer-reviewed medical literature. I considered mentioning it to Frank, but that would have confirmed for him, at last, that I was fucking nuts.

On the mental side, deciding to pursue this project was the best thing I could have done. When you're on the dole, public or private, the easiest thing in the world is to put off something until the next day.

There's always tomorrow. I'd spent the better part of two years following that philosophy. If you look hard enough, you can always find something that will get in the way of what you want to accomplish. Building this addition, which was in no way necessary for me or my daughter to live a comfortable life, required that I use my brain. I had to get up every morning, look at what I'd done the day before, and make a reasonable estimate of what I could accomplish in the next eight to ten hours. Owing to my pathetic short-term memory, most days I was surprised at what I (or some invisible nocturnal laborer, but I was pretty sure it was me) had accomplished the day before. That part never ceased to amaze me.

If I didn't finish up where I expected to at the end of the day, I felt like a lazy fat ass, so I tended to be conservative in my daily estimates. As I grew more confident that I could make my work quota, I got faster at doing tasks, especially the repetitive ones, so I could increase my estimates without fear of failing. Most importantly, I had to work on one step and forget about the next step until I was done. "Little by little, one travels far." I'd never thought much about that saying, but now I was living it on a minute-by-minute basis.

When I finally finished up and received the COO (Certificate of Occupancy), my daughter was just about out the door, headed for college. In retrospect, the project was a waste of money. She didn't get to benefit from it the way I'd planned. On the other hand, I came out of it with some semblance of control of my angina and the confidence that I could plan, execute, and complete a task. I still couldn't cook a piece of fish without under- or overdoing it, but this was the best I'd felt about myself since before my surgery.

148. WINE, WOMEN AND SONG, MINUS THE LATTER TWO

I met my first non-medical employer in thirty years at a Christmas party in 2010. He lived to the east of Scottsdale, in a bedroom community called Fountain Hills. The town is named for a big fountain, the world's fourth largest, in the middle of the town. The guy who built la fontana, Robert McCulloch, also reconstructed the London Bridge in Lake Havasu City. When he built the fountain in 1970, it was the world's tallest. It has three pumps. Usually only two pumps are used, sending the plume of water over three hundred feet into the air. On special occasions, when all three pumps are used, the fountain jet reaches five hundred sixty feet, about five feet higher than the Washington Monument. Every day it erupts for fifteen minutes on the hour between 9 A.M. and 9 P.M. On St. Patrick's Day, the town throws in green dye. I don't know how they get rid of it the next day.

With my daughter out of town, by 2012 I was ready for a change. His vineyard and winery are about four hours southeast of my place; at an elevation over four thousand feet, there is none of the dreadful heat wave that tortures Phoenix from June through September. Nights down there are usually in the low fifties, as opposed to around ninety in the metroplex. It may surprise you to learn that arriving in summertime Phoenix is not exactly the same as happening upon Shangri-la. That is, unless your idea of Paradise is a populace in a perpetual battle with dehydration. A potent combo, hot dry climate and some of the hardest, most calcium-laden water on the face of the earth, keeps us neck-and-neck with Riyadh, Saudi Arabia for supremacy as the kidney stone capital of the world.

I agreed to come down and work full-time from mid-August through Halloween. He warned me the work would be hard, farm work with a lot of lifting. Other than that I'd undergone heart surgery in the past, I didn't mention my health issues; after all, I'd framed the addition to the house without cashing it in, and that turned out to be a huge boost to my confidence and to my health. Learning the rudiments of a new craft and helping out someone in need would be good for me. At least there wouldn't be any ladders or joists involved on the crush pad.

Wine tasting can be oh so romantic: the brilliant ruby clarity, the complex bouquet, the fruit forwardness on the palate, the yeasty aroma of the tasting room, the cute little clouds of drosophila melanogaster (fruit flies) circling your head and falling into your tasting glass. Oh and let's not forget the babbling bullshit that piles higher and deeper (Ph.D.) as the tasting day wears on.

The winemaking process, however, has nothing to do with romance. It is merely the combination of two distinct but intertwined processes: farming and chemistry. The farming is tricky because you are raising a very fragile crop. Grapes are not potatoes. One sub-Biblical plague of locusts or one five-minute hailstorm and you are done for the year--no revenue, no profit, no product, no fun. All you have to show for your time, money and effort are bushels of damaged or rotten grapes and one enormous tax write-off.

The chemistry is tricky too. You are orchestrating enzymatic processes involving a living organism--yeast. Too much or too little warmth, acid or sugar and you have ruined what might have been a world-class petite sirah. A pinhead of the wrong kind of bacteria can turn a barrel of beautiful cabernet sauvignon into three hundred bottles of very pricey red wine vinegar.

The nice thing about working a small winery is the variety of tasks you get to sample on a continuous basis. Prepping in the morning with the sanitizer gets old after the second blast of toxic chemicals scours your lungs, but everything else comes along at just about the right interval to keep the routines fresh in your mind. The boss had to re-instruct me on every step in the process at least three or four times. By the second month, I was retaining enough to pretend that I knew what I was doing and why. Other than planting and picking, which were done by a local crew of legal Hispanic immigrants who really did know what they were doing, I participated in every step in the process, from spraying weeds and training vines, destemming and pressing grapes, punching down the cap, and filtering the must, to filling, corking, labeling and boxing the final product, the bottle of wine.

The toughest thing about spending so much concentrated time down there was the isolation. Most days it was just he and I. On a big day there was a trip to the gas station--twelve miles--or a visit from the UPS guy. Willcox, a farm town to the north, as desolate a burg as you will find on I-10, is about forty-five miles away. To get to Bisbee, an old mining town down on the border which boasts nice bars and restaurants, quaint B&Bs and an olive oil boutique, you drive south through farmland for sixty miles. After an afternoon or an overnighter there, it was not easy to head back north to nowhere.

Cochise County will never be confused with Napa or Sonoma or any other winemaking area of California, Oregon or Washington. The closest metro area is Tucson, one hundred miles away. In general, Tucson is not much of a market for thirty-dollar bottles of wine, especially Rhone varietals. The closest large wine-purchasing metro area is Phoenix/Scottsdale, over two hundred miles away. Like the denizens of San Francisco or the East Bay who take a day trip up to St. Helena or Healdsburg, Phoenicians may make the two-hour trip to the Verde Valley wine region near Sedona, but an eight-hour round trip to Cochise County for a wine country experience is pretty much out of the question. Adventurous cuisine, hip music venues, quaint bed and breakfasts, tony delis doling out cute picnic lunches, those may eventually find their way to the area, but probably not any time soon.

There are more cattle and horses per square mile of Cochise County than there are people. Nevertheless, it offers reasonably-priced farmland graced by a climate favorable to Rhones. More than one Californian with big dreams and bigger suitcases full of cash has come east to buy land and make wine. The real estate market is surprisingly vibrant, with retirees of means seeking the good life away from the big city buzz. Some have been known to take up one expensive hobby or another.

Four years prior, in the spring of 2008, I went on a Lower San Juan river trip with a bunch of friends. Normally the drop from 4200 feet at Mexican Hat to 3700 at Clay Hills at the origin of the San Juan arm of Lake Powell allows for a nice easy seven-day float with a few rapids sprinkled in for excitement. Because of the high flow, I had almost no trouble rowing for several hours at a time, even upwind on the flat spots. Most of the short hikes were no problem either.

One day a friend and I decided to climb up to the top of the canyon. It was merely a half-hour of gentle switchbacks up to about 5000 feet or so. I was doing fine until I got within a hundred yards of the summit. All of a sudden I experienced that same old upper back pain. I had to stop and go back down the trail about one hundred feet. The pain resolved within five minutes. I tried going up again, and the pain returned. My friend went on up to the top; I made some excuse and waited for her to come back down. I tucked the altitude in the back of my mind.

Because it had been so predictable for over six years, I was usually pretty comfortable dealing with my angina. I'd reached the point where, except for tense situations, I could almost ward it off. There was some strange feeling, perhaps a palpitation or two, that warned me to stop what I was doing if I wanted to avoid having an episode. If I was lifting something, I'd put it down and walk for a minute or two. If I was bent over, planting or weeding, I'd stand up and take a few deep breaths. Almost nobody knew I still had any angina at all. During my biannual nuclear stress tests, I'd stop when I felt the warning, before I experienced angina. As long as I didn't bend forward too much, I could go for eight or nine minutes with no EKG changes or reversible defects on the images. The readings invariably came out as normal, with substandard exercise tolerance.

Chores on the crush pad, be it sanitizing vats, racking barrels, moving barrels or lifting cases, is basically heavy static lifting work. Much of the work, especially first thing in the morning, is done bent forward-- cleaning out various tanks, pushing heavy items around on carts or pallet jacks, pushing heavy items around without carts. When added to excellent food, I started putting on what I call my construction body; increased muscle mass, especially in my shoulders, but a bit of a gut from lack of aerobic activity. I was still having angina two or three times per day when I arrived from Phoenix.

The vineyard is situated at about 4200 ft. elevation The first couple of weeks almost killed me; I became short of breath at the drop of a hat and felt exhausted at the end of the day. My episodes of angina increased back up to three or four per day and they were lasting a good ten minutes, rather than the usual five. None of my methods of warding that shoulder pain off were working. When the pain came on, I'd dabble around until it resolved. The winemaker, who prefers to work in long bursts of heavy activity, would occasionally give me the eye when I had to stop working. I didn't mention the angina; I just said I needed a break. This wasn't going to cut it. There was a ton of work to do in a short span of time, and if I had to stop and rest frequently, the work day would grow from eight hours to twelve or more and everything would go to hell in a handbasket.

On a rare trip back to Phoenix, I went out and bought a cheap mountain bike at a local shop. The vineyard access road is rutted dirt with occasional protruding rocks. The bone-rattling ride would have destroyed my antique road bike in no time. Each day at 5:30 A.M. I'd get up and pedal for a half-hour, slow and steady, up to the junction to wave at the Border Patrol guys waiting in their vehicles to change shifts. After doing the ride for about a week or so, I realized there were the makings of a pretty good novel about the area, vis-a-vis immigration, winemaking, Indian history and spectacular rock formations.

Concentrating on plot and characters during my daily ride took my mind off my medical woes. Within a few weeks, I noticed my anginal episodes were decreasing in frequency, severity, and duration. My time on the crush pad became more enjoyable and I could work for hours without having to stop to rest or catch my breath. My exercise tolerance on the bike was way up as well. I could make the round-trip ride almost twice as quickly as when I started.

After about a month of riding, I realized that, for the first time in almost seven years, I was angina-free. Even in tense situations, and down in Cochise County there weren't many, I felt no pain whatsoever. Pushing heavy loads on the pallet jack went more easily. Even lifting barrels was no problem. I'd pretty much resolved that I would have chest and back pain the rest of my life, so this was a stunning change. My meds were the same. Owing to the bike riding at that higher altitude, my lungs were in their best condition in years. My best guess is that I grew some collaterals to supply the ischemic portion of my heart. The other feature about life on the farm, I mean life at the winery, is the absence of melodrama. As long as I completed whatever tasks we had that day, everything was hunky dory. The lack of tension removed one of my biggest anginal instigators from consideration.

The stay down there made me grow some collaterals and made me appreciate living in a metropolitan area. I came away with no doubts about what I could handle physically. It was, even more so than building the addition, a confidence booster. And, no, working in a winery did not give me even the slightest urge to buy land and start making wine. I stuck with the romantic part--sipping it out of a glass, swirling it in my mouth, furrowing my brow, and pontificating ad nauseam.

149. WITH FLYING COLORS

It was November 2014, time for my biannual nuclear stress test. On the last one, almost two years prior, I'd made it a little ways into stage 4, a total of ten minutes, and had no signs of ischemia. Since then I'd been riding my bike up and down some local hills every day; in the summer I swam laps a few times a week and switched to hiking in the nice weather. I still hadn't experienced any angina since my stint at the winery in late 2012, and I was now more active than I'd been at any time since my first surgery nine years ago. I was fairly certain this nuke tread wouldn't show anything, certainly nothing that was going to land me on a cath table.

The first couple of these follow-up stress tests are a real challenge, and you hope to God nothing turns up. After the second or third time around, you're pretty much into a routine, and the idea of stressing yourself to the point of exhaustion doesn't seem so daunting. You can look at them either of two ways. You can consider it a check-up; if you pass, you have a green light for the next two years. Or you can consider it an unnecessary pain in the ass, especially if you've been physically active with no symptoms. Although the last one cost me some serious dinero out of pocket, I didn't begrudge the cardiology group making a few bucks every couple of years. And it is nice to get through it and find that you continue to defy the odds. On the other hand, as active as I was without symptoms, I didn't see how a nuke tread was going to change what I did, which is to live my life and come in every six months to check the EKG, the vital signs, and the cholesterol levels.

This time Frank decided to throw in a carotid ultrasound.

"What for?" I asked. I wasn't having any TIAs or other neurological symptoms, my spells were mostly a thing of the past, and I wasn't excited about looking for trouble elsewhere. Should there be some blockage, I sure as hell didn't want anyone wandering into my brain via a CT or MRI to see if I'd had a stroke or two. I figured that there was no malignant brain tumor up there, or I'd be dead already. I had no interest in their finding a benign mass, like a meningioma or an aneurysm, that would land me on the table with Jethro Bodine poking around in my squash.

"We're finding that patients with coronary disease develop carotid disease as well. It is basically the same disease process. The last time we looked at yours was in 2005, just before you went in to surgery. So it's time to take a look."

"Okay." What are you going to say?

I rolled through everything with flying colors. I made it to twelve minutes on the treadmill and could have gone another minute or so, but I was bored, the tech had other cardiac fish to fry, and it was a beautiful day outside.

150. ANTHONY'S LAMENT

Car keys. My life is nothing but car keys. Do you have any idea what it's like to have incredible power, the power to influence men's minds, and be left with nothing but car keys? Of course you don't. Take it from me, it was suh-weet. In the old days, I mean. I covered lost kids, jewels, riches beyond imagination, incredible responsibilities. In the last few decades, my realm of influence has shrunk. Total lack of respect. Let me give you an example.

Back in the 60s there was this surgeon, Raimundo Trasini. He operated out of this particular hospital outside of Philadelphia. Holy Macarius Hospital. The locals called it Holy Mackerel. A fair number of famous people were born there over the years, but HIPAA prevents me from sharing those names with you, ha-ha. Anyway, on a Saturday in June, a guy shows up at the hospital with excruciating rectal pain and a swollen abdomen. This surgeon, this Trasini, lives right across the street, so they give him a call.

On this particular Saturday in June, Ray is planning to take the kids to the Phillies' game. Nonetheless, he figures, *What the hell, I'll examine the guy, probably has diverticulitis or a perirectal abscess, admit him to the hospital, start some antibiotics, and check on him after the game. With any luck, he'll need a drainage procedure or a colostomy.* Can't blame a surgeon for wanting to cut. That would be like blaming a lawyer for wanting to screw somebody over. As the young people say these days, no problem. Apparently "No problem" means the same as "You're welcome", because every time I thank a waiter, that's what I get. I mean, I'm glad it's not a problem for them, but I never expected it would be. That's why I like Italy. They still say "Prego" there.

Back to Trasini. He checks out the guy, who is in his early thirties, kind of young for diverticulitis. He says he's had the pain since the night before, hasn't been able to pass gas or move his bowels. No fever, his belly is soft, he's got good bowel sounds, something is not adding up. Trasini figures he'll take a quick peek with the straight sigmoidoscope, see what's up, ha-ha, and maybe get a better idea whether this guy has to be admitted to the hospital. The guy is not wild about the idea, wants to know whether having a shiny steel tube shoved up his butt is going to hurt, but gives his consent and off they go.

Trasini sticks the sig in and immediately bumps up against something firm and immobile. He asks the guy if he's ever had this problem before, thinking that something is not quite right here. The guy says no. Then he asks him if he is in the habit of sticking things in his butt. The guy says no. Then Trasini thinks, maybe this guy is a tad cagey, so he asks him if anyone else put something in his butt. Like my friend Peter, for the third time the guy says no. Now Trasini is up against a dilemma. He can't leave this guy with a rectal obstruction, but he promised his kids they would all go to the game. So he twists the scope ever so slightly and pulls it out.

On the end of the scope is some yellow-orange fibrous material, like vegetable matter. Again he asks the guy, and again the guy says no. So he sticks the scope in and starts curetting out the yellow-orange stuff. Time is getting short, it is a laborious process, and the kids are waiting. So what does he do? He starts praying to the twins. Over and over in his head. Because it's a "lost cause". Whoop-de-doo.

After about an hour, he has ninety percent of the stuff out of the guy, and he can get the straight sig pretty much all the way in. The patient finally admits he stuck a sweet potato up there the night before. The guy feels much better. Just to be on the safe side, Trasini admits him to the hospital. For the admitting diagnosis, he writes, "The Case of the Jammed Yam."

On the way back to the house, Trasini says a prayer of thanks to the twins, Simon and Jude this, Simon and Jude that, blah-blah-blah. Then he starts singing, "Dear St. Anthony, please come around. Something is lost and cannot be found." That's my cue, the only guy up here with his own jingle. I spring into action for...car keys. He's misplaced his fucking car keys.

151. EPILOGUE

Just like a Quinn Martin production.

In May 2015, I sold the red Benz convertible to a guy who was buying it for his not-quite sixteen-year-old son. That's a lot of car for a first-time driver. I advised the kid that cops would be climbing up his ass every time he went one mile per hour over the speed limit, especially at night.

In November 2015, I sold my house to a developer. He planned to put three or four big stuccos, those silly pseudo-Tuscans, on the lot. The older adobe part came down in minutes, reduced to nothing but dirt and termites. The concrete block addition, on which I had so lovingly toiled for two and one-half years, took about three hours. I was asked incessantly whether it felt bad to see it torn down. In truth, it was easier to walk away after twenty years knowing that nobody would ever live there again. It felt like the end of a chapter.

As far as activity goes, I've been riding my bike every day for the past four years. I do the same route, up and down some hills. It takes a little less than an hour. Once in a while I go off-road in the Squaw Peak recreation area, but I don't do that often because the only thing I hate worse than walking my bike home with a flat tire is fixing said flat tire out in the wilderness. Occasionally I load my bike into my truck, drive somewhere, and ride a different route. Often I get lost, or at least I think I'm lost. Lost is usually a function of time, as in, *I don't know where I am, and I have to be somewhere else at a certain time, and if I don't get un-lost soon, I won't be able to get where I'm supposed to be by the time I'm supposed to be there*, rather than simply space, as in, *I don't know where I am*.

My short-term memory is still crummy, but it's not getting any worse. I've done all the online memory helper sites, but they don't seem to make a difference. That worm still crawls at his leisure through my brain, bringing answers minutes to hours after the question has been asked. I'm not bothered by this impairment as much as I once was. Maybe that's because most of my contemporaries are complaining of the same memory problems. In terms of mental incompetence, they seem to be catching up with me. I miss my co-workers, but not the day-to-day of working in an E.R. Most E.R.s are so congested with uninsured primary care patients that the sick ones often get diverted to other places. Besides, working night shifts in that environment is a young person's game, not for the elderly, frail of heart and mind.

My medical knowledge continues to fade. I still retain an impressive collection of random facts in my brain, but the matrix behind them, the beautiful structure that supports them and provides an orderly symmetry, is gone forever.

Here is a real-life example of the effectiveness of statins and niacin. Every day since 2006 I have been taking 4000 mg. of niacin, four fiber capsules, 5000 mg. of fish oil, all of which have been shown to effectively lower your LDL-C, and a single statin tablet, Vytorin, which contains 10 mg. of Zetia (ezetimibe) and 20 mg. of Zocor (simvastatin). Ever since I started this regimen, my HDL-C, initially in the low twenties, has run above 80 mg/dl (that's good), my total cholesterol below 170 mg/dl (also good), and my LDL-C below 70 mg/dl (good cubed). I let my prescription for Vytorin lapse for about three months. Don't ask why. Before I restarted it, my HDL-C was still above 80 mg/dl (good), but my total cholesterol was up to 257 mg/dl (bad), and my LDL-C rose to 160 mg/dl (very bad). Six weeks. That's all. From a perfect cholesterol profile to a high-risk one. Because my HDL-C was so high, I knocked the niacin down to 1000 mg. three times daily; six months later, my HDL-C is still 80 mg/dl.

Speaking of niacin. As expected, I developed a mild case of gout about two years ago. I thought about getting off the niacin, but the thought of another ruptured coronary plaque scares me much more than gouty arthritis. So allopurinol was added to my daily regimen. It seems to be working.

I got to see my daughter graduate from grade school, high school, and, last summer, from college. She loves her entry-level job on Capitol Hill which hopefully will lead to a career in fundraising. I still haven't had anyone come around to collect on all those deals I struck to stay alive, and I have yet to come face-to-face with my day to die. Who knows? I may be able to stick around until I'm a father-in-law and a grandfather. I try to tempt fate as little as possible.

Frank Surdakowski shed the lead and sold his practice to his partners a few years ago. Now he and Maryann see office patients in the lair of the dreaded archenemy against whom he waged business war for decades. Time softens everyone. They see me every six months in an effort to keep me out of harm's way, for which I am truly grateful.

That cold numbness that consumed me after my second surgery is finally starting to thaw. For the first time in years, I seek and enjoy the company of other humans. I'm still not much of a conversationalist, at least I don't think I am. However, people keep talking with me. They look at me funny, but they don't run away. I delude myself into thinking that they find me interesting. Without our delusions, could we even get up in the morning?

Every so often I get that morning sickness feeling for a day or two. Even after fasting for eight hours or more, I don't ever feel hunger, just weakness from an empty gut and perhaps a trace of hypoglycemia. Despite all that, I've managed to return to the environs of my preoperative weight.

In the winter, I hike a few times a week. It is hilly where I live, so that works me pretty well. When I had a pool, I swam a few times a week during the summer. In early 2016, I decided to add running to my exercise regimen. I ran about a mile each day for eight days. Although I used to run on a regular basis, my form was never anything but painful to watch, certainly not Salazarian. After the eight days, my knees felt like they were being squeezed in a vice. Real runners advised me to follow the RICE regimen. Rest, ice, compression and elevation. I tried that but it didn't help that much. Not running for two weeks helped a lot. I think I'll try not running for two years.

Using the Bruce protocol as a guide, for two months in the summer of 2016, I practiced on a treadmill three times a week. In October, I made it through stage 5 for my nuclear treadmill test. Fifteen minutes on the dot. No angina, no significant EKG changes, no imaging defects. I felt elated. A couple weeks later, Frank showed me the report. It concluded, "The patient's exercise capacity was **average**." Really? Average for whom? Salazar? Next time I'm shooting for 18 minutes.

Owing to all this exercise, I am in the second-best physical shape of my life. My best shape ever? One week before that plaque ruptured in my left main in August, 2005.

Alberto Salazar, whose birthdate is exactly four years after mine, suffered a heart attack in 2007. You can out eat an exercise program, you can out eat a gastric bypass, but you cannot outrun your genetics, especially when it comes to heart disease. Unlike Jim Fixx, he survived.

What shall I do now? Maybe I'll run for president.

When I was in fifth grade I read Lou Gehrig's biography. At the time, there were two things I didn't understand. One was his love of his mother's pickled eels. The other was his farewell speech, where, despite being forced to quit baseball because of ALS, he considered himself the luckiest man on the face of the earth. I still don't get the eel thing, but the latter? I feel like the luckiest man on earth. Every single day.

Book printing and bindery by

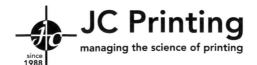